THE Prevention.
ULTIMATE GUIDE TO
WOMEN'S
HEALTH
AND
WELLNESS

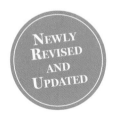

NEWLY REVISED AND UPDATED

ACTION PLANS FOR MORE THAN
100 WOMEN'S HEALTH PROBLEMS

RODALE.

© 2002, 2011 by Rodale Inc.

Prevention is a registered trademark of Rodale Inc.

Portions of this book were previously published by Rodale Inc. in 2002.
Revised and updated edition published August 2011.

Printed in the United States of America

Rodale Inc. makes every effort to use acid-free ♾, recycled paper ♻.

Book design by Carol Angstadt
Photo credits can be found on page 537.
ISBN 13: 978-1-60961-085-2

Library of Congress Cataloging-in-Publication Data is on file with the publisher

2   4   6   8   10   9   7   5   3   1   hardcover

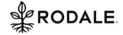

We inspire and enable people to improve their lived and the world around them.
For more of our products visit **prevention.com** or call 800-848-4735.

Contents

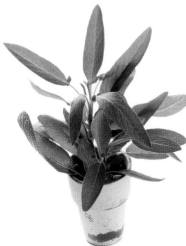

PART ONE: The Savvy Woman's Health Planner

PART TWO: Your Stay Well, Stay Young "To Do" List

PART THREE: Primary Care: Essential Protection

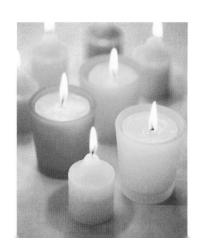

PART FOUR: Hormonal Wellness: The Best-Ever Life-Stage Strategies

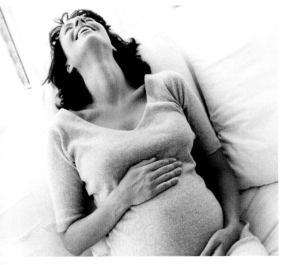

PART FIVE: Doctors' Best Symptom Solvers

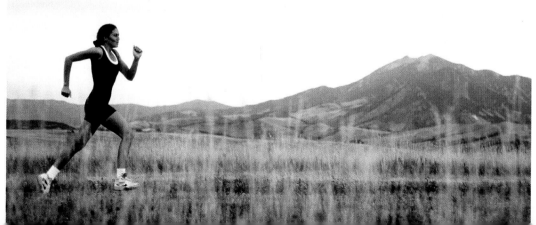

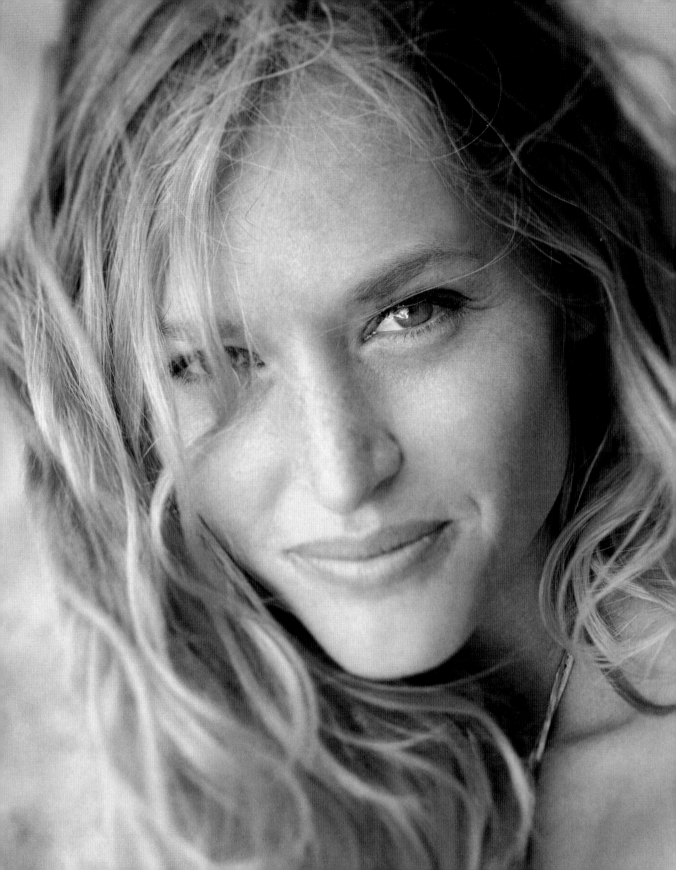

PART ONE

THE SAVVY

WOMAN'S

HEALTH

PLANNER

The Female Body, Decade by Decade

If there's a 21st-century poster child for aging well it's Olympic swimmer Dara Torres. In 2008, at the age of 41, she became the oldest swimmer ever to place on the U.S. Olympic Team, winning silver medals in three events. Even more remarkable, this was Torres's fifth Olympics. She's the only one of a small, elite group of Olympians to medal in five games. All told, she's brought home 12 Olympic medals—four of them gold—since she first competed as a teenager in the 1984 Summer Olympics in Los Angeles.

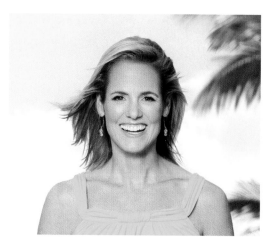

Dara Torres has made a habit of breaking records and shattering myths about the "inevitable" decline that comes with age. At 40, 15 months after giving birth to her first child, she won gold in the 100-meter freestyle at the US nationals; a few days later, she set a new American record in the 50-meter freestyle. To do that, she had to break the record she set 26 years before at the age of 15.

It should come as no surprise, then, that Torres has her sights set on the 2012 summer games in London. She'll be 45 years old—potentially 20 years (or more) older than most of her teammates.

If you're thinking that deserves a fist pump, you're right. But not just for Dara Torres. Even if you don't train like an Olympian, making some other smart moves can help you grow better, not just older—with toned muscles, a healthy heart, glowing skin, sharp eyes, and a memory so reliable you'll be trouncing the smarties on *Jeopardy* every night.

It's easier than you might think. Start right here, with our checklists for every stage of a woman's life—from high school graduation through career, marriage, kids, menopause, retirement, and beyond.

At each life stage, you'll start with the building blocks of wellness: Self-Care Checklists, which cover a healthy diet and nutritional solutions to problems that you may encounter along the way, such as weight gain, high blood pressure, or hot flashes, plus Your Doctor's Office Checklists, with special attention to conditions to watch for and medical screening tests that can help you detect and manage small problems before they become big and unmanageable.

Part 2, Your Stay Well, Stay Young "To Do" List will show you, age by age, the best exercises, food and supplements, and preventive steps you need to take as well as step-by-step action plans to customize medical advice.

If you don't think these strategies can make a difference in 20 or 30 years, ask Michael Lichtenstein, MD, geriatrician at the University of Texas Health Science Center in San Antonio and principal investigator for the National Institutes of Health's Positively Aging educational program. "People who have lifelong health maintenance habits like exercising and eating healthy will live long and healthy lives," he says.

Who knows, maybe you'll be breaking some records that *you* set at 15.

AGES 18 *to* 35

On the road to Olympic gold—or to a healthy life over the decades—a young woman is in training camp. Measures you take now will make the difference in everything from your fertility to your longevity, and you have every reason to expect to be dandling great-grandchildren on your knee some day. Women's life expectancy has increased by nearly 52 percent in the last 100 years, from 53.2 years in 1910 to a projected 80.8 in 2010. The number of centenarians—people who live to be 100—is increasing by as much as two-thirds every 10 years in the United States, and 85 percent of them are women. Credit improved nutrition, the discovery of antibiotics that controlled infectious diseases, advances in screening and treatment for killer ailments such as heart disease and cancer, and better health habits. It was not so long ago that a cancer diagnosis meant a slim chance of survival. But now, thanks to improved methods of prevention, detection, and treatment, two-thirds of the 11 million Americans who have cancer are outliving the disease.

The regimen of your training camp: a base of healthy habits that continue throughout your lifetime.

The medical screenings you'll find here help detect cancer and other diseases early, when they're easier to treat, or even cure. You'll find nutrition advice that will help you prevent disease in the first place: for instance, recommendations for feasting on fruits and vegetables that contain phytochemicals, substances that actually fight cancer, diabetes, heart disease, and even Alzheimer's; whole grains that provide fiber, lowering your risk for diabetes, heart disease, and cancer; and omega-3 fatty acids in foods such as fish and avocados, which are good

for the heart and also help lift your mood.

Now is the time to make sure you're at your ideal weight. Your metabolism tends to slow as you age (though the good news is it's for largely preventable reasons) so it only gets harder to whittle off the consequences of fast-food lunches and pizza dinners. Being obese—more than 30 percent over your ideal body weight—puts you at greater risk for a host of diverse conditions, from cancer, diabetes, high blood pressure, and heart and artery disease to sleep disruptions, varicose veins, osteoarthritis, and complications during pregnancy and surgery. If you're overweight, the nutritional guidelines here will help you get started on a healthy eating plan. For a more thorough program on losing weight, see Chapter 6.

Even if you don't have a weight problem, eating healthfully throughout your lifetime is still vital. Good nutrition will help you stave off the diseases of aging, increase your energy levels, improve your mood and, when you're pregnant, could help you avoid birth defects in your baby. It's also the foundation of young skin for life.

Following training camp rules in the kitchen will help you from the starting line right on to the finish. Now's the time to stick to the plan. It's never going to be any easier.

"Most of us have eating patterns that were formed when we were very young," says Terri Brownlee, MPH, RD, former nutrition director of the Duke University Diet and Fitness Center in Durham, North Carolina, and now regional director for Bon Appetit Management Company in Charlotte, North Carolina. "Even at 20 years old, it's difficult to make changes. But it's certainly harder the longer you wait. If you wait until you're 50 or 60 years old, bad habits are much harder to break."

Studies on people who have adopted a healthy diet and continued with it for years have shown that lifestyle changes are actually the only way to do it.

Your Self-Care Checklist

○ **Multivitamins and mineral supplements.** To be extra sure you're getting the vitamins and minerals you need, get in the habit of taking a multivitamin and mineral supplement that provides 100 percent of the Daily Value for most nutrients, including vitamin A or beta-carotene, vitamin D, vitamin B_6, copper, iron, and zinc.

If you're not a fan of citrus or greens—major sources of vitamin C—consider taking a separate supplement of 200 mg daily. You may also want to take up to 400 IU of vitamin E, which is found in wheat germ, nuts, and fortified cereal. Both are antioxidants, counteracting the natural effects of aging and environmental damage at the cellular level. Caution: Don't apply the "more must be better" precept to vitamin E. Recent studies have found that those who took more than 400 IU a day were more likely to die than those who took less.

If you're not eating enough calcium-rich foods, consider a supplement.

Also, make sure your multivitamin has a USP (United States Pharmacopeia) label on it. It means the manufacturer guarantees the supple-ment contains the amount of vitamins listed on the label.

○ **Calcium and vitamin D.** For all women under 50, *Prevention* recommends 500 mg of calcium in addition to eating plenty of low-fat dairy. This is the time in your life when you should be banking calcium in your bones so you don't come up short when you hit midlife. You should be getting at least 1,000 mg every day when you're under 50. Never take more than 500 mg of calcium at one time: Your body can't absorb it in higher quantities and you'll just lose it. One type, calcium carbonate, should be taken with meals, but you may take calcium citrate on an empty stomach. Make sure you're also getting 600 IU of vitamin D, which helps your bones absorb calcium. Recent research on the sunshine vitamin—so called because it's made in our skin with the help of the sun's ultraviolet rays—suggests it may also help protect from some cancers as well as type 1 and type 2 diabetes.

○ **Folate/folic acid.** The B vitamin folic acid (the supplement form of folate) prevents neural tube defects—birth defects of the brain and spinal cord—in babies. Women who plan to become pregnant should get 400 micrograms of folic acid daily, from a supplement only if you're not getting enough from your diet. While pregnant, your doctor may advise you to increase your intake to 600 mcg.

Along with your supplements, eat two folate-rich foods a day, such as spinach, kidney beans, or oranges.

One caveat: Emerging research has suggested that getting too much folic acid—as little as 1 mg daily—may increase the risk of some cancers. Because so many grain products, from rice to bread to cereal, are fortified with folic acid, there is a real possibility that you can get too much. Once your childbearing days are over, consider dropping the supplement.

◯ **Iron.** One out of five premenopausal women doesn't get the Daily Value of 18 mg of iron, which your body uses in the process of delivering oxygen to your cells. Without enough iron, you'll feel tired and have trouble concentrating; you can even become anemic.

To battle that fatigue, eat iron-rich foods such as extra-lean meat, legumes, and dark green leafy vegetables. Consuming vitamin C, such as a glass of orange juice, with iron-rich foods boosts absorption.

◯ **Good-mood foods.** Women in their thirties who battle mood problems may be reacting to the food they eat, the nutrients they're missing, or the drugs they take.

■ Premenstrual symptoms may be worse if you're not getting enough calcium, so make sure you're eating three servings of dairy that add up to 1,000 mg of calcium a day, from milk, yogurt, or calcium-fortified orange juice. This will help minimize PMS mood swings.

■ Women who take birth control pills are often low on vitamin B_6, which helps manufacture the mood-boosting brain chemical serotonin. Make sure you're getting enough by eating bananas and

extra-lean meat. You don't need an extra supplement as long as your diet is rich in B_6 foods; what you get in a multi should be enough.

Your Doctor's Office Checklist

◯ **Dental checkups.** Go to the dentist at least every 6 months to help prevent cavities, gum disease, and other oral problems.

◯ **Eye exams.** If you haven't already done so, get an initial comprehensive eye exam that tests your vision and looks for signs of glaucoma, cataracts, and macular degeneration. Follow up with your eye doctor if your vision changes. You'll need more frequent checkups when you're in your forties.

◯ **Serum ferritin test and transferrin saturation test.** If waning energy makes you suspect you're getting too little iron, talk to your doctor about getting a serum ferritin test, a blood test that measures the amount of iron in the body. Iron deficiency is the most common known form of nutritional deficiency, and it's highest among women of childbearing age, largely because iron is lost in menstrual blood. Twelve percent of nonpregnant women ages 16 to 49 are deficient in iron, and 3 to 5 percent have iron deficiency anemia.

Iron overload, or hemochromatosis, is also a common genetic disease, in which too much iron builds up in the body, damaging tissue and organs. Get screened for it at age 18 with a serum ferritin test and a transferrin saturation

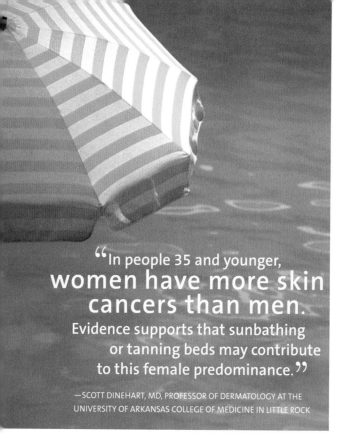

"In people 35 and younger, **women have more skin cancers than men.** Evidence supports that sunbathing or tanning beds may contribute to this female predominance."

—SCOTT DINEHART, MD, PROFESSOR OF DERMATOLOGY AT THE UNIVERSITY OF ARKANSAS COLLEGE OF MEDICINE IN LITTLE ROCK

test, especially if you're frequently fatigued or have liver disease, diabetes, arthritis, or a family history of hemochromatosis. If you have it, you may need to make frequent blood donations.

○ **Skin exam.** Just one or two blistering sunburns in youth can set the stage for skin cancer later in life. Though it can take decades for the signs to surface, it's not unusual for young women to get skin cancer. In fact, the rate of skin cancers—along with the tanning bed trend—among young women rose by 50 percent between 1980 and 2004. Today, melanoma, the deadliest kind of skin cancer, is the number one cancer in the 25 to 29 age group. More than 1 million cases of skin cancer are diagnosed each year in North America, but most are curable if detected early enough.

Starting at age 18, examine your skin at least once a year for signs of skin cancer. "Check your

birthday suit every year on your birthday," says Ira Davis, MD, assistant professor of dermatology at New York Medical College in Valhalla.

Use a mirror or ask someone to check those hard-to-see places and look for:

▪ Pearly white bumps or spots that may bleed, break down, or don't heal, usually on the face or the arms (but they can appear anywhere on the body)

▪ Red and scaly bumps that resemble a scar and are shallow in the middle, usually on the face or the arms (but they can appear anywhere on the body)

▪ Dark spots that are asymmetrical, have irregular borders, have more than one color, and are bigger than the size of a pencil eraser, usually on the legs and trunk (but they can appear anywhere on the body), and may be flat or elevated.

You should also see a dermatologist every 3 years for a skin examination. If someone in your family has had melanoma and you're at risk for skin cancer (you've spent a lot of time in the sun, you've had many sunburns, you have fair skin, or you have many moles), get examined twice a year. If skin cancer runs in your family but you don't have risk factors, get checked once a year.

○ **Tetanus shot.** This may seem like stuff for elementary school kids, but everyone needs a tetanus shot every 10 years to stay immune to the rare but fatal disease. Tetanus is caused when bacteria in an open wound attack the central nervous system.

◯ **Blood pressure check.** This is usually standard screening every time you see your family doctor or gynecologist. Make sure your blood pressure is checked at least every 2 years or more frequently if it's above 120/80, which is considered a normal reading. High blood pressure is a side effect of oral contraception in some women, so have your pressure checked when you start the Pill, and again a few months later.

◯ **Complete blood lipid profile.** Today experts are seeing evidence of atherosclerosis (blood vessels with unhealthful deposits of cholesterol and other fats) in teenagers, which is why regular cholesterol checks are so important. With just one blood test, your doctor can measure your total cholesterol, HDL ("good") cholesterol, LDL ("bad") cholesterol, levels of triglycerides, and total/HDL ratio. Get this test done every 5 years, starting at age 20. If the results are abnormal, go every 4 months.

Healthy results are:

- Total cholesterol of 199 mg per deciliter or below

- HDL 50 mg/dl or above

- LDL less than 100 mg/dl

- Total/HDL ratio of 4 or below

- Triglycerides levels less than 150 mg/dl

◯ **Thyroid-stimulating hormone test.** Many doctors don't recommend thyroid screening until age 40 or 50 unless you have risk factors, such as a family history of thyroid problems or

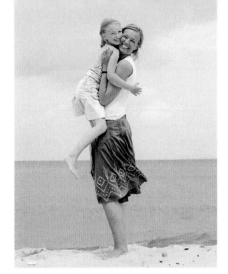

"Women should get in the habit at a very young age of not bending over at the waist to pick up anything, especially heavy children.

This helps prevent ruptured disks and back strain

as well as reduce the chance of spinal fractures. Bending at the knees and squatting down strengthens the muscles around the hip, which not only gives you a nice shape but reduces your risk of hip fractures from osteoporosis later in life."

—MARJORIE LUCKEY, MD, MEDICAL DIRECTOR,
ST. BARNABAS OSTEOPOROSIS AND METABOLIC BONE DISEASE
CENTER, LIVINGSTON, NEW JERSEY

autoimmune disease, but *Prevention* suggests getting screened at age 20 and every 5 years thereafter. Because 5 to 7 percent of women under age 35 have mild thyroid dysfunction, and because the test is inexpensive and simple, get this screen at the same time you get your cholesterol checked.

Thyroid problems can raise cholesterol levels, which put you at greater risk for heart disease, or cause conception problems or low birth weight or miscarriages. Other symptoms include fatigue, weight gain, and cognitive problems. Even subclinical thyroid deficiency can cause symptoms.

◯ **Fasting glucose test.** While the majority of women who develop type 2 diabetes don't do so until they are over 45, the incidence of the disease among younger women is rising and doctors are concerned about a precursor called "prediabetes," in which your fasting glucose levels are high (more than 100 mg/dl), but not high enough to warrant a diabetes diagnosis. Even without prediabetes, your body may not be using the insulin it produces properly, a condition called insulin resistance or metabolic syndrome. Too much sugar (glucose) in your blood can cause organ and tissue damage. If you're at high risk, get tested now and every 3 years.

Risk factors for diabetes include:

■ A family history

■ Being from an at-risk ethnic group, such as African American, Hispanic, Native American, Asian, or Pacific Islander

■ Obesity

■ High cholesterol

■ A history of gestational diabetes

■ Low HDL cholesterol and high triglycerides

Risk factors for metabolic syndrome include:

■ Borderline blood sugar readings (fasting blood glucose levels 100 mg/dl or above)

■ Excess weight around the waist (waist measurement 35 inches or more)

■ High blood pressure (130/80 or above)

■ High triglycerides (150 mg/dl or above) and low HDL cholesterol (below 50 mg/dl)

◯ **Pelvic exam, Pap test, and HPV screening.** Since 1970, the incidence of and death rate from cervical cancer have gone down by 40 percent, thanks in part to early detection with the Pap test. Starting at age 21, or about 3 years after starting sexual intercourse, see your gynecologist every year for a pelvic exam and a Pap test until you reach 30. The American Cancer Society recommends a Pap test every other year if your physician uses a liquid-based Pap test. After 30, you should have a Pap every 2 to 3 years if three previous Pap tests were negative, and a screening for human papillomavirus (HPV), a sexually transmitted disease that causes about 70 percent of all cervical cancers.

During the pelvic exam, the doctor examines the genitals, vagina, and cervix for infections, rashes, or abnormal growths. She also checks the size and position of the ovaries and uterus to make sure they're not enlarged.

She'll also take a sample of cells from your cervix for the Pap test. This screens for cervical cancer. She may use those same samples or take a second sample to test for HPV. If you or your partner has multiple sexual partners, you should be tested for other sexually transmitted diseases as well.

If you haven't already done so, and are between the ages of 9 and 26, talk to your gynecologist about a vaccine to prevent 4 types of HPV, two of which are linked to cervical cancer and two to genital warts.

◯ **Clinical breast exam.** Recent studies have called into question the benefit of breast self-exams. Statistically, there's no survival benefit and, since most lumps are benign, finding one can lead to an unnecessary biopsy. However, *Prevention* still recommends that you give yourself a monthly check because many women detect their own breast cancers. But it's more important to get a clinical breast exam from your doctor every 3 years, too. With her expertise, she might be more likely to detect a tumor at an early stage before it spreads.

Symptoms to watch for: breast lumps, thickening, swelling, distortion, tenderness, skin irritation, dimpling, nipple pain, discharge, or scaliness.

Though breast cancer in younger women accounts for a small percentage of cases, there are more than 250,000 women in the United States who were diagnosed before the age of 40. Unfortunately, many of them were diagnosed at a later stage than older women, so it's vitally

important to be vigilant about breast health no matter what your age.

◯ **Genetic testing.** If a close family member has had breast cancer, especially when premenopausal, or ovarian, prostate, or colon cancer, consider seeing a genetic counselor to determine if you carry a gene that might predispose you to cancer. Women with what are called BRCA mutations may be at risk for breast, ovarian, or colon cancer and need to follow a different screening plan than other women. For example, when you reach 30, you may need to have a pelvic exam, a transvaginal ultrasound with color Doppler, and a CA-125 blood test (a chemical that can signal ovarian cancer) every 6 months to look for ovarian cancer. You may need more frequent mammograms with an MRI and clinical breast exams.

◯ **Flu shots.** Until recently, vaccine experts recommended flu shots only to the very young, pregnant women, people with chronic conditions, health care workers, and those over 50. While those remain the high-risk populations, in 2010 the Centers for Disease Control and Prevention recommended universal flu shots to expand protection against the flu to more people. Get one as soon as they become available, usually in early fall. The flu season runs from September to late winter or early spring, and usually peaks in January. Do not get a flu shot if you're allergic to eggs or to influenza shots or if you've had Guillain-Barre syndrome within 6 weeks of getting a flu shot.

AGES 35 *to* 40

You're in the race now and you can't backpedal on any of the good health habits you've kept up through young womanhood. But as you approach midlife, there are subtle changes occurring in your body that you need to be aware of, and some lifestyle changes to consider.

For one, you may start to experience perimenopausal symptoms (they can occur as early as age 35!). You may still be getting your monthly periods, but your levels of estrogen and other female hormones wane gradually as your body inches closer to menopause. You might experience irregular menstrual periods (shorter, longer, or skipped altogether), hot flashes, night sweats, insomnia, mood swings, and vaginal dryness.

Not surprisingly, it can be harder to become pregnant. About 20 percent of women wait until 35 to start a family, and the risk of miscarriage increases to about 50 percent by the time you're 45. Women in their forties also have a higher risk of pregnancy complications such as premature labor, stillbirth, and the need for cesarean section. As you age, the eggs produced by your ovaries are more likely to have chromosomal damage. For example, your risk of having a child with Down syndrome is 1 in 1,250 when you're 25 but jumps to 1 in 106 at 40.

More than ever, exercise is essential to keeping muscles toned and your bones intact. Beginning in their thirties, women lose 1 to 2 percent of their muscle mass per year; fortunately, exercise can reverse the process and keep your metabolism revved up so you don't develop "meno-pot"—excess weight around your waist. Redouble your efforts not to gain weight now because once you reach 40, it won't be as easy to drop 5 or 10 pounds at will.

Along with losing muscle, you can also lose bone. During childhood and puberty, your skeleton built more bone than it broke down. But by the time you reach 35, the process reverses itself. Weight-bearing exercise, such as walking and lifting weights, will strengthen your skeleton and help you avoid osteoporosis, a bone-thinning disease that can lead to fracture.

Your Self-Care Checklist

○ **A fertile weight.** Obesity affects ovulation and could make it hard to get pregnant or carry a baby to term. In one study, a group of women who had a 75 percent miscarriage rate lowered that rate to 18 percent after eating a healthy diet, exercising, and losing weight. If you're infertile and overweight, losing weight may help.

On the other hand, being underweight increases your risk for miscarriage, cesarean deliveries, or premature birth. A healthy weight is your best bet for maintaining fertility.

○ **Folic acid/folate.** Folic acid (the supplement form of folate) is recommended for all women of childbearing age because it plays a role in preventing neural tube birth defects that affect the brain and spine of your baby. Once you get pregnant, your doctor may advise you to

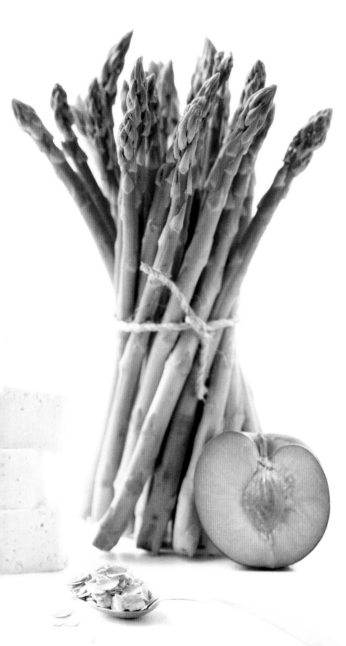

increase your intake to 600 mcg. But even if you're not pregnant, getting at least five servings of folate a day from food (including fortified grain products) may decrease your risk of getting colon cancer later on. Folate, which is found in fruits and vegetables such as spinach and legumes, works on your DNA to keep it normal. Your suggested Daily Value is 400 mcg. If you're deficient in folate, you're more likely to develop the type of DNA damage that can lead to cancer.

○ **Vegetables and calcium.** You should already be exercising and getting enough calcium (DV is 1,000 mg) to keep your bones strong, but you should also be eating plenty of vegetables. Research shows that the nutrients in fruits and vegetables—zinc, magnesium, potassium, fiber, and vitamin C—decrease the risk of having low bone mass.

Your Doctor's Office Checklist

○ **Dental checkups.** Schedule them twice a year, or more often based on your dentist's advice.

○ **Eye exams.** If you have never had one, schedule an initial comprehensive eye exam. Then see an eye doctor if you notice any changes in your vision. Otherwise, you don't need regular exams until you turn 41.

○ **Serum ferritin test and transferrin saturation test.** You should have had a serum ferritin test and a transferrin saturation test when you were 18 to screen for hemochromatosis. If you didn't, do it now, especially if you're frequently fatigued or have liver disease, diabetes, arthritis, or a family history of hemochromatosis. Talk to your physician about the most current recommendations regarding these iron tests.

◯ **Skin exam.** Continue getting a skin examination from a dermatologist (studies show they're better at spotting cancer than a general practitioner) every 3 years if you're not at high risk for skin cancer, every year if your only risk is family history, and twice a year if you're at high risk, as described on page 7. If you have lots of moles (50 or more), you are at higher risk of melanoma; talk to your dermatologist about the frequency of clinical screenings you need.

◯ **Tetanus shot.** If it's been 10 years, get another one.

◯ **Flu shot .** Get yours in September or earlier if they're available.

◯ **Blood pressure check.** Continue to have it checked at least every 2 years, or more frequently if it's been abnormal. See page 8 for normal values.

◯ **Complete blood lipid profile.** If your lipids have been normal, you've been getting a complete lipid profile every 5 years. Now's the time to step it up to every 2 years. Abnormal results should be rechecked every 4 months. See page 8 for normal values.

◯ **Thyroid-stimulating hormone test.** Have this done every 5 years.

◯ **Fasting glucose test.** If you're at high risk of diabetes or prediabetes, as described on page 9, get tested now and every 3 years thereafter.

◯ **Pelvic exam, Pap test, and breast exam.** Continue getting a pelvic exam every year, do monthly breast self-exams, and have a clinical breast exam every 3 years then every year once you reach 40.

◯ **Mammogram.** If two or more close relatives had breast cancer, particularly if they were diagnosed before they turned 40, start getting annual mammograms in your thirties. If, after genetic testing, you learn you have a mutation in your genes known as BRCA1 or BRCA2, you should also have an MRI each year along with your mammogram. In one study of 236 women, MRIs found 77 percent of cancers compared with 36 percent detected by mammography. That gene profile may also predispose you to ovarian and colon cancer, which would require you to have more frequent screenings.

◯ **Bone-density test.** If you're at high risk for osteoporosis because of another illness or a medication, talk to your doctor about getting a baseline bone density scan prior to menopause. (For example, some medications to treat conditions such as rheumatoid arthritis, endocrine disorders, seizure disorders, and gastrointestinal diseases may damage bone and lead to osteoporosis.) *Prevention* recommends the dual energy x-ray absorptiometry (DEXA) scan, the gold standard for diagnosing osteoporosis. If you don't have osteoporosis but a precursor called osteopenia, you can now take measures—more calcium and vitamin D, weight-bearing exercise, or medication—to halt bone decline. Otherwise, wait until menopause for the test. You're at risk for osteoporosis if:

- You broke a bone after the age of 35 from low trauma (falling from a standing height or less)

- You have a family history of osteoporosis or hip fractures

- You weigh less than 127 pounds, even if you're short

- You smoke cigarettes or drink excessive amounts of alcohol

- You have taken steroids for 3 months or longer for conditions like asthma

- You have a chronic disease that increases your risk for osteoporosis (both before and after menopause), such as seizure disorders, inflammatory bowel disease, chronic liver disease, kidney disease, or celiac disease

AGES 40 *to* 50

You're now in hot flash territory, but you have a choice: You can think of yourself as a victim of your dwindling estrogen, or you can be a "red hot mama" who regards a hot flash as a power surge. In fact, studies show that women who approach menopause with a great attitude actually experience fewer symptoms.

Almost all women—85 to 90 percent—experience some symptoms of perimenopause, when the ovaries slow down their production of estrogen and hormone levels fluctuate. The most common of these symptoms is irregular periods.

"Anything is possible," says Margery Gass, MD, professor of obstetrics and gynecology and director of the University Hospital Menopause and Osteoporosis Center at the University of Cincinnati College of Medicine. Your periods could be completely normal and regular up until menopause, or they might move closer together or further apart, skip cycles, or become heavier.

"Although more frequent periods are most common, it's important to stay in touch with your physician to figure out what's normal for you during this time," Dr. Gass says. "Heavy bleeding, irregular bleeding, periods every 2 to 3 weeks, and breakthrough bleeding are always worrisome symptoms that should be checked by your doctor. They could be signs of cancer, polyps, fibroids, infections, or miscarriages."

Other symptoms include:

- Hot flashes, night sweats, and extreme sweating (with or without chills)

- Vaginal dryness

- Changes in sexual desire

- PMS symptoms

- Mood changes

- Frequent urination

- Achy joints

- Difficulty concentrating

- Headaches

- Insomnia

- Early wakening

You may get one or two, you may get them all; some may bother you, others not so much. A lot depends on your emotional state. As you enter midlife, your life and your body undergo many changes. You could be facing an empty nest, for instance. Though studies suggest most women are happy finally to have the time to focus on their own interests, you may feel sad that one phase of motherhood is over. Even longtime marriages may crumble: A study by the American Association of Retired People (AARP) in 2007 found that divorce rates among people ages 40 to 79 was on the rise, and that women were more likely than men to make the break when the reason for staying together–the kids–was gone. You may trade caring for your kids for caring for an aging parent (though since many women wait until they're in their thirties before having children, you could be caring for both simultaneously).

The death of a parent or other older relative may make you more conscious of your own mortality, and of the diseases that could alter the course of your life. In fact, this is the time of your life when it's important to take a look at both your family and personal history and focus on reducing your risks of disease, which go up as we age.

Together, the physical and life changes you face might leave you feeling as though you're going through puberty all over again. But there's plenty you can do to ease yourself through the 2 or 3 years it typically takes to make this transition and to lay the groundwork for living to a ripe, healthy old age.

Your Self-Care Checklist

○ **Exercise, exercise, exercise.** First and foremost, continue to rev up your metabolism with exercise. Researchers have found that women tend to gain about 1 pound a year in their forties, and the hormonal changes you're going through make it more likely that you'll be depositing extra fat around your abdomen where it can do the most damage to blood sugar, cholesterol levels, and blood pressure. Called visceral fat, it does more than make a bulge in your little black dress. It's biologically active, making and secreting hormones that affect other body tissues including your heart, colorectal organs, breasts, and even your brain.

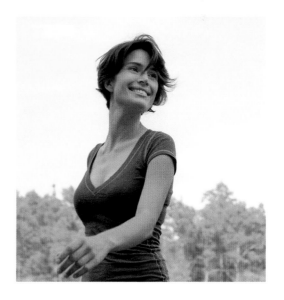

It's easy to blame all your weight gain on your changing hormones, but recent studies have found that something else that happens around menopause is the major culprit: We stop moving. Peri- and menopausal women, perhaps because they no longer have children to run after or pick up, are less active than younger women. Since women's risk for heart disease goes up after menopause and having more body fat could exacerbate the risk, work on keeping your weight down now by eating healthy and exercising. Make sure you add weight training to your regular aerobic exercise regime. Lean muscle burns more calories than fat (since men have more of it, they lose weight faster than women). Keep up a daily walking program; it's a great exercise for building and maintaining bone.

○ **Calorie control.** With slower metabolism, you're likely to find you're gaining weight even if you haven't changed your eating habits. But training the scale not to budge is as simple as eating one bite less at every meal. That adds up to about 100 fewer calories a day, the number of calories you should cut from your daily diet each decade.

○ **Hunger signals.** Studies by researcher Brian Wansink at the Cornell University Food and Brand Lab always garner headlines because they prove what most of us suspect: We don't eat because we're hungry. We eat because there's food in front of us. Wansink even found that people would overeat stale popcorn if it were served in giant bowls. You'll be able to keep your weight in control if you stop eating mindlessly and stay tuned into your hunger and satiety signals. Take small portions, eat slowly, and chew more carefully, paying attention to taste and how the food makes you feel. It takes about 20 minutes before your brain gets the message that your belly is full, so don't gobble past fullness.

○ **Fiber.** Women should be getting 25 grams of fiber daily by eating whole grain bread and cereals and fruit and vegetables. A high fiber diet has been shown to reduce the risk of heart disease, and may help lower your risk for some cancers.

○ **Low-fat dairy.** Another great way to stay slim and have healthy bones: Choose low-fat and fat-free cheeses and yogurt. They have all the calcium and other nutrients their high-fat counterparts carry—without the saturated fat.

"They're nutritional powerhouses without the guilt," says Leslie Bonci, MPH, RD, director of nutrition at the Center for Sports Medicine at the University of Pittsburgh and spokesperson for the American Dietetic Association.

Continue supplementing with 500 mg of calcium (up to 1,000 if you don't eat dairy) and 600 IU of vitamin D to protect you from osteoporosis and cancer.

○ **Unprocessed foods.** Since women need fewer calories as they get older, avoiding processed foods—which are usually low in vitamins, minerals, and fiber, and high in fat and sugar—will give you the nutrients you need at a discount: fewer calories.

Your Doctor's Office Checklist

◯ **Dental checkup.** Continue to go to the dentist every 6 months, unless your dentist advises more trips.

◯ **Eye exams.** If you have never had one, schedule an initial comprehensive eye exam now. Then see an eye doctor every 2 to 4 years or sooner if you notice a change in your vision.

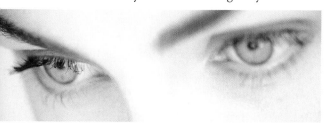

◯ **Serum ferritin test and transferrin saturation test.** If you're frequently fatigued or have liver disease, diabetes, arthritis, or a family history of hemochromatosis and haven't gotten these tests, get them. Talk to your physician about the most current recommendations regarding these iron tests.

◯ **Skin exams.** Until age 40, you've been getting checked every 3 years. Now let your dermatologist look you over annually.

◯ **Tetanus shot.** Repeat every 10 years.

◯ **Blood pressure check.** The risk of developing hypertension tends to increase as we get older, so get checked at least every 2 years, but preferably every time you see the doctor. See page 8 for normal values.

◯ **Complete lipid profile.** Continue getting this done every 2 years if results are normal, and every 4 months if they're abnormal. See page 8 for normal values.

◯ **Thyroid-stimulating hormone test.** Get screened every 5 years for an underactive or overactive thyroid.

◯ **Stress-echocardiogram test.** If you're 40 or older and at high risk for heart disease (you have high blood pressure, high cholesterol, a strong family history of heart disease or early heart attack, have a personal history of bypass surgery, or have had a heart attack or angioplasty) get a stress echocardiogram test. This noninvasive test allows your doctor to see via ultrasound how your heart responds to stress–in this case, walking on a treadmill. A stress echo is also a smart move if you're about to embark on a vigorous exercise program and you've been virtually sedentary.

◯ **Flu shot.** Get a flu shot in September or October of every year.

◯ **Bone-density test.** If you're at high risk for osteoporosis, as described on page 13, or at the first signs of menopause, get a bone density scan.

◯ **Pelvic exam, Pap test, and breast exam.** If you've have three normal Pap and/or HPV tests, you only need to be tested every 3 years. But you should still see your gynecologist for a pelvic exam and clinical breast screening yearly. This is the time to talk to your doctor about any signs of perimenopause you might be experiencing. Symptoms to watch for: heavy bleeding, bleeding longer than 7 days (or 2 or more days longer than usual), having fewer than 21 days between periods, spotting between periods, and bleeding after intercourse. They could indicate a hormone imbalance, misuse of birth control pills, pregnancy, fibroids, thyroid dysfunction, abnormalities in the uterine lining, cancer, or bleeding outside the uterus (such as in the vagina or cervix). Many women also experience incontinence at this time—even if it's just when they laugh or lift a heavy bag. Your doctor can tell you about treatments for this.

○ **Pelvic ultrasound.** Women at high risk for ovarian cancer (several family members had breast or ovarian cancer or you have a mutated BRCA gene) will probably be advised to have a pelvic ultrasound and a CA-125 test, a blood test that looks for cancer markers in the blood.

Women with BRCA1 and BRCA2 mutations are also at higher risk for ovarian, breast, and some other cancers. If you know you have a gene that could give you cancer, you may want to be tested every 6 months.

Symptoms to watch for: Enlargement of the abdomen is the most common sign of ovarian cancer, but it's not always present. A large tumor could make you look 5 months pregnant. Another sign is persistent digestive problems, such as unexplained stomach discomfort, gas,

and abdominal swelling. In rare cases, abnormal vaginal bleeding will occur. Though ovarian cancer is often called a "silent" cancer, studies have found that most women diagnosed with the disease noticed subtle symptoms that they communicated to their doctors months before their diagnosis. Ovarian cancer has a low survival rate because the symptoms aren't taken seriously; when caught early, it can have a 90 percent survival rate.

○ **Mammogram.** You've been doing monthly breast self-exams and getting an annual clinical breast exam, but once you reach age 40, it's time to start getting an annual mammogram. A mammogram is a low-intensity x-ray that can confirm whether lumps you or your doctor found are in fact tumors. It can also detect tumors when they're too small to feel with your hand. When tumors are found early, they're easier to treat and could be cured because the cancer hasn't spread to other parts of the body.

Symptoms to watch for: breast lumps, thickening, swelling, distortion, tenderness, skin irritation, nipple pain, scaliness, or dimpling.

AGES 50 *to* 62

For some women, life begins—again—at 50. Careers are solid, the kids are flying out of the nest, and for the first time in your life you can enjoy sex without birth control. Perimenopausal symptoms—hot flashes, insomnia, headaches, night sweats, and mood swings—

gradually ebb when estrogen production and menstruation cease. In fact, postmenopausal women are the least likely of all women to be depressed–thanks to a well-deserved sense of well-being.

If you've had 12 straight months without a period, you've reached menopause. It could happen anywhere between the ages of 40 and 58, but the average age is 51. Women who smoke usually go through menopause about a year and a half earlier than women who don't, and women with a higher body mass index (see page 98) or who have had more than one pregnancy usually experience later-than-average menopause. You'll probably reach menopause at the same age your mother did.

In the past, doctors thought a decline in health after menopause was a normal part of aging. Although the rates of chronic and killer diseases do go up as we age, we know that a healthy lifestyle now more than ever can keep us going like Energizer bunnies. Good thing, too, since many women spend at least one-third of their lives after menopause.

Of course, menopause does bring new health challenges. Women can lose between 2 and 5 percent of bone mass on average per year in the first 3 to 5 years after menopause. Your risk of dying from breast cancer, too, rises with age (although it's still a distant third behind heart disease and lung cancer for women in general). When you were 35, your chance of getting breast cancer was only one in 622. By age 60, the relative risk is one in 24 (although the risk varies greatly from woman to woman). And while estrogen protected you in younger years from heart disease, losing it in menopause raises LDL ("bad") cholesterol levels, and by the time you're 60, your risk will have increased to equal a man's. Estrogen also kept your blood vessels naturally elastic. Without it, the risk of heart disease and stroke increases.

When Calcium Isn't Good

Calcium supplements can help preserve bone density, protecting you from fractures. But did you know that taking calcium just before a bone scan might blur your bone density test results?

The very best test for measuring bone density in the spine and hip—dual energy x-ray absorptiometry, or DEXA—works by reading how much calcium is present, not only in the bone but also within a cross section of the body. Poorly absorbed calcium can linger in the intestines and mimic dense bone on a spine scan, obscuring telltale signs of thinning bone, says Jeri Nieves, PhD, director of bone-density testing at Helen Hayes Hospital in West Haverstraw, New York.

This rarely happens, but it could at least cause inconvenience: If your doctor notices an odd reading, she may suggest a second scan. "Don't quit taking supplements or cancel your DEXA," says Dr. Nieves. Instead, use a calcium supplement labeled "USP"—meaning it's met the U.S. Pharmacopeia's standard for dissolving. And don't take any calcium supplement within an hour of a DEXA, adds Dr. Nieves. ∎

Again, these risks are relative and within your control. That's why a healthy diet and screening are extra important at this age. Calcium and vitamin D help fight bone loss, but if a bone density scan finds that you have low bone mass, your doctor can put you on protective therapy early to fight it. If a breast tumor is found with a mammogram or breast exam, the earlier it's detected the easier it is to treat and cure. In the meantime, you can eat food associated with low breast cancer risk. Eating a low-fat diet, getting exercise, and not smoking can lower your odds of getting heart disease.

The scale presents another challenge. It may get harder and harder to keep your weight down, unless you watch what you eat and stay active. Increasing your muscle mass with exercise will help you burn calories.

Your Self-Care Checklist

○ **Calorie reduction.** To compensate for slower metabolism, cut another 100 calories from your diet daily. Cut down on the size of your meals instead of completely eliminating a food group, such as carbohydrates like bread. To fill your plate without overeating, use a salad plate for dinner and you won't feel deprived.

○ **Mini-meals.** One of the best ways to keep your metabolism going strong is to eat. Your body burns up to 15 percent of your daily calories just digesting food. It's called the thermic effect of eating. Now would be a good time to ditch the usual three big meals and eat six smaller ones of about 250 calories each throughout the day. Researchers have found that women who eat larger meals may burn 60 fewer calories per day than women who eat mini-meals—the equivalent of 6 pounds a year.

○ **Portion control.** To make sure you're not eating double or triple portions of snacks, crackers, and other packaged foods, check the serving size on food labels, and limit yourself to single servings, not the whole amount provided.

○ **Low-fat, high-fiber diet.** A diet low in fat and high in fiber has been associated with a lower risk of both heart disease and cancer. Reach for fruit, vegetables, whole grain breads and cereals, legumes, soy foods, and low-fat or fat-free dairy foods.

○ **Calcium and vitamin D.** Postmenopausal women get only half the calcium they need, yet they need more calcium than ever. Without estrogen, you've lost some protection from bone loss, so increase your daily calcium consumption to 1,200 mg.

You don't have to drink three glasses of milk a day. Instead, you may take calcium supplements equal to 700 mg toward that Daily Value. *Prevention* recommends that for better absorption you spread the dose out over the day, and take no more than 500 mg at one time. Though you need to take calcium citrate, with meals, you may take calcium citrate on an empty stomach. Look for a calcium supplement formula with vitamin D, calcium's little helper (it totes calcium to your bones, where you need it). You may need more D than what your daily multi provides.

◯ **Vitamin B$_{12}$.** Women need only 6 mcg per day of vitamin B$_{12}$ to fight heart disease, but after age 50 it's harder for us to absorb the vitamin when we get it from food because we have less stomach acid. Take it in a multisupplement or in fortified foods.

◯ **Leafy greens.** Lutein and zeaxanthin, antioxidants found in spinach, may protect the retina from age-related macular degeneration, a leading cause of blindness. Eat spinach or another dark leafy green with olive oil once a day, since fat promotes lutein absorption.

◯ **Fall prevention.** As you approach age 60, step up your efforts to prevent falls, to guard against wrist and hip fractures. Keep electrical cords away from through traffic areas of your home, use night-lights, arrange for handrails (and nonskid tape) to be installed in the shower, clean up spills in the kitchen right away, wear sturdy, rubber-soled shoes, and put rubber mats under throw rugs to keep them from sliding under your feet. If you're having balance problems, consider tai chi, a meditative form of the Chinese martial arts that has been found in studies to improve balance (and also to provide relief in people with arthritis).

◯ **Baby aspirin.** If you're over 55, ask your doctor if you might benefit from taking a low dose (81 mg or a baby aspirin) every day. Though aspirin therapy has not been shown to

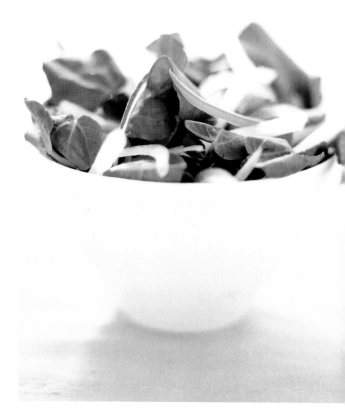

help prevent heart attacks in women, it does reduce risks of strokes caused by arterial blockages. However, it may increase your risk of strokes caused by the bursting of blood vessels in the brain. Aspirin can also cause bleeding. You and your doctor will need to weigh the risks and benefits.

Your Doctor's Office Checklist

◯ **Height measurement.** You should be getting your height measured every time you're at the doctor's office, or at least once a year. Over your lifetime, a gradual loss of about 1.5 inches is normal. But if you've lost more height than that—or you've lost 1.5 inches in 10 years or less—it could indicate vertebral compression fractures as a result of osteoporosis.

◯ **Bone-density test.** Get a bone-density measurement if you're in menopause or past menopause and you've never had the test. Out of the 25 million Americans who have osteoporosis, 80 percent are women.

The best measurement for women is a DEXA scan of the spine and the hip, the two places that usually have the most serious fractures. The spine is also where the first bone loss most often occurs after menopause. Some rural areas don't have the machine. In that case, an ultrasound of the heel or a dual or single x-ray of the arm or finger will measure your bone density.

◯ **25-hydroxy vitamin D serum level check.** If you're older than 49, especially if you're at risk for osteoporosis, have your level of vitamin D checked. Vitamin D helps calcium get absorbed in the body. Your levels should be over 20 nanograms per liter.

◯ **Dental checkup.** Go to the dentist every 6 months, or more often if you experience pain or other problems.

◯ **Eye exams.** Go for a comprehensive eye examination, if you have not already done so. You should be getting an eye exam every 2 to 4 years, or sooner if you notice a change in your vision.

◯ **Serum ferritin test and transferrin saturation test.** Women are often tested at age 18 for hemochromatosis, an iron overload disease. After menopause is a good time to get tested again. Talk to your physician about the most current recommendations regarding these tests.

◯ **Skin exams.** Don't let up on those annual skin exams. One in five Americans is diagnosed with skin cancer over the course of a lifetime. Between 40 and 50 percent of Americans who live to be 65 will be diagnosed at least once.

◯ **Blood pressure check.** Get your blood pressure checked at least every 2 years, and more often if it's abnormal. See page 8 for normal values.

◯ **Complete lipid profile.** Now more than ever, it's important to have your cholesterol checked at least every 2 years, or every 4 months if it's abnormal. Women typically get cardiovascular disease 10 to 15 years later than men, when they experience the postmenopausal loss of estrogen. Also, cholesterol levels change after menopause. "Bad" LDL cholesterol levels go up, while "good" HDL cholesterol levels go down, putting postmenopausal women at greater risk for cardiovascular disease. See page 8 for normal values.

◯ **Thyroid-stimulating hormone test.** Don't forget to get screened every 5 years for an underactive or overactive thyroid.

◯ **Pelvic exam, Pap test, and breast exam.** Menopause doesn't mean you should stop your yearly gynecologist visit. You may still need a Pap test (once every 3 years if the previous three were normal) and are at higher risk of some cancers at this stage of life. Even if you've had a hysterectomy and your ovaries were removed, you still need a pelvic exam, says Dr. Gass. The pelvic exam can be helpful in finding and treating other problems, such as incontinence, genital itching, sores, or painful intercourse.

◯ **Mammogram.** Continue to get an annual mammogram.

◯ **Colorectal screening.** Colorectal cancer is the third most common cancer among American women, but it's almost always curable if found early enough. If everyone started getting regular screenings for colon cancer at age 50, about 25,000 lives a year could be saved.

Make sure your annual pelvic exam includes a digital rectal exam, starting at age 50. Also, get a colonoscopy at age 50 and every 10 years thereafter.

Risk factors for colon cancer include:

■ A family history

■ A genetic predisposition

■ Chronic inflammatory bowel disease

■ A previous history of colon polyps or colon cancer

Watch out for rectal bleeding, blood in stool, or a change in bowel habits.

> "Studies show that **aspirin reduces the growth of polyps** that lead to colon cancer. The dose and frequency are not clear, but talk with your doctor about taking either regular or baby aspirin at least every other day."
>
> —HAROLD FRUCHT, MD, DIRECTOR OF GASTROENTEROLOGY AT FOX CHASE CANCER CENTER IN PHILADELPHIA

◯ **Low-dose CAT scan.** Lung cancer kills more Americans than any other cancer, and it's usually not diagnosed until it's too far along to treat. Annual low-dose CAT scans in women 60 or older who smoke now or smoked in the past may be able to detect tumors while they are small enough to be treated. A 2010 study by the National Cancer Institute found that having a low-dose CAT scan reduced deaths by 20 percent among more than 50,000 people who are or were heavy smokers.

◯ **Flu shot.** Everyone over age 50—except those allergic to eggs or the flu vaccine—should get a flu shot each September or October. If you're healthy, the shot can prevent illness, and if you have a chronic medical condition, such as asthma, it can reduce the flu's severity and risk of serious complications.

◯ **Fasting glucose test.** All women 45 and older should have their blood sugar tested every

3 years to screen for diabetes. If results are abnormal or if you're at high risk for diabetes, get tested more often.

The signs of diabetes are unexplained weight loss, unusual thirst, frequent desire to urinate, extreme fatigue, extreme hunger, irritability, frequent infections, blurred vision, slow-healing cuts and bruises, tingling or numbness in the hands or feet, or recurring skin, gum, or bladder infections. If you have prediabetes—your fasting blood glucose levels are elevated though not enough for a diabetes diagnosis—you may not experience any of these symptoms, but the glucose circulating in your blood may already be causing damage to your arteries and organs. Almost everyone who has this precursor develops full-blown diabetes within 10 years and is at increased risk of cardiovascular disease.

◯ **Tetanus shot.** Two out of three people over age 60 haven't gotten a tetanus shot in the past 10 years, which means they're not immune to tetanus. If you're one of those people, make sure you get the shot.

AGES 62 *and* OLDER

About one in eight Americans has reached the age of 65, and 20.2 million of them are women. By year 2030, one in four Americans will be over 65, and most of them will be women.

There's no doubt about it: We're living longer than ever before—and these years bring unique health concerns.

Screens for colon cancer and mammograms are absolutely necessary now. Colorectal cancer is nearly 100 percent curable if discovered early. While women over 65 who have had several negative Pap tests don't have to get them anymore, it's still important to see your gynecologist for pelvic exams and clinical breast exams.

Getting exercise should also be high on your list of priorities. You want to stay active and independent for years to come, so go for walks, garden, dance. Spend a minimum of 30 minutes most days of the week doing weight-bearing aerobic exercise. (New exercise guidelines suggest being active for an hour a day.) Every other day, lift weights for 15 or 20 minutes, suggests Michael Lichtenstein, MD, geriatrician at the University of Texas Health Center in San Antonio and principal investigator for the National Institutes of Health's Positively Aging educational program. You'll burn extra calories and strengthen your bones and muscles so you can lift your own grocery bags and those precious grandchildren. It can also help you maintain your balance.

Even if you have low bone mass or osteoporosis, lifting weights is safe if you start with a light weight of no more than 5 pounds and go slowly, he says. To avoid injury, give yourself a day to rest between strength-training sessions. Besides keeping you strong, exercise, along with a sensible eating plan, can help you lose any excess weight, which can ease any aches and pains from osteoarthritis, the wear-and-tear kind that strikes about half of us when we're 65 and older.

But your muscles and skeleton shouldn't be the only thing you should be exercising, say health experts. Filling up your social calendar, connecting emotionally with friends and family, and staying stimulated also keep you happy and healthy.

"There's no question that people who remain intellectually active and socially engaged in older years do better," says Eugenia Siegler, MD, professor of clinical medicine at Weill Cornell Medical College of Cornell University in New York City. Use this time to travel, learn new things, take classes at a local college, volunteer, and connect to friends and family.

Most retired Americans are already active. The proportion of retired American women who are sedentary fell from 44 percent in 1985 to 39 percent in 1995.

Women are challenging themselves by going back to school or work, volunteering, and making use of the Internet. In one survey, 37 percent of older adults said continuing their edu-

cation was important in retirement. "Learning-in-retirement" programs have even popped up around the United States, from local community colleges to Harvard, and many of them are free.

Attitudes toward these years have changed, too. Compared with a generation ago, today fewer Americans over age 65 say poor health, loneliness, few job opportunities, and too little money are problems for people in their age group.

Your Self-Care Checklist

○ **Nutrient-dense food.** As you age, your basal metabolic rate—the amount of calories you need to breathe, keep your heart beating, and digest your food—decreases and your caloric needs drop with it, while your nutritional needs are rising. Make every calorie count by eating whole grains, beans, low-fat dairy foods, fruits and vegetables, and small amounts of extra-lean meats—a diet that can help you avoid heart attack, stroke, some cancers, macular degeneration, perhaps even Alzheimer's disease. Take a multi supplement just to make sure you're getting all your nutrients, but choose one without iron.

○ **Antioxidant-rich food.** Antioxidants found in fruits, vegetables, and whole grains stimulate your immune system and help you avoid infections like the flu or pneumonia. So polish off your vegetable stir-fry with a bowl of berries.

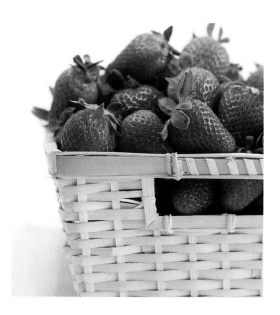

◯ **Calcium and vitamins D and B₆.** You should be getting 1,200 mg of calcium through food or supplements, along with 600 IUs of D until you reach 70. when you should increase it to 800 IU. That will not only promote bone health; studies have found that getting sufficient vitamin D may help prevent heart disease and even depression in older people. Many older people don't get enough D the usual ways—via dairy products and sun exposure. You should also be getting 1.5 mg of B₆ daily, as low levels have been linked to impaired immunity in older people. Foods rich in B₆ include fortified cereals, bananas, salmon, turkey, chicken, potato, and spinach.

◯ **Drink plenty of water.** As you get older, your thirst signals wane so waiting until you feel thirsty to grab a cold one isn't going to get you all the fluid you need. Remind yourself to drink 6 to 8 cups of water or other fluid every day to guard against dehydration and constipation.

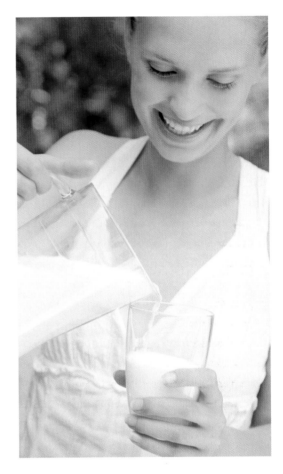

Your Doctor's Office Checklist

◯ **Flu shot.** Continue getting a flu shot in September or October of every year. If you have a chronic medical condition, the shot might not prevent the flu, but it could make your illness less severe if you do get it, and lower your risk of complications.

◯ **Pneumococcal vaccine.** Get the vaccine for pneumococcal pneumonia at least once after age 64. You'll want to avoid the trip to the hospital or the infections that could result from pneumonia.

◯ **Dental checkups.** Continue going to the dentist every 6 months, and don't ignore gum pain, swelling, or bleeding.

◯ **Eye exams.** After you turn 65, start going to the eye doctor every 1 to 2 years if you haven't been already. If you have diabetes, go to the ophthalmologist every year to make sure you don't get diabetic retinopathy, a disease in which tiny blood vessels in the eye weaken and leak, causing blurred vision or even blindness.

◯ **Skin exams.** This is no time to slack off on skin care, especially if leaving the workforce affords you more time in the outdoors. Continue getting tested annually for skin cancer.

◯ **Tetanus shot.** Two out of three people over age 60 aren't immune to tetanus, a disease in which bacteria enter an open wound and attack the nervous system, causing muscle spasms, lockjaw, difficulty swallowing, rigid muscles, fever, sweating, and an accelerated heart rate. Get vaccinated every 10 years.

◯ **Bone density test.** You should be getting a DEXA scan regularly by now. Nine out of ten women have osteoporosis by age 75, so being screened regularly is essential.

If your test results are normal, go back for another scan every 3 to 5 years. If you have low bone mass and you're on therapy to treat it, go back in 2 years to track your progress. After that, your doctor will put you on your own screening schedule to see if you're progressing from the therapy.

◯ **Blood pressure check.** Continue getting your blood pressure checked at least every 2 years, or more often if your readings are abnormal.

◯ **Complete lipid profile.** Keep getting this test every 2 years if results are normal, and every 4 months if abnormal.

◯ **Fasting blood plasma glucose test.** Screening for diabetes is still important, so get a fasting blood plasma glucose test every 3 years.

◯ **Colon cancer screening.** Continue getting a digital rectal exam every year and a colonoscopy every 10 years, along with a yearly fecal occult blood test.

◯ **Thyroid-stimulating hormone test.** You should still be getting screened every 5 years for thyroid disease.

◯ **Pelvic exam, Pap test, and breast exams.** Many women think they don't need regular gynecological exams after menopause, but women's risk for reproductive cancers goes up after menopause, so make and keep that appointment. It's also a good time to talk to your doctor about any problems you may be having, such as incontinence or pelvic pain.

◯ **Mammograms.** Don't forget your yearly mammogram. To help you remember, schedule it on your birthday.

WAITING ROOM

Get the Most Out of Your Next Doctor's Appointment

It will come as no surprise that two-thirds of people looking for health information look to their computer rather than their doctor. However, those same people say their most trusted source for such information is their personal physician. Doctors know. In recent decades, they've become accustomed to patients arriving with computer printouts or pages ripped from magazines. There's even a French term for it: *La maladie du petit papier* . . . the sickness of the little paper. We have arguably become better informed than ever.

What that means is that health care, now more than ever, has become a partnership between doctors and their patients—and women don't hesitate to ask questions or even suggest their own therapies. But forming that partnership takes time, and time is a precious commodity in the era of managed care.

Visits with doctors have always been shorter than they should be, and the rise of HMOs has made them even shorter, says Mary Jane Minkin, MD, clinical professor of obstetrics and gynecology at Yale University School of Medicine. "There's not a heck of a lot you can discuss with somebody in 5 minutes," says Dr. Minkin.

Fortunately, those short visits may be getting slightly longer. According to the National Center for Health Statistics, we're now spending about 20 minutes with our doctors these days, compared to barely 17 minutes 20 years ago.

Still, that's not a lot of time to get all your questions answered and concerns addressed. Make the most of your time by following this advice from some of our experts and advisors, the same strategies they use when they themselves are the patients.

Your Routine Checkup

This is your chance to discuss recent health problems as well as any physical or emotional changes that have occurred since you last saw your doctor. Routine checkups also give your doctor the opportunity to do comprehensive physical exams. To get the most out of the visit:

Know your family history. Many illnesses (and risk factors for illnesses) are influenced by a woman's family history. Before you arrive for your checkup, take a few minutes to jot down what you know about the health of your grandparents, parents, siblings, and children. You'll probably be asked to fill out a form and give details about your family's experience with heart disease, diabetes, and other conditions. A family history of some illnesses, such as heart disease and breast or colon cancer, may require you to have more frequent screenings, so your doctor needs to know about them.

Bring medical records. Give your doctor a copy of any medical records that he doesn't already have. These might include reports of mammograms, Pap tests, colonoscopies, or other tests you've had within the past year. If you don't have copies of these reports, you can

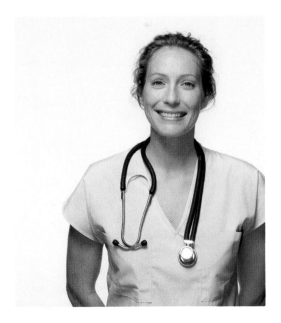

get them (usually free of charge) from the clinics or hospitals where they were performed.

Make a list of current health concerns. It's easy to forget things when you're in the doctor's office. To make sure nothing gets missed, make a "cheat sheet" that lists symptoms or problems that are worrying you, such as a persistent cough, nagging joint pain, or difficulty sleeping, advises Marianne Legato, MD, director of Partnership for Women's Health at Columbia University in New York City. Try to avoid what doctors call "doorknob complaints:" Your doctor thinks he's taken care of all your concerns and once his hand is on the doorknob you say, "Oh, by the way," and proceed to ask about something you may have forgotten, were too embarrassed to mention, or just couldn't get in edgewise because your doctor interrupted

you. Doorknob complaints may not be adequately addressed. The problem is, your doctor may have mentally moved on, says Melissa Piasecki, MD, associate professor of psychiatry at the University of Nevada and author of a handbook for doctors on how to improve their patient communication skills. "They can come back and re-engage, but they've already signaled to you that they've got time pressure, and it's not going to be the same kind of conversation as before the hand touched the doorknob."

Be firm. "Doctors can get intimidating, they get going fast, and patients feel it's inappropriate to interrupt, then all of a sudden the doctor is gone and there are two things they haven't talked about," says Robert C. Smith, MD, professor of medicine at Michigan State University and author of *Patient-Centered Interviewing*, a manual for

Time-Management Tips

doctors and patients agree: There simply isn't enough time in the average visit to get everything done. Here are a few ways to cope with the time crunch.

Find a doctor with time. Every doctor spends different amounts of time with patients. If you're choosing a new doctor, call the office and ask how much time they allot for new-patient visits, annual physicals, and regular doctor visits. One doctor might allow 5 or 10 minutes; another might allow 30. For a fee (which can range from $400 to $3,000), concierge practices allow greater access to your primary care doctor day or night via house calls, phone or e-mail, or same-day appointments, and sometimes

offer discounted services such as screening tests.

See other health professionals. Physician's assistants and nurse practitioners are totally qualified to treat most common problems, and they usually spend more time with patients than doctors do, says Dr. Minkin.

Discuss the main topics first. Before walking into your doctor's office, prepare a list of key points you want to bring up—and start with the most important ones. When researchers looked at 264 patient-physician interviews, they found that the doctors tended to interrupt after a patient had been talking for an average of 23 seconds. That doesn't give you a lot of time, so plan on starting with the three or four issues that are most important. ■

doctors. Be firm without being pushy—"assertive without being aggressive," says Dr. Smith.

Talk about tests. In the preceding chapter, you learned about health issues that affect women at different stages of life. After reviewing the information, you may want to ask your doctor if you're due for important screening tests, such as a cholesterol test or a mammogram.

Your Annual Pelvic Exam

No one looks forward to it, but the yearly pelvic exam is essential for a woman's long-term health. Here's how to make the most of this important appointment.

Think beyond reproductive health. Your gynecologist needs to know about all your health issues, not only those that appear to involve the reproductive organs. Many common symptoms—fatigue, for example—may be linked to a woman's hormones. Your gynecologist can't provide comprehensive care unless she knows about any and all symptoms that may be troubling you, says Dr. Legato.

Don't hold back. It's not uncommon for women to make an appointment to see their gynecologists then neglect to discuss personal or intimate details. Don't let embarrassment hold you back. If you're experiencing low sex drive, for example, tell your doctor. Are you having trouble controlling urine? Talk about it. The issues may be uncomfortable, but this is your chance to find out if something's wrong—and what you can do to resolve it, says Dr. Legato.

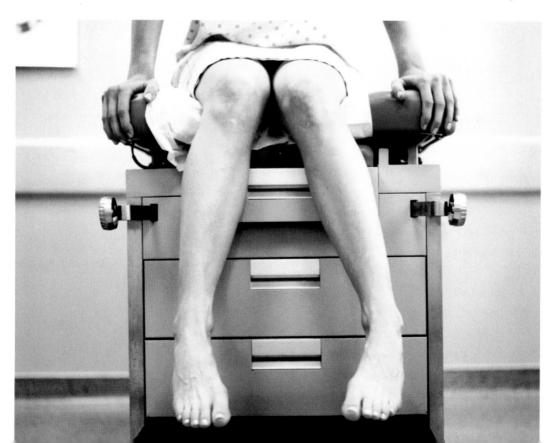

If you're uncomfortable, speak up. No one feels completely comfortable during a pelvic exam, but you shouldn't be in pain. Always let your doctor know if the exam is more uncomfortable than usual. She can probably reduce the discomfort, by using a smaller speculum, for example, or applying less pressure to the abdomen.

> "Patients have taught me a substantial amount of what's important to me in medicine. **The story of a patient's illness** as told by an intelligent and sensitive patient is **invaluable** because it tells you how the disease is experienced."

—MARIANNE J. LEGATO, MD, DIRECTOR OF PARTNERSHIP FOR WOMEN'S HEALTH AT COLUMBIA UNIVERSITY IN NEW YORK CITY

When You're Sick

Doctors aren't mind readers. Whether you're seeing your doctor because you have been fatigued, have a persistent discharge, or simply aren't feeling well, he won't know where to begin unless you describe your symptoms clearly.

"In at least 80 percent of cases, we can diagnose the illness before any laboratory testing—if the patient communicates effectively," Dr. Legato says.

To communicate clearly:

Describe your symptoms exactly. If you have pain in a joint in your elbow, don't tell your doctor that you're feeling achy. If you have a cough, tell your doctor if it's "wet" or "dry," or if it's painful or merely irritating. The more specific you are in describing symptoms, the easier it will be for your doctor to figure out what's going on, says Dr. Legato.

One woman told Dr. Legato that she felt as though blood couldn't get through her right calf. "That happens to be a perfect description of deep-vein thrombosis, which is exactly what she had," the doctor says.

Some other good rules to follow when describing symptoms:

- Point to what hurts. Is the pain deep or superficial? Does it radiate?

- Score it. On a scale of 1 to 10, 10 being the worst pain you've ever had, rank your pain.

- Time it. Does the symptom come and go, last for minutes, hours, days? Does it happen periodically, during a certain season, or time of day? What were you doing when you had the dizzy spell or suddenly had to run to the bathroom? Does it happen in a certain place, such as the office, at home in the morning or evening, on the weekends, while you're walking, running, or sitting?

- Explain how it affected you. This is very useful for doctors, says Dr. Piasecki. "For example, 'I was so tired I started taking the elevator instead of walking up five floors. I was so tired I didn't get out of bed all weekend except to use the toilet.'" For many psychological problems, the symptom has to interfere with your daily life before your doctor can diagnose you with a condition.

- Don't neglect to discuss physical symptoms, even those that appear to be vague or minor.

Leave the diagnosis to your doctor. Patients often walk into their doctors' offices and tell them what they think is causing their symptoms—often something horrible they read about on the Internet or saw on the latest episode of *House* or *Grey's Anatomy*. Self-diagnosis is unlikely to be accurate and can waste valuable time by leading your doctor in the wrong direction. You're better off simply telling your doctor your symptoms, says geriatrician Helen K. Edelberg, MD, senior director of the therapeutic strategy unit in aging at Sanofi-Aventis and former adjunct clinical assistant professor at Mount Sinai School of Medicine in New York City.

Brown-bag your medications. Both prescription and over-the-counter medications could contribute to your symptoms or affect the treatment your doctor recommends. Put all the medications, supplements, and herbal treatments you've taken or are taking in a paper bag and bring them to the doctor's office with you. Or you can make a written list—just remember to write down the dosages.

Don't leave until you completely understand your diagnosis. If you're not sure what the diagnosis is, ask your doctor to repeat it. Make sure you also fully understand what your doctor says about test results, future plans, and treatment options. You won't be able to take proper care of yourself if you don't clearly understand what's happening with your health, says Barbara Korsch, MD, professor of pediatrics at Children's Hospital, USC Keck School of Medicine, and author of *The Intelligent Patient's Guide to the Doctor-Patient Relationship*.

Make sure you understand your instructions. Before leaving your doctor's office, take a moment to repeat everything you were told to do: what medicines to take, the proper dosage, and so on. Doctors often advise men and women alike to bring a notepad so they can jot things down while the information is still fresh.

Bring backup. If you're anxious or get a frightening diagnosis, you may not be able to remember all your symptoms or everything the doctor tells you. "I've talked to people who say 'I

When to Go to the Emergency Room

most illnesses and conditions can wait until you're able to see a doctor, but some symptoms require emergency attention. They include:

- Chest or upper abdominal pain or pressure
- Difficulty breathing or shortness of breath
- Any sudden or severe pain
- Unusual abdominal pain

- Uncontrolled bleeding
- Coughing or vomiting blood
- Sudden dizziness, weakness, numbness, or a change in vision, ability to speak, or balance
- Severe or persistent vomiting or diarrhea to the point of fainting from dehydration
- Marked changes in mental function, such as confusion
- Suicidal feelings ∎

wasn't having problems,' but the family member behind them is nodding and saying, 'No, he had huge problems,'" says Dr. Piasecki. Have someone with you whose job it is to prod your memory and take down notes for you. It won't hurt to have emotional support either.

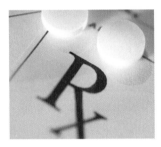

Discussing Treatment Options

More than two-thirds of all doctors' visits end with a prescription being written, making medication the most common form of intervention.

Whether your doctor is recommending medications, physical therapy, or surgery, you have to be sure that you fully understand the implications of the treatment. Here are some questions everyone should ask.

What are the benefits? People often undergo treatments without really understanding what they stand to gain. Once you know why your doctor has recommended a particular course of action—taking a pill to "thin" the blood, for example, or using physical therapy to relieve pressure on a spinal nerve—you'll be more likely to stick with the plan. It's also important to discuss with your doctor the alternatives to treatment, including the anticipated results if treatment is not initiated. Sometimes people do get well on their own, says Dr. Korsch.

What are the side effects? Doctors are often reluctant to mention a medication's side effects because some people will report anything from itchy teeth to stools that glow in the dark, jokes Dr. Minkin. But you need to know if the medications you'll be taking are likely to cause problems—and you'll be more likely to keep taking them when you're sure that side effects are rare or insignificant, says Dr. Legato.

"My greatest disappointment is when a patient says, 'I didn't fill the prescription because I was afraid of the side effects,'" she adds. "That means I didn't give the patient enough time to express concerns."

How soon will it work? Treatments don't always work right away, and it's important to know what to expect. An antibiotic will relieve symptoms within a day or two, while some antidepressants won't be fully effective for weeks. Physical therapy for back problems may take months. Knowing the time frame ahead of time makes it easier to gauge the effectiveness of treatment, says Dr. Minkin.

Get the Most from Tests

Diagnostic tests are essential for your health. Consider colonoscopy: If everyone—men and women alike—had this test at age 50 and regularly thereafter, there would be 25,000 fewer deaths annually from colon cancer.

No one likes getting tested. It can be nerve-wracking, especially if you have a strong family history. And it can be uncomfortable—and certainly inconvenient. Don't let your fears hold

"Doctors' visits are **emotionally charged.** When you're in that type of situation and you're without power, you're not in a state to listen. So **prepare for the visit** so you don't get overwhelmed."

—BARBARA KORSCH, MD, HEAD OF GENERAL PEDIATRICS AT CHILDREN'S HOSPITAL OF LOS ANGELES AND AUTHOR OF *THE INTELLIGENT PATIENT'S GUIDE TO THE DOCTOR-PATIENT RELATIONSHIP*

you back. For most women, screening tests catch serious illnesses early enough to make them curable. Here are a few ways to calm your nerves.

Learn the details. Tests are scariest when you don't know what to expect. Ask your doctor to describe the test in detail. Will there be pain? How long will the discomfort last? How long does it take to get results? The more information you get, the less nervous you are likely to be.

Also, don't hesitate to ask other women, including women in the doctor's office, about their experiences with the tests, and what helped them relax and reduce the discomfort. Just be aware: Everyone's pain/fear/annoyance tolerance is different. Some people will tell you that their colonoscopy was the worst experience they ever had; others will just shrug it off as no big deal.

Know what's normal. When your doctor gives you test results, ask for the normal range. For example, if you're premenopausal and you score a 55 on a follicle-stimulating hormone (FSH) test, your doctor should tell you that you're 25 points above the normal premenopausal score of 30. She'll also explain what this means, and how the numbers affect your long-term health.

Discuss a plan of action. If your test results are normal, your doctor might tell you to keep doing what you're doing. But if they're not, make sure you fully understand what you need to do in the days, months, and years ahead.

How to Ask for Psychological Help

Many women assume that their gynecologists or family doctors are concerned about solely their physical health. But your doctor is also trained to recognize and treat psychological problems. She has to: More than two-thirds of all doctors' office visits are precipitated by psychological concerns, says one study. And some common physical ailments—from headaches to backaches to high blood pressure—can have an emotional component.

Explain any emotional or psychological changes you have experienced lately. If you're having trouble remembering things, give your doctor specific examples: maybe you've been misplacing keys or important papers, or can't remember once-familiar parts of town. Tell your doctor if you're crying more frequently, or, if you're having anxiety attacks. Maybe your palms sweat or your heart races. Details provide important clues about the underlying causes of your feelings.

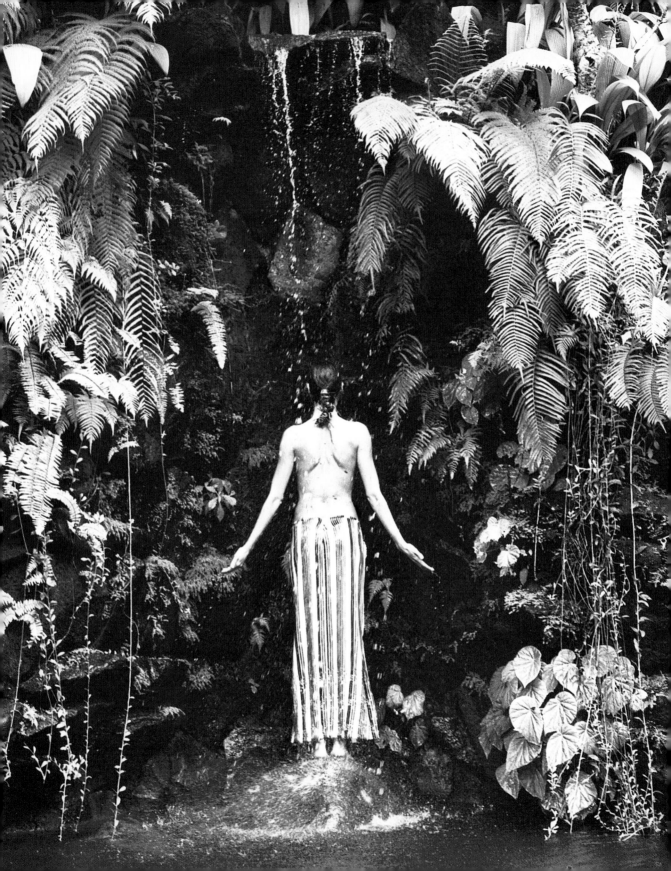

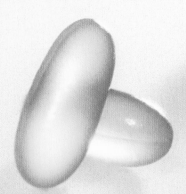

Nutrition: Your Complete Plan

Did you know that fewer than one in five women ages 51 to 70 meets the current minimum daily recommendation for vegetable and fruit consumption? And only 11 percent meet their quota in other age groups. Even women who are conscientious about healthy eating will occasionally fall short on essential nutrients, particularly calcium, vitamin D, and fiber.

Some surveys have shown that only 32 percent of American adults—women included—eat five servings of fruits and vegetables daily. Even that's probably not enough: Many experts advise that for optimal health protection, women should eat as many as nine daily servings of fruits and vegetables, depending on their calorie intake.

And you should get as many of your nutrients from food as you can. In the last decade, new studies have found that some supplements—notably antioxidants such as vitamin A, beta-carotene, vitamin E and selenium, particularly in high doses—may not be beneficial and in some cases may lead to increased mortality, not better health. One study even found that high doses—10 to 100 times more than is consumed in the diet—could actually contribute to cancer. Consider folate. This nutrient has been shown to reduce the risk of heart disease as well as certain birth defects and even cancer. It's abundant in many vegetables and, in the United States, is added to grain products, from cereal to bread.

Yet a 2009 study in Norway found that folic acid and vitamin B supplementation was associated with more cancer cases and more deaths from cancer. Since the jury is still out, only women of childbearing years should take a supplement—400 micrograms of folic acid—to help prevent birth defects, but stop when they've completed their family. There are some nutrients that are hard to get via diet. Only nuts and vegetable oils have appreciable amounts of vitamin E and they're high in calories, which is why government nutrition surveys find that women

only get about 9 to 12 IU of vitamin E daily (the Daily Value is 22 IU of natural E, 33 IU of the synthetic version).

Studies show that getting at least 100 IU daily is associated with a reduced risk of heart disease and it's tough to get that much without supplementing. "It's in a lot of foods but in small amounts," says Maret Traber, PhD, professor and director at the Oxidative/Nitrative Stress Core laboratory at the Linus Pauling Institute at Oregon State University in Corvallis. You would have to eat a mixing bowl full of spinach to get enough, though a handful of almonds or a bowl of vitamin-fortified cereal would just about do it. If you can't get it through your diet, then capping the amount of vitamin E you take at 400 IU—the point at which it may change from helpful to harmful—is the wisest move.

Another reason *Prevention* recommends eating well as the best way to get all the nutrients you need: Many experts now suspect that the health benefits once ascribed to individual constituents of a food (such as vitamins and minerals) may be from the hundreds of chemicals, called phytonutrients, specifically in plant foods, and the kinds of fats and fatty acids in meat, poultry, and fish. "Many of the components of food work synergistically, so it's much better to have the food than it is to isolate one component and give it to people in larger amounts," says Jerianne Heimendinger, PhD, RD, a scientist at the AMC Cancer Research Center in Denver who studied the antioxidant effects of fruit and vegetables.

Nutrition: Where to Start

These days, for good nutrition guidelines, we look to the Mediterranean. *Prevention* recommends what's known as the Mediterranean Diet, a way of eating that emphasizes plenty of vegetables and fruit, good fats, whole grains, with smaller amounts of lean protein, mainly from poultry and fish. People who follow this diet live longer, have a lower risk of cardiovascular disease, cancer, diabetes, and Alzheimer's disease, are thinner, more fertile, and have healthier babies than people in the United States and other parts of the world. The diet may also protect against asthma, chronic diseases such as arthritis, and depression.

Surprisingly, the Mediterranean Diet is higher in fat than it might have been. But most of it is heart-healthy monounsaturated fats from foods like olive oil and nuts. It is lower in saturated fat–found in meat and full-fat dairy products–than the average American diet and falls within the guidelines for a healthy heart established by the American Heart Association. It is also heavy with vegetables and fruits. Meats are downplayed and likely to be a condiment rather than star of a meal. Dairy products are eaten in moderation and sweets just once in a while. After-dinner treats are more likely to be a fresh pear or a bowl of strawberries in season than a dish of creamy tiramisu.

Best of all, a Mediterranean diet is easy to stick to. Because it's high in fiber, it's filling, and the variety–including red wine–makes it enjoyable.

Here's how to eat healthy and well:

Calories. Calorie needs vary from woman to woman depending on height, weight, age, and body composition, and whether she's on a weight loss diet. A very muscular woman might need 2,500 calories per day, and a woman with less muscle might only need 1,800 calories. But a good rule of thumb, if you're not trying to lose weight, is to eat no less than 10 times your body weight in calories, says Leslie Bonci, MPH, RD, director of nutrition at the Center for Sports Medicine at the University of Pittsburgh and spokesperson for the American Dietetic Association. "And for women who weigh less than 100 pounds, no fewer than 1,500 calories per day," she says.

Fruit and vegetables. Aim for at least 2 cups of fruit and $2\frac{1}{2}$ cups of vegetables daily if you're eating around 2,000 calories (servings are measured mainly in $\frac{1}{2}$ cups, so that's four servings of fruit and five servings of vegetables). That will give you a good helping of antioxidants–substances that protect your DNA, the genetic information in every cell of your body–from cancer. (See page 51.) You'll also reap the benefits of the high-fiber content of plant foods, not to mention essential nutrients, like folate, potassium, vitamin A, and vitamin C, abundant in fruits and vegetables.

If you're not accustomed to eating so many fruits and veggies, you need to increase your intake slowly or risk gas pains, Bonci says. Or you can jump right in but use an enzyme product called Beano, which helps digest the undigestible portions of some carbs in your intestines. Start out by tossing a handful of chopped onions

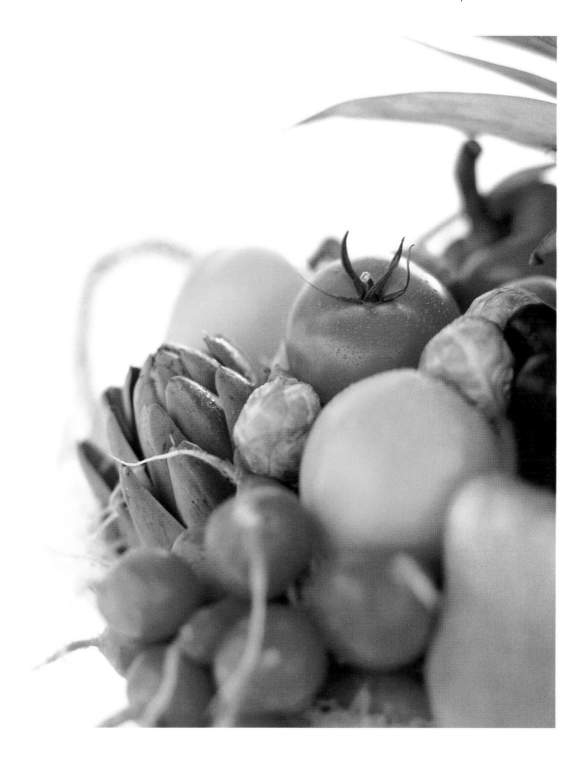

or mushrooms into your spaghetti sauce or morning eggs. Substitute grilled eggplant parmigiana made with low-fat cheese for chicken parmigiana with cheese high in fat. Bake an apple with cinnamon for dessert. Bonci sneaks in two extra servings of vegetables while she makes dinner by snacking on hummus or another bean dip and baby carrots.

To get the best health protection, choose from a variety of colors and botanical families rather than sticking to the same old fruits and veggies every week. Have blueberries, grapes, bananas, and kiwi fruit on hand for snacking or fruit salad. Then mix apples and oranges. The rainbow of colors reflect a variety of phytochemicals that are good for you. For example, carrots and squash get their red-yellow color from alpha- and beta-carotene. A 2010 study found that people who have high blood levels of alpha-carotene are less likely to die of heart disease and cancer than people who have less. Juicy red tomatoes and watermelon are rich in lycopene, which gives them their color. Lycopene in the diet has been linked to protection from heart disease and some forms of cancer. Red-purple fruits such as blueberries, grapes, cherries, blackberries, cranberries, and plums, and purple veggies such as cabbage and beets contain anthocyanin, a pigment that's a potent antioxidant. In studies, it has been shown to improve memory, reduce inflammation (which may account for its heart attack, cancer, and Alzheimer's protection), and protect cellular DNA from ultraviolet light damage, making it the sunscreen you can actually eat.

Whole grains. Get three to six servings whole grain, such as whole wheat bread and bran cereal every day. Whole grains provide all

Extra Help for Smokers

the smoke from cigarettes does more than damage the lungs. It also triggers the formation of free radicals, which "use up" vitamin C in the body. That's why smokers are advised to get 110 mg of vitamin C daily, compared with 75 mg for nonsmokers.

There's another reason smokers may need greater amounts of vitamin C and other nutrients. If you smoke, your diet may not be as good as it should be—in part because nicotine suppresses appetite, and also because smokers are more likely to light up than to enjoy nutritious snacks, says Michael Fossel, MD, PhD, clinical professor of medicine at Michigan State University in East Lansing and author of *Reversing Human Aging*.

The best thing, of course, is to quit smoking. But in the meantime, be sure to take a vitamin C supplement daily. You also may want to get extra amounts of vitamin E and selenium, which will lower levels of free radicals in the body. ■

the nutrients from the grain, like fiber, that are taken out of refined products. They're also satisfying. "We feel like we're really eating something, and we feel fuller when we're finished," Bonci says.

To make sure you're eating the real deal, check the label. Don't be fooled by the brown color or the words "made from wheat"–even the whitest bread is made from wheat. "Whole wheat" should be listed first in the ingredients of bread and crackers, and "100 percent whole grain" should be included on your box of cereal.

Lean protein. You should be getting 10 to 15 percent of your calories from lean protein, such as beans and peas, nuts, fish, skinless chicken and turkey and lean red meat (if you eat meat), and low-fat or nonfat milk, cheese, and eggs (only one a day). Don't be fooled by meat labeled "lean," Bonci says. Check the fine print, and take note of how many grams of fat the meat really contains. Don't buy it if it has more than 10 grams of fat per serving.

Fish. Make sure to have two servings of fatty fish such as salmon, mackerel, halibut, or albacore tuna every week. These fish are rich in omega-3 fatty acids that, research suggests, may reduce inflammation and lower risks of chronic diseases such as cancer, heart disease, and arthritis. A steady supply of omega-3s may also protect against memory problems, dementia, and Alzheimer's. Fish oil also lowers triglycerides, another dangerous blood fat.

Unfortunately, fatty fish also tends to be high in mercury and other toxins. To avoid overexposure to heavy metals and chemicals, don't eat the same fish twice in one week. Having a variety means you're not going to miss any of the important nutrients, but you're not likely to get too much of something that's bad," says Walter Willett, MD, Fredrick John Stare professor of epidemiology and nutrition at the Harvard School of Public Health and one of the leaders of the Nurses' Health Study. You can also choose "safe" fish such as wild Alaskan salmon, albacore tuna from the United States or Canada, Pacific halibut caught in Alaska or Canada, and haddock caught by hook and line (as opposed to net). You can also take fish oil capsules, or get your omega-3s from nuts (walnuts), flaxseed, olive oil, pumpkin seeds, and soybeans.

One easy, vegetarian way to get omega-3s (along with fiber) is by using flaxseed. Add a tablespoon of ground flaxseed a day to your diet in addition to your two servings of fish a week. Because the seeds come in hard shells, you'll be able to digest flaxseed better if you grind it in a blender or food processor and store it in the fridge or freezer. Then sprinkle the ground seeds on salad, oatmeal, or muffins. Another option: Buy flaxseed oil and use it in place of other oils in your cold dishes. But don't cook with flaxseed oil, because heat changes its structure. Store the oil in the refrigerator as soon as you bring it home.

Dairy. Eat two or three servings of low-fat dairy products a day–or 1,000 mg of calcium. Low-fat and fat-free milk, yogurt, and cheese are excellent sources of calcium, which helps keep your bones strong.

By the time you reach your early thirties,

your body begins to lose more bone than it builds. That's why it's so important to start banking calcium when you're young. The recommended 1,000 mg of calcium is the equivalent of about three servings of a dairy food; for example: 1 cup of fat-free milk, 8 ounces of yogurt, and 2 ounces of part-skim mozzarella cheese. If you have trouble getting calcium from dairy food, try calcium-fortified food, like orange juice or cereal. Some vegetables also have calcium: Cooked broccoli contains 180 mg a cup; raw arugula, 125 mg a cup; and cooked spinach contains a whopping 240 mg, though

some of it may not be absorbed because of other phytochemicals in spinach.

Fat. You probably already know that you're supposed to eat fat and sweets "sparingly." That means no more than 25 to 30 percent of your total calories should come from fats and almost all of them should come from monounsaturated fats: olive oil, canola oil, peanut oil, and avocado. Monounsaturated fats bring down total cholesterol and bad cholesterol (LDL) without affecting HDL ("good") cholesterol levels—a strong asset, given that researchers have detected high cholesterol levels even in teens. Monos also reduce

A Vegetarian's Guide to Supplements

doctors agree that a vegetarian diet is a healthy choice. But even if you're careful to eat well—ideally a vegetarian diet will include fruits, vegetables, legumes, and whole grains with almost every meal—it may be a challenge to get all the essential nutrients you need.

If you're a vegan—one who avoids eggs and dairy as well as meats—you'll have to work harder to get adequate amounts of all vitamins and minerals. Doctors usually advise vegetarians to take a few key supplements, including:

- Iron. Menstruating women who eat meat are advised to get 18 mg of iron daily. Women who are vegetarians need almost twice as much—33 mg daily—because the iron in plant foods is less easily absorbed. If you're in your childbearing years, choose a multi supplement that contains 18 mg of iron. If you're postmenopausal, you may not need supplemental iron unless

you are anemic or have a very low dietary intake.

- Vitamin D. It's found mainly in fish and dairy foods. If you're a strict vegetarian, you will almost definitely need to take a vitamin D supplement.

- Vitamin B$_{12}$. Vitamin B$_{12}$ is found in animal products and milk but is not generally found in plant foods. Vegetarian women should make sure they get at least 2.4 mcg daily by taking a multivitamin.

- Calcium. Even though plant foods contain some calcium, they can't compete with the amounts found in milk, yogurt, or other dairy foods. If you're premenopausal, aim for 1,000 mg a day; after menopause try to get 1,200 mg per day. Women who don't get that much in their diets, which includes most of us, should make up the rest with a supplement. ■

inflammation, now considered a risk factor for heart disease, cancer, and even Alzheimer's disease.

Polyunsaturated fats–like safflower, sesame, and sunflower seeds, corn and soybeans, and other nuts and seeds and their oils–are also good choices. These fats also bring down cholesterol levels. In one Dutch study, researchers found that when carbs were replaced by polyunsaturated and monounsaturated fats, harmful LDLs fell while beneficial HDLs rose.

Foods high in saturated fat and trans fatty acids (processed fats that resemble saturated fat) should be eaten sparingly, if at all. Both raise cholesterol levels and contribute to heart disease. Saturated fat is found in animal products, like beef, whole milk, and ice cream, as well as in so-called tropical oils: cocoa butter, coconut oil, palm oil, and palm kernel oil. Trans fats are manufactured by adding hydrogen to polyunsaturated fats to make them more solid. Also called hydrogenated oils, they have been the primary fat in most vegetable shortenings, crackers, desserts, snacks, chips, and some margarines. However, since January 2006, when the US government required food manufacturers to list trans fats on product labels, many have found substitute fats and some of these foods are now trans fat free. Still, read the labels and reject products containing trans fats and hydrogenated oils.

Fiber. Women should get 22 to 28 grams of fiber a day or 14 grams for every 1,000 calories consumed. Government surveys show that we often fall far short. "Studies show that the number one source of fiber in the American diet is

veggies, especially French fries, and grains from things like hot dog and hamburger rolls," says Joanne Lupton, PhD, Regents professor at Texas A&M University. "These are not high-fiber products but we eat a lot of them."

The better way to get the fiber you need: high-fiber foods such as beans and legumes (the latest dietary guidelines recommend at least 3 cups a week), whole grain cereal and bread, vegetables, fruit, and nuts. Fiber helps lower cholesterol and the risk of heart disease–and you feel full so you eat less. Look for products that contain at least 5 grams of fiber per serving, which is the only way a product can call itself high fiber.

Sodium. Eating food naturally low in sodium, such as fresh fruit and vegetables, and avoiding excessively salty food–like smoked, cured, or processed meat; regular soy sauce; garlic salt; regular canned soup; some frozen meals; and salty crackers, chips, pretzels, popcorn, and nuts–may help lower your blood pressure. Try to get fewer than 800 mg of sodium per meal, or 2,400 mg a day, the equivalent contained in 1 teaspoon of table salt. Have high blood pressure? The gold standard for lowering blood pressure and cholesterol is what's called the DASH diet ("Dietary Approaches to Stop Hypertension"). While people on the diet lowered their blood pressures just by following an eating plan similar to the one we're recommending here, those who cut their sodium down to 1,500 mg a day saw their pressures drop even further.

Alcohol. For women, having up to three drinks of wine, beer, or distilled liquor a week raises HDL ("good") cholesterol levels, prevents blood clots, and interferes with cell growth in the blood vessels, all factors that lower risk of heart disease. Even better news: The effects are most apparent in people over age 50 or people with risk factors for heart disease. It's best to limit yourself to no more than one drink a day, however. Drinking more than that may be a risk factor for breast cancer.

The Superfoods

No food or nutrient is a guarantee of optimal health, but recent research suggests there are some foods that do double or triple duty in preventing disease. Here are a few that *Prevention* recommends as part of a woman's regular menu.

Barley. Studies have found that this grain, when added to a heart-healthy diet, reduces total cholesterol, as well as LDLs (the bad cholesterol), raises beneficial HDLs, and knocks down the lesser known but most dangerous small cholesterol particles called Very Low Density Lipoproteins (VLDL).

Barley's fiber is a boon—it can keep you regular and promote colon health, and feeds the friendly bacteria in your gut, keeping everything moving and in tip-top shape. It may also help protect you from heart disease. After menopause, a woman's risk for heart attack and stroke go up, largely because she loses the protection of estrogen. In one study of postmenopausal women, those who ate at least six servings of whole grains every week slowed their progression of atherosclerosis—the buildup of plaque that narrows the arteries—and what's

called stenosis, the abnormal narrowing of arteries.

If you have or are trying to avoid type 2 diabetes, barley may lower your body's glucose and insulin responses—which drive up blood sugar. In fact, in one study, barley reduced glucose response in a group of overweight women by up to 65 percent, while oats only lowered them by up to 36 percent. And only barley had any effect on insulin reactions, dropping them by up to 56 percent.

There's also some evidence that barley and other whole grains may protect against breast cancer. Like other grains, barley contains plant lignans, which are converted in the body into a breast-protective chemical called enterolactone. One study found that women who eat the most whole grains have more of this chemical than others.

Beans. When the United States Department of Agriculture (USDA) published a list of the top-scoring antioxidant foods a few years ago, the number one spot was held by a surprise contender: red beans. This humble ingredient of "red beans and rice" and chili should be on your plate at least 3 times a week.

Beans and other legumes may decrease the risk of type 2 diabetes by helping maintain control of blood sugar and decreasing insulin secretion (which occurs in response to elevated blood sugar). This, in addition to beans' fiber content (one cup contains a whopping 13 grams of fiber), can also help control hunger, making beans a must for any weight loss diet. A 2010 Finnish study also found that people who ate the most legumes, berries, and fish had dramatically lower risk of developing metabolic syndrome, a collection of symptoms that can include high LDL and triglycerides, high blood sugar, and high blood pressure, which can lead to diabetes or heart disease or both.

Beans have other pluses. Black and red beans, for example, contain anthocyanin, the same anti-oxidant phytochemical found in red-purple fruits and veggies that protects against heart disease and cancer. Kidney beans are high in vitamin B_1, which may preserve your memory and brain function as you age. Other studies have found that beans may also protect against high blood pressure, as well as breast and colon cancer.

They're also handy for busy women who don't have time to cook. Canned beans are just as nutritious as dried and can be mixed with canned tomatoes and cut-up frozen vegetables to make a quick bowl of chili. Just make sure to rinse them thoroughly before cooking to remove excess sodium, or buy low-sodium beans.

Berries. Blue, black, red—no matter what their color or size, berries are a powerhouse food. Wild blueberries hold the number two spot on the top antioxidant foods list and high bush blueberries (they're the larger ones) are no slouch in the health department either. In the long-running Nurses' Health Study, which looks at the nutrition and lifestyles of more than 87,000 women, it was found that those who ate the most anthocyanin-rich foods (mainly blueberries and strawberries) had an 8 percent reduction in their risk of high blood pressure.

Another long-term look at women's nutrition, the Iowa Women's Health Study, revealed that women who consumed a high flavonoid diet (flavonoids are a class of antioxidant) were the least likely to die of heart disease. Strawberries were specifically associated with cardiovascular disease protection.

Blueberries may also be your best choice for maintaining a memory that allows you to juggle work and family schedules like an air traffic controller. Studies have found that blueberries damp down inflammation and improve memory; one 2010 study from the University of Cincinnati found that older people with early memory changes who drank wild blueberry juice daily did better on memory tests after 12 weeks, and had fewer depression symptoms too.

The research is still new, but animal and lab studies now suggest that berries, which also contain the phytochemical ellagic acid, may also protect against cancer. In one 2010 study at the James Graham Brown Cancer Center at the

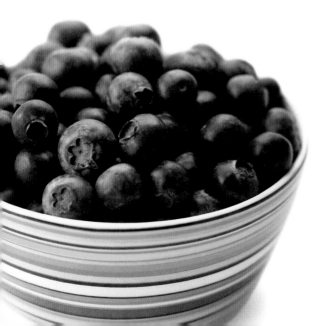

University of Louisville, rats given juice from black raspberries and blueberries along with ellagic acid had fewer tumors than rats in control groups that didn't get the berry cocktail.

Toss some berries into your morning high-fiber cereal, swirl them into yogurt, or make a mixed berry fruit compote for dessert.

Broccoli. This dark green, tree-like plant is the star of a celebrated family of vegetables called crucifers, which also includes cauliflower, cabbage, kale, and brussels sprouts. Broccoli and its siblings contain isothiocyanates, which target and kill cancer in several ways, including de-activating cancer-causing compounds, whisking them out of the body, and preventing tumors from setting up a system of blood vessels to nourish themselves. Studies have linked intake of crucifers to lower risk of colorectal and breast cancers.

Scientists at Johns Hopkins University isolated a compound in broccoli called sulforaphane that appears to reduce cancer risk by stimulating the production of anticarcinogenic enzymes that are part of the body's own detoxification system. Studies also suggested that it may eradicate the *Helicobacter pylorum (H. pylori)* bacteria linked to peptic ulcer and stomach cancer, protect the skin from harmful ultraviolet rays, protect arterial cells from inflammation and reduce the risk of atherosclerosis.

For a major dose of sulforaphane, try BroccoSprouts, a proprietary product developed by Johns Hopkins researchers that contains 20 times the concentration of the chemical than broccoli itself. Like other sprouts, they're perfect in salads, sandwiches, and wraps.

Cinnamon. Cinnamon improves glucose metabolism and may lower your risk of diabetes. Specifically, it slows the rate at which your stomach empties so that your blood sugar remains stable after you eat, and it also helps increase the ability to respond to insulin in people with type 2 diabetes.

But this spice, which has been used as a medicine for centuries, does even more: It helps prevent the clumping of blood constituents called platelets. You need platelets to clump if you've just sliced your finger with a knife, but if they clump too much, they can cause the kinds of clots that trigger a heart attack or stroke.

Just stir a quarter to a full teaspoon into orange juice, coffee, or oatmeal every day.

Cranberry. You probably already know that cranberry juice can prevent urinary tract infections by preventing bacteria from sticking to the walls of the urinary tract. It may also help prevent gum disease by making your mouth too slippery for bacteria to cling to teeth and gums.

But its bacteria-fighting power extends even further. Studies suggest cranberry in juice form or as dried fruit can eradicate *E. coli*, the bacteria that can cause antibiotic-resistant infections.

There's also some evidence that drinking cranberry juice regularly may promote healthier arteries. Like other berries, cranberries contain anthocyanin, the pigment that gives them their red color, and may work like other berries—and even red wine—to reduce levels of bad cholesterol.

Dark chocolate. In 2010, the National Heart, Lung, and Blood Institute released an interesting finding from its long-running Family Heart Study. People who ate candy had a 49 percent higher risk of coronary heart disease—unless it was chocolate. The chocolate eaters had a 57 percent lower risk.

That was great news for chocoholics. Though that study didn't determine what kind of chocolate the participants were eating, previous research suggests the greatest cardiovascular benefit comes from eating dark chocolate, which is richer in heart-protective flavonoids than milk or other kinds of chocolate. Dark chocolate may help lower blood pressure, bad cholesterol, and even blood sugar.

You don't need a lot. Along with those healthy flavonoids, chocolate packs a wallop of sugar and calories. In most studies, people had about an ounce a day.

Flaxseed. These tiny seeds contain lignans, a group of chemicals that may protect the body from hormone-related cancers by mimicking the action of estrogen and preventing it from attaching to cells, where it can cause the damage that leads to cancer. In laboratory and animal studies, it prevented breast tumor growth and spread; in human trials, it reduced tumor growth in postmenopausal women.

Because of its estrogenic effects, flax may also work on menopausal symptoms: In one study, 40 grams of flaxseed taken daily worked as well as hormone replacement therapy for mild symptoms such as hot flashes, vaginal dryness, and moodiness.

But flax may be better known as a nonfish source of omega-3 fatty acids, which protect the heart. Flax doesn't actually contain omega-3s, but it is rich in alpha-linolenic acid (ALA), an essential fatty acid that is converted into an omega-3. The body absorbs omega-3s from fish more readily, and it takes more flaxseed or flax oil to get the same effect, but it can be a good alternative to fish or fish oil.

Studies do show that people who eat ALA-rich foods like flax are less likely to die from a heart attack. ALA diets seem to improve the function of blood platelets (making them less likely to stick together as a clot), promote healthy arteries, and decrease the risk of arrhythmias, which are irregular heartbeats.

Nuts. A handful of nuts to help you lose weight? Given their calories (249 in 1½ ounces of dry-roasted peanuts and 245 in the same amount of almonds), you might think they would do just the opposite. But a number of studies have found a strong link between eating nuts in moderation and weight control, with an added bonus—better heart health.

Nuts may help you watch your waistline because even small amounts are so satisfying they curb your hunger. Since you don't fully digest nuts, not all their calories are absorbed, and there's evidence that they may rev up your metabolism, burning off some of the calories that you do absorb—and they certainly do your heart good. Nuts are a rich source of protein and monounsaturated and polyunsaturated fats; one kind, the English walnut, also contains good amounts of omega-3 fatty acids. A 2010 study that put two groups of people on weight reduction diets—one munching 240 calories worth of pistachios as an afternoon snack, the other eating the same amount of calories in salted pretzels—found that both lost weight, but the pistachio group experienced positive cardiovascular changes, including lower triglycerides.

Other studies have found that people with metabolic syndrome (see page 47) have improved insulin sensitivity when they eat a 1-ounce snack of mixed nuts or almonds daily.

Just remember that one ounce is roughly a quarter cup and should fit in the palm of your hand.

Oats. The high levels of fiber in oats, specifically, beta-glucon, accounts for their ability to lower bad cholesterol.

In one study, people with mild to moderately high levels of cholesterol who ate a heart-healthy diet that contained beta-glucans from oats had a greater drop in blood fats (33.3 percent vs. 8.4 percent) and LDL to HDL ratio (42.1 percent vs. 13.3 percent) than people on the same diet who got most of their fiber from whole wheat bread.

Oats can also be part of a healthy weight-loss regimen. A 2010 study in the *Journal of the American Dietetic Association* found that overweight and obese people who ate two servings of whole-grain oat cereal a day (containing 3 grams of beta-glucan) on a low-calorie diet had the expected improvements in their LDL cholesterol and also lost more than 3 inches around their waists. Why that's important? New studies show that belly fat is linked to increased risk of heart disease and diabetes, cancer, osteoporosis, and even early death, because it sits in and around internal organs, producing hormones and chemicals that create body-wide inflammation and increase cholesterol and triglycerides.

A USDA study also found that oats contain compounds called avenanthramides that quell inflammation and prevent blood cells from sticking to arteries.

There's also evidence that oatmeal's fiber slows down digestion so the food you eat moves through your digestive system more slowly, keeping you feeling full longer. It also means that blood sugar remains stable, which tells your brain that you're no longer hungry and may help protect you from type 2 diabetes by keeping blood sugar on an even keel.

Pomegranate. This strange fruit is a rising star, both as a health food and a versatile ingredient (in everything from salads to desserts to martinis). One reason: It's a powerful antioxidant, on par with red wine and green tea, and is being studied for its potential to fight cancer, brain degeneration, and diabetes.

Most studies are in their infancy, conducted in the lab or on animals, yet already pomegranate has been shown to protect against breast, colon, and skin cancer.

Other studies in people with type 2 diabetes suggest that drinking about 6 ounces of pomegranate juice every day may help prevent cardiovascular complications of the disease. People with diabetes have a higher risk of heart attack and blood vessel disease (atherosclerosis) than healthy people. When people with serious atherosclerosis were put on a daily dose of pomegranate juice—this time for 3 years—they saw an improvement in their condition. The thickness in their carotid artery—one of the main vessels carrying blood to the brain—went down by 35 percent and their blood flow increased by 44 percent. They also experienced a 21 percent drop in their systolic blood pressure (the top number in the reading, a measure of how strong the pressure is in the vessel while the heart is beating).

Tea. A drink made from the leaves of the *Camellia sinensis* plant, tea could be classified as an herbal remedy just as easily as a food. There are three kinds of tea—black, green, and oolong—and the difference is mainly in their processing. They're all high in powerful antioxidants called polyphenols that help protect your DNA from the kind of damage that can cause cancer. Evidence from population studies says drinking black or green tea may help protect against various forms of cancer. In one study, women in the early stages of breast cancer who drank at least 5 cups of tea every day before they were diagnosed were less likely than non-tea drinkers to have recurrences after they finished treatment. In another study, women under 50 who drank 3 or more cups of any kind of tea were 37 percent less likely to develop breast cancer.

Other research in both humans and animals suggests that green and black tea can lower total cholesterol and raise good HDL cholesterol; it may work by blocking the intestinal absorption of dietary cholesterol. Green tea may also help boost your metabolism and burn fat.

Yogurt. It may sound hard to believe, but eating bacteria can be good for your health—if it's the good bacteria found in yogurt and other fermented milk products. Yogurt is a probiotic, meaning it contains live, active cultures of bacteria that colonize our digestive systems, basically leaving no room for the bad bacteria to take up residence. If you're taking antibiotics, you know that these are take-no-prisoners drugs, killing good bacteria with bad. Eating yogurt can prevent the wholesale slaughter. There's even some research suggesting that yogurt may help prevent colon cancer by keeping healthy cells from changing into cancerous ones. It may be helpful with other gut issues too, including lactose intolerance (even if you can't drink milk you can eat yogurt), inflammatory bowel diseases, and *H. pylori* infections.

The Antioxidant Edge

Most of the power foods you just read about get their might from antioxidants. Vitamins C and E are among the best-known (and best-studied) antioxidants, but many other vitamins and minerals have similar effects. Because antioxidants are so important to your overall health, it's worth taking a moment to explain what these nutrients are and how they protect against dozens (if not hundreds) of illnesses and conditions, many common among women.

As your cells work, they use oxygen to create energy. But during normal metabolic processes, some oxygen molecules lose an electron and become unstable. These molecules, called free radicals, careen around your body, trying to stabilize themselves by stripping electrons from other molecules. When they succeed, they create still more free radicals—and damage healthy tissues in the process.

Every day, your body faces thousands of assaults from free radicals. Free radical damage is what causes low-density lipoprotein (LDL, the "bad" cholesterol) to stick to artery walls and impede or block the flow of blood. When free radicals damage the DNA in cells, the result can be cell mutations that lead to cancer. Free radicals can damage tissues in the eyes and cause cataracts or macular degeneration, the leading

Menus with the Most

there's nothing wrong with using supplements as extra insurance against nutritional deficiencies, but you don't want to depend on them. Experts agree that you'll get the best nutritional bang for your buck when you get most of your nutrients in their natural form—from deliciously wholesome foods.

"Supplements are like seat belts," says Jeffrey Blumberg, PhD, professor of nutrition at Tufts University in Boston. "You don't buckle your seat belt and drive through red lights. You wear one for added security."

Even though supplements can make up for shortfalls in your diet, foods always provide a greater range of health benefits because they provide protein and fiber, along with a host of protective plant chemicals called phytonutrients.

Unfortunately, even women who try to eat a nutritious diet don't always succeed. The average American diet is often deficient in such nutrients as calcium, iron, and vitamins A and C, says Leslie Bonci, MPH, RD, director of nutrition at the Center for Sports Medicine at the University of Pittsburgh and a spokesperson for the American Dietetic Association.

To get the optimal amount of vitamins and minerals from your diet, here's what she advises.

Think plant-based. As long as your diet consists primarily of plant-based foods, such as fruits, vegetables, and whole grains, you'll almost automatically get enough nutrients and fiber.

Color your plate. Foods that are colorful are often the most nutritious. The colors in plant foods come from phytochemicals, plant-based chemical compounds that are among the most healthful things you can eat. When you have a whole grain cereal, for example, top it with red strawberries or dewy blueberries. Add snow peas to rice dishes, or mustard greens to meat dishes. The more colors you get, the healthier your diet will be.

Give desserts a nutritional kick. There's nothing wrong with enjoying rich desserts on occasion. But why not make them healthier? Topping a slice of chocolate cake with flavorful berries or adding fruit slices to a bowl of ice cream will provide important nutrients along with the sweet tastes you crave. ■

causes of vision loss in the elderly. Many scientists believe that free radicals are the prime force behind aging itself.

There's no way to completely eliminate free radicals. As we've seen, they're a normal by-product of the body's metabolism. They're also formed by exposure to such things as sunshine, pollution, tobacco smoke, and simple everyday wear and tear.

Nature anticipated the harmful effects of free radicals, and created a number of counter-measures. Just as your body produces free radicals, it also produces antioxidants, enzymes that "voluntarily" give up their own electrons to the marauding molecules. In other words, they essentially come between free radicals and your body's cells, preventing potential damage. These antioxidant enzymes can do only so much, however. In fact, they can easily get overwhelmed by the sheer volume of free radicals. That's when women need to call in the reserves—the antioxidant nutrients found in foods and many supplements.

In any discussion of antioxidants, you'll come across a lot of references to vitamins C and E, simply because they're the ones scientists have studied most. But it's worth keeping in mind that they're only a small part of a massive army of protective compounds. For example, the minerals zinc and selenium, which are included in most multi supplements, act as potent antioxidants. So do many of the B vitamins, as well as minerals such as magnesium.

Even though the individual antioxidants are effective on their own, they perform best when they're working together. Vitamin E, for example, is one of the most powerful antioxidants ever discovered, but it's quickly exhausted in the body. When you get vitamin C at the same time, it "recharges" vitamin E and allows it to protect your body longer. The greater the variety of antioxidants you consume, the more protection you get.

Nutrition for Life

The complete nutrition action plan that follows will make it easy for you to eat well at every decade of life. A woman in her twenties who's thinking of getting pregnant, for example, requires different nutrients (and amounts of nutrients) than a woman who's entering menopause. The vitamins and minerals you need to watch for in your thirties and forties aren't necessarily the same ones that you need to focus on in your fifties and sixties.

Your Twenties

Build strong bones. Now is the time to start building up bone mass, when your body is still under construction—a strong skeleton can prevent osteoporosis, when you're older. One of the simplest things that you can do is make sure you get enough calcium and vitamin D.

In one study, women who took 500 milligrams of calcium and 700 IU of vitamin D daily for 3 years were able to reduce the loss of supportive bone throughout their bodies. This was impressive enough—but the most important

What You Need During Pregnancy

a woman's body changes dramatically during pregnancy. Everything gets larger and more active: The uterus and its supporting muscles enlarge, the joints get more flexible in anticipation of childbirth, and blood volume increases by as much as 60 to 80 percent.

Even if you eat a nutritious diet, it's not always possible to get enough vitamins and minerals to supply your needs as well as those of the baby-to-be. That's why doctors usually advise women to take prenatal supplements during pregnancy, says Bruce K. Young, MD, professor of obstetrics and gynecology at New York University's Langone Medical Center in New York City.

Every woman needs different kinds of supplements, depending on her diet, says Dr. Young. A woman who's a vegetarian, for example, may need a supplement with higher-than-usual amounts of iron or vitamin B_{12}. On the other hand, a woman who eats a lot of meat or seafood will want to avoid high-iron supplements because she'll probably get more than enough of this mineral in her diet.

If you're pregnant now or are planning to get pregnant, here are a few nutrients you'll need to pay attention to.

- **B vitamins.** You don't have to worry about getting too much of the B vitamins during pregnancy because these nutrients do not accumulate in the body. Two B vitamins to focus on are folate and vitamin B_{12}. Folate prevents birth defects called neural tube defects, and vitamin B_{12} aids in fetal metabolism and maintains healthful levels of red blood cells. Foods high in folate include fortified cereals, bread, and legumes. Foods high in vitamin B_{12} are meats and fish. Your doctor may recommend a plasma folate test, which will determine whether you need to supplement your diet with extra folic acid. If you've already had a baby with neural tube defects and you're planning another pregnancy, your doctor may prescribe taking up to 4,000 mcg of folic acid daily.

- **Vitamins A and D.** Unlike the B vitamins, your body accumulates vitamins A and D over time. The amount of these nutrients you should get in your prenatal supplement will depend on the amount you get in your diet. Foods high in vitamin A include squash and carrots; vitamin D–rich foods include fatty fish and fortified milk.

- **Calcium.** Women who are pregnant often have low levels of calcium, which is essential for strengthening fetal bones.

- **Iron.** Women who are pregnant are sharing their blood supply with the growing fetus, and they require a large amount of iron in order to keep up with the increased demand for red blood cells. Even if you have a healthful diet, you have a high risk of becoming anemic during pregnancy, says Dr. Young.

Before your doctor gives you a prescription for prenatal nutrients, be sure to mention whether you're eating a lot of iron-rich foods, such as red meat, liver, or green leafy vegetables. This will help your doctor determine how much additional iron you'll need. ∎

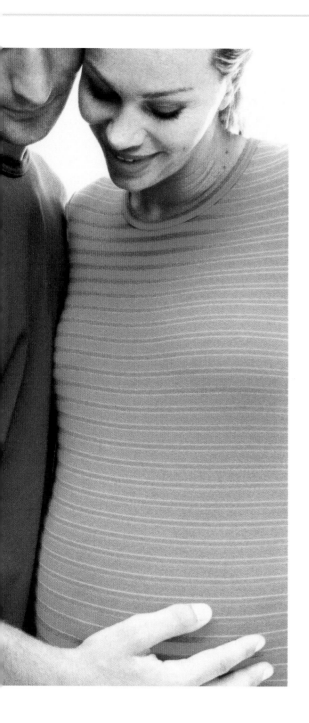

lesson occurred after the study ended. About a third of the participants quit taking the supplements, and within 1 year they lost all of the bone density gains.

You should be getting 1,000 mg of calcium every day. About half of all women fall short, mainly because we're not a nation of milk drinkers. But milk isn't the only way to get calcium. While only 3 cups of milk will do it–plus give you 300 IU of vitamin D–you can get about the same amount of calcium in 12 ounces of milk from 8 ounces of fat-free yogurt, or 2 to 3 ounces of low-fat cheese. These days you can also get your calcium dairy free–in fortified orange juice. An 8-ounce glass provides 35 percent of your daily requirement and 25 percent of your D needs.

Big bonuses: One study found that people who ate more low-fat dairy products had a lower risk of type 2 diabetes. And as little as 500 mg of calcium may also reduce PMS symptoms, though other studies suggest that an extra 1,000, taken as a calcium carbonate supplement, helps. Don't take more than 500 mg of calcium at a time. That's all your body can absorb.

Get relief from PMS. There is some evidence that taking a multi containing B$_6$ and magnesium may help relieve symptoms such as bloating, anxiety, and mood swings. Also consider taking an herbal supplement called Vitex, containing chasteberry, which may work on opiate receptors in your brain to relieve mood swings and painful cramps.

Protect your baby. Even if you're not pregnant, you should pay attention to folic acid intake. You'll find this B vitamin in legumes, leafy greens, and citrus. Studies have found that it can help reduce the risk of birth defects. Since pregnancy can sometimes happen by surprise, many experts recommend that all women in their childbearing years try to consume at least 400 micrograms every day.

Dodge diabetes. There's a good reason to take action against diabetes right away. Women in their teens and twenties are increasingly being diagnosed with this lifestyle disease, often triggered by weight gain. In the past, this condition usually affected women after age 45.

If you are used to pushing produce to the side of your plate, start piling it on. Studies show that people who eat five to nine servings of veggies and fruit daily have a lower risk of diabetes. If you already have diabetes, eating a rainbow of produce every day will help you bring your disease under control. Make sure some of them are leafy greens: A 2008 study in *Diabetes Care* found that women who ate more salad greens as well as fruit had a lower risk of developing diabetes. And leafy greens are high in vitamin E. One study of more than 10,000 people found that those with the highest levels of vitamin E were the least likely to become diabetic. Make sure your multivitamin contains vitamin E, and look for one that also contains chromium and magnesium—both minerals have been shown to make cells in the body more sensitive to insulin's effects, thereby reducing the risk of developing full-fledged diabetes.

Keep your gums healthy. Young women who don't get enough vitamin C and calcium in their diet are more likely to develop periodontal disease, an infection of the gums and other tissues that support the teeth. Take a multi supplement that contains at least 60 mg of vitamin C, and floss daily. Unhealthy gums are linked to increased risk of heart disease because inflammation in the mouth can literally spread like wildfire throughout the body. Inflammation is now considered a major cause of cardiovascular disease, some forms of cancer, and Alzheimer's disease. For calcium, women in their twenties should take a supplement that provides 500 milligrams daily.

Keep up your strength. A menstruating woman loses an average of 15 to 20 mg of iron every month. If you're not getting enough iron, you won't just feel fatigued, you could be at risk of developing iron deficiency anemia, a condition in which your body doesn't have enough healthy red blood cells to deliver oxygen to your tissues. Get your iron from lean red meat, fish, and poultry. There are plant sources too—green leafy vegetables, potatoes, whole grain and fortified grain products. Have a glass of orange juice with your iron-rich food; the vitamin C will help you absorb it.

Your Thirties

Build up your immunity. Women in their thirties are often juggling careers and family responsibilities. The nonstop stress makes the body vulnerable to upper respiratory infections—especially when children come home from school with sneezes and runny noses.

On average, Americans get two to six colds a year and as much as 20 percent of the population will come down with the flu. Make sure your diet is full of these immune-boosting foods to help your body fight off infection.

■ **Sweet potatoes, carrots, dark leafy greens, eggs and fortified milk.** They contain significant amounts of vitamin A, a powerful antioxidant that maintains the frontline of defense against bacteria and viruses by strengthening the skin and mucosal cells that line the airways and the digestive and urinary tracts.

■ **Citrus fruits.** They're high in vitamin C, which helps support many of your immune system's disease fighting cells. Though many people believe that vitamin C enhances immunity—and even prevents the common cold—the jury is still out. But C's antioxidant power does seem to protect the integrity of immune cells when under assault.

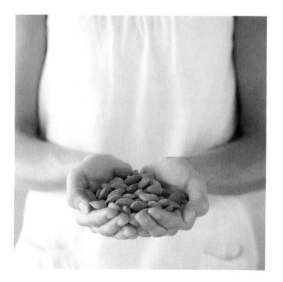

■ **Whole grain products, wheat germ, seeds and nuts.** Rich in vitamin E, these foods may help prevent the common cold.

■ **Lean red meat, poultry, beans, nuts, and fortified cereal.** These foods contain zinc, an immune system supporter than has also reduced the incidence of lower-respiratory infections such as pneumonia, though it may be most effective in people with a zinc deficiency.

To be sure, take a multi with 100 percent of these vitamins and minerals daily.

Protect your heart. One in three women under age 40 will eventually develop heart disease. The best way to protect your heart is to eat a diet low in saturated fat—with lots of vegetables and fruit (five to nine servings daily could lower your heart disease risk by up to 40 percent) and omega-3 fatty acids from fish or other foods, exercise daily for 30 to 60 minutes, maintain your ideal weight, and, if you smoke, stop.

■ **Folic acid (folate).** This nutrient, which is abundant in fortified breads and cereals, legumes, and leafy greens such as spinach, may help protect the heart by tamping down an amino acid called homocysteine. Elevated levels have been identified as a risk factor for heart attack and stroke. The chemical appears to impair the vasomotor function—the ease with which your blood flows through your body—by damaging the inner lining of blood vessels (called the endothelium). Fortunately, mandatory fortification of grain foods in the United States has decreased the prevalence of folate deficiency in middle-aged and older adults. Two other vitamins—B_{12} and B_6—also help lower homocysteine levels.

As a bonus, a diet rich in folate also may lower your risk of cancer, particularly colon cancer. Both are available in fortified cereals. You'll find vitamin B_6 in potatoes, bananas, poultry, and oatmeal. B_{12} is usually found in animal products such as lean meat. There is no evidence that taking extra supplements of these three vitamins will protect your heart.

■ **Omega-3 fats.** Have two servings of a fatty fish such as salmon, mackerel, halibut, or albacore tuna each week to keep up your stores of omega-3 fatty acids, essential nutrients you need to get from your diet. If you absolutely hate fish, you can substitute foods such as flaxseed, walnuts, or beans, but the preponderance

of evidence showing that omega-3s protect the heart comes from studies in which fish or fish oil capsules were consumed. Fish oils lower triglyceride levels, may help reduce high blood pressure, and may reduce the risk of premature death from all causes—cardiovascular disease in particular.

To keep your heart in tip-top shape, you need to keep a balance of omega-3s and another essential fatty acid called omega-6, which is found in margarine and vegetable oils. Americans eat 10 times more omega-6s than omega-3s. You should be eating one omega-3 for every two omega-6s in your diet.

■ **Magnesium.** The halibut you're eating for the omega-3s also has 90 mg of magnesium in it, and that may help you prevent both heart attack and stroke as well as lower your blood pressure. Other magnesium-containing foods include tree nuts (almonds and cashews, for instance), soybeans, spinach, and fortified oatmeal. You'll also find potassium in fish, fruits, vegetables, and legumes.

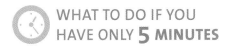

WHAT TO DO IF YOU HAVE ONLY **5 MINUTES**

Set aside a little time to decide what you can do to improve your health today, suggests Irwin H. Rosenberg, MD, dean for nutrition sciences at Tufts University in Boston.

Think about the nutritious foods you'll eat at lunch or the exercise you'll get before the day is done, he says. Even if you achieve only part of what you planned, you'll still be on the road to better health.

Your Forties

Keep your thyroid healthy. More than one in five women ages 40 to 60 don't get enough iodine in the diet. Low levels of iodine can result in goiter, a swelling of the thyroid gland at the front of the throat. Iodine deficiency can also cause a decrease in thyroxine, a thyroid hormone that regulates energy production.

Most of the salt in the United States is iodized (fortified with iodine). If you don't use a salt shaker, you may be getting iodine-laden salt through breads, cheese, saltwater fish, even yogurt and other dairy products. Make sure your multi provides the Daily Value of 150 micrograms. But don't go over that; too much iodine can cause or worsen thyroid disease.

Fight cancer. Studies show that women who get an abundance of fruits and vegetables have a lower risk of cancer. Some of the credit for this goes to folate, which is found in fruits, vegetables, and other plant foods. Studies also suggest that women who don't get enough folate in the diet have a higher risk for developing cancers of the cervix, colon and rectum, lung, esophagus, brain, pancreas, and breast.

The body uses folate to synthesize DNA. If you don't get enough folate in your diet, DNA becomes more vulnerable to damage, which can increase cancer risk. Doctors advise women to get 400 mcg of folic acid (the synthetic form of folate) daily. In addition, be sure your multi supplement contains vitamin B_{12}. This nutrient is necessary for folate to function in the body.

Another cancer-preventing nutrient is calcium. One study found that people who got 1,200 mg of calcium daily (the Daily Value for women) were less likely to develop recurring polyps, growths in the colon that often precede the development of cancer.

Vitamin D may help too. Scientists have noticed that deaths from colon cancer are more common in parts of the United States that have the lowest amounts of sunshine. The sun's ultraviolet rays trigger the production of vitamin D in the body. This is important because

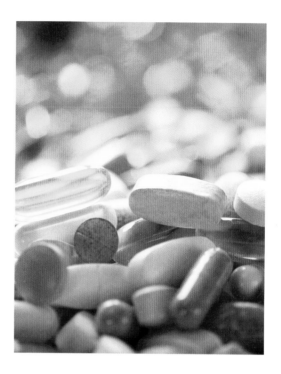

vitamin D has been shown to suppress tumor growth.

You can get both of these essential nutrients in one package: a carton of fortified milk. Three glasses of low- or nonfat milk supplies 900 mg of calcium and 345 mg of vitamin D. Or you can take supplements. Just don't take more than 500 mg of calcium at one time because your body can't absorb it and will excrete it in your urine.

Reduce joint pain. By the time women reach their forties, their joints start to rebel against a lifetime of flexing. Osteoarthritis, also known as "wear and tear" arthritis, occurs when tissues in the joints begin to break down over time. Several nutrients may help ease arthritis pain, including omega-3 fatty acids from fish, flax, or nuts; selenium, a trace mineral that also acts as an antioxidant and is found in whole-grain wheat products and shellfish; and vitamin D, which may work as an immunosuppressant to reduce the risk of rheumatoid arthritis, an autoimmune disease in which the body attacks healthy tissue as if it were a foreign invader. Another way to reduce joint damage from arthritis is to take a supplement that provides 600 IU of vitamin D.

Sharpen your eyesight. Cataracts and macular degeneration are the most common causes of vision loss in older people. Cataracts occur when proteins in the lenses of the eyes are oxidized, or damaged, by free radicals. Macular degeneration is a disorder of the macula, a part of the retina, the thin layer of tissue at the back of the eye that changes light and images entering the eye into nerve signals sent to the brain. When it's damaged, you lose sharp central vision and eventually it can lead to blindness. Though you may have grown up thinking carrots helped your vision, the truth is that it's carotinoids—specifically those found in leafy green foods such as kale, spinach, and collard greens, as well as eggs, oranges, and peas. They contain two antioxidant phytochemicals, lutein and zeaxanthin, that have been shown in large studies to help neutralize the free radicals that cause eye damage.

Your Fifties

Maximize your immunity. The immune system becomes less effective over time, which is why older women may be more susceptible to infections as well as cancer. If you don't already, consider putting these foods on your menu daily.

- **Yogurt.** Studies have found that people who supplement their diets with the healthy bacteria in yogurt take fewer sick days. Eat two 6-ounce servings of yogurt with live active cultures.

- **Oats or barley.** The beta-glucan in these power foods are more potent antioxidants and antimicrobials than the herb echinacea, says one study.

- **Garlic.** In one British study, people who took garlic extract for 12 weeks were two-thirds less likely to catch a cold than people taking a placebo. Studies also suggest that eating garlic lowers the risk of colorectal cancer by 30 percent and of stomach cancer by 50 percent.

- **Tea.** Harvard researchers found that people who had 5 cups of black tea daily for 2 weeks had 2 times the amount of a virus-fighting chemical called interferon in their bodies. The immune booster in both green and black tea is L-theanine, and it's in decaf too.

- **Lean beef.** Beef and other foods rich in zinc (fortified cereals, yogurt, poultry, and milk) may help "beef" up your immune system by helping develop white cells, the ones that seek out and destroy bacteria, viruses, and other foreign invaders.

- **Sweet potatoes, carrots, and squash.** Their vitamin A protects your frontline—the skin and mucus membranes of your respiratory system.

- **Mushrooms.** Exotic ones like shiitake, maitake, and reishi make your white blood cells more aggressive when confronting invaders.

Strengthen your memory. You're not the only one who walks into a room and forgets why you're there. Nearly everyone has "senior moments" as they age. Some of these lapses are normal, others may signal something more serious, such as Alzheimer's disease. You can boost your brainpower with these foods.

- **Berries.** These powerful antioxidants—may protect brain cells from free radical damage and inflammation.

- **Fatty fish.** A 2006 study found that those who ate the most fish had the highest levels of DHA in their blood, which cut their risk of dementia by 47 percent.

- **Avocados, olive oil, nuts, and sunflower seeds.** These foods have vitamin E in common. People who ate moderate amounts (2 ounces of almonds, for example) daily lowered their risk of Alzheimer's by 67 percent.

Your Sixties and Beyond

Stay regular. It's not unusual to experience more constipation as you get older. Most Americans don't eat enough fiber—barely 14 gm when they should be getting 25 or more. As you age, you may rack up a few more risk factors for constipation: You may become less active, drink less fluid (studies show our thirst mechanisms are sometimes impaired as we age), and need medi-

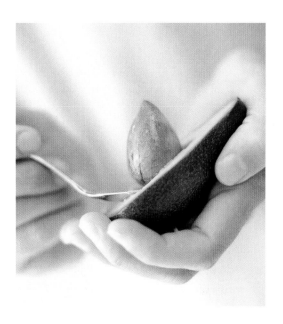

cations that cause constipation, such as antacids, pain medication, or antidepressants. Increasing fiber seems like a simple solution, but the aging digestive system may not be able to handle a major influx of roughage. Gradually add more fiber from whole grains, vegetables, and fruits to your diet. If you have a problem, consider using an enzyme product called Beano that will help you digest fiber.

Eat smart. If you're deficient in three of the B vitamins—folate, B_{12} and B_6—you can experience problems with both learning and memory, according to studies done at the Jean Mayer USDA Human Nutrition Research Center on Aging. You can also become depressed. Boost your intake of foods rich in these nutrients (see page 58). And serve up a big bowl of blueberries regularly. Studies tell us that these berries can not only protect your brain, but also help with balance and coordination, another casualty of aging.

Protect your eyes. One in three people over the age of 75 will develop age-related macular degeneration. Treatments for the condition, which can rob you of your sight, cannot restore lost vision but can slow or prevent severe vision loss if begun early enough. Be sure to get regular eye exams, and get tested for macular degeneration if you start noticing shadowy spots or fuzzy vision. To keep it at bay, keep up your intake of foods rich in lutein and zeaxanthin, including spinach, corn, eggs, oranges, and peas. Have some fish too. Studies show that omega-3 fatty acids like those found in fatty fish can help your body absorb lutein.

Go nuts for your heart. Make your midafternoon snack a handful of almonds. A Tufts University study found that people who munched on 2½ ounces of nuts a day had lower markers for oxidative stress, the metabolic process in which free radicals cause damage to your tissues and that is a risk factor for heart disease. Other studies have found that nuts can lower your cholesterol too.

Take calcium and D. Consuming foods high in calcium and vitamin D, such as fortified milk, is linked to lower risk for type 2 diabetes. Women in the Nurses' Health Study who had the most calcium in their diets had a 21 percent lower risk of developing the disease, while those with the most vitamin D in their diets had a 13 percent lower risk.

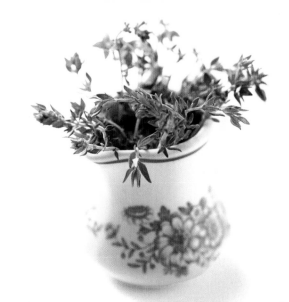

Using Herbs Wisely

From echinacea for colds to evening prim-rose oil for premenstrual syndrome and ginkgo for memory problems, women often turn to herbal remedies to solve everyday health problems. Long before the development of prescription and over-the-counter drugs, herbs were commonly employed to fight infection, reduce pain, soothe anxiety, and relieve menopausal or menstrual discomfort.

Scientists have learned that herbs contain dozens or even hundreds of chemically active compounds. In fact, the active ingredients in many of the drugs you buy at pharmacies are very similar (or even identical) to the chemicals in herbs.

Unfortunately, shopping for medicinal herbs can be a challenge. Herb manufacturers in the United States are prohibited from making health claims on the labels; nor are they allowed to give advice on how to use herbs to treat medical problems. Without medical guidance, it can be difficult to know which herbs are most effective for treating different conditions, or how to use them to get the best results. And because the herb industry isn't strictly regulated, some unscrupulous manufacturers use ingredients that aren't effective or tout herbal combinations that don't work, says Douglas Schar, PhD, a medical herbalist and researcher in Washington, DC, and Florida. Used as directed, the herbs suggested in this book can be very effective. When taken correctly, they're often less likely than drugs to cause side effects. They're often milder than drugs, yet still have beneficial effects. But because herbal medicines are sold over the counter, you become the doctor and pharmacist. It's important to have the same respect for herbs that you do for prescription drugs.

In the following pages, you'll find a comprehensive guide to dozens of important medicinal herbs used for women's wellness. *Prevention*'s experts explain which herbs are best for different conditions, tell you how to take the herbs, and offer information on possible side effects or interactions. Dr. Schar provides some dosage recommendations; others come from the medical literature. However, the physician or experts that you consult for specific conditions may recommend slightly different amounts.

THREE THINGS I TELL EVERY FEMALE PATIENT

DOUGLAS SCHAR PhD, *a medical herbalist and researcher in Washington, DC, and Florida, who specializes in preventing disease with herbal medications, offers this advice to women who use herbs.*

1

DON'T ASK THE CLERKS IN HEALTH FOOD STORES FOR ADVICE. *They're not medically trained, and they rarely have expertise in the actions and interactions of herbal medicines. Instead, consult a professional herbalist, or a physician who incorporates medicinal herbs in her practice.*

2

READ LABELS CAREFULLY. *The best products contain a single herb. Those that contain multiple herbs are less likely to be effective because the dosages will rarely be high enough to be therapeutic.*

3

TRUST YOUR INSTINCTS. *When manufacturers make claims that seem too good to be true, they probably are. Does the label "guarantee" you'll lose 20 pounds a month? Save your money. The manufacturer is more interested in marketing the product than in protecting your health.* ∎

How Herbs Heal

We have dozens of healing herbs at our disposal, but their active ingredients can all be grouped in a few chemical families. These chemicals, which occur in herbs in varying proportions, give herbs their healing powers. They include:

Bitters. These bitter-tasting chemical compounds stimulate bile flow and digestive juices.

Flavonoids. They're among the most important antioxidants. They strengthen blood vessel walls, and reduce water retention, inflammation, and muscle spasms.

Volatile oils. They give herbs their unique scents, and they also have a mild antiseptic action. When inhaled, volatile oils relieve stress. They may also enhance appetite, stimulate circulation, and reduce water retention associated with the menstrual cycle.

Alkaloids. They've been shown to fight bacterial and fungal infections.

Gums and resins. They bind to lipids (fats) in the blood. Herbs that contain gums and resins are often used to lower cholesterol.

Mucilage. This slippery substance helps relieve constipation, soothes irritated mucous membranes in the throat, intestine, and other parts of the body.

Saponins. These have cough-relieving properties. They also regulate women's hormones, reduce stress, and strengthen blood vessels.

Tannins. These promote skin healing. They also help speed the healing of mucous membranes (as with sore throats).

Anthraquinones. These stimulate bile production and help strengthen and restore proper liver function.

Cautions and Caveats

Men and women alike often assume that because herbs are natural, they're inherently safer than synthetic drugs. Nothing could be further from the truth. Many familiar drugs, from aspirin to morphine, were once derived from plants. Even the most natural products can have powerful side effects. For the most part, herbs are safe as well as effective, but only when you use them properly. Here's what doctors advise.

Avoid herbs during pregnancy. Your doctor may recommend certain herbs if you're pregnant, but the information here is designed for women who aren't pregnant or nursing.

Don't double dip. Some herbs have similar actions as prescription or OTC drugs. If you elect to take herbs suggested for various ailments discussed in this book, don't combine them with medication. If you're taking a sedative medication such as diazepam (Valium), for example, it might be harmful to combine it with a sedative herb such as kava kava. The same is true of antidepressants: Prozac, for example, shouldn't be combined with Saint-John's-wort, an herb commonly taken for depression. See the chart beginning on page 66 for specific herb-drug interactions.

Stick to one herb. Just as it may be harmful to combine herbs and drugs that have similar actions, it can be risky to take two similar herbs.

Know which plant parts you need. The medicinal part of echinacea is the root, but that doesn't stop unscrupulous manufacturers from selling the leaves. In the chart below, we've included information on the parts of herbs that are most effective.

Avoid creative but misleading product names. Products with intentionally misspelled names, such as "Clenze," "Nutra-mune," or "Staminex," are unlikely to be effective herbal medicines, Schar says. Also, avoid products that say "pro," "combo," "max," "turbo," or "plus" on the label.

Know when to quit. Herbs act more slowly than drugs, but you should still notice an improvement in your condition within a few weeks to a month. If an herb doesn't seem to be helping, stop taking it and get professional advice, Dr. Schar advises.

Your Personal Herb Guide

Allergies

Herb and Standard Doses	What It Does	General Cautions	Drug Interactions
NETTLE *(Urtica dioica)* Three times daily: 20 drops 1:1 tincture or 1 tsp 1:5 tincture. Use only the plant, not the root.	Relieves allergies, allergic skin rashes, hay fever, and seasonal rhinitis. 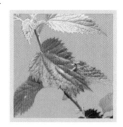	May lower blood pressure and blood sugar and interfere with blood's ability to clot.	Do not take with blood-thinning, antihypertensive, diabetes, or diuretic drugs.

Anxiety

Herb and Standard Doses	What It Does	General Cautions	Drug Interactions
KAVA KAVA *(Piper methysticum)* 150–300 mg , 1–3 times daily, standardized to contain 30–70 percent kavalactones; dried kava root 2–4 gm as a decoction (boiled in water) up to 3 times daily.	Treats nervous anxiety, insomnia, and restlessness, similar to Valium.	Don't take more than the recommended dose. Use caution when driving or operating equipment. Do not take if you have a history of liver disease. Discontinue use if you experience symptoms associated with jaundice, such as nausea, fever, or dark urine.	Do not take with alcohol, prescription or OTC drugs, particularly antianxiety medicines. Kava may cause liver damage, though the side effect is rare and may be related to interactions with drugs.

Herb and Standard Doses	What It Does	General Cautions	Drug Interactions
PASSIONFLOWER (*Passiflora incarnata*) 3–4 cups of tea a day for anxiety (steep 1 tsp in 1 cup boiling water for 10 minutes, strain, and cool); for insomnia, drink 1 cup an hour before bedtime. Take 10–30 drops of fluid extract (1:1 in 25% alcohol) 3 times a day, or 10–60 drops of tincture (1:5 in 45% alcohol) 3 times daily.	Treats insomnia and anxiety.	None.	Don't take with sedatives, sleeping pills, or antianxiety medication, or if you are pregnant or breastfeeding.
RHODIOLA (*rhodiola rosea*) 100 mg twice a day	Affects mood-altering brain chemicals, reducing depression and anxiety, particular generalized anxiety disorder (GAD).	None.	None known.
VALERIAN (*Valeriana officinalis*) Two 200-mg root tablets 3–4 times a day for anxiety. For insomnia, take 1–2 hours before bedtime or up to 3 times a day. Pour 1 cup of boiling water over 1 tsp of dried root, steep 5–10 minutes. May take several weeks before you feel the effects.	Reduces nervousness and insomnia, similare to Xanax and Valium. Reduces digestive discomfort.	None.	Don't take with sleep-enhancing or mood-regulating medications, alcohol, antihistamines, statins (cholesterol-lowering drugs), and some antifungal drugs. Valerian might increase the effectiveness of anesthesia so tell your doctor you're taking it.

Cancer Protection

Herb and Standard Doses	What It Does	General Cautions	Drug Interactions
GARLIC (*Allium sativum*) 2–4 gm fresh minced garlic clove daily (1 clove = 1 gm); 600–1,200 mg aged garlic extract daily; 200 mg freeze-dried garlic tablets, 2 tablets twice daily.	Garlic may strengthen the immune system and reduce side effects from chemotherapy.		A blood thinner, should not be taken with aspirin or other blood-thinning drugs or protease inhibitors used to treat HIV.
GREEN AND BLACK TEAS (*Camellia sinensis*) 1 cup green or black tea 3 times daily.	Green and black tea act as antioxidants, reducing cell damage that may lead to cancer. Also reduce joint inflammation in those with arthritis.	The caffeine in green and black tea may result in anxiety or insomnia.	Very high dosages found in green tea supplements may interfere with drugs affecting blood clotting such as aspirin and alter the way the body metabolizes some drugs.

Cancer Protection *(continued)*

Herb and Standard Doses	What It Does	General Cautions	Drug Interactions
MAITAKE MUSHROOM *(Grifola frondosa)* 600 mg twice daily or 30–60 drops of tincture 2–3 times a day.	Improves immune system's ability to recognize or destroy damaged cells. Stimulates production of white blood cells.	May lower blood sugar and interfere with blood-thinning medications.	Do not take with blood thinners or hypoglycemic medications.

Cardiovascular Disease and High Blood Pressure

Herb and Standard Doses	What It Does	General Cautions	Drug Interactions
GARLIC *(Allium sativum)* 400 mg 2–3 times daily. Use supplements with standardized amounts of alliin or allicin. (Avoid garlic oil gel caps.)	Acts as an antioxidant. Lowers blood pressure, cholesterol, and the risk of cardiovascular disease.	A blood thinner: discontinue 2–3 weeks prior to surgery, and for 2 weeks after surgery. Do not use if you are having dental work or have a bleeding disorder. May increase stomach acid production.	Do not use if you're on blood-thinning medications or saquinavir, an HIV drug
GUGGUL *(Commiphora mukul)* 500 mg standardized guggul extract twice daily.	Reduces cholesterol levels and eases joint inflammation.	In rare cases, may cause diarrhea, restlessness, apprehension, or hiccups. Avoid this herb if you have hypothyroidism.	None known.
HAWTHORN *(Crataegus oxycantha, C. laevigata, C. monogyna)* Two or three times a day: 20 drops 1:1 tincture; or 1 tsp 1:5 tincture. Use only the berries, flowers, and leaves.	May relieve symptoms of coronary artery disease, such as angina and congestive heart failure.	If you already have a cardiovascular condition, don't take without medical supervision. Use with caution if you have low blood pressure.	May necessitate lower doses of blood pressure and other medications.
ELDERBERRY *(Sambucus nigra)* Three times daily: 1 tsp syrup or 1 tsp 1:5 tincture. Use only the ripe berry and flower.	Acts as a powerful antiviral agent that minimizes coughs, colds, and flu.	None.	None.

Colds and Flu

Herb and Standard Doses	What It Does	General Cautions	Drug Interactions
AMERICAN GINSENG *(Panax quinquefolius)* 400 mg a day; supplements should use roots only.	May prevent, lessen symptoms of colds.	People with hyper- or hypotension should not take ginseng unless supervised by a doctor; not recommended for people with bipolar disorder because it increases the risk of mania. Pregnant and breastfeeding women or women with a history of breast cancer should not take ginseng.	Could interfere with the effectiveness of diabetes drugs, blood-thinning medications; increase side effects when taken with MAOI antidepressants; increase effectiveness of antipsychotic drugs; increase stimulant effects; and block the painkilling effects of morphine.
ECHINACEA *(Echinacea purpurea)* 300 mg, 3 times a day (root only); 1–2 gm of dried roots in tea, 3 times a day; 2–3 ml of standardized tincture extract, 3 times a day. Take for 7–10 days.	Could reduce risk of colds by more than half and duration of colds by a day and a half.	Can cause allergic reactions, sometimes life-threatening, in some people. Should not be taken by people with autoimmune diseases.	Do not take if you are on immunosuppressant drugs.
ELDER, OR ELDERBERRY *(Sambucus nigra)* 3–5 gm of elderflower steeped in one cup of boiling water for 10–15 minutes, 3 times a day. Follow dosage recommendations on label for proprietary elderberry products Sinupret and Sambucol.	May reduce symptoms of colds and flu, possibly by reducing congestion and making you sweat.	Unripe or uncooked elderberries can be poisonous.	May lower blood sugar dangerously when taken with antidiabetes drugs. Do not take with laxatives; elderberry has laxative properties. May reduce the effectiveness of theophylline, an asthma drug, and interfere with immunosuppressants.
GARLIC *(Allium sativum)* One or two cloves of garlic 3 times a day or standard dosage of Allimax Liquid and Capsules supplements, the brand used in the colds study.	Helps prevent and reduce symptoms of the common cold.	Whole garlic can cause bad breath, heartburn, and upset stomach in some people; can increase the risk of bleeding.	Do not take with blood-thinning medications or aspirin.

Constipation

Herb and Standard Doses	What It Does	General Cautions	Drug Interactions
FLAXSEED *(Linum usitatissimum)* 2 Tbsp ground flaxseed daily.	Contains soluble fiber to keep you regular.	Grind before eating and take with at least 8 oz water. Don't take if you have a bowel obstruction or diverticular disease. May interfere with the absorption of drugs so take 1 hour before or 2 hours after taking medications.	Flaxseed acts as a blood thinner so don't take with blood-thinning medications unless you talk to your doctor. Talk to your doctor if you take antidiabetes medicine (including insulin) or are on oral contraceptives or hormone replacement therapy; flaxseed may alter hormone levels.

Depression

Herb and Standard Doses	What It Does	General Cautions	Drug Interactions
GINKGO *(Ginkgo biloba)* Standardized extract (40–80 mg) 3 times a day. 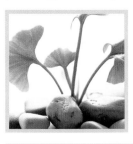	Reduces depression, possibly by making the brain more receptive to mood-lifting chemical serotonin. May also improve cognitive function and increase blood flow in people with reduced blood flow to the legs (intermittent claudication).	People with epilepsy and women who are pregnant or nursing should not take ginkgo.	May reduce the effectiveness of anti-convulsive medications; increase the risk of serotonin syndrome, a potentially fatal condition in people taking selective serotonin reuptake inhibitors (SSRIs); and cause bleeding when taken with blood thinners. Lowers blood pressure so check with your doctor If you're taking blood-pressure-lowering drugs.
SAINT-JOHN'S-WORT *(Hypericum perforatum)* 300 mg capsules 3 times a day; 40–60 drops of liquid extract (1:1) twice daily; or 2–4 tsp of dried Saint-John's-wort in 8 oz of hot water, steeped for 10 minutes, 3 times a day.	Improves mood and symptoms of depression, psychological symptoms of premenstrual syndrome and meno-pause, and seasonal affective disorder, when used with light therapy. An antibacterial, it prevents wound infection when applied topically.	May cause sensitivity to light. May cause gastrointes-tinal symptoms, allergic reactions, and fatigue.	Interacts with many drugs, including antidepressants, antihistamines, dextro-methorphan cough medicines, immuno-suppressants, HIV drugs, sedatives, oral contra-ceptives, migraine drugs (triptans), theophylline (for asthma or bronchitis), blood thinners, statins, some blood pressure medications, and antifungal drugs.

Fever

Herb and Standard Doses	What It Does	General Cautions	Drug Interactions
ANDROGRAPHIS (*Andrographis paniculata*) 6 gm daily as a tea; take for 7 days.	A traditional Chinese remedy, it reduces symptoms of colds, sore throats, and fever.	Do not use if you have gallbladder or an autoimmune disease, or are pregnant or trying to get pregnant.	None known.

Headaches

Herb and Standard Doses	What It Does	General Cautions	Drug Interactions
BUTTERBUR (*Petasites hybridus*) 50–75 mg of standardized extract twice a day.	May reduce the frequency and duration of migraine attacks and possibly tension headaches.	Use only products marked "PA-free," which have a liver-damaging chemical removed. Pregnant and nursing women should not take this herb.	None known.
FEVERFEW (*Tanacetum parthenium*) 100–300 mg capsules up to 4 times daily, standardized to contain 0.2–0.4% parthenolides. Use only fresh or freeze-dried feverfew leaves. Or take 20 drops 1:5 tincture, or 10 drops 1:1 tincture.	Prevents migraine and cluster headaches.	Chewing fresh leaves can cause mouth sores in some people.	May interact with blood-thinning medications.
WILLOW BARK (*Salix*) Three to four cups of tea (1–2 tsp of dried bark in 8 oz of water, steeped for ½ hour) daily; 60–240 mg of standardized salicin a day in powdered herb capsules or liquid.	Eases pain and reduces inflammation of headache and back pain.	Do not take if you are aspirin-sensitive or have asthma, diabetes, gout, gastritis, hemophilia or stomach ulcers. Do not take if pregnant or nursing.	A blood thinner; should not be taken with other blood thinning drugs, beta blockers, diuretics, or nonsteroidal anti-inflammatory drugs. May increase levels of Dilantin in the body, resulting in toxicity.

Inflammatory Bowel Disease and Other Stomach Problems

Herb and Standard Doses	What It Does	General Cautions	Drug Interactions
CHAMOMILE (*Matricaria recutita*) Pour 1 cup boiling water over 2 to 3 tsp dried herb, cover, and let steep for 10–15 minutes. Drink 3–4 times a day. Use only the flowers.	Relaxes muscles in the stomach. Eases indigestion, irritable bowel problems, diverticular disease, and colitis. A mild sedative, it can also help with anxiety and sleep.	Causes allergic reactions in rare cases. Those who are allergic to related plants, such as ragweed, asters, and chrysanthemums should drink the tea with caution.	None known.

Inflammatory Bowel Disease and Other Stomach Problems *(continued)*

Herb and Standard Doses	What It Does	General Cautions	Drug Interactions
CRANBERRY *(Vaccinium macrocarpon)* 400 mg twice a day.	May inhibit *H. pylori*, the bacteria associated with peptic ulcer.	None.	None known.
PEPPERMINT *(Mentha piperita)* Pour 1 cup boiling water over 1–2 tsp dried herb, cover, and let steep for 10–15 minutes. Use only the leaves. Or enteric-coated 0.2–0.4 ml pills, taken 3 times a day.	Helps ease indigestion, gas, cramping, and nausea of irritable bowel syndrome and symptoms of peptic ulcer.	None.	None known.
CRAMP BARK *(Viburnum opulus)* Three times daily: 1 gm dried-bark capsules, or 20 drops 1:1 tincture, or 1 tsp 1:5 tincture.	Relaxes intestines.	Safe.	None.

Insomnia

Herb and Standard Doses	What It Does	General Cautions	Drug Interactions
CHAMOMILE *(Anthemis nobilis)* 400–1,600 mg of standardized extract daily; or steep chamomile flowers in a cup of boiling water for 10–15 minutes and drink.	Promotes relaxation and sleep.	Don't use chamomile if you're allergic to flowers in the daisy family.	None known.
RHODIOLA *(Rhodiola rosea)* Standardized extract 100–600 mg daily.	Acts on the same brain chemicals that influence mood and sleep.	May paradoxically cause insomnia and anxiety in some people.	None known.
VALERIAN *(Valeriana officianalis)* 200–400 mg standardized extract 1–2 hours before bedtime or up to 3 times a day. Pour 1 cup boiling water over 1 tsp of dried root and steep 5–10 minutes.	Has a calming effect, working much like benzodiazepine drugs such as Valium and Xanax.	Should not be used while driving or during other activities that require alertness. Some people may become anxious and restless after taking. Pregnant and nursing women should not take it.	Can increase the effect of sedative drugs, alcohol, and tricyclic antidepressants. May interact with drugs broken down by liver enzymes, such as statins, antihistamines, and antifungals; may increase the effects of anesthesia.

Low Energy

Herb and Standard Doses	What It Does	General Cautions	Drug Interactions
ASIAN GINSENG (*Panax ginseng*) 100–300 mg twice a day (only tablets that contain the root).	Acts as a mild stimulant and mood enhancer. Also acts as an antioxidant. May reduce the risk of some cancers.	Don't take if you have high blood pressure, with caffeine or other stimulants, or when under acute stress. May cause menstrual irregularities or intensify menopause symptoms. May cause headaches, nervousness, and insomnia in women under age 45.	Talk to your doctor if you take ACE inhibitors or calcium channel blockers for high blood pressure, blood-thinning medications, diabetes drugs, other stimulants including ADHD drugs and caffeine, or MAOI inhibitors for depression. May block the effects of morphine.
SIBERIAN GINSENG (*Eleutherococcus senticosus*) 500–3000 mg daily as tea or in capsules, 100–200 mg of standardized extract twice a day. Use only the root bark.	Similar properties to Asian ginseng.	Do not take if you have high blood pressure, obstructive sleep apnea, narcolepsy, or are pregnant or nursing.	May raise blood levels of the heart drug digoxin, interact with blood thinners and increase the risk of bleeding, and may increase the effects of sedatives.

Macular Degeneration

Herb and Standard Doses	What It Does	General Cautions	Drug Interactions
BILBERRY (*Vaccinium myrtillus*) Pour 1 cup hot water over 1–2 Tbsp dried whole berries (or 2–3 tsp crushed berries). Steep, covered, for 10 minutes, then strain. Drink 1 cup daily. Commercial tea bags are also available. Or take 80–480 mg tablets in 2 divided doses of standardized bilberry extract (25% anthocyanidin).	Contains flavonoids, which may help prevent and treat macular degeneration, a leading cause of blindness.	Don't take in large quantities over an extended period because of the risk of muscle spasms, severe weight loss, and even death.	May interfere with blood-thinning drugs and medications for diabetes because it appears to lower blood sugar.
GINKGO (*Ginkgo biloba*) 15 drops extract dropped into a sip of water, once or twice daily for 1 month. Or take 160–240 mg a day.	Slows vision loss in people with macular degeneration.	In very rare cases can cause headaches, digestive upset, and skin reactions. Thins blood, so don't take it 2–3 weeks before or after surgery. Can cause skin inflammation, diarrhea, and vomiting in doses larger than 240 mg. May cause internal bleeding.	Don't take with MAOI inhibitors, aspirin, or other nonsteroidal anti-inflammatory drugs; diabetes medications; antihypertensive or blood-thinning drugs, such as warfarin (Coumadin).

Memory

Herb and Standard Doses	What It Does	General Cautions	Drug Interactions
GINKGO *(Ginkgo biloba)* One 240 mg tablet standardized to 24 percent ginkgo flavone glycosides, 3 times daily.	Improves memory in people with memory deficits, concentration, and alertness. As effective as prescription medication in treating intermittent claudication, pain caused by reduced blood flow to the legs.	In very rare cases ginkgo can cause headaches, digestive upset, and skin reactions. Thins blood, so don't take it 2–3 weeks before or after surgery. Can cause skin inflammation, diarrhea, and vomiting in doses larger than 240 mg. May cause internal bleeding.	Don't take with MAOI inhibitors, aspirin, or other nonsteroidal anti-inflammatory drugs; diabetes drugs; antihypertensive or blood-thinning drugs, such as warfarin (Coumadin).
LEMON BALM *(Melissa officianalis)* 60 drops a day of tincture made from leaves; 300–500 mg of dried lemon balm 3 times a day.	Improves cognitive function and decreases agitation in people with Alzheimer's disease. May also promote calmness and sleep.	Pregnant and nursing women should not take lemon balm.	May interact with sedatives or thyroid medications.

Menstruation and Menopause Problems

Herb and Standard Doses	What It Does	General Cautions	Drug Interactions
ANGELICA *(Angelica sinensis, also dong quai)* Take 3 times daily: two 500 mg tablets or 20 drops 1:1 tincture or 1 tsp 1:5 tincture. The root is the most effective part.	May relieve hot flashes; relaxes and stimulates uterine muscles, reduces pain, dilates blood vessels.	Use for short periods of time. Don't take it if you have estrogen-dependent cancer or a bleeding disorder. Increases sun sensitivity. Safety of this herb has not been determined.	Don't take if you're on blood-thinning medication or hormone therapy, or are undergoing cancer treatment; avoid it when taking Saint-John's-wort because it intensifies sensitivity to light.
BLACK COHOSH *(Cimicifuga racemosa)* 40–80 mg a day standardized to 1 mg of 27-deoxyactein or 2–4 ml 3 times a day in water or tea. The root is the most effective part.	May relieve menopausal symptoms, such as thin vaginal tissue, vaginal dryness, memory loss, depression, mood swings, and hot flashes.	Don't use longer than 6 months. Avoid this estrogenic herb if you have estrogen-dependent cancer. May cause occasional gastric discomfort. Teas are less effective at relieving symptoms than capsules.	Don't use if you're on hormone replacement therapy.
EVENING PRIMROSE *(Oenothera biennis)* 500–1,000 mg daily or 2–8 gm of EPO daily, standardized to contain 8% gamma-linolenic acid (GLA).	Reduces physical and emotional symptoms of premenstrual syndrome.	Rarely causes nausea, headache, stomach pain, all signals the dose is too high.	May interact with some blood-thinning drugs and herbs, as well as schizophrenia medications.

Herb and Standard Doses	What It Does	General Cautions	Drug Interactions
FLAXSEED *(Linum usitatissimum)* 1 Tbsp ground flaxseed 2–3 times daily, taken with a lot of water; or 1–2 Tbsp of flaxseed oil, 1–2 capsules daily, or 40 gm flaxseed.	Reduces mild meno-pausal symptoms such as hot flashes, mood disturbances, and vaginal dryness. May decrease risk of osteoporosis, fight cholesterol and protect against some cancers.	Take with at least 8 oz of water several hours before or after other medications or supplements. Don't use if you have diabetes, breast cancer, or schizophrenia, without doctor supervision.	May interfere with the absorption of drugs, increasing effects of blood thinners, altering hormone levels and so the effects of oral contraceptives and HRT, and altering blood sugar levels, changing your need for diabetes medications.
SAGE *(Salvia officinalis)* 4 heaping Tbsp dried leaves steeped 4 hours in 1 cup boiling water. The leaves are the most effective part.	Helps reduce and even eliminate night sweats.	May contain plant estrogens so should be taken with caution or avoided by those with breast cancer.	Can increase sedative side effects of drugs.
VITEX *(also called chasteberry) (Vitex agnus-castus)* Twice daily: two 500 mg tablets or 60 drops 1:5 tincture or tablets containing 250 mg 4:1 extract. The seeds (also called the berries) are the most effective part.	Relieves premenstrual symptoms. Helps treat irregular, painful, and heavy periods.	See your gynecologist if you experience bleeding between periods. Contains precursors of steroids including progesterone, testosterone, and androstenedione, and may have estrogenic properties. Avoid or use with doctor supervision if you have a hormone-sensitive disease.	May lower the effectiveness of birth control pills and interfere with the action of drugs that work on dopamine receptors, such as haloperiodol.

Skin Problems

Herb and Standard Doses	What It Does	General Cautions	Drug Interactions
ALOE *(Aloe barbadensis)* Apply 3 times daily to injured area. Buy pure (clear) aloe gel or squeeze from the leaves of a live plant.	Heals sunburn and minor burns and wounds. Also treats chronic skin disorders such as psoriasis, eczema, and acne.	Don't use on surgical incisions or deep wounds and don't take internally. May cause an allergic rash.	None known.

Skin Problems *(continued)*

Herb and Standard Doses	What It Does	General Cautions	Drug Interactions
GUGGUL *(Commiphora mukul)* 500 mg twice a day.	In one study, was as effective as tetracycline antibiotic in treating acne.	Don't take if you're pregnant or nursing, or have a hormone-related cancer or a family history of one.	May interact with blood thinners, oral contraceptives, herbs with estrogenic effects, or tamoxifen, a breast cancer drug.
GOTU KOLA *(Centella asiatica)* Apply externally as needed.	Triterpenoids in herb aids wound healing. Eases pain of insect bites, poison ivy, and sunburn. Improves acne, acne rosacea, eczema, and psoriasis, and varicose veins.	Not recommend for those under 18; should not be used for more than 6 weeks because of potential liver damage.	May interfrere with cholesterol-lowering drugs, diabetes medications, diuretics, and sedatives.
TEA TREE OIL *(Melaleuca alternafolia)* 5% gel applied to skin.	May reduce acne-causing bacteria, inflammation, and improve symptoms as well as OTC acne medications.	Very few side effects.	None known.

Urinary Tract Problems

Herb and Standard Doses	What It Does	General Cautions	Drug Interactions
GREEN TEA *(Camellia sinensis)* 250–500 mg of standardized extract daily or drink in tea form (the leaf only, 1 tsp per cup).	Promotes healthy urinary function. 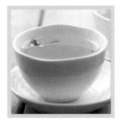	Contains caffeine, which may cause sleeplessness and anxiety.	May interfere with drugs affecting blood clotting such as aspirin and alter how the body metabolizes some drugs.

The Ultimate Ladder of Fitness

Remember that old Confucius saying about the journey of 1,000 miles that starts with one step? It's time to take it. And follow it with another and another and another. Regular physical activity is one of the best lifestyle changes you can make to ensure a long, healthy, active life. Research has found that people who are active just 7 hours a week—an hour a day—have a 40 percent lower risk of dying early than those who are active less than 30 minutes a week.

And those smart, healthy, active women aren't all running marathons. Some of them are walking, others are dancing, and others are at their local gym at spinning class or dancing to the Latin beats of Zumba, one of the latest trends in aerobic exercise that combines traditional moves with salsa. But they all started with a first step—maybe a walk around the block, then nudging past the block until they were competing in their first 5K; poking along on the stationary bike for 20 minutes until they were fit enough to spin at top speed; testing out their dance moves in one class, and signing up for three more when they realized how good it made them feel. Regular exercise will make you fit and more. Studies have shown that it lowers anxiety, reduces the risk of heart disease, and even improves the frequency and quality of sex (yes, walkers, runners, bikers, and swimmers do it better).

And it all starts with the first step. That's why *Prevention* experts created the Ultimate Ladder of Fitness—a six-step plan for gaining mobility, burning calories, and trimming inches off your waistline. You'll also discover ways to make exercise a lot more fun, which is the real key to making it part of your life.

Exercise: You Need It

When it comes to your health, exercise isn't an option. It's a necessity.

We all know that being a couch potato increases the risk of heart disease and other serious health threats. Yet surveys show that more than 60 percent of Americans don't get regular physical activity—and women are more likely than men to skip the workouts. Of those who do exercise regularly and moderately, only 15 percent do it 5 days a week for 30 minutes or longer.

What, exactly, can you gain from exercise? Here's why you need exercise.

■ It reduces your risk of heart attack and stroke. Exercise lowers blood pressure, slows resting heart rate, lowers cholesterol, and burns abdominal fat. In one study, menopausal women who exercised only a little more than 3 hours a week saw their total cholesterol and triglyceride levels drop—and gained more bone mass to boot.

■ Studies have shown that exercise protects against colon cancer. It may lower the risk of breast, lung, and endometrial cancers as well.

■ It helps maintain steady blood sugar levels, reducing the risk of type 2 diabetes. In one study, people who exercised only 150 minutes a week had a 58 percent lower risk of developing the disease, with a 71 percent lower risk if they were over 60. Exercise also improves insulin sensitivity.

■ It boosts immunity and can prevent colds and other infectious diseases. One 2010 study found that the most physically fit exercisers had 46 percent fewer respiratory infections during cold and flu season than less physically fit, sedentary people.

■ It strengthens bones. Older women who are active are less likely to develop osteoporosis and suffer fewer bone fractures than women who don't exercise.

WHAT WORKS FOR ME

With work, family, and constant travel vying for their time, some of our favorite health professionals are every bit as swamped as the rest of us, yet they still manage to work out most days of the week. Here are their secrets for practicing what they preach!

Use your weekend. "I confess, when I'm seeing patients from 7:00 a.m. to 7:00 p.m., I don't exercise. But on weekends (including most Fridays), it's priority number one. I take an hour on these days just for me and have a quality run or workout. Then I find a smaller chunk of time 2 more days of the week. The trick is preparation: I always have my gym bag with me. So if I suddenly have 30 minutes free, I'm out the door for a walk or jog!" says Mary Jane Minkin, MD, clinical professor of obstetrics and gynecology at Yale University School of Medicine and coauthor of *What Every Woman Needs to Know about Menopause.*

Have a plan B. "I start the day with an exercise plan. But as a doctor, my plans are routinely disrupted. So I have a plan B and plan C. For instance, I always carry exercise bands. If I can't make it to the gym, I can do resistance training at home, in my office, or in my hotel room. I also carry my sneakers. If I have lots of meetings, I take short walks in between to clear my head. Every 5 seconds counts!" says Pamela Peeke, MD, assistant clinical professor of medicine at the University of Maryland School of Medicine in Baltimore and author of *Fight Fat after Forty.*

Make it a family affair. "I have three school-age kids, so my life is out of control. I still exercise at least 4 days a week, but I don't lock myself into a routine. I take advantage of my children's desire to play outside. I run while they bike, I play tennis with my son, or we all play soccer. It's so much better than watching TV," says Miriam Nelson, PhD, associate chief in the physiology laboratory at Tufts University in Boston and author of *Strong Women, Strong Bones.*

Focus on the benefits. "I practice what I preach: I exercise every day or almost every day. One way I keep myself on track is by focusing on the rewards of my efforts: That time spent exercising will help reduce my risk for heart disease, control my weight, and handle stress more effectively—and I can eat dessert now and then without worrying or feeling guilty!" says James Blumenthal, PhD, professor in the department of psychiatry at Duke University in Durham, North Carolina.

Give it top priority. "It would be easy to put off working out until the house is clean, more writing is done, or I've gone through the mail. But I still put on my shorts and get going. The endless household and work duties will always be there. And if my exercise actually helps me live longer—I'm gaining time," says Christiane Northrup, MD, cofounder of the Women to Women Healthcare Center in Yarmouth, Maine, and author of *Women's Bodies, Women's Wisdom* and *The Wisdom of Menopause.*

- It burns fat, builds muscle, and may lower levels of leptin, a hormone linked to appetite that has been implicated in weight gain.

- It helps you live longer. A study of 14,000 women and men showed that moderate levels of physical fitness increased life span. In fact, walking just 2 miles daily could potentially add years to your life, keeping you active and independent as you age.

- It can help you sleep better. In a Stanford University study, middle-aged and older volunteers with sleep problems who exercised moderately over a period of 12 months reported fewer awakenings at night, falling asleep faster and feeling more rested in the morning than a control group who just attended a health education program.

It's clear that exercise can improve the long-term quality of your life. But what will it do for you right now? Research shows that women who exercise may have less menstrual discomfort and are less anxious or depressed (possibly because exercise increases feel-good chemicals called endorphins and may stimulate brain chemicals affecting mood). They have less pain overall since exercise tamps down pain perception, and more self-confidence.

Convinced? Let's get started.

Step 1: Make the Change

If you haven't exercised regularly in the past, getting started can be a challenge. Your muscles won't be primed for action, and you won't have the force of habit to help you along. But once you get out the door and get moving, it won't be long before exercise feels natural and comfortable. In fact, you may find yourself craving it.

Before you do anything else, get a checkup and let your doctor know about your plans to start exercising. Women who have been sedentary can easily injure themselves if they start out too quickly, says Alan Mikesky, PhD, professor in the department of physical education at Indiana University–Purdue University in Indianapolis.

Look for exercise opportunities. Anything that gets your body moving counts as exercise. It could be walking the dog, working in the garden, or raking leaves. Even cleaning house can give you a decent workout if you move quickly.

"There are many ways to sneak in exercise," says Martha Coopersmith, owner of the Bodysmith Company in New York City. "We all have to go places, so park a couple of blocks away and walk the rest. Take the stairs instead of the elevator. Or pace while you talk on the phone."

Make it more like play. The problem with formal exercise is that it can easily feel like one more responsibility in an already hectic day. But it shouldn't be like that. Exercise is any physical activity that you enjoy. Coopersmith suggests indulging in some of the activities that you enjoyed when you were young–but with a twist.

Used to climb trees? Try rock climbing–in the wild or on the "rock wall" at a local health club. Are you a dancer? Zumba might be the ticket. For that matter, swing, salsa, or line dancing can give you quite a workout, Coopersmith says. One study found that older dancers can boost their aerobic fitness, bone mass, strength, flexibility, and gait. And anyone can burn 200 calories an hour or more by getting out there to boogie.

Set reasonable goals. One reason so many women start an exercise program and then give it up is that they don't feel they're making progress. Don't set impossible goals for yourself; keep things simple. Try to walk 10 more minutes than you usually do. Do one extra pushup. Lift the weights 2 more times. Studies have shown that people who believe they can achieve a goal—any goal—are much more likely to stick with the program.

Step 2: Stretch Those Muscles

Stretching is an integral part of any fitness plan. It improves your range of motion, helps you stay flexible, improves coordination, and helps prevent muscle strains and other injuries. Start with the stretches that begin on page 82, recommended by Carol Espel, MS, national director of group fitness programming for Equinox Fitness Clubs in New York City.

Step 3: Work in Regular Aerobic Exercise

What does aerobic mean? It simply means you're moving fast enough to increase your heart and respiratory rates. When you exercise aerobically, the heart pumps more blood, and the lungs fill the blood with more oxygen. Aerobic exercise makes the heart work harder, which makes it stronger: It pumps more blood with each beat, which means that it beats less often. In other words, aerobic exercise lowers your resting heart rate. Aerobic exercise can also result in drops in blood pressure because the blood moves more easily through arteries and veins.

You don't have to be an exercise fanatic to get impressive gains from aerobic exercise. *Prevention* recommends that you accumulate 30 to 60 minutes of moderate activity 4 to 5 days a week to stay healthy and fit.

One more point about aerobic exercise: Don't waste time doing something you don't enjoy very much. For years, women felt that they had to run in order to be aerobically fit. But a lot of them hated running, and therefore didn't do it for very long. You have to do something that you like doing, says Dr. Mikesky. It could be tennis, bicycling, swimming, using the stairclimber, or even country dancing.

Step 4: Add Strength Training

The next time you go to the health club, take a look at the folks lifting weights. Chances are, most of them are men. That's unfortunate, because weight lifting, also called strength training, is among the best workouts for women.

For starters, strength training makes your muscles stronger and more compact, so you look trimmer. It also helps you lose weight. Muscle tissue is more active metabolically than fat. When you lift weights and build muscle, you'll burn more calories, even when you aren't exercising—even while you sleep!

After age 40, women can lose half a pound of muscle and gain a pound of fat every year. By the time a woman reaches her 65th birthday,

(continued on page 86)

Learn to Stretch
Your Muscles

Stretching is most effective when it's done before and after every workout. If that sounds like too much work, it's fine to do your stretches after exercising. Don't stretch when your muscles are cold; you're more likely to get injured. These stretches, recommended by Carol Espel, MS, national director of group fitness programs for Equinox Fitness Clubs in New York, hit every major muscle group in the body. For each one, hold the stretch for 10 to 30 seconds, breathing deeply all the time.

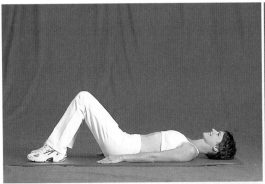
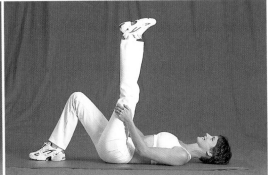
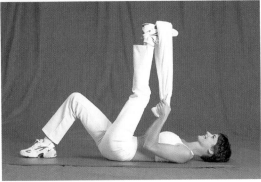

Hamstrings

Lie on your back with your legs bent and both feet on the floor (top left). Straighten and raise your left leg. Gently pull your thigh toward your body and hold (above). If you can't reach your leg, loop a towel under your foot and, with a slight bend at the knee, gently pull your leg toward your chest (bottom left). Repeat with the right leg.

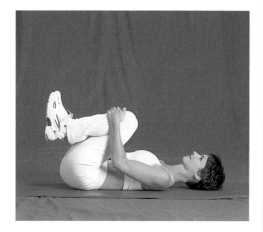

Lower Back

Lie on your back and pull both knees to your chest. Keep your upper body relaxed on the floor.

Calves

Stand facing a wall, with your right foot about 18 inches from wall, and your left foot about 2 feet behind it (below). Place your hands against the wall for support and lean forward while pressing your left heel to the floor. Switch legs.

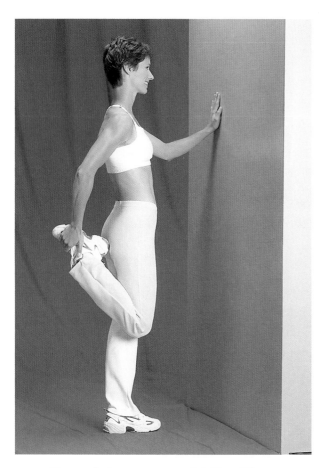

Quadriceps and Hip Flexors

Put your left hand on a wall (above). Bending your right knee, bring your right foot toward your buttocks; hold it in place with your right hand. Keep your knees together and do not arch your back. Repeat with the left leg, putting your right hand on a wall.

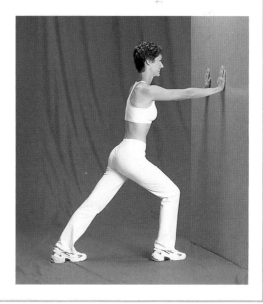

(continued)

Learn to Stretch Your Muscles

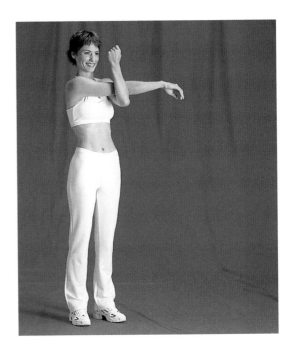

Upper Back and Shoulders

Cross your right arm in front of your chest (right). With the opposite arm, gently pull your right arm toward your body, and hold. Repeat with left arm.

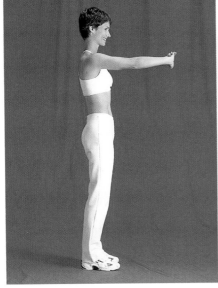

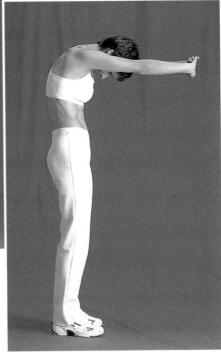

Upper Back

Clasp your hands in front of you with your palms facing away (above). Round your back, drop chin to chest, relax your shoulders, and press your hands forward (right).

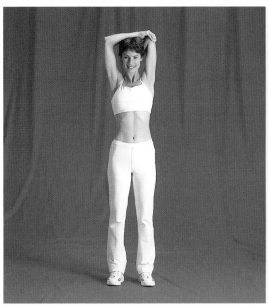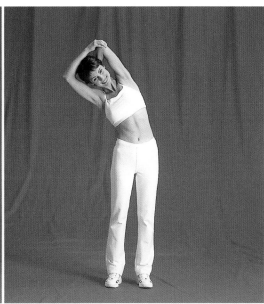

Triceps and Sides

Stand straight and raise your left arm over your head; bend the elbow, and drop the hand toward the middle of your back (left). With your right hand, gently pull your left elbow to the right. Tilt your body to the right (right) to stretch the muscles in your side. Keep your stomach tight. Repeat with your right arm.

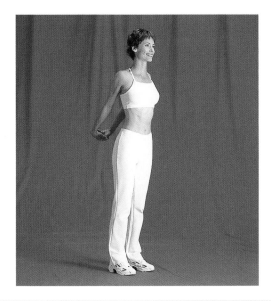

Chest

Stand with your feet shoulder-width apart and knees slightly bent. Clasp your hands behind your back with your palms facing in toward your body. Slowly push your chest forward, keeping your back and abdomen stable. (If this movement is uncomfortable, do the stretch without your hands touching.) You can lean forward slightly, but don't allow yourself to become pitched forward.

she could have lost half of her muscle tissue—and her slower metabolism means she burns 200 to 300 fewer calories daily than when she was younger.

Strength training boosts metabolism and reverses muscle loss. In fact, women who lift weights or do other forms of strength training twice a week for a few months can replace between 5 and 10 years of "lost" muscle tissue.

It may surprise you to know that strength training can also make your bones stronger, which is critically important for women. After a woman reaches menopause, she can lose up to 20 percent of her bone strength. Strength training literally adds mass to the bones, which makes them stronger and helps prevent fractures.

It has other benefits too. In one Tufts University program, people with knee arthritis experienced a 43 percent reduction in pain and relief from symptoms after just 16 weeks. People with diabetes who do strength training have better control over their blood sugar and lose weight too. Strength training also improves self-esteem and confidence, relieves symptoms of depression, and, surprisingly, boosts aerobic fitness.

To ease you into this vital part of exercise, we've created a customized strength-training plan (see pages 86–90) for women.

Step 5: Increase the Intensity

When you've being doing the same exercises for a while, you'll find that they get easier. This is because your body has adapted to the workload and is no longer feeling the strain. This is satis-fying, in a way, because it means that you've made progress. But it also means that you won't progress further until you push your body a little harder.

To keep your workouts at maximum pitch, increase the intensity. In other words, lift more weight, run faster, and generally exercise harder 2 or 3 times a week. The boost in intensity can have substantial health and fitness benefits. One study found that people who regularly pushed their workouts to the limit had higher levels of high-density lipoprotein (HDL, the "good" cholesterol) than those who exercised at lower intensities.

To boost the intensity of your workouts, try:

Exercise longer. Suppose you're currently exercising for 30 minutes. To increase the intensity, kick it up to 35 minutes. Keep it at that level for a few weeks, then add another 5 minutes, and then another. Exercising hard for 45 minutes will quickly add up to impressive fitness gains.

Try interval training. Instead of going all-out all the time—or, conversely, coasting along at a comfortable pace—shake things up with interval training. For example, exercise at a moderate pace for 4 minutes, then switch to high intensity for 4 minutes. Interval training will keep your body challenged without exhausting your muscles and lungs, says Wayne Westcott, PhD, fitness research director at the South Shore YMCA in Quincy, Massachusetts, and author of 20 fitness books.

Add new exercises. Remember the strain you felt when you first started exercising? It's

(continued on page 93)

Strength
Training

Plan on repeating each of the following exercises 8 to 12 times. For those that involve weights, choose weights that are heavy enough so that you can barely complete the set of 12. To get the most benefits from each exercise, do two or three sets of 12, resting for a few minutes in between. Repeat the exercises 2 or 3 times a week, but not on consecutive days, Martha Coopersmith, owner of the Bodysmith Company in New York City, advises.

Remember to do your stretches when you're done.

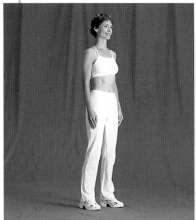

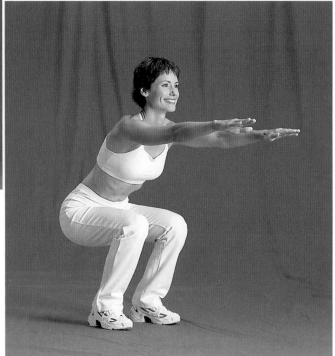

Squat

Stand with your feet shoulder-width apart (above). Bend your knees and squat as though you're sitting; hold your arms in front for balance (right). Make sure that your knees don't extend beyond your toes. Then return to the starting position.

(continued)

Strength
Training

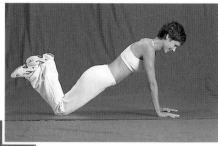

Pushup

Start on hands and knees, hands in line with shoulders. Your hips should be extended so that your body forms a straight line from head to knees. Cross your ankles in the air (left). Push yourself up (above), then return to the starting position. Repeat.

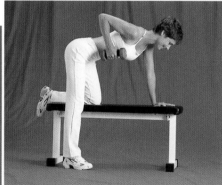

One-Arm Row

Put your left knee and left hand on a bench or a chair, keeping your back flat. Hold a weight in your right hand with your right arm straight and the weight hanging toward the floor, parallel to the bench (left). Raise the weight, keeping it close to your body, until it's even with your waist; your elbow should be pointed toward the ceiling (above).

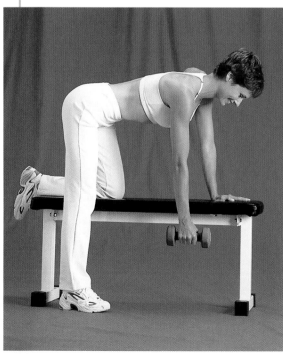

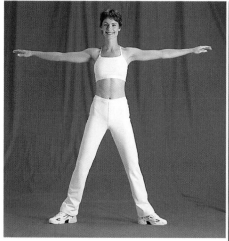

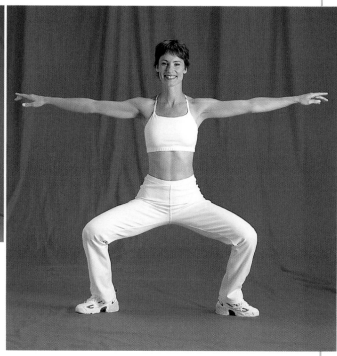

Plié

Stand with your feet about 2 feet apart; your legs should be turned out (above). With your back straight, lower your body (right). Then, as you straighten your legs, squeeze your inner thighs. Your knees should be in line with your ankles. Return to the starting position.

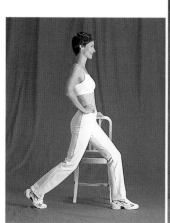

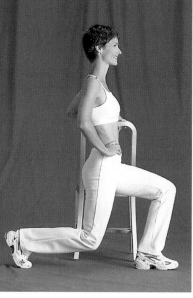

Lunge

Lightly place your left hand on the back of a chair for balance. Step forward with your left foot (far left). Your knee should be above your left foot, not sticking out past your toes. Lower your body by bending your knees and dropping your hips straight toward the floor (near left). Return to the starting position, then repeat with the other leg.

(continued)

Strength
Training

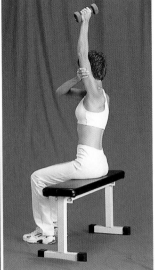

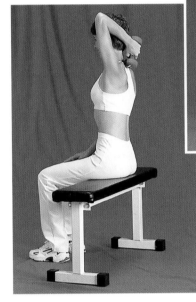

Triceps Extension

Sit on a bench or a chair while holding a weight in your left hand with your palm facing in. Bend your arm and raise it over your shoulder; your elbow will be pointing toward the ceiling, and the weight will be behind your head (near right). Hold your left elbow steady with your right hand, and raise the weight until your arm is straight (far right); return to the starting position.

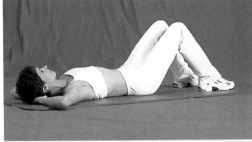

Abdominal

Lie on a mat with your knees bent, your feet flat on the floor and hip-width apart, your hands behind your head, elbows out to the sides (left). Contract your abdominal muscles and raise your shoulder blades off the ground about 30 degrees (below). Return to the starting position.

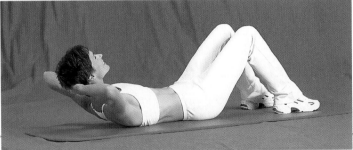

Military Press

While sitting, hold a weight in each hand. Start with the weights at shoulder height; your palms should be facing forward (near right). Raise the weights above your head without bringing them together or locking your elbows (far right), then bring them back down to your shoulders.

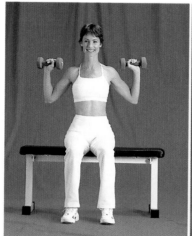

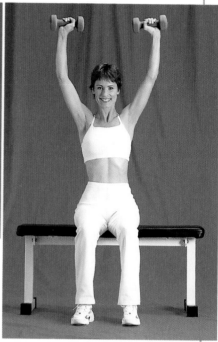

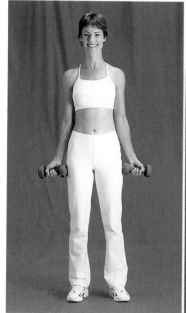

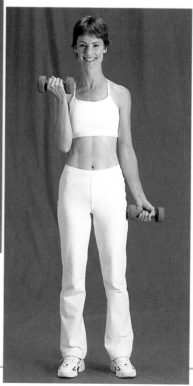

Biceps Curl

Stand straight and hold a weight in each hand, palms facing forward (far left). Keeping your elbow close to your body, bend your right arm and lift the weight toward your shoulder near left). Return to the starting position, then repeat with the other arm.

Prevention's
STEP UP
TO FITNESS

If you haven't been active in the past but are getting ready to start, you may be wondering what types of activities you'll enjoy most, and what the fitness benefits will be.

Prevention magazine's Ladder of Fitness makes it easy. You'll find dozens of exercises—from "formal" workouts to recreational activities and hobbies— along with the number of calories they burn (based on a 140-pound woman who exercises for 15 minutes). You're sure to find some that will satisfy your interests as well as your fitness goals.

The activities at the bottom of the ladder are low intensity. As you go up the rungs, the exercises become more intense.

140 CALORIES

Mountain biking, hiking a moderate-to-difficult grade, snowshoeing in soft snow, running a 10-minute mile, running up stairs, karate or tae kwon do, kickboxing, jumping rope, swimming vigorously, using a stair-climber or a ski machine

120 to 139 CALORIES

Running a 12-minute mile, singles tennis, volleyball on the beach, downhill skiing, rock climbing, swimming laps, water jogging, having a snowball fight

95 to 119 CALORIES

Backpacking, doubles tennis, racewalking, briskly walking uphill, jazz and modern dance, basketball, racquetball, soccer, high-impact aerobics, using a stationary rower, bicycling at a moderate pace, ice-skating, sledding, shoveling snow

70 to 94 CALORIES

Golf (carrying your clubs), downhill skiing on beginners' slopes, gardening, calisthenics, step aerobics, walking at a brisk pace, dancing (country, polka, or disco), playing tag, washing the car, using a snowblower, kayaking, mowing the lawn with a push mower

40 to 69 CALORIES

Lawn and lane bowling, badminton, croquet, dancing (cha-cha or swing), tai chi, golf (using a cart), mowing the lawn on a riding mower, raking leaves, playing catch or Frisbee, walking the dog good to repeat the experience periodically because it puts a beneficial load on your whole body. As you challenge different muscles, your heart and lungs will work harder, and that's the cornerstone of boosting overall fitness. Called cross training, this "must" for athletes is just as important for you.

Exercise to music. Sure, it's a good way to make the time go quickly, but music—as long as it has a fast tempo—also promotes impressive fitness gains. In one study, 24 men and women cycled to music. But the intensity of their cycling increased when they listened to music with a fast beat, possibly, the study's authors speculated, because the music distracted them from how tired they felt. Another study found that moving to a good beat—think Queen or the Red Hot Chili Peppers—increased exercise endurance by 15 percent in a group of treadmill users.

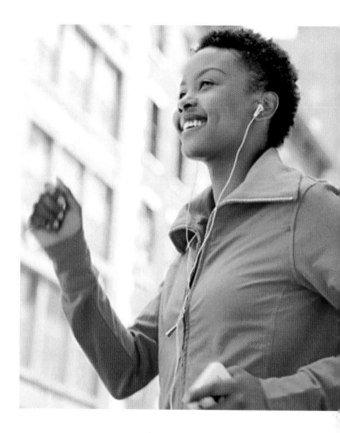

reality *check*

Her Goals Kept Her Motivated

As a lawyer in New York City, Claudia Cohen, 35, knows what it means to be really busy. She spends long days at the office, and for a long time the idea of getting in a quick workout during the day, or even after work, seemed out of the question.

Her feelings changed, however, when she decided it was finally time to put herself first and lose some weight. So she started exercising— and she did it with a vengeance.

Cohen exercises 5 days a week, for at least an hour each time. Sometimes she rides an exercise bike or uses the treadmill at her health club. Other days, she works out with weights at home with a personal trainer.

Boredom hasn't been a factor, Cohen says, partly because she's always setting goals for herself. When she's doing pushups, for example, she mentally challenges herself to do just one more. Striving for and achieving small goals keeps her focused and motivated, she explains.

Of course, she also wears a smaller dress size than she used to, and few things are more motivating than that. ∎

Step 6: Keep Yourself Motivated

We've talked about how hard it can be to launch into an exercise program when you haven't been active lately. What's even harder is sticking with it: Researchers have found that many people who take up strength or aerobic training will slack off or stop altogether within a few months.

Men and women alike offer all sorts of reasons for giving up their workouts. Not enough time. Too much work. Family responsibilities. They're all valid reasons, but what about those women with fast-paced careers, growing families, and a lot of outside interests who still find time to exercise?

What it usually boils down to is this: Women quit exercising because they aren't sufficiently motivated, says Dr. Westcott. It's a common problem, which is why creating motivation is an essential part of any training plan. Here are some things you may want to try.

Test yourself often. Dr. Westcott often advises women to keep exercise logs, in which they record how long they exercised, the distance covered, the amount of weight lifted. With every workout, you should try to push yourself just a little bit harder. Setting goals and then reaching them is among the strongest motivators, he explains.

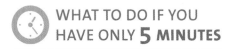

WHAT TO DO IF YOU HAVE ONLY 5 MINUTES

You don't have to do "formal" exercise to get a great workout: All you have to do is move, says Martha Coopersmith, owner of the Bodysmith Company in New York City.

"Jump rope, walk up stairs, dance, or play tag with the kids," she says. "Just keeping moving—while you wait for a pot of water to boil, for example, or when you're waiting for the laundry to dry."

Show your competitive side. Some women do their best work—and their best workouts—when they're in competition with someone else. You may want to ask a like-minded friend to exercise with you and keep a friendly competition going to see who improves the most in a certain period of time.

Push past the doldrums. We all have times when the idea of lifting weights or even going for a walk seems like just too much work. Unfortunately, if you skip one workout, coming back to the routine will be that much harder.

When you find your motivation flagging, mentally force yourself to be active, even if it's only to take a quick walk. Once you get off the couch and start moving, you'll find that you enjoy the way you feel—and you'll probably keep going.

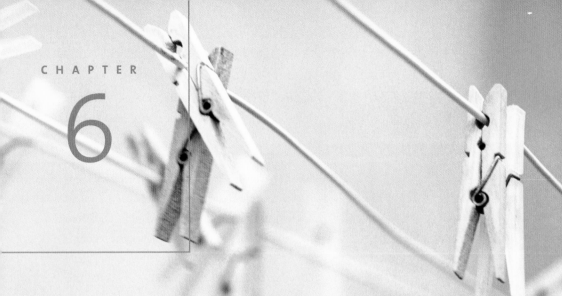

Prevention's Guide to Your Perfect Weight

A hundred years ago, only about 10 percent of adults were overweight. Today an estimated 62 percent of Americans are overweight or obese.

Yet we have the same genes as our ancestors. What's changed isn't our genes but our lifestyle.

It took great-grandmother hours to make dinner from scratch. She scrubbed clothes clean with her own hands. And without a car, she walked everywhere.

Today we take a whirl through the drive-thru to feed the family. We load the washing machine to clean clothes. And a short car ride takes us to work, the store, or a friend's house.

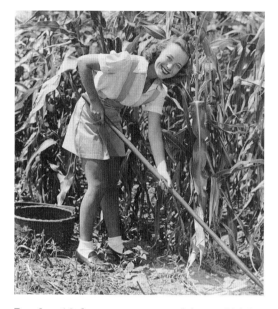

In the 19th century, machines did 70 percent of the work on farms and factories. Men and women did the rest. Now machines do 99 percent of the work, and many of us earn a living sitting at a desk or computer. Cars have taken the place of walking or cycling. We burn rubber instead of calories. And computers, cell phones, and fax machines help make life more fast-paced and stressful, which can send added pounds straight to our middles.

Superimpose stress and inactivity on a world where it's practically impossible not to come face-to-face daily with food that makes us fat and it's easy to see why so many more women (and men) have a weight problem today than did our ancestors.

Yes, a few people genuinely have a genetic disposition toward overweight. Children of obese parents have an 80 percent chance of being obese themselves, while children of normal-weight parents have less than a 10 percent

chance. Even adopted children tend to follow their biological parents' weight patterns. Recent studies have identified a number of genes that may play a role in obesity. One, also linked to diabetes, may be responsible for up to 22 percent of all cases of obesity.

Does this mean you were born to be fat? Genes may predispose you to obesity or other conditions, but they don't doom you. Although you may have a tougher time peeling off pounds, your behavior ultimately determines the number on the scale.

"The only way to gain weight is to eat more than you burn," says John P. Foreyt, PhD, director of the Behavioral Medicine Research Center at Baylor College of Medicine in Houston and coauthor of *Living without Dieting.*

Your Healthy Weight

Reaching or maintaining a healthy weight pays off in many ways. It lowers your risk for heart disease by lowering your blood pressure, cholesterol levels, and triglyceride levels. In fact, weight loss works better than drugs at lowering blood pressure in women with and without hypertension. Losing weight also helps you become more sensitive to insulin, which will help you avoid type 2 diabetes. These effects are especially beneficial to women after menopause, when they're more vulnerable to heart disease.

Because obesity contributes to five of the leading causes of death in the United States—heart disease, stroke, high blood pressure, cancer, and diabetes—losing weight can even help us live longer.

Regardless of the major health benefits, slimming down also improves quality of life. Think about it. Losing extra pounds will help you:

- Breathe more easily

- Sit more comfortably in movie theaters and airplane seats

- Get into and out of your car with ease

- Wear belted skirts and slacks

- Tie your shoes effortlessly

- Wear a swimsuit and enjoy going to the beach without feeling self-conscious

- Give you the confidence to try new things, like rock climbing

- Live to see your great-grandchildren and great-great-grandchildren

- Improve your sex life and overall energy level

As you slim down, you'll probably discover other, personal benefits of your own.

Here's everything you need to know to lose weight and keep it off, once and for all.

Overweight? Get Your Thyroid Checked

about 11 million people in the United States have hypothyroidism, an underactive thyroid. More than half of all women experienced three or more symptoms of hypothyroidism in the past year. If you're one of them, it could be why you're overweight.

The butterfly-shaped thyroid gland wraps around the front of the windpipe just below the Adam's apple and produces a hormone that regulates metabolism and organ function. It influences every organ, tissue, and cell in the body.

When the thyroid doesn't produce enough of the hormone—often because the immune system creates antibodies that damage or destroy it—you could experience:

- A weight gain of 10 pounds or less of fluid

- Fatigue

- Mood swings

- Dry, coarse skin or hair

- Hoarseness

- Forgetfulness

- Difficulty swallowing

- Intolerance to cold

Women are at higher risk than men for an underactive thyroid. But just being overweight and feeling tired doesn't mean you have thyroid dysfunction.

"I think a lot of us hope that when we gain weight, it's because of our thyroid," says Gay Canaris, MD, assistant professor of internal medicine at the University of Nebraska College of Medicine in Omaha.

So how do you know if you should get tested? Talk to your doctor about your symptoms. Fatigue could be caused by other disorders, such as anemia, cancer, depression, or sleep disorders. It could also result from too much work.

Even if you don't have symptoms, though, get screened at age 20 and every 5 years thereafter. There are no general screening guidelines for the public, and many doctors recommend screening at age 40 or 50, but since so many women could have dysfunction without knowing it and the test is so inexpensive, it can't hurt to get screened. ■

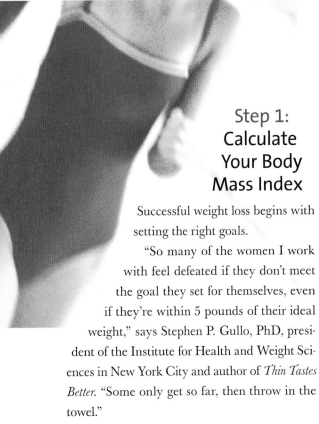

Step 1: Calculate Your Body Mass Index

Successful weight loss begins with setting the right goals.

"So many of the women I work with feel defeated if they don't meet the goal they set for themselves, even if they're within 5 pounds of their ideal weight," says Stephen P. Gullo, PhD, president of the Institute for Health and Weight Sciences in New York City and author of *Thin Tastes Better.* "Some only get so far, then throw in the towel."

Others hope to reach whatever weight they were in high school or on their wedding day. But that might not be realistic. A better strategy is to set a goal based on your body mass index (BMI), a ratio of weight to height.

Along with waist circumference (discussed in Step 2), body mass index is a more accurate indication of total body fat than body weight alone.

To calculate your BMI:

1. Multiply your weight in pounds by 703.

2. Divide that number by your height in inches.

3. Divide that number again by your height in inches, and you'll have your BMI.

You can also use the BMI calculator at www.nhlbisupport.com/bmi/bmicalc.htm, the Web site of the National Heart, Lung, and Blood Institute. You can also download a BMI app to your iPhone.

A BMI of between 18.5 and 25 is considered healthiest. You're considered overweight if your BMI is 25 or over, and you're considered obese if it's 30 or over.

"When someone has a BMI of 25, their risk for disease goes up because their blood pressure, cholesterol, blood sugar, and risk for diabetes may all go up," Dr. Foreyt says. "We've also found that at a BMI of 30, three-fourths of all people have at least one risk factor for heart disease, such as type 2 diabetes or hypertension."

But don't let your BMI go below 18.5—that's too low because it's unhealthy to be that skinny.

If you're very muscular, are under 5 feet tall, or are older, your BMI may not be a good measure of the amount of fat on your body.

Step 2: Measure Your Waistline

Because abdominal fat is associated with a greater health risk than fat carried in the hips, backside, or thighs, your waistline is also a better gauge of your weight than total number of pounds. It's also a good way to double-check your weight if your BMI, measured in Step 1, isn't considered high, but it's obvious that you're heavier than you should be.

There's a right and a wrong way to measure

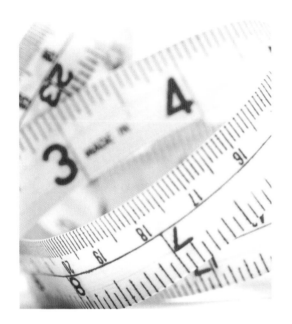

your waist. Hold a measuring tape horizontally around the abdomen at navel level, parallel to the floor. The tape should be snug, but not pulled tight. Breathe out, and note your waist measurement.

For women, a waist circumference of 35 inches or higher is unhealthy.

Step 3: Set a Starting Date

Once you know where you really stand weight-wise, your next step is to set your goals and commit yourself to them. If you don't set a starting date, you could fall into the "tomorrow syndrome," Dr. Gullo says.

Make sure you're ready. Before you "X" your calendar, make sure this is really the right time to start a weight-loss program. You might

WHAT WORKS FOR ME

MARY JANE MINKIN, MD, *clinical professor of obstetrics and gynecology at Yale University School of Medicine, shares her secrets of weight control.*

I love to eat! I've never been skinny, and I've always gained weight easily. I was the first kid on my block whose mother served skim milk; I was drinking a quart of milk a day! Now I eat a sensible, low-fat diet that includes lots of fruits, veggies, and whole grains, and I still love my milk.

My fanaticism about exercise is what saves my life—and my waistline! Three or four times a week, I run 5 miles or do the equivalent on the stairclimbing or rowing machine, or I bike for an hour. This helps me indulge my passion for food but still be able to wear a size 12.

As a child, I was never encouraged by my parents to exercise. It wasn't until I got to medical school that I adopted the exercise habit to relieve stress and get more energy. When I gained 30 pounds during my residency—who had time to work out?—exercise finally helped me to lose it. Now I shoot hoops regularly and play soccer with my kids. I'd like to add strength training to my routine next.

Getting up earlier to exercise in the morning works for me. You don't have to go to a gym, either. I tell women that taking the stairs rather than the elevator and walking short distances frequently during the day all adds up. ∎

want to wait if other responsibilities consume your life right now, such as a new job or a family illness.

Avoid holidays. You've probably heard that most people gain 5 pounds from November to January. With so many holiday dinners and parties, trying to lose weight during this time is a lofty goal. Instead, try to maintain your weight, and plan to start losing after the holidays.

Mark your calendar. Once you've established the best time to begin, make an appointment with yourself. Use the time from now until your start date to fill your kitchen with healthy foods, find a walking partner, and prepare for an exercise routine. "There's a reason races have a starting point," Dr. Gullo says. The more you prepare for your goal, the better you'll perform.

Step 4: Determine Your Real Calorie Needs

Eating too much food makes you overweight, but eating too little lowers your metabolism because your body instinctively interprets a dearth of calories as a famine and shifts into low gear to conserve calories. The solution: Balance what you eat with your activity. Here's a point system that makes it easy.

Consider your activity level.

- If your job or lifestyle involves a lot of sitting and you exercise rarely, give yourself 12 points.

- If you get more daily activity than light walking and you exercise aerobically for 45 to

WHAT TO DO IF YOU COULD CHANGE **ONLY ONE THING**

To jump-start your weight-loss program, eat more fruits and vegetables, says Kristine Clark, RD, PhD, nutrition consultant to the United States women's soccer team. Besides all the nutrients that produce contains, it also plays a role in weight loss. Fruits and vegetables fill you up for a small number of calories.

60 minutes 3 times a week, give yourself 15 points.

- If you get more daily activity than light walking and you get 45 to 60 minutes of aerobic activity at least 5 times a week, give yourself 18 points.

Multiply your points by your goal weight in pounds to get your daily calories. For example, if you're a 140-pound active woman and you want to lose 10 pounds, multiply 15 by 130 and get 1,950 calories.

To lose fat instead of muscle, you need to eat at least 1,200 calories a day. Problem is, the typical American woman eats an average of 3,800 calories a day—many more calories than she needs. If you eat just 500 extra calories a day—the equivalent of a Snickers bar and a medium Coke—you'll be getting 3,500 more calories a week than you need. That adds up to a new pound of fat on the scales.

Step 5: Keep a Food Diary

People tend to underestimate what they eat by 20 to 50 percent, particularly when they eat out. Along with restaurant meals, our calculations are clouded by drinks and foods we deem healthy or low-fat. In one Cornell University Food and Brand Lab study, people who were offered low-fat chocolate consumed 89 more calories on average—46 percent more than they did when given food that wasn't low-fat. To take stock of what you're really eating, write down your foods and portions every day for a week, making note of calorie counts on food labels. Then review what you've eaten.

Your diary will help you see your eating patterns for workdays and weekends (and holidays) and pinpoint when you tend to overeat. Once you know when those periods of overeating are, you can either make sure you have a healthy snack ready or schedule an activity to keep yourself away from the fridge.

And don't give up the food journaling. Studies suggest that keeping track of what you consume can keep you from eating mindlessly, which can rack up hidden calories.

Count what you drink. "A lot of people don't realize how many calories they take in from beverages," says Ellen Albertson, RD, owner of Cook2 Communications in Boston, Massachusetts. When people drank an extra 450 calories a day in one study (two gin and tonics or a cup of eggnog), they gained weight. But when they ate those extra calories in food, they ate less later in the day and lost weight. Don't sip your weight-loss goals away. Here's how to make your drinks work for you.

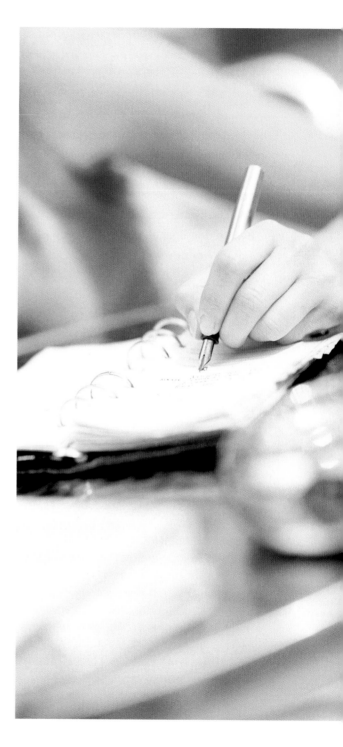

Drink water. There's no better thirst quencher. Water has zero calories, it fills you up, and it keeps your metabolism running more efficiently.

Watch the alcohol. When you choose wine over water, you don't only get extra calories in the drink. In fact, one study found that people ate 200 more calories in food at dinner. When compared with people who drank water, those who drank alcohol ate faster, took longer to feel full, and continued eating after being full.

Even if you don't drink with food, look at how alcohol can stack up the calories.

- 5 ounces of wine: 106 calories
- 12-ounce wine cooler: 220 calories
- 1½-ounce cocktail: 100–250 calories
- 3 ounces of sherry or port: 123 calories
- 12 ounces of regular beer: 150 calories
- 12 ounces of light beer: 99 calories

Add a mixer. Combine your favorite juice with sparking water. You can cut up to 85 calories per glass and lose up to 5 pounds a year. Halve your wine intake by adding sparkling water too.

Drink green tea. The antioxidant compounds in this popular drink combine with caffeine to increase your calorie burn.

Step 6: Eat More Plant Foods, Fewer Animal Foods

"Eat food. Not too much. Mostly plants" is good advice whether you're trying to lose weight or just want to stay healthy. The quote, from *New*

THREE THINGS I TELL EVERY FEMALE PATIENT

STEPHEN P. GULLO, PhD, *president of the Institute for Health and Weight Sciences in New York City and author of* Thin Tastes Better, *offers this advice to people he counsels about weight loss.*

1 **KNOW YOUR BEHAVIORS, NOT JUST YOUR CALORIES.** If you find that you're constantly regaining weight you've lost by abusing the same types of foods, either stop buying them or find replacements for them, such as a frozen chocolate sorbet instead of a big bag of M&Ms.

REMEMBER THAT WEIGHT LOSS IS ABOUT LIBERATION, NOT DEPRIVATION. It's about a change in perspective. Eat fewer calories and

2 cut down the amount of fat you eat in the spirit of liberating yourself from the discomfort of the pounds that you've been carrying, instead of depriving yourself from certain foods.

3 **DON'T FORGET THAT BEING THIN IS A LIFE MANAGEMENT SKILL.** It's normal to experience setbacks and periods of feeling defeated. But in the future, when you turn 40 or 50 or 60 at a healthy weight, it won't be by accident, because aging well is not an accident. It's the gift that those who care deeply give to themselves. It will be because you planned and honed your skills at weight management. ∎

York Times bestselling food/environment writer Michael Pollan, was his synthesis of decades of nutrition advice for maximizing your health, and losing weight plays a part in that. Here are some proven ways to attack excess pounds.

Eat more, weigh less. Low energy-dense foods like fruits, vegetables, broth-based soups, potatoes, fish, oatmeal, and whole wheat pasta are typically low in fat and high in water and fiber, and carry fewer calories per mouthful so they make satisfying meals. Eating them instead of high-energy-density foods like cheesecake could help you eat 20 percent fewer calories.

Make fruits and vegetables the main attraction of your meal. Instead of a sandwich with four slices of meat, crackers, and cookies for lunch, eat just two slices of meat and add sliced tomato, cucumber, and fresh spinach. Follow it with a piece of fresh fruit and a cookie. Instead of ordering veal parmigiana at an Italian restaurant, order a large bowl of minestrone soup, a salad, and half of a portion of pasta with marinara sauce.

In fact, one study found that one particular food—broth-based soup—made women feel so full that they ate 100 fewer calories at a buffet than women who had had an appetizer of chicken rice casserole. If you follow the same logic and start eating broth-based soup before your meals, you could drop 10 pounds in a year. (Subsequent studies found that any food that contains lots of fluid—including salads—can keep your daily calories down.)

Stress protein. That doesn't mean piling meat on your plate. But studies have found that since the body takes a longer time to digest protein—

> **"Drink** eight glasses of water daily. None of your body parts, from your **brain to your toes**, work well without adequate **hydration."**

—JANE BRODY, HEALTH COLUMNIST FOR *THE NEW YORK TIMES*

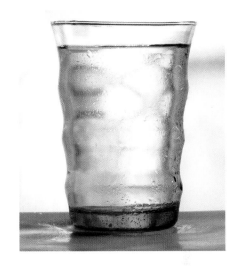

which is found in meat, poultry and low-fat dairy, as well as legumes and nuts—you stay fuller longer. For example, one study found that people who ate an egg breakfast ate less at subsequent meals than people who ate a bagel. The egg-eaters lost 65 percent more weight than the bagel noshers. As a bonus, the body also expends more calories digesting protein, so you boost the burn (called the thermic effect of food).

Eating more fiber, too, could help you lose weight. Your body will quickly absorb the calories from a breakfast made of white flour

"Switch to **whole grain** carbohydrates such as **whole wheat bread** and **brown rice**. High intakes of refined carbohydrates and sugar are the main sources of calories in the U.S. diet, and thus a major contribution to being overweight."

—WALTER WILLETT, MD, CHAIRMAN, NUTRITION DEPARTMENT,
HARVARD SCHOOL OF PUBLIC HEALTH

and sugar, and you'll feel hungry again soon after your meal. But the calories in a bowl of bran cereal with no added sugar are absorbed slower and will keep you full longer. The same is true for fiber in other foods.

Fiber also helps move other food out of the body before the body has a chance to absorb them. For every gram of fiber you eat, you'll absorb about 4 fewer calories than if you ate simple carbohydrates.

Triple your fiber intake. Most people eat 13 grams of fiber a day. But if you eat about 3 times that amount—40 grams—you could block the absorption of 160 calories a day.

Start hearty. One study found that people who had eaten high-fiber oatmeal for breakfast ate 30 percent fewer calories at lunch than people who had eaten cornflakes.

Grab beans. Beans are a sure way to get fat-fighting fiber, so add them to salads, soups, chili,

and other dishes. Chili has nearly 10 grams of fiber per serving, three-bean salad with balsamic vinegar has 12½ grams, and red beans and brown rice has a whopping 18 grams.

Eat whole grains. Whole grains not only have fiber but also have more micronutrients, like folate, magnesium, and vitamin E, than their white-flour counterparts. Enjoy whole grain products such as brown rice; whole wheat or whole grain bread; whole wheat flour; whole grain and multigrain cereals; oatmeal; oat bran; whole wheat pasta and couscous; and whole wheat, whole grain, and rye crackers.

Aim for nine. Fruits and vegetables are naturally high in fiber, low in fat and calories, and full of healthy nutrients and antioxidant vitamins—like A, C, and E—that are important in preventing heart disease and cancer. You've probably heard advice to eat five a day, but because so many studies link diets high in fruits and vegetables with less cancer, heart disease, diabetes, and osteoporosis, *Prevention* recommends nine

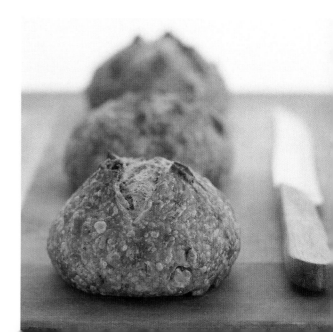

servings a day. And since they have all the components to help you lose weight, eating nine a day should be part of your weight-loss program, too. Try this trick to increase your veggie and fruit intake: When you scoop a serving onto your plate, scoop a second right away. A Penn State University study found that people who doubled up on veggies and fruit in a meal ate fewer calories and were more likely to leave more calorie-dense meat and grains on the plate.

Stay low on the GI. The glycemic index (GI) ranks foods on how much they raise your blood sugar. "The body uses insulin to bring down blood sugar," says Yunsheng Ma, MD, PhD, an assistant professor of medicine at the University of Massachusetts Medical School. Your body stores that excess sugar as fat, and as soon as the sugar leaves your blood stream, you're going to be hungry again—that's how low blood sugar makes you feel. Dr. Ma, who studied the eating patterns of 572 people, found that those who ate foods high on the glycemic index—white bread, potatoes, sweets, snack foods—weighed significantly more than those who didn't. "There's about a 10-pound body weight decrease for every 10-point drop in the glycemic index of all the food a person eats each day," he says. Eat lower on the GI by trading potatoes for sweet potatoes, whole wheat bread for white, grapes for raisins, and pasta for pizza.

Step 7: Scale Back Your Fat Intake

Fatty foods are more packed with calories than are low-fat foods. One gram of fat has 9 calories and a gram of carbohydrates has only 4 calories. So with fewer bites of a high-fat food, you'll get a lot more calories.

Fat may also affect the appetites of overweight people. In one study, overweight men who had had a high-fat meal before eating at a buffet ate 56 percent more than lean men who had eaten the same high-fat meal. But when the overweight men had eaten a low-fat meal, they ate the same amount at the buffet as the lean men, who'd also eaten a low-fat meal. It appears that the appetite switch of some overweight people is turned off slower from fat because it takes longer for their bodies to detect that fat has been ingested.

To lose weight, try to get 25 percent of your calories from fat. Here are some satisfying ways to do it.

> "Eliminate all foods containing partially **hydrogenated** oils. There's growing evidence that these **unnatural fats** are not good for us, and avoiding them and the **processed foods** that they come in would be a huge step to improving nutritional health."
>
> —ANDREW WEIL, MD, DIRECTOR OF THE PROGRAM IN INTEGRATIVE MEDICINE AND CLINICAL PROFESSOR OF MEDICINE AT THE UNIVERSITY OF ARIZONA COLLEGE OF MEDICINE IN TUCSON AND AUTHOR OF *8 WEEKS TO OPTIMUM HEALTH*

Choose lean meat. Choose meat that's naturally low in fat, such as turkey breast or skinless chicken. And when you're buying any type of meat, make sure it has no more than 10 grams of fat per 3-ounce serving.

Look for low-fat cheese. Another great way to lower your fat consumption is to choose low-fat and fat-free cheeses and yogurt. They carry all the calcium and nutrients of the full-fat varieties.

Bake instead of fry. If you have a recipe that calls for frying–such as potato wedges for french fries–try this instead: Coat the potato wedges with nonstick spray and bake in the oven at 450°F to 475°F until they're brown and crisp.

Downsize dessert. Sweet, satisfying desserts don't have to include astronomical grams of fat. Here are some tips on making them healthier.

- Use mini chocolate chips in dough and batters. They'll spread out more, so you use fewer.

- Use at least half of the baking chocolate squares your brownie recipe calls for, and replace the rest with cocoa powder, which is much lower in fat.

- Use phyllo dough instead of puff pastry or strudel dough; it's fat-free. Use nonstick spray instead of butter to moisten the sheets.

- Sweeten recipes with applesauce or prune puree to cut down on refined sugar consumption.

Step 8: Bone Up on Portion Size

You could count a heaping bowl of spaghetti as one portion, but your body knows how many calories you're eating. Get to know portion sizes, and you'll always have a mental picture of how much you should eat.

- ½ cup of fresh or cooked vegetables, or about a rounded handful

- 1 cup of raw or leafy vegetables, or the size of a baseball

- 1 medium piece of fresh fruit, also the size of a baseball

- ½ cup cooked or canned fruit, about a rounded handful

- 1 slice of bread

- 1 ounce of ready-to-eat cereal could be anywhere from ½ cup to 1¼ cups, so check the nutrition label

- ½ cup cooked cereal, about a rounded handful

- ½ cup cooked rice or pasta, about a rounded handful

- 3 ounces of cooked fish or meat (4 ounces raw), the size of a deck of cards

- ½ cup cooked dried beans, about a rounded handful

- ⅓ cup nuts, about a level handful

- 1½ ounces of cheese (or 2 ounces processed); 1 ounce is the size of four dice

You can also follow the serving size listed on the nutrition label of your food. It should be equivalent to the USDA's standard serving size.

Another tip: Measure out your servings a few times and make a mental note of how much it covers the plate or bowl.

Step 9: Eat All Day

If you plan to skip breakfast to save on calories, your scheme will backfire. One study found that the metabolisms of people who skipped breakfast were about 5 percent lower than those of people who ate three or more meals a day. A 5 percent boost in metabolism could help you lose 10 pounds in a year. One of the characteristics of people in the National Weight Control Registry—an ongoing study of people who've lost at least 30 pounds and kept it off—is that they're breakfast eaters. Their typical morning meal is cereal and fruit.

It's also important to keep it up throughout the day. Eating more often—without increasing the amount of food you eat—will keep you full. In two studies, men who had eaten breakfast in small portions throughout the morning had a 27 percent smaller lunch than men who had eaten breakfast as a single meal.

Another good reason to avoid long stretches without food: After 4 hours, blood sugar drops, and you'll crave sweets instead of healthier foods.

Try these healthy snacks for fewer than 175 calories each.

- Half of a whole grain bagel with jam or low-fat cream cheese

- A handful of baby carrots with a dip of ¼ cup salsa and ¼ cup low-fat sour cream

- A cup of instant bean soup

- ½ cup whole grain cereal

Step 10: Sweat a Little

More than one-third of people who are overweight say they get no physical activity. Almost 60 percent say they don't exercise enough. But working out for 30 to 40 minutes could help you burn between 250 and 500 calories an exercise session. You could also burn as many as 50 or 100 calories more for the rest of the day after exercising.

Working out routinely can change your body's

Watch the Sweets, Sugar

eating reasonable amounts of sweets is one thing, but making sugar the main attraction of your eating plan won't help you lose weight.

Sugar may not have fat, but it sure has a lot of calories, and we're not skimping on it. On average, sugar makes up about one-third of women's diets—that's 62 pounds a year and 151,840 calories. But it's more than extra calories that squelch weight-loss efforts: Sugar also makes you hungrier. It's digested faster and its calories are stored quickly, so you'll get hungry again sooner than if you had a high-protein snack.

To get down to the 7 teaspoons of sugar you should be eating a day (rather than the 19 women typically get), try to eliminate or lower your consumption of the five biggest offenders: nondiet soda, baked goods, ice cream, sweetened fruit drinks, and candy. If you have the willpower to cut them out completely, you could save 78,000 calories a year and lose more than 20 pounds. ■

composition. Exercise helps you lose more fat, gain more muscle, and regain less weight. Women who exercise also tend to follow their eating plans more closely than women who don't exercise.

And if you're one of those people with a lagging metabolism, exercise is a great way to speed it up. For more information about establishing a regular exercise program, see Chapter 5.

Work it in. So you say you don't have time to exercise. Sandra Adamson Fryhofer, MD, clinical associate professor of medicine at Emory University in Atlanta and member of the American Medical Association's Council on Science and Public Health in Atlanta, hears that all the time from her patients, but she doesn't accept the excuse. "There's always something you can do," she says. If you watch the morning news before work, do it while you're walking on the treadmill. "Every little bit of exercise helps."

If you take just 15 minutes to walk the dog in the morning, 10 minutes to walk to the deli for lunch, 5 minutes in the afternoon to stretch at your desk, 15 minutes to weed the garden when you get home from work, and 15 minutes after dinner to play tag with the kids, your activity adds up to 1 hour–and 300 extra calories burned that day.

Fidget. For some people, feeling antsy in their chair keeps them thin. Scientists gave 16 normal-weight people 1,000 extra calories a day for 8 weeks, but the amount of weight they gained varied between 3 and 16 pounds. The ones who gained the least weight burned up to 692 calories a day doing everyday activities, such as walking, climbing stairs, household chores, sitting up straight, standing up straight–and fidgeting. Can you train yourself to be a more active person naturally? "Sure, if you make a conscious attempt at it," Dr. Fryhofer says.

Try adding these habits to your life:

- Stand up to answer to the phone.

- Do a household chore during commercials on television.

- Tap your feet against the floor or rotate your ankles when you're sitting.

- Dance to music as you do the dishes, iron, or fold clothes.

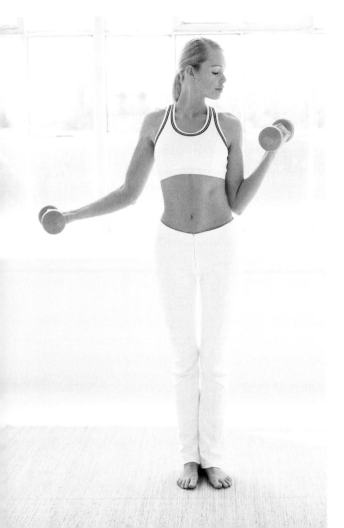

Turn off cravings. While you work out, your body suppresses digestion and releases glucose and fatty acids into the blood for energy. You won't feel the urge to eat until you reach a state of rest and your energy fuels are back in storage. Some recent studies have found that brisk exercise may help you tap into your body's own hormonal appetite suppressants. The next time you find yourself hungry out of boredom, get up and take a walk, work in the garden, or do housework. You'll curb your craving and burn some extra calories.

Turn off the TV. If you gave up one television show a day and took a 2-mile walk for 30 minutes instead, you'd burn enough calories to lose 18 pounds in a year.

Don't stop. Once you start an exercise program, you'll probably like it so much you won't want to stop—and that's good news when it comes to weight loss. Research shows that people who manage to maintain weight loss exercise the equivalent of walking 3 to 4 miles a day.

Other Helpful Strategies

If you're doing everything "right" and still not losing weight—or losing it more slowly than suits you—these additional strategies can help get you unstuck.

OUTSMART RESTAURANT FARE

The average American eats four meals a week away from home. Even when you choose the healthy options at family-style restaurants, that's a weekly total of about 3,000 calories and 73 grams of fat.

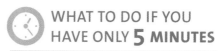

WHAT TO DO IF YOU HAVE ONLY **5 MINUTES**

You can still get in a workout for 5 minutes a day—and see health results. Follow this plan by Glenn A. Gaesser, PhD, director of the Healthy Lifestyles Research Center at Arizona State University in Phoenix and author of *Big Fat Lies: The Truth about Your Weight and Your Health.*

Spend 5 minutes a day doing an exercise, but vary what you do from day to day. One day, walk, go up stairs, or do some other aerobic exercise for 5 minutes. The next, strength train for 5 minutes, with or without weights. And the next, stretch for 5 minutes. (For examples of exercises, see Chapter 5.)

If you continue on this exercise schedule—or, better yet, do a little more—you'll probably lose weight, improve your health, and start enjoying exercise.

That was the result of Dr. Gaesser's study of 40 people, mostly women, who didn't like to exercise. They did 15 sessions a week for 10 minutes at a time at least every other day while eating a sensible diet. In 3 weeks they lost 3 pounds, improved their strength and endurance, increased their flexibility, improved their cholesterol levels, and admitted that they actually liked exercising.

You can start out with 5 minutes a day, Dr. Gaesser says. If you find more time for these exercises, you'll benefit even more.

Calories in restaurant meals stack up quickly because restaurants typically serve more than 3 times the amount of one serving of food. In one 2007 study, researchers asked a group of executive chefs to describe the portion sizes in their restaurants. Although 76 percent of them thought they served "regular" portions, the portions of steak and pasta were actually 2 to 4 times larger than serving sizes recommended by the government's leading nutrition experts. The typical serving sizes of penne pasta were anywhere from 4 to 8 ounces, while the USDA recommends 1 ounce. Eight out of ten of the chefs served strip steaks that were more than twice as large as the 5.5 ounces nutrition experts recommend. Restaurants have even increased the size of their standard plate from 10½ to 12 inches to accommodate the excess food, says Melanie Polk, RD, director of nutrition education at the American Institute for Cancer Research in Washington, DC.

But you still get a healthy meal in a restaurant if you take control. You can ask for your food at restaurants to be specially cooked with no or less oil, request a nutrition guide from the restaurant, check the nutritional content of their menu foods online, or choose healthy foods at a buffet or party.

Wrap it up. According to a survey by the American Institute for Cancer Research, 26 percent of people dining out say they eat everything that's put in front of them. That's a good reason to have your waiter wrap up half of your meal before it even makes it to your table.

Share with friends. Since restaurant meals are usually two or three servings anyway, ask

> " Watch your **portion sizes**. Most of us eat far more food than we really need, and there are many reasons to eat less, including **slowing** the **aging** process. "
>
> —KATHLEEN JOHNSON, RD, DIRECTOR OF THE NUTRITION PROGRAM AT CANYON RANCH HEALTH RESORT IN TUCSON

your dinner partner if she wants to share an entrée with you.

Get what you want. Don't even open your menu at a restaurant. Instead, think about what you want to eat, such as whole wheat toast and scrambled eggs, and ask the waiter for it. But don't stop there. Tell the waiter you don't want sausages or hash browns, or else he might bring it.

Think small. Polk uses an old standby when she's at a buffet. She takes small portions of her favorite foods and refuses to go up for seconds. She takes her time and eats it slowly so she's not left watching everyone else eat when she's finished.

Really party. You don't have to stuff yourself to have fun. Instead of celebrating a birthday or holiday at a restaurant, stay home and shift the emphasis from food to fun, with charades, board games, or music and dancing.

LEARN TO TAKE YOUR TIME

Give yourself plenty of time to eat, rearranging your schedule if you have to. After looking at high-tech images of the brains of 21 adults while they ate, researchers found that their appetite switch turned off 10 minutes after they started their meal. The more time you take to eat, the fewer calories you'll inhale in the first 5 minutes of dinner, so try to spend 20 minutes at the dinner table.

Getting pleasure from your food can actually help you lose weight, says Albertson.

"I find that people gain weight when they're not focusing on their food—when they're at their desks, in their car, or in front of the television," she says. But a great way to lose weight is to make a fantastic dinner and sit down and truly enjoy it. Once you get pleasure from your food this way, you probably won't need so much to feel satisfied.

CHIP AWAY AT STRESS

When you're under stress, your body releases a hormone called cortisol, which sends fat to your abdomen, where it can increase risk for heart disease. It also suppresses growth hormone and testosterone, which protect you against heart disease and gaining abdominal fat. These effects are even more dangerous after menopause, when women's estrogen levels drop.

You may find that you eat more when you're under stress. That's because food helps some people to relax. Stress activates your sympathetic nervous system and makes you feel on edge. Eating may activate natural painkillers in your brain, helping you to feel relaxed.

reality *check* Joining a Church Sent Her Weight Plummeting

When Marilyn Rozsnaki set out to lose 20 pounds, she didn't know that going to church would help.

At 5 feet 2 inches and 150 pounds, Marilyn first changed her diet. She started eating less meat and fat, and more vegetables.

In 3 weeks she lost 6 pounds, and then hit a plateau. So she started a walking program, but she wanted to get more active in other ways, too.

Before she started eating better and exercising, lack of energy and insecurity from being overweight kept her from getting more involved with her church. But once the scale slipped down, she had more confidence and energy to spend more time at church. It worked. The time she spent in Bible studies class, at service, and helping out families in need was time she was away from her kitchen—and snacks. She also prayed for the strength to eat well and exercise consistently.

"I knew I couldn't do it alone, so I asked for help," she says.

The spirituality of worship—along with keeping busy—keeps her from worrying about problems that could send her to the cookie jar.

She even found an exercise partner at church. A neighbor who attends her church became interested in Marilyn's weight loss, and now they walk up to 3 miles 4 or 5 times a week.

Marilyn's new lifestyle sent her weight plummeting. In 5 months, she had surpassed her 20-pound goal and was 25 pounds thinner.

"My then-10-year-old son told me I look like an 18-year-old chick," she says. ■

"Control your calorie intake, get no more than 20 percent of your calories from fat, and be sure to get five to nine servings of fruits and vegetables daily."

—MOSHE SHIKE, MD, DIRECTOR OF THE CANCER PREVENTION AND WELLNESS PROGRAM AT MEMORIAL SLOAN-KETTERING CANCER CENTER IN NEW YORK CITY

Anxiety can affect your behavior in other ways, too. Stress from financial problems, relationship issues, or just being overworked is often followed by a period of depression. And whenever you're depressed, you're probably going to eat more and be less motivated to exercise, says Dr. Fryhofer. You're also more likely to grab comfort foods, which are usually higher in fat.

A study of 1,300 people found that those who were cynical and had high levels of anxiety had the most abdominal fat. Depression also ranked high among women with the most abdominal fat.

Keeping stress under control should be part of your weight-loss strategy. Here are some ideas on how to do it. (For more on stress, see Chapter 7.)

Accept imperfection. The house can't be completely clean, you'll miss a deadline once in a while, and your kids probably won't get straight A's. Trying not to control every aspect of life may help you lose extra flab.

Take care of you. If you make sure you are well rested, get enough exercise, and eat well, you'll feel better and hold on to positive emotions.

Catch the negative self-talk. For one day,

pretend you have a cartoon bubble over your head and catch everything you say to yourself, suggests Sandra Haber, PhD, a psychologist in private practice in New York City. Write it down a read it back to yourself. Negative self-talk stresses you out. "Keep saying you're fat and lazy and it's little wonder that you hide away and feed yourself junk," she says. Instead, offer yourself the same kind encouragement you'd give a friend.

Turn on the radio. Listen to some soothing music, and you may ease your anxiety and even your blood pressure and heart rate under very stressful situations.

Shake, shake, shake. If you get up and dance, you'll burn calories and release endorphins in your brain, which will elevate your mood and erase stress.

Tell a joke. Humor helps ease anxiety. One study found that people who performed a stressful task after watching an episode of *Seinfeld* had lower blood pressure and heart rates than people who hadn't watched the television show.

Have a cuppa. Black and green tea contain theanine, an amino acid that increases levels of relaxing chemicals in the brain.

Get at least 7 hours sleep. Not only will you feel refreshed, you may lose weight. Researchers at the University of Chicago found that people who weren't getting enough sleep had lower levels of hormones that control appetite. "The research suggested that short sleep durations could be a risk factor for obesity," says James Gangwisch, PhD, an epidemiologist from Columbia University Medical Center. His follow-up study of 9,588 Americans found that women who slept 4 hours or less a night were

234 percent more likely to be obese than those who slept more hours. The key number for most people is 7 hours or more a night, he says.

GET SUPPORT

Pay attention to the small gains you make along the way and congratulate yourself for them. Even if you don't lose weight as fast as you wanted, remind yourself that you can bound up the stairs and not lose your breath or that you cook meals that make you feel good and keep your body healthy. Even if it's 5 pounds, celebrate every step you take to better health.

Lose together. A friend may be the perfect motivator to get out of the house for a brisk walk or to inspire you to eat low-fat meals at restaurants.

Send for reinforcements. "Long-term weight loss requires support," says Marion

---

Forget Fad Diets

The best advice you'll ever get when it comes to dieting: "Quit!"

Whether you're pigging out on pork rinds or living on 800 calories a day, diets that don't include a variety of healthy foods or that severely restrict calories aren't good for long-term weight loss or your health. Some fad diets are actually more damaging to your health than obesity.

It's hard to keep up a diet low in calories, for obvious reasons: It's uncomfortable to be hungry. Think of starving as holding your breath underwater—you can do it for only so long before you gulp for air.

"Starving has nothing to do with losing weight," says Stephen P. Gullo, PhD, president of the Institute for Health and Weight Sciences in New York City and author of *Thin Tastes Better*. "Hunger pangs are a sign that you're doing something wrong. Succeeding at weight loss doesn't mean you have to give up fine taste in food. It means you have to be a selective gourmet."

When you lose weight from starving, your metabolism may decrease as a result. This means that even though you're eating fewer calories, you're also burning off fewer calories. It also means that instead of losing weight, you lose muscle. When you go back to eating foods higher in fat or calories, you're more likely to gain fat instead of muscle. With this new efficiency, you may regain weight quicker, and it may take longer to lose weight in the future. Yo-yo dieting also may put your health at risk if you already have health problems. A diet of only 800 calories a day could result in lower immunity, an irregular heartbeat, irregular menstruation, a lower sex drive, lower metabolism, loss of lean body tissue, headaches, fatigue, dry skin, and sleeplessness.

But even when a diet allows you to eat plenty of just a few types of food, your health will suffer. Anytime you eliminate food groups, you lose out on the nutrients they provide, such as the calcium in dairy foods, fiber and vitamin E in grains, and carotenoids and phytochemicals in vegetables. And some diets require you to eat foods high in saturated fat, which isn't good for your heart.

Your best bet is to stick to eating plans that include reasonable amounts of a variety of foods and don't allow you to lose more than 2 pounds a week. A satisfying meal of hearty portions of vegetables has fewer calories than some meals recommended by fad diets. ■

Franz, RD, a nutrition consultant in Minneapolis. Her study found that people who met regularly with a dietitian or attended reinforcement meetings were more likely to maintain their weight loss than those who didn't. It also helps to announce your weight loss intentions so friends can support you, she says.

Go online. Inspiration may lie on the other side of a Web site link. Some research shows that weight-loss Web sites can help women lose weight. Check out a few chat rooms, calorie counters, and exercise logs to see if this type of support is for you. Look for sites that include food diaries, personal feedback, weekly lessons, and emotional support.

Trade chores. If cleaning the kitchen puts you too close to the cookie jar to avoid temptation, head outside and rake leaves, shovel snow, or garden. Ask your spouse to pick up the indoor chores.

Work together. If you want to join a support group like TOPS (Take Off Pounds Sensibly) or Weight Watchers and your spouse could use a lesson on nutrition, join together and get extra support.

Hide temptation. Don't keep temptation right on the counter. If you're likely to overeat certain snacks, ask a family member to hide them on a high shelf, in the back of the cupboard, in a closet, or somewhere else you won't find them easily.

Lose a Little Weight—At First

If your BMI is 25 or higher, start out by aiming to lose between 5 and 10 percent of your body weight, says Dr. Foreyt. For example, if you're 5 feet 4 inches and weigh 180 pounds, your BMI is 31. To get it down to 25, you'd need to lose 35 pounds. At first, concentrate on losing the first 10 or 15 pounds. Moderate weight loss will give you lower blood pressure, lower lipids, lower blood sugar, and more self-esteem, and it's an easier goal than trying to lose 35 pounds (or more) at once.

Pace yourself. People who lose 5 to 10 pounds in a week lose water, not fat, so try to lose a pound or two a week. Depending on how much you have to lose, it could take as long as 6 months to lose 10 percent of your body weight in a healthy way, but that means you're more likely to maintain your new weight.

Look for other evidence. It may take a while to see results on the scale, but you'll feel your body getting stronger and healthier immediately after you start to eat well and exercise.

If you lose weight but your body mass index doesn't budge, measure your waist again. Your abdominal fat may disappear—a benefit—even if your total weight or BMI doesn't budge. It will also help keep you motivated when your weight seems to be stuck in the same 5- to 10-pound range despite your efforts to reduce.

Work on maintenance. Once you lose your initial goal of 10 percent, maintaining it for 6 months will continue to improve your health and make it easier to avoid weight regain.

Do it again. If you have more to lose after your first 10 percent, continue to set the same goals until you've reached a healthy BMI.

A Real-Life Guide to Stress Relief

As comic Lily Tomlin once put it, "Reality is the leading cause of stress among those in touch with it." And what's reality for American women? We have more on our plates than ever before. At work, we skip lunch and put in overtime. At home, we're in charge of most of the housework and child care. (Research has found that women put in 17 hours of housework before having kids, and 28 hours after they become moms.) And who takes care of parents and in-laws when they get sick? Seventy-five percent of all unpaid caretakers in the United States are women. We do it all.

The result? Women are often overwhelmed and feel out of control. The unrelenting stress disrupts our peace of mind and also damages our health, says Margaret A. Caudill-Slosberg MD, PhD, adjunct professor of medicine at Dartmouth Medical School and an expert in stress and pain management. Two-thirds of American workers—and more women than men—say that work has a significant impact on their stress levels. And stress follows women home. Research has found that even American women who are highly satisfied with their jobs have significantly elevated levels of stress hormones during and after work, resulting from work and home responsibilities. After the economic downturn of 2008, women—particularly baby boomers—bore the brunt of economic stress, says a survey done by the American Psychological Association. But Gen X women and those between 18 and 29 also reported greater than normal stress over money and housing costs in a survey that found that 83 percent of women were worried about finances. That anxiety was being translated into unhealthy behaviors and emotional and physical symptoms from depression to headaches. Stress in moderation isn't necessarily a bad thing. The stress response—tightened muscles, racing heart, pumping blood pressure, the flow of adrenaline—is designed to help protect us from physical danger, to make us jump out of the way of the careening car or duck an oncoming fist. A little stress can help us produce chemicals that help us learn and remember, boost our immune system, and even improve our mood. But that "fight-or-flight" process isn't supposed to stay in the on position indefinitely. When stress becomes chronic, it can damage relationships, steal restful sleep, wear out the arteries, and set the stage for a host of diseases.

It doesn't have to be this way. Stress isn't really something objective—the deadline, the traffic jam, or the uncooperative teenager. Stress is how you react to those things. That's why one woman who sees a long line at the supermarket may feel her temper rising out of control, while another simply relaxes and browses through a magazine while she waits. That's good news, because it means that control of stress is in your hands. You may not be able to change the circumstances of your life all the time, but you can change how you respond to them.

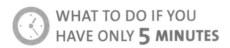

WHAT TO DO IF YOU HAVE ONLY **5 MINUTES**

Find a quiet place to close your eyes. Tune out the rest of the world and rest your mind, says Pamela Peeke, MD, assistant clinical professor of medicine at the University of Maryland School of Medicine in Baltimore and author of *Fight Fat after Forty*. "Or go for a walk around the block if you're a physical type of person."

Even a short break from stress will help you feel better physically as well as emotionally, she explains.

Your Body on Stress

While we tend to view stress as toxic to our minds, we generally don't consider its potentially harmful effects on the body. But the physical effects of stress are profound.

During times of stress, the nervous system triggers the release of stress hormones: adrenaline, norepinephrine, and cortisol. They stimulate virtually every system in the body. For example, they cause sugars and fats to pour into the bloodstream for quick energy. Blood pressure rises, and the heart beats faster in order to boost circulation to muscles in the arms and legs. Respiration increases, which supplies the muscles with more oxygen. The blood clots more easily as a precaution against injury, and perspiration increases in order to cool the body in this energized state.

The stress response happens very quickly. It's designed to save your life in emergency situations. Once the danger is past, your body gradually returns to its normal state.

Most days, of course, stress isn't a physical threat. Stress is time pressures, traffic, and the weight of responsibilities. They don't always go away and their effects on the body may be profound, says Dr. Caudill-Slosberg.

Stress can depress your immunity, which is why people who are under pressure a lot of the time tend to experience more infections, such as colds or flu. One study found that women who cared for relatives with Alzheimer's—which can be an emotionally draining full-time job—had weaker immune responses than those who weren't caregivers.

Depression, which can be a major response to stress, is considered a risk factor for cardiovascular disease, particularly in women. A 2009 study involving more than 63,000 women from the long-running Nurses' Health Study found that even relatively healthy women who were severely depressed were more than twice as likely to die of sudden cardiac death and coronary heart disease. A 2010 study based on findings from the Women's Health Study—the largest-ever study of women's health—revealed that women in demanding jobs were up to 56 percent more likely than other working women to have a heart attack or other forms of cardiovascular disease.

WHAT WORKS FOR ME

MARGARET A. CAUDILL-SLOSBERG, MD, PhD, *adjunct associate professor of anesthesiology at Dartmouth Medical School in Manchester, New Hampshire, has just as much stress in her life as the patients she counsels. Here are her tricks for staying calm.*

I teach stress management, so I have the luxury of doing what I teach. I'm always aware of my comfort and happiness levels. If I find myself saying, "I don't want to do this anymore," I listen closely to the cue, examine what needs to be changed, and take care of it.

I also exercise, even though I've never been an exercise enthusiast. In fact, I hated exercise in the past, so I have to do it on my own terms. I tell myself that I only have to put in 10 or 15 minutes on the treadmill every morning. While I exercise, I listen to books on tape or National Public Radio.

Exercise gives me the energy to face stress later in the day. It also helps me distance myself from problems so I can see them objectively, which gives me new perspectives. ■

How does stress hit the heart? Feeling stressed raises blood pressure, which damages the linings of blood vessels. At the same time, substances that are released during times of stress, such as fatty acids, are trapped in the damaged areas of the blood vessels. This leads to the development of plaques, fatty deposits that can block blood flow, increase

Restoring Sleep

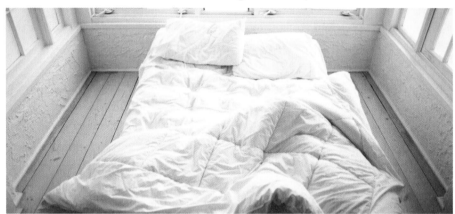

Women are feeling increasingly stressed-out—and they are losing sleep over it.

In a sleep census poll of more than 1,000 Americans, 62 percent said they had a hard time sleeping, and more women than men reported symptoms of insomnia. Americans as a whole lose almost 5 hours of sleep a week because of sleep deprivation. Do that every week, and you'll lose 260 hours by the end of the year—more than a week and a half.

What's behind all this tossing and turning? Stress tops the list.

When you're stressed, your muscles are tense, you have high levels of stress hormones that arouse instead of relax the body, and your mind is full of troubling thoughts.

You might think you can get away with less sleep, but getting fewer than 7 or 8 hours of sleep a night affects your concentration, judgment, reaction time, memory, and physical performance.

Here are a few ways to ensure you get the sleep you need.

Establish relaxation rituals. Every night, take a warm bath. Or read a magazine or watch TV. Everyone should do something relaxing before going to bed. If you do this every night, your body will naturally start preparing for sleep.

Avoid stimulants. The caffeine in coffee, chocolate, soda, tea, diet drugs, and some pain relievers may keep you awake. If you smoke, the nicotine in cigarettes can lead to early-morning awakenings because the body is demanding the next "hit." Now might be a good time to quit smoking. You'll get better sleep if you do.

Stick to your workouts. People who exercise sleep better. But to avoid being too pumped up at bedtime, finish exercising 5 to 6 hours before then. ■

the risk of clots, and possibly lead to heart attacks.

Fat also heads to your middle during times of stress. The stress hormone cortisol, produced by the adrenal glands, tells the body to deposit fat around your waist. Having an apple shape is more closely linked to heart disease and other conditions than having a pear shape, with fat around the hips and thighs. Studies have also found that women in particular tend to eat during times of stress, which also contributes to unhealthy weight gain, a risk factor for diabetes, heart disease, and some cancers. A 2010 report on women's health found that obesity among women had risen more than a percentage point since 2007, as had the incidence of diabetes and hypertension, two consequences of both obesity and stress. Researchers have identified dozens of physical symptoms that are associated with stress overload. They include:

- Fatigue
- Frequent headaches or migraines
- Frequent colds or flu
- Asthma or wheezing
- Poor sleep
- Muscle tension and aches
- Nausea
- Reduced sex drive
- Hair loss
- Eating too little or too much

Apart from physical changes, constant stress also affects the emotions. You might notice frequent feelings of:

- Anxiety
- Sadness
- Frustration
- Irritability
- Anger

No matter how much stress you experience, and regardless of the physical or emotional tolls you're currently paying, you can do something about it. Once you identify the causes of stresses in your life and recognize the danger signs, you can start taking steps to reduce them with this six-step action plan.

Step 1: Identify Your Boiling Point

Why do some women get frazzled and irritated when they're stuck in traffic, while others stay cool even during catastrophes? Two things make the difference: the amount of control that you feel you have over your life, and your basic personality.

If you're responsible for the care of your ill mother, on top of being a mom and a full-time employee, you'll understandably be stressed. A lot of things are happening in your life, and you really can't control the outcome.

"Think of Supreme Court justices," says Deborah Belle, EdD, professor of psychology at Boston University and author of *Lives in Stress: Women and Depression.* "They have what seem to be extremely stressful jobs, they have a heavy workload, and they make extremely important decisions."

But they seem to live forever. Why?

"I think it's because they have the best law clerks in the country working for them, they can choose which cases to hear, they have the esteem and admiration of many people, and they can take lavish vacations to recuperate," Dr. Belle says. "On the other hand, their secretaries have a heavy workload without much control. They're probably under much higher levels of stress."

Then there's personality. Women with hostile, type A personalities—they snap at restaurant waiters for making mistakes, tailgate cars on the highway, and blow up at coworkers—have a higher risk of cardiovascular disease resulting from stress. In a study at the University of Pittsburgh, of 276 healthy men and women, those who were less agreeable had higher blood pressures and levels of stress hormones than those who were calmer and more easygoing.

Other personality types, too, are vulnerable to health damage. In the same study, people who were introverted also tended to have high blood pressure and elevated levels of stress hormones.

Many women share a personality trait that may increase their risk for depression: rumination. Women who are introspective and passive and tend to dwell on their problems—which often makes problems seem worse than they really are—generally experience depression and unnecessary levels of stress.

"All of the complexities that make people human affect the stress response," Dr. Caudill-Slosberg says.

Does that mean you're stuck with your personal and perhaps genetic stress response? Not if you learn resilience, the ability to rebound from whatever life tosses your way. Some people are naturally resilient, but it's a trait you can learn by adopting a few important strategies.

Identify and play to your strengths. Give yourself credit for all the times you triumphed over adversity (or, at least, just got through tough times). Do what you can in any given situation. "Resilient people focus on what they can influence and they don't spend time on what they can't," says Robert Brooks, PhD, assistant clinical professor of psychology at Harvard Medical School and coauthor of *The Power of Resilience.*

Accentuate the positive. A vast body of research in the field of positive psychology has found that people who keep their sunny side up—no matter what's going on in their lives—are happier and healthier and even more successful than those who approach life with negativity. How do you turn that frown upside down? One way is to keep a log of all the things that have gone right for you every day. One study found that people who did that had a better attitude and were happier than people who didn't. By listing all the good things that happened—even on a bad day—"You're training yourself to reverse your focus from what you did wrong to what you did right," says Carol Kauffman, PhD, assistant clinical professor of psychology at Harvard Medical School. Making a point to express gratitude—to the guy who held the door for you, the motorist who waved you across the intersection, the third grade teacher who made you feel special—is another upper. "Gratitude is an affirmation of the goodness in one's life and the recognition that the sources of this goodness lie at least partly outside the self," says Robert A. Emmons, PhD, professor of psychology at the University of California Davis. "It's a very social experience, and it's restorative in times of stress."

Do good. Helping others gives us as sense of mastery over life. If you have the ability to help, then you're likely to think of yourself as strong rather than vulnerable. There's another benefit to tending to others. Landmark studies by UCLA neuroscientist Shelley Taylor have found that in times of stress, women respond differently than men. Instead of poising ourselves to fight or flee, we "tend and befriend." This nurturing response involves different body chemicals than fight–or–flight: endorphins, which the body secretes to relieve pain, and oxytocin, a female reproductive hormone that promotes bonding. There's nothing better to help us get through a stressful time than love and people who support us—and women come by that naturally.

Step 2: **Recognize the Triggers**

Sometimes the source of stress is obvious: Driving behind a school bus or garbage truck that makes several stops en route is making you late for work, for example. Other times, it's not always clear if you're freaked out by being late, or if it's your job, problems with the kids, financial worries, or all of the above.

You can't begin to control stress if you're not sure what's behind it. At the first sign that something's wrong, try to get to the bottom of it. One way to do that is by keeping a journal.

Sit down for a few minutes every day to write about issues that concern you. Stressing out because you have to stand in line at the grocery store is probably just a symptom of what's really bothering you says Dr. Caudill-Slosberg. You may be on overload—too much to do and too little time—and waiting a few extra minutes is just the last straw. At that point, you can start problem solving. Make a list of some of your options: getting household help, researching a new job, talking to a counselor, and so on.

Once you can identify your stress triggers and consider solutions, you'll feel a sense of control you didn't have before, and that's one of the best ways to combat stress, says Dr. Caudill-Slosberg.

It's not uncommon for women to feel so tired and burned out that they can't begin to muster the energy that's required for problem solving, she says. In fact, stress actually interferes with your ability to come up with solutions. At that point, it makes sense to see a therapist right away. You'll learn more about yourself and also discover practical ways to bring additional calm to your life.

Step 3: **Practice the "Calm Response"**

We've already talked about the physical changes that accompany stress. Even though these changes are a necessary part of survival, they can make life really uncomfortable a lot of the time.

Here are a few ways to control the symptoms of stress and bring additional calm into your life.

Breathe deeply. Try to make a fist while taking a deep breath. You probably can't maintain the tension for very long because breathing naturally eases tension, Dr. Caudill-Slosberg says. It's common, however, for people to breathe shallowly when they're experiencing stress, which can make them feel even more stressed out.

Studies have found that deep breathing—pranayama breathing, as it's known in yoga and meditation—flicks a switch in the body that moves breath control from the sympathetic nervous system, which orchestrates arousal, to the parasympathetic system, which calms you down. Bonus: Deep yoga breathing has been linked to increased immunity (something stress can depress) and control of hypertension, asthma, and stress-related disorders, including tension headaches and back pain.

To help you remember to breathe deeply, place some reminders around the house, office, and in your car. Write "Take a deep breath" on sticky notes and put them where you can see them. Every time you see one of these cues, take a moment to drop your shoulders, breathe deeply, and let go of some of the tension, Dr. Caudill-Slosberg advises.

Go to Maui—in 30 seconds. Warm sand beneath your bare feet. A cool breeze against your face. The sound of a crashing ocean in your ears. Your body tenses at the perception of stress, so calm it down by thinking of something serene. Keep a favorite vacation photo on your desk or use a calming image as your computer screensaver so you can let it take you away in times of angst.

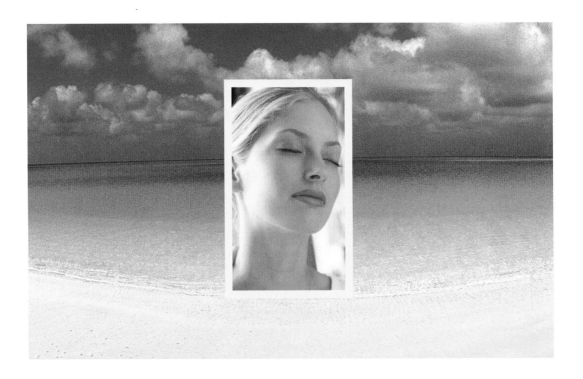

Bend with stress. When life's pressures are getting to you, put your imagination to work. Imagine that you're a strong oak tree. The trunk of the tree is your inner core, and no amount of wind will affect it. "But your branches bend for you," says Pamela Peeke, MD, assistant clinical professor of medicine at the University of Maryland School of Medicine in Baltimore and author of *Fight Fat after Forty*. When you're faced with a traffic jam, for example, tell yourself that your core is strong and sustainable. You don't have to get upset about it.

Get some sun. Even if you don't think you have the time, get outside for a few minutes. Exposure to sunlight increases levels of serotonin, a natural brain chemical that reduces stress and imparts feelings of calm and well-being.

Take mini-breaks. If you let your mind rest for at least 5 minutes every hour, you'll find it easier to stay calm and focused. Close your eyes and think peaceful thoughts, or stand up and stretch. Better yet, walk briskly for a few moments: It stimulates the release of endorphins, body chemicals that neutralize stress hormones

Distract yourself. Filling your free time with activities you love will help keep your mind off the stress of tomorrow. "Humans are wonderful at distracting themselves," Dr. Belle says. "And we need to feed our souls this way."

Find the off switch. Your BlackBerry or iPhone shouldn't be an extension of your arm, says Helen L. Coons, PhD, clinical associate professor of psychiatry at Drexel University College of Medicine. "Make a point of not looking at your e-mail or texting all night when you come home from work," she says. "Learn to put

work away." Create a no-work zone during your evening commute, a barrier that reminds you that work is done and home is about to start. Listen to soothing music in the car or a relaxation tape on the bus or train, she suggests.

Turn drama into comedy. When you find yourself believing that a bump in the road is a true catastrophe, take a new perspective. Your roof sprang a leak and the car transmission blew up on the same day? Instead of blowing your lid, laugh at the irony.

"Turn life into a comedy instead of a drama," say Loretta LaRoche, an international stress management consultant in Plymouth, Massachusetts, and author of the audiocassette *Life Is Not a Stress Rehearsal*.

Studies have found that laughter can actually reduce your body's production of cortisol, a stress hormone that suppresses your immune system.

Have regular meals. Make sure you always eat breakfast and don't let work keep you from getting lunch, says Dr. Coons. "Plan a 4 p.m. healthy snack so your blood sugar stays stable." Blood sugar spikes can leave you fatigued and irritable and less able to cope with stress.

Go a little Zen. Countless studies have confirmed the benefit of meditation to relieve stress. One way it works is to help you find a core of calm inside you that you can retreat to when there's chaos around you. With meditation, you actually build up a tolerance for stress, a boon if you're temperamentally vulnerable. Experienced Zen meditators literally tune out the chaos. In fact, a recent study found that "tuning out" can actually help you reduce your sensitivity to both physical pain and emotional pain. You don't have to take a course, but it helps. Simply find a quiet place once or twice a day, close your eyes, and pay attention to your breath as you inhale and exhale, calmly pushing your thoughts away. You won't find inner peace right away, but you'll get better with practice.

Step 4: Accept What You Can't Change

Stress is never going to go away. Women have to accept that. But remember, stress isn't the issue—how you react to it is. Here are a few ways to unwind, no matter what life throws at you.

Go with the flow. Some types of problems that give you stress defy solution. Breathing or taking a mental vacation might help, but nothing will take away the heartache of watching a relative become ill, or the grief over the death of a parent. You need to get comfortable with those feelings, not try to force them away.

"Stay in touch with the complexity of the situation, and do your best to heighten the quality of the days you have," Dr. Belle says.

This is the kind of stressor that mindfulness meditation targets best. While you're usually inclined to try to avoid the full experience of this kind of trouble in your life, with mindfulness you learn to tune into it without being overwhelmed by it. In mindfulness, you focus on your breath as you inhale and exhale, gently ushering out the thousands of thoughts you have without being judgmental. You can also focus on various parts of your body, how tense you are, and relax muscle by muscle. In "loving-kindness" meditation you focus on wishing yourself peace, happiness, and health, then expand that to others. Studies have found that loving-kindness meditation can increase social connectedness—a feeling of positivity and closeness toward others, even strangers, which is linked to better mental and physical health.

Be imperfect—and calmer. When you try to achieve the unachievable—as so many women tend to do—you'll feel frustrated, anxious, or depressed. So concentrate on your strengths, instead of obsessing over your flaws. The second a negative thought enters your mind, replace it with "I'm doing the best I can" or "I'm fine and happy and fulfilled."

Acknowledge your mistakes and move on. Because so many people depend on them, women often feel as though they have to make the right decisions every time. It doesn't work that way, of course. Everyone makes mistakes, and the worst thing you can do is berate yourself and dwell on them. In studies, rumination—dwelling on the negative—is associated with depression, particularly in women, and impairs your ability to solve problems creatively.

Here's a better approach: Remind yourself that within every mistake is an opportunity for growth and renewal. You can't change what's already happened, but you can take the lessons you learned and apply them to the next challenge that comes along.

Step 5: Stay Socially Engaged

One thing women do well is bond with other women. As Shelley Taylor's research suggests, women may be hardwired to "tend and befriend," to protect themselves and their children by building a social network that they can rely on for help. The chemicals we release are the ones associated with bonding and breastfeeding, which allow us to feel calm and centered

"We're social creatures," Dr. Belle says. "We're healthiest and happiest when we're part of a supportive group."

Talking to friends about what's bothering you might help you see things in a different light. It also helps to get reassurance from friends that you're still loved and supported, despite how crummy you feel, Dr. Belle says.

If things are really bad, schedule a girlfriend getaway. You don't have to go far–maybe just to the bowling alley or the corner coffee shop.

Step 6: Practice a Lower-Stress Life

If you establish certain habits every day, even when you're not under stress, you'll naturally be a little calmer when things do get crazy.

Exercise regularly. It's one of the best ways to reduce anxiety, tension, apprehension, depression, and fatigue. Study after study has shown that moderate exercise reduces cortisol, the stress hormone that triggers the runaway stress response.

You don't have to be an athlete to get the benefits of exercise. Walk in the morning and again in the evening. Go to the health club three or four times a week. Spend some time weeding the garden or raking leaves. Any kind of physical activity releases "feel-good" endorphins, which will help you feel calmer and more relaxed.

reality *check* She Discovered Calm in a Life of Chaos

Amy Mitrani of Miami has worked in a notoriously stressful job for years: sales. The phone is always ringing off the hook. Clients are difficult. And the pressure to be "on" all the time takes a toll. Mitrani, who's in her thirties, admits that her stress levels rose out of control.

She didn't want to change careers, but Mitrani knew that she had to bring some calm to her life. So she started taking yoga classes. At the same time, she began keeping a journal, and every morning she repeated this affirmation to herself: "I live in harmony and balance."

They were simple strategies, but they completely changed how Mitrani handled stress. In the past, for example, she would lose confidence when she failed to get a sale. Today she doesn't let it bother her. Her trick, she says, is like "changing the channel on a TV."

When negative thoughts start coming into her mind, she quickly replaces them with positive ones. Sometimes, for example, she'll find she is attacking herself for what she could have done better. Now she turns things around by thinking of what she did that was positive and what she has learned for her next prospect.

Mitrani has more confidence than ever before. She's happier, and she says her newfound calm has made her more successful on the job. ■

Have a plan B. Preparing backup plans is a great way to increase control over your life. Suppose you have to drive your daughter to soccer practice after work, but you always worry that you'll get stuck in traffic. Make plans with one of the parents to share driving responsibilities in a pinch. You'll worry less because you'll know that everything is covered "just in case."

Get involved in your church or temple. In one study by the California Department of Health Services, researchers looked at more than 2,600 people over 30 years. They found that those who attended religious services regularly were less likely to suffer from depression. They also engaged in activities that naturally reduce stress, such as attending social gatherings and staying physically active.

Get a pet. Many studies have shown that having a dog, cat, or other pet reduces stress. Pet owners even have lower cholesterol and blood pressure than those without pets. But if you don't like animals or can't face another responsibility, skip this. You don't want to add another stressor to your life.

Put pleasure on your schedule. You can't be a great mother, wife, or friend if you're burned out and exhausted. So think about what you can do for yourself. Do you want to read the paper on Sunday mornings? Enjoy a long bath in the evenings? Put it on your schedule—actually write it down. It will make you much more likely to actually keep the "appointment."

Keep healthy finances. Debt—credit card bills in particular—may be linked to high blood pressure, insomnia, and other physical prob-

lems. When researchers surveyed more than 1,000 people, they found that those with higher credit card debts were more stressed and had the most health complaints. Get your finances in order now, and you'll enjoy better health.

Get regular massages. One study found that several weeks of massage therapy could reduce levels of the stress hormone cortisol by nearly a third on average and triggered the production of feel-good chemicals dopamine and serotonin.

Keep a low-maintenance house. Dirt won't stress you out if you can't see it. Buy rugs, couches, and chairs in earth tones, which hide stains. Choose easy-to-clean wood or linoleum floors. Put washable gloss or semigloss paint on the walls—they'll be easier to wipe down. And buy low-care plants and shrubbery: Less work in the yard means more time for the things that are important to you.

Spend some time at the playground. If you have young children, head to the playground or join a playgroup to give you some adult time. You might also consider babysitting for other mothers so everyone gets a break. Women without children often find that it's a real kick to spend time with nieces, nephews, or grandchildren. It's hard to take life too seriously when you're making up rhymes, talking in a silly voice, or pushing a swing. It's a great distraction from life's stress.

Cherish life. A warm breeze in the summer. The beauty of nature. The rush you feel as you ride your bike. If you believe you deserve pleasure from life, you'll be much more likely to achieve all the things that you need to be happy.

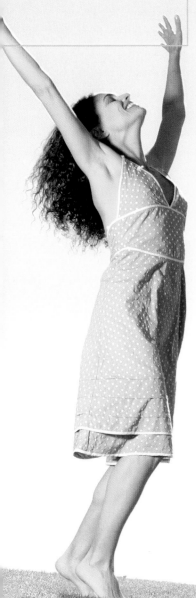

A Quit-Smoking Program That Can't Fail

After 27 years of smoking cigarettes, Susannah Hayward crushed her last butt. Once she got over the withdrawal symptoms, she felt reborn.

"Everything smells and tastes better, my skin is pink and healthy, I can run without wheezing, and I have more energy overall," Hayward says. "I'm also more relaxed. I don't feel agitated anymore in a nonsmoking environment."

The best part for Hayward? Higher self-esteem.

"If I can give up smoking, I can do anything," she says. And she did. She wrote a book about quitting smoking, called *Breathe Easy*.

Despite the fact that tobacco use is the single most preventable cause of disease in the world, as many as 18 percent of the women in the United States light up regularly. Smoking is directly responsible for 80 percent of all lung cancer deaths in women in the United States; in 1987, lung cancer surpassed breast cancer as the leading cause of cancer death in the United States. Smoking also can cause heart disease, stroke, and cancer of the larynx, mouth, bladder, cervix, pancreas, and kidneys. Women who smoke have weaker bones and more wrinkled skin. Smoking increases the risk of infertility, preterm delivery, having a low-birth-weight baby, and sudden infant death syndrome (leading causes of infant mortality).

Scary? Unfortunately, if scare tactics worked, no one would smoke. The fact is, nicotine is just as addictive as heroin, 10 times more potent than cocaine, and 1,000 times more powerful than alcohol. No wonder it's so hard to quit.

But it's never too late. Successfully quitting almost erases the damage of moderate cigarette smoking, especially if you quit before age 35—which is when ailments, such as bronchitis, emphysema, periodontal disease, and circulatory disorders, first start appearing in cigarette smokers. The positive changes happen almost immediately. Within 24 hours of stopping, your blood vessels start to recover. After a year, your risk of heart attack goes down by 50 percent. And within 15 years, your risk of heart disease is about that of a lifelong nonsmoker. Quitting may even extend your life; smokers tend to die 7 years earlier than nonsmokers.

Why Smokers Smoke

Seven to 10 seconds after you inhale the 4,000 or so chemicals found in tobacco smoke, one, nicotine, releases super-normal amounts of norepinephrine and dopamine, brain chemicals that give you pleasure. You'll feel more satisfaction than you do from laughing, watching the sun set, or drinking cool water on a warm day, says Linda Hyder Ferry, MD, MPH, associate professor of preventive and family medicine at Loma Linda University in California and the originator of the first FDA-approved treatment for smoking cessation using the antidepressant bupropion (Zyban).

But after a while, your body depends on nicotine for the release of these chemicals, and it takes more nicotine to feel the same amount of pleasure, says Dr. Hyder Ferry. But on their way to your brain, the components of tobacco smoke also:

- Narrow your arteries, some of which are no bigger than a pencil lead, and allow less blood

If you smoke 15 to 30 cigarettes a day, your skin can't repair itself from exposure to the sun's ultraviolet rays. Some doctors say they can tell whether or not a woman smokes just by looking at her face.

flow to your heart. That constriction causes blood to move faster, which traumatizes the lining of vessels.

- Rob your heart and blood vessels of oxygen hours or days after you smoke because of the effect of carbon monoxide's attaching to hemoglobin cells, which transport oxygen.

- Lower HDL ("good") cholesterol levels while raising LDL ("bad") cholesterol, which leads to a buildup of plaque and lipids in already damaged arteries.

- Trigger an irregular heart rhythm or heart attack if the heart becomes completely starved of oxygen.

- Interfere with bone rebuilding, contributing to osteoporosis.

- Damage the tiny air sacs in lungs, reducing oxygen exchange.

The effects are immediate. It's hard to breathe, let alone exercise. If you keep it up for 15 or 20 years, you'll lose 40 to 50 percent of your lung function, called chronic obstructive pulmonary disease, and may become short of breath when taking a shower or walking to your car.

Smoking a pack a day also causes 5 to 10 percent bone loss by menopause, a significant loss considering smokers reach menopause up to 4 years earlier than women who don't smoke.

If you're a smoker with a pack-and-a-half-a-day habit (about 30 cigarettes), you're getting roughly 300 nicotine hits to your brain a day. It's easy to see how quickly you can become addicted. A few hours after you crush out your

Prevent Bronchitis and Emphysema

If you smoke and you've had a persistent cough for more than 2 years, don't dismiss it as nothing more than "smoker's cough." A consistent cough with mucus could be chronic bronchitis.

While nonsmokers can and do get bronchitis, smoking is by far the most common way to get bronchitis because smoke causes the bronchi to become inflamed and interferes with airflow. But it's also possible to get it from a bacterial or viral infection, air pollution, or industrial dusts and fumes. Bronchitis may lead to or accompany emphysema.

By all means, if you have bronchitis and you smoke, quit. Exercise may also indirectly help by strengthening the heart and body, but because exercise could make breathing even harder, consult your physician before beginning a new exercise program, recommends Linda Hyder Ferry, MD, associate professor of preventive and family medicine at Loma Linda University in California.

Like bronchitis, emphysema is accompanied by cough and shortness of breath. If the diseases occur together, they're called chronic obstructive pulmonary disease. And as with bronchitis, smoking is the biggest cause of emphysema. Cigarette smoke damages the air sacs in the lungs so that they have trouble transferring oxygen to the blood. You'll probably notice you can't exercise as well. Even a brief walk could make you lose your breath. Quitting smoking can halt emphysema's progression in its tracks. ■

stub, you'll start having cravings for that plea-sure blast. If you don't have a cigarette, you may have withdrawal symptoms—irritability, anxiety, depression, attention problems, cravings and increased appetite. But half of addiction may depend on your genes. A recent study found that having a variant in a gene that affects nicotinic receptors more than doubles addiction risk among smokers and makes them more vulnera-ble to lung cancer and arterial damage.

Women Take the Biggest Hit

The more than 21 million American women who smoke experience more wheezing, cough-ing, breathlessness, and asthma than men who smoke, even if they light up less often, says Jill Siegfried, PhD, chair of lung cancer research in the department of pharmacology and chemical biology at the University of Pittsburgh. Among

men, death from lung cancer is decreasing; for women, rates doubled between 1975 and 2007.

Researchers don't know exactly why damage is more severe in women, but estrogen may play a role. Researchers think estrogen releases chemicals in the lungs that cause cells to divide. That in turn thickens the airways and stimu-lates cells with mutations to form tumors, says Dr. Siegfried. Estrogen may also help convert chemicals in cigarette smoke to carcinogens.

If you quit now, in the years to come you will erase almost all that damage. Your skin will look better and you'll breathe easier. Your risk of can-cer will go down, and after 4 years your heart attack risk will dwindle to that of a never smoker, says Dr. Hyder Ferry. When it comes to lung cancer, however, you'll always have higher risk than never smokers. But risk will decrease every year to nearly a nonsmoker's level of risk.

If you've tried to quit before and couldn't,

reality *check* Once She Quit, She Could Laugh Again

Judy Lin-Eftekhar, a writer and editor in Santa Monica, California, started smoking at 19 to look cool, avoid eating, and feel less anxious. But after 15 years, smoking almost two packs a day made it hard for her to breathe. Then one morning she woke up with the flu, and the thought of lighting a cigarette made her feel even sicker. She knew this was her chance to quit forever, so she did.

Judy made a list of reasons to quit—"to be healthy again" and "so my clothes don't stink"—

and taped them to her refrigerator. She imag-ined herself as a happy nonsmoker and exercised every day. She also felt a spiritual awakening and let a higher power guide her.

She realized that she had used ciga-rettes to suppress negative feelings toward her job and relationship. But instead of going back to smoking, she found a new job and broke off her relationship.

Soon Judy felt like a new person. Now she breathes deeper. Her skin looks more vibrant. She's thinner from exercise. And without a cigarette to puff, she laughs more often. ■

you're not beat yet. On average, it takes five or six tries to quit for good. Today, smokers have more options to quit than ever before. If one strategy didn't work for you in the past, another will. Here's a step-by-step action plan from experts who have studied smoking habits of women.

Step 1: Get Screened for Depression

Researchers estimate that one-fourth to one-third of all smokers experience anxiety or depression. They may be self-medicating with cigarettes. Since women are twice as likely as men to experience depression, they're more likely to fall into this group of smokers, claims Dr. Hyder Ferry.

"I screen all my female patients for depression and anxiety before they quit smoking, and I ask them how they are feeling after they quit so they can get treated if they have mood changes," she says. (For more on the symptoms of depression, see page 374.)

Step 2: Set a Quit Date

Commit to a quit date that falls sometime in the next 7 to 10 days, and get rid of all your cigarettes and ashtrays by then.

"Like anything, if you don't plan exactly when you're going to do it, it doesn't get done," says Kenneth Perkins, PhD, professor of psychiatry, at the University of Pittsburgh School of Medicine and author of *Cognitive-Behavioral Therapy for Smoking Cessation*.

The worst time to quit is during the second half of your menstrual cycle because PMS could make withdrawal worse. In one study, women who quit in the first 2 weeks after their period and attended group sessions experienced less severe withdrawal symptoms than women who quit later in their cycle.

Do whatever it takes to quit successfully. Studies show that women are less likely to try to quit and more likely to relapse partly due to the fear of weight gain (usually around 5 to 10 pounds) but possibly also because withdrawal may be more intense. Don't think you have to "man up"–choose a way that makes it easiest for you.

Step 3: Choose Your Weapon

Going "cold turkey" is the least effective way to quit–only about 2 to 5 percent of smokers can do so. Most others need help of some kind. If one method doesn't work, try another, recommends Dr. Hyder Ferry. Here are your options.

Consider nicotine replacement therapy. Although it's less effective in women than in men, nicotine replacement therapy provides enough nicotine to keep you from going into withdrawal while you break the habit of reaching for a cigarette–which takes about 5 to 10 weeks, says Dr. Hyder Ferry. Nicotine replacement therapy is available over the counter in the form of the patch (which could cause a mild skin rash) or gum. Prescription versions include an inhaler and a nasal spray. It can even be used during pregnancy, but talk to your ob/gyn before using anything.

If you tried nicotine replacement therapy before and felt miserable, you probably didn't use a high enough dose of nicotine or you stopped using it too soon, Dr. Hyder Ferry says.

For best results, talk to your doctor about which therapy and dose is best for you.

Ask your doctor about bupropion. Like nicotine, the prescription compound bupropion (Zyban) is used as an antidepressant and stabilizes the levels of norepinephrine and dopamine, two brain chemicals responsible for feelings of well-being. But while nicotine causes the chemicals to spike and then fall, bupropion releases a smaller, steady stream without causing any addiction. That means withdrawal symptoms won't bother you as much.

A 2004 study found that buproprion was highly effective in women, especially when combined with behavioral counseling. Another study found that when 4,000 people took bupropion with or without nicotine replacement therapy and had professional counseling, 40 to 60 percent of them remained smoke-free for at least a year. Consider signing up for some weight counseling too. University of Pittsburgh Medical Center researchers found that when women took buproprion and participated in a cognitive behavioral therapy program focused on weight gain issues, they were more likely to quit and avoid a relapse than women who had the same counseling but didn't take the drug.

Phase out cigarettes. Gradually decrease the number of cigarettes you smoke until you're down to 5 to 10 a day—just enough to keep from going into withdrawal. Then quit completely.

For instance, if you smoke a pack of cigarettes a day, allow yourself to smoke only half of each cigarette for a week. The next week, throw three cigarettes out before you start the pack. Continue to reduce at this pace for 4 to 6 weeks before you quit completely.

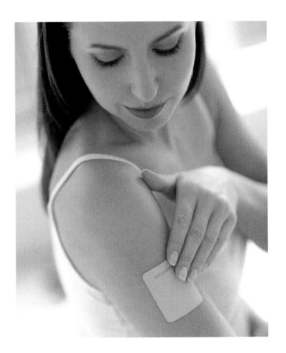

Try hypnosis. Through hypnosis, you might increase your motivation, lower your cravings, and keep from lighting up. A study done at North Shore Medical Center in Salem, Massachusetts, found that patients hospitalized with cardiopulmonary problems were more likely to be nonsmokers 6 months later after only one hypnotherapy session than patients who used nicotine replacement therapy or who went cold turkey. To request referrals for hypnotherapists, send a self-addressed, stamped envelope to the American Society of Clinical Hypnosis at 130 East Elm Court, Suite 201, Roselle, IL 60172.

Look into acupuncture. This ancient Chinese health practice involves puncturing the skin with hair-thin needles at particular locations—usually the ear for nicotine addiction. Although there's little research that proves acupuncture works, some women who try it may experience milder withdrawal symptoms. To find a certified acupuncturist in your area, call the American Association of Acupuncture and Oriental Medicine at (888) 500-7999.

Step 4: Increase Exercise

The average smoker weighs 6 to 11 pounds less than a nonsmoker but gains roughly that amount of weight after quitting. Ten to 15 percent of women who quit gain more than 28 pounds. That's because nicotine curbs hunger, decreasing between-meal snacking. The elimination of nicotine reverses the weight-suppressing effect, causing women to eat more after quitting.

Research shows it's just too hard to diet and quit smoking, but you can exercise. Women who smoked 10 or more cigarettes a day and joined a smoking cessation program that involved weekly behavior modification sessions and about 50 minutes of exercise three times a week gained less weight and were more likely to stay smoke-free than women who didn't exercise.

Even if you do gain weight, you'd have to put on more than 100 pounds to cancel out the benefits to health of quitting, says Dr. Perkins.

Step 5: Quash Cravings

If you eat more to make up for not smoking, your weight will be harder to control. Here's how to deal with those cigarette cravings during and after therapy.

Change your routine. Cues can make you want a cigarette all day long, and women may be more susceptible than men. The most common cues are the smell of cigarette smoke and drinking coffee. But there are other situations that you may not think about, such as talking on the phone, opening a beer, or unwinding after work. The solution: Change your routine to miss the urge. Drink tea instead of coffee, take public transportation to work if you have access, and visit a nonsmoking friend instead of talking on the phone. Go for a walk when you feel a craving coming on, and keep hard candy, sugarless gum, and lollipops handy. If possible, take a vacation from work the week you quit.

Avoid bars and alcohol. Until you've learned to cope with the craving-inducing sights and smells and the easy availability of cigarettes, stay away from bars and alcohol. Whenever possible, avoid people who smoke. A recent study found that 25 percent of quitters took up

THREE THINGS I TELL EVERY FEMALE PATIENT

LINDA HYDER FERRY, MD, *associate professor of preventive and family medicine at Loma Linda University in California, says, "Quitting smoking was your first step to minimize aging and slow down the skin wrinkling process."*

Here are some other strategies that she emphasizes.

1 Eat a diet high in natural antioxidants, which you'll get from fruits and vegetables.

2 Use a mild cleanser that exfoliates your skin.

3 Wear a UVB/UVA spectrum sunscreen with an SPF of at least 15 every day. ∎

cigarettes again when they spent time with other smokers.

Breathe deeply. When you get the urge to smoke, take deep breaths to help you relax.

Give yourself a 2-minute massage. A study at the University of Miami found that a 2-minute hand or ear massage cut cravings, reduced anxiety, and improved mood. Try these.

- Pinch your ear from the top down to your earlobe.

- Gently tug your earlobe.

- Use your thumb to massage the palm of your hand in a circular motion.

Step 6: Join a Support Group

Researchers found that people were more successful when they went to group programs offering behavior techniques and mutual support than when they quit with little or no help. Maybe that's because just when you think you can't go another day without smoking, your group knows exactly how you feel. Quality of sessions varies, so if you don't like one, try others.

Step 7: Prepare for Withdrawal

Withdrawal symptoms vary from person to person, depending on how much you smoke and your method of quitting, says Dr. Hyder Ferry. Knowing what to expect will help you get through it. Here's a day-to-day guide.

Days 1 and 2. Physically, you'll feel a unique combination of withdrawal symptoms. You might have a headache, increased irritability, or anxiety, and you'll feel uncomfortable. You might also have trouble sleeping at night and concentrating during the day.

Days 3 through 7. Your withdrawal symptoms peak on day 3 and then stabilize. Many give up at this point, but as soon as you get over this hump, you'll feel better—promise!

Days 8 through 13. Your symptoms may begin to improve.

Days 14 through 365. Physically you feel back to normal. For the first several months, you might crave a cigarette occasionally, and you may have trouble sleeping. But studies show that going cigarette-free for a full year increases your chances of staying that way.

Step 8: Give Yourself a Year of Rewards

Make it easier to get to that year mark. Treat yourself to a new book or theater tickets after the first day, first week, first month of not smoking. Make the reward greater as time goes by.

Not only will your health improve, but your sense of taste and smell will be heightened, you won't have to clean up ashes, your clothes won't smell like smoke, and you'll have more free time In addition to pocketing the cash you would have spent on cigarettes, you'll probably save money on health insurance. Best of all, you won't have to rely on smoking to feel good. And remember: One slip doesn't mean you're a smoker again, so don't quit quitting.

9

Sun-Proof (and Age-Proof) Your Skin

The sun can do a lot of good. It regulates sleep cycles, stimulates the body's production of vitamin D, and enhances feelings of well-being. But there's also a downside: Exposure to sun can lead to wrinkles, age spots, and skin cancer.

In fact, sunshine is considered the single biggest cause of visible aging. But you aren't at the mercy of the sun's damaging rays. Even if you haven't been sun savvy in the past, it's never too late to start protecting your skin, says Darrell S. Rigel, MD, clinical professor of dermatology at New York University School of Medicine in New York City.

For starters, every woman should eat a diet rich in fruits and vegetables. They contain antioxidant compounds that reduce the damaging effects of sunshine. If you smoke, stop. Cigarette smoke contains hundreds of skin-damaging free radicals that affect not only your face but, according to a 2007 study from the University of Michigan, the skin on your entire body, even the parts you protect from the sun. But the most important thing you can do is shield your skin from the sun. As long as you use sunscreen, take advantage of shade, and wear the right clothing, you can enjoy your favorite outdoor activities without worrying about the damaging rays.

How Sunshine Ages Skin

Every time the sun strikes your skin, the skin produces pigment called melanin that scatters and absorbs the rays. The resulting tan may look great to you, but it means your skin is defending itself from harmful radiation.

But a tan can do only so much. Over time, the ultraviolet A (UVA) and ultraviolet B (UVB) radiation in sunshine can weaken the lower layer of skin, known as the dermis, and promote wrinkles, brown spots, and the development of skin cancer.

One in five Americans will develop skin cancer over the course of a lifetime. That means that as many as 50 percent of all Americans who reach the age of 65 will have skin cancer at least once. The most common (and least aggressive) form of skin cancer is basal cell carcinoma. About 2.8 million basal cells cancers are diagnosed every year. This skin cancer begins in the top layer of skin, the epidermis, and generally doesn't spread any further. While another form—squamous cell carcinoma—often remains at its original site, it is more likely spread to

Treat Psoriasis with Sun—Safely

most people are advised to avoid the sun, but doctors have found that sunshine is among the best treatments for psoriasis, a skin condition that results in itchy red patches or silvery scales on the face, elbows, knees, and other parts of the body. The sun's ultraviolet rays kill T cells, which are a type of white blood cell that triggers the unattractive flare-ups.

To get the benefits of ultraviolet light while minimizing the risks, here's what doctors advise.

Cover unaffected areas. Apply sunscreen to areas that aren't affected by psoriasis. Since your face and hands get an abundance of sunshine naturally, wear gloves and put a towel over your face during "light therapy" sessions, suggests Gerald Krueger, MD, professor of dermatology and Benning Presidential Endowed Chair at the University of Utah in Salt Lake City. Light therapy sessions are prescribed by a dermatologist and involve using a tanning bed or a home ultraviolet light system to treat psoriasis.

Stick to the schedule. Some ultraviolet light is helpful, but excessive amounts can needlessly damage the skin. Your dermatologist will prescribe how much light you should be getting. ■

other parts of the body. Both basal cell and squamous cell carcinomas can be cured if detected early, though the surgery to remove them can be disfiguring. However, melanoma—a cancer that starts in the skin's pigment cells and readily spreads to other organs—can be deadly. It causes 75 percent of all deaths from skin cancer, though it too is easily curable if caught early.

How can you protect yourself from the sun's harmful rays? This four-step action plan will make all the difference.

Step 1: Determine Your Risk Profile

There's no way to accurately predict whose skin is most likely to show premature signs of aging or who is more likely to develop skin cancer, says Dee Anna Glaser, MD, professor and vice chairman of the department of dermatology at St. Louis University School of Medicine.

You should schedule a skin exam with your dermatologist at least once a year after the age of 40. If skin cancer runs in your family, you may want to start earlier than that. In addition, it's important to do self-exams once a month. Have someone else check the parts of your body that you can't see. Most skin cancers occur on the face, neck, arms, and trunk, but can also occur on the tops of the ears, the back of the legs, and in places where you get little sun. Signs of trouble include:

- Small pearly white bumps, or sores on the skin that bleed and don't heal.

- Reddish patches or irritated areas that may itch, hurt, or crust.

- Red, scaly bumps that resemble a scar and have a depression in the middle.

- Shiny bumps that are pearly or translucent, and may be white, pink, or brown.

- Dark spots that are asymmetrical, have irregular borders, have more than one color, and are bigger than the size of a pencil eraser. These spots may be flat or elevated.

- Any existing wart or mole that changes in size, shape, color or other trait.

Anyone can get skin cancer, but some people have a much higher risk than others. The risk factors include:

- Fair skin. It doesn't contain as much of the natural pigment called melanin that scatters the sun's rays. People with light eyes and hair may also be at special risk since the three often go together.

- Multiple (50–100 or more) moles or "beauty marks." Melanoma cells are more abundant in moles and freckles. The more beauty marks you have, the greater the risk that cancer cells will be present.

- A history of sunburns. Even if you've had only one blistering sunburn in your life, you have a higher risk for developing skin cancer.

- A tropical address. The ozone layer, which blocks ultraviolet light, is thinner in tropical regions. Ultraviolet radiation is stronger in the southern United States than it is in the north.

- A family history. Heredity plays a role in melanoma in particular. About one in every 20 people diagnosed with the disease has a family member who has also had it.

Step 2: Choose (And Use) the Right Protection

Wearing sunscreen is essential. You should use it every day during every season especially when you're spending time outdoors. To get the most benefits from sunscreen, here's what Dr. Glaser advises.

Choose products with a high SPF (30 or more). It stands for "sun protection factor," and it's a measure of how well sunscreen protects your skin. SPF refers to the length of time that sunscreen protects the skin. Suppose your skin naturally starts to burn in 20 minutes. If you use sunscreen with an SPF of 15, you won't begin to burn for 5 hours–15 times longer.

Apply it often. In real life, sunscreens aren't always as effective as the SPF would indicate, says Dr. Glaser. If you're swimming, sweating a lot, or rubbing your skin with a towel, the sunscreen, even if its label says it's water resistant, is going to dissipate. Reapply it every 2 hours—more often if you're swimming or perspiring a lot, or if you're around water, sand, or snow, which can reflect the sun's UV rays.

Buy a broad-spectrum sunscreen. These help block UVB and UVA rays. UVB light is the primary cause of sunburns, and protecting skin against UVA light plays an important role in preventing wrinkling and signs of aging. Choose a product containing zinc oxide, titanium dioxide, or avobenzone, also known as Parsol 1789.

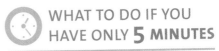

WHAT TO DO IF YOU HAVE ONLY **5 MINUTES**

Use a moisturizer that provides UVA and UVB protection, advises Alan Kling, MD, assistant clinical professor of dermatology at Mount Sinai School of Medicine in New York City. It may not block radiation as completely as regular sunscreen, but it provides good protection, and it's fast and convenient to apply. Most cosmetics companies make facial moisturizers with UVA and UVB protection. Check the label to be sure.

Apply it with your makeup. If you use moisturizers or other skin products in the morning, it's fine to apply sunscreen at the same time. First, apply topical medications if you use them. Let them dry, then apply alpha hydroxy acid or other antiaging creams if you use them. Be sure to follow with a moisturizer, especially if you're using alpha hydroxy acids, which may have a drying effect on the skin. Then apply the sunscreen, followed by any makeup you're going to wear.

Give it time to work. In general, sunscreen is most effective when it's absorbed into the skin. Rub it on about 20 minutes before you go outside, says Dr. Glaser.

Use the right amount. It takes about an ounce of sunscreen to cover the average person's body. That's about the amount that would fill a shot glass. "You should feel messy after putting it on," Dr. Glaser says.

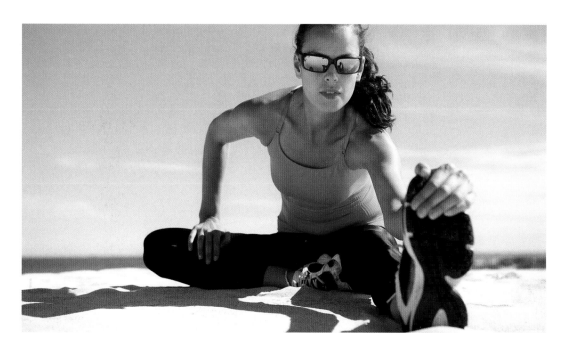

Step 3: **Add Extra Protection**

Wearing sunscreen helps to decrease the incidence of wrinkles and prevent the development of skin cancer. But sunscreen isn't enough by itself. Here are some additional ways to protect the skin.

Always wear shades. Sunglasses protect the delicate skin around the eyes from wrinkles. They also help prevent cataracts and macular degeneration, the leading causes of vision loss in the elderly. Wear shades whenever you go outside, even on hazy days, says Phillip Calenda, MD, an ophthalmologist at the Westchester Medical Practice in Cortlandt Manor, NY.

The best sunglasses block 99 to 100 percent of UVA and UVB rays—look for ones that have labels claiming 100 percent or total UV protection.

WHAT WORKS FOR ME

TOBY SHAWE, MD, *a dermatologist at SkinSmart Dermatology in Glenside, Pennsylvania, knows all too wel l what happens with excessive sun exposure— which is why she's careful to protect her own skin.*

I always use the best sunscreens I can find. I look for sunscreens that contain transparent zinc oxide, like SkinCeuticals Ultimate UV Defense SPF 30, which contains 7 percent transparent zinc oxide.

When I know I'll be spending some time outside, I wear a sunscreen with an SPF of 30. But when I'm going to be inside most of the day, I use a sunscreen with an SPF of 15. ■

WHAT TO DO IF YOU COULD CHANGE **ONLY ONE THING**

Stop associating a tan with beauty and health, says Dee Anna Glaser, MD, professor of dermatology at St. Louis University School of Medicine. It may take time to become accustomed to a paler complexion—but not having a tan means that you're healthier.

Wraparound sunglasses and styles that fit close to the eye are especially good because they prevent the sun's rays from coming in through the sides.

Wear a hat. A tightly woven hat made of canvas, with a 4-inch brim all the way around, helps shade your face, ears, and the back of your neck.

Wear long-sleeve shirts. And wear long pants. They offer the best protection from the sun's burning rays.

Buy clothing with tight-knit weaves. It's best to buy tight-weave clothes, some of which have SPF ratings just like sunscreen. Companies that sell high-SPF clothing include Sun Precautions, Solarveil, and SunGrubbies.com.

Step 4: **Protect Yourself Year-Round**

Sun protection shouldn't stop at the end of summer. Skiing without protecting your skin can be just as damaging as lying on the beach. To protect your skin in all seasons:

Check the UV index. The National Weather Service and the United States Environmental Protection Agency publish information about the daily UV index—the amount of ultraviolet radiation that is expected to reach the earth's surface when the sun is at its highest point. You'll find the index on the weather page of newspapers and on television or radio news. Ultraviolet radiation between zero and 2 is considered minimal and between 3 and 4 is low. It's moderate at 5 to 6, and high at 7 to 9. A UV index rating above 10 is considered to be very high. You should protect yourself from sun damage every day of the week—even if you can't see the sun—but on days the UV index is ultra-high, you may want to avoid prolonged time outdoors.

Avoid midday sun. Whenever possible, stay out of the sun between the hours of 10:00 a.m. and 4:00 p.m., when the rays are strongest.

Stay in the shade. Enjoy the outdoors from underneath a tree or umbrella—and even then, use sunscreen because UV rays bounce around a lot. You can get burned even when you're in the shade.

Forget about tanning booths. For some people, the UVA rays in tanning booths can produce a tan faster than the sun can. That's because the rays are intense—and damaging. But new research has found that indoor tanning increases melanoma risk by 74 percent—and more young women than ever are being diagnosed with this deadliest form of skin cancer. Instead, opt for a "sunless tan," using products that temporarily darken the skin, or sunless tanning booths, which spray on a realistic tan. A recent study found that women who used sunless tanners (and got a primer on skin cancer) were 33 percent less likely to sunbathe.

Beauty Products That Rejuvenate

The next time you browse the cosmetics counter at the pharmacy or department store, take a moment to check out some of the "anti-aging" lotions and potions. You'll be amazed at how many there are. Cosmetics companies have developed hundreds of products for protecting and preserving the skin. A few may even reverse some of the visible signs of aging, such as wrinkles and age spots.

Before reaching for specific skin-care products, you should keep in mind that your skin reflects your life.

If you smoke, bake in the sun for a tan, eat junk food, gain too much weight, or experience a lot of stress, your skin will pay for it. If, on the other hand, you relax often, eat healthful meals, and generally maintain positive lifestyle habits—as outlined in chapters throughout this section—you'll be rewarded with skin that's smooth and firm, even in your later years.

Drinking a lot of water—at least eight glasses daily—is especially important because it helps plump the cells of the skin, making them look smoother and younger, says Kathy A. Fields, MD, clinical instructor of dermatology at the University of California, San Francisco. Equally important to making the skin look plump, she adds, is good humidity in the air around you.

Sunscreen, of course, is essential. It's the only way to prevent future damage because it blocks the sun's ultraviolet radiation. This is important because sun exposure accounts for about 90 percent of all skin cancers. Doctors advise applying sunscreen lavishly after your moisturizer but at least 30 minutes prior to sun exposure and reapplying every 2 hours. Choose products that block both UVA and UVB rays and that have a sun protection factor (SPF) of at least 15. (For more information about sunscreens, see Chapter 9.)

Wearing sunscreen and generally taking care of your health are just the beginning for healthy-looking skin. The skin naturally breaks down over time, especially after menopause, when declines in estrogen cause the skin to lose elasticity. Genetic factors also play a role: If the men and women in your family have a lot of wrin-

kles, you have a higher chance of developing them, too.

This doesn't mean that you're at the mercy of time, however. In the past few years, cosmetics companies have created hundreds of rejuvenating products that really can protect the skin, reverse wrinkles, and generally make you look younger.

Some products have been exhaustively tested and proven to work. Others look good in the bottle, and the labels make them sound effective, but there's little evidence that they make a difference. The only way to know which products to take seriously is to understand a little bit of the science behind them. To make things easy, we've created a quick six-step plan to show you which products to look for and how to use them to get the best results.

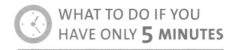

WHAT TO DO IF YOU HAVE ONLY **5 MINUTES**

Rather than experiment with dozens of antiwrinkle products, go straight to Renova, which has been proven to work, says Lisa Kates, MD, a dermatologist at Cook County Hospital and in private practice in Chicago.

Available from dermatologists, Renova is a better moisturizer than Retin-A because it is in an emollient base, and it works just as well at removing fine wrinkles, she says.

Step 1: **Start with a Cleanser**

The skin needs to be clean to be healthy, so it's important to use cleansers to gently wash away dust, makeup, and surface oils.

Use nonsoap cleansers. They're much less drying than regular soaps. David J. Leffell, MD, chief of dermatologic surgery at Yale University School of Medicine and author of *Total Skin*, recommends Neutrogena Extra Gentle Cleanser, Aquanil, or Cetaphil.

Exfoliate after age 40. The skin naturally sheds its top layer, uncovering the fresh, youthful-looking layer underneath. In women under 40, this shedding occurs every 30 days. After age 40, it slows to every 60 days, which dries the skin, enlarges and clogs the pores, and makes the skin dull and sallow. You can, however, speed up the process with a scrub soap.

Scrub soaps contain tiny polyethylene beads, which gently remove dead cells and moisturize the skin. Don't bother with scrub soaps that contain pits from almonds or walnuts, Dr. Fields advises. They can actually damage the skin.

If you're 40 or older, you can use gentle scrub soaps every day, says Dr. Fields. If you're under 40, use them only once a week or as needed.

Always wash at night. "The most important time to wash your face is before you hit the sack," says dermatologist Doris Day, MD, who practices in New York City. Leaving dirt, germs, and makeup can irritate your skin, clog your pores, and even trigger breakouts. If you're over

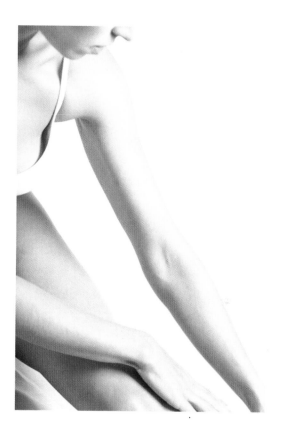

40, don't cleanse in the morning. Oil production declines with your hormones at midlife and twice-daily cleansings can dry out your face and make wrinkles look pronounced. Freshen up in the morning with lukewarm water.

Step 2: **Use a Moisturizer**

Before using any antiaging skin product, it's worth giving moisturizers a try, says Dr. Fields. They add moisture and plumpness to cells on the surface, which makes the skin softer.

Use oil-free products on the face. They contain an ingredient called dimethicone. It's a type of silicone that gives moisturizers a light feel, Dr. Fields says. A good example would be Oil of Olay. Try moisturizers with sunscreen for added protection. You can use oil-containing products on other parts of the body, like elbows, knees, hands, and feet. Look for products containing alpha hydroxy acid for tough areas like feet and elbows.

Keep your moisturizers simple. If you have sensitive skin, avoid moisturizers loaded with fragrances and extracts. Check the label: It should list fewer than 10 ingredients, says Dr. Fields. Cetaphil is a good choice as a moisturizer for sensitive skin, as well as Eucerin and Almay products.

If you still want the luxurious feel of moisturizers made with green tea or other extracts but you aren't sure how your skin will react, test them on a small area on your neck near the ear. Apply the moisturizer a few nights in a row. If you don't have any irritation, redness, or itching, you can use it on your whole face.

Moisturize after showers or baths. The moisturizer will form a barrier over the moisture that's already on your skin, which gives it time to be absorbed by the cells, says Dr. Leffell.

Eat some moisture. Eating olive oil, avocados, nuts, and fish, which contain essential fatty acids, may help protect your skin from UV damage. Since EFAs are also part of the cell membranes that hold in moisture, you'll be replenishing your cell's best protection.

Step 3: Fight Wrinkles Naturally

Many antiaging products claim to "erase" wrinkles and make the skin look years younger. Some of this is marketing hype, but there's good evidence that products that contain natural

THREE THINGS I TELL EVERY FEMALE PATIENT

KATHY A. FIELDS, MD, *is a clinical instructor of dermatology at the University of California San Francisco. She offers women the following advice for achieving fresher and younger-looking skin.*

ALWAYS USE SUNSCREEN. Choose a product that blocks both UVA and UVB light. Don't be afraid to use too much. Apply a thick, even layer 30 minutes before you go outside, and reapply every 2 hours if you are in the sun all day.

1

USE AN EXFOLIANT SCRUB. It's fine to use regular soap on your hands, but for your face, use a gentle scrub. Use it once a week or as needed if you are under 40 and every day if you are over 40. It is safe to use daily and makes your skin glow.

2

USE A MOISTURIZER DAILY. It's among the best ways to keep the skin looking healthy. You may want to buy a moisturizer that contains either alpha hydroxy acids, retinol, or kinetin, which will remove old skin cells and brown spots and hydrate the skin. ∎

3

acids (alpha or beta hydroxy acids from milk, fruit, or sugarcane) really can erase fine lines or brown spots, at least temporarily. They work by exfoliating the superficial layers of skin and can stimulate collagen production, which plumps up the skin and makes it look softer and fresher, says Lisa Kates, MD, a dermatologist at Cook County Hospital and in private practice in Chicago.

Alpha hydroxy acids come in moisturizers, eye creams, and many other products. Terms to look for on labels include glycolic acid (derived from sugarcane), lactic acid (from milk), tartaric acid (from grapes), citric acid (from citrus fruits), malic acid (from apples), and mandelic acid (from walnuts). You may want to look for products that contain salicylic acid, which is a beta hydroxy acid. Be aware that some of these products can be irritating to sensitive skin.

Use a mild product first. Over-the-counter products can have acid concentrations up to 10 percent, while stronger versions, usually available by prescription only, have concentrations up to 30 percent, says Ira Davis, MD, assistant professor of dermatology at New York Medical College in Valhalla. The acids can be irritating, so it's a good idea to start with a low-concentration product, then move up to something stronger if you need to. Be patient. It may take 6 to 8 weeks to see a difference.

Products with alpha or beta hydroxy acids make the skin more sensitive to sunshine because the top layer of skin is thinned, which allows more ultraviolet radiation to penetrate.

The New Wrinkle Fighters

talk to your dermatologist about the latest weapons in the fight against lines and wrinkles.

Botox. Made from purified botulism toxin, it eases fine lines and wrinkles by blocking nerve impulses and temporarily paralyzing the muscles into which it's injected. It's the main treatment for easing forehead frown lines. Each treatment typically lasts 4 to 6 months. Botox is also effective for migraines and other conditions.

Dermal fillers. Injections of fat, collagen, hyaluronic acid (in products such as Restylane and Juvederm), and other materials can fill in fine lines as well as deeper wrinkles or repair acne scars. This minimally invasive procedure, which has little or no recovery time, can restore a youthful fullness to your face and soften facial creases and wrinkles. For that reason they're often called "liquid facelifts." You can use fat from your own body for the injections, though you'll be adding another procedure—liposuction—to the process. But it does eliminate the risk of rejection or allergic reaction. A PMMA (polymethylmethacrylate) filler is composed of tiny microspheres suspended in purified collagen gel and is considered semipermanent (it can be removed).

Laser skin resurfacing. Using one of two types of lasers (CO_2 and erbium lasers), the doctor sends short, concentrated pulsating beams of light at damaged skin, which removes the skin one layer at a time. It's especially effective for acne scarring. ∎

Although other factors, such as the amount of melanin, also affect the skin's tendency to reflect or absorb harmful rays, it's essential to use a sunscreen and avoid excessive sun exposure when using these products, says Dr. Davis. Chemical-free sunscreens, such as those containing titanium dioxide or zinc oxide, may be the best choice since other sunscreen ingredients may irritate the skin.

Use furfuryladenine. It's a plant compound that moisturizes the skin, and research suggests it can help improve fine lines or even out skin tone. Look for products that contain N6-furfuryladenine or kinetin (its chemical name), says Dr. Fields. Kinerase and Almay Kinetin are two brands you may find at your local drugstore.

Try something stronger. OTC aging products usually have such low concentrations of active ingredients that the benefits may be minimal, says Dr. Fields. To change the structure of the skin, you may want to try prescription products that contain tretinoin, such as Renova or Retin-A, a version of vitamin A. "It's medically proven that retinoids are the strongest thing you can use to slow the aging process," says Francesca Fusco, MD, a dermatologist

who practices in New York. "They diminish fine lines, increase cell turnover to give a youthful glow, and lighten brown spots." Products with tretinoin can dry or irritate the skin, so start slowly, using it just 2 or 3 nights a week, and increase to nightly as tolerated, advises Dr. Fields.

There are prescription products that contain lower strength retinoids, and drugstores also carry OTC products with retinol, which is lower in strength than tretinoin and generally well tolerated. Retinol is converted to active retinoids in the skin and is an excellent start for improvement in texture, tone, and pore size.

Step 4: Bleaches for Skin Spots

After decades of sun exposure, nearly everyone will develop pigment-related problems, such as age spots or freckles. It isn't always possible to eliminate them completely, but they can almost always be faded to the point of invisibility with bleaching creams.

These products contain active ingredients such as hydroquinone or kojic acid, which interfere with pigment formation, Dr. Kates

---

WHAT WORKS FOR ME

LESLIE BAUMANN, MD, *is director of the Baumann Cosmetic and Research Institute in Miami, Florida. Here's how she keeps her skin looking young.*

I use Retin-A at night, and Eucerin Q10 Anti-Wrinkle Sensitive Skin facial moisturizer underneath my sunscreen. Eucerin's active ingredient, coenzyme Q10, is an antioxidant. There haven't been enough solid studies to show whether it offers real benefits topically. Still, I love how it feels as a moisturizer. ∎

says. For the most part, it doesn't work as well as hydroquinone. Prescription-strength hydroquinone tends to give better results than OTC products.

Hydroquinone is available in prescription as well as in OTC products, such as Porcelana. It's very effective at fading most age spots and must be used with a good UVA and UVB sunscreen, says Dr. Fields. To get the best results, she advises using prescription hydroquinone in combination with OTC products containing kojic acid. Use daily or twice per day as tolerated and avoid the sun, or the brown spots and age spots will return within hours.

Step 5: Freshen Up with Masks or Peels

Over the centuries, women have used an incredible number of natural products to make masks—skin-coating slurries—that remove oils from the skin. Masks leave your face feeling clean and refreshed. Peels are somewhat different. They remove the top layer of skin, as well as lighten some brown spots.

Choose the right mask. When you're shopping for mask products at the cosmetics counter, it's important to find one that matches your skin type. If you have dry skin, buy a hydrating mask. For oily skin, use clay masks or deep cleansers. For acne, use a sulfur or purifying mask.

Make your own. If you enjoy the feel of fresh ingredients on your skin, it's easy to make your own masks. One you may want to try is

Prevention's Tropical Fruit Masque. It includes pineapple and papaya, natural sources of alpha hydroxy acids.

To make the mask, use a blender or food processor to puree 1 cup of fresh pineapple and 1 to 2 cups of slightly green fresh papaya. Add 2 tablespoons of honey, and mix thoroughly.

Test a small amount on your inner arm to be sure you aren't sensitive. Leave it on for 20 minutes. If your skin doesn't get red or itchy, go ahead and apply. Wash your face thoroughly, spread the mixture evenly over your face, avoiding the eye area, and leave it on for 5 minutes. Then rinse with cool water. You can repeat the treatment once a week.

Get a glycolic acid peel. Performed by dermatologists, this is sometimes called the "lunchtime peel" because it works so quickly. The dermatologist will apply glycolic acid to your face, which removes dead cells and quickly uncovers the younger, smoother skin underneath. The peel tingles, but it isn't uncomfortable, says Seth L. Matarasso, MD, associate clinical professor of dermatology at the University of California San Francisco, and a dermatologist in San Francisco. Peels cost between $75 and $2,000 per treatment, depending on the type you get and who performs it, and you can get them as often as once a month. Much cheaper are the facial peel kits you can buy in the drugstore for about $25. They contain low concentrations of alpha or beta hydroxy acids. You'll get a healthy glow, but unlike professional peels, they don't improve wrinkles, sun damage, or brown spots.

Try a chemical-free peel (microderm-abrasion). Your dermatologist or aesthetician uses a wandlike tool that uses high pressure to slough dead skin and vacuum it away. "The combination of abrasion and suction stimulates collagen production, helping improve fine lines and minor scars," says Debra Jaliman, MD, clinical professor of dermatology at Mount Sinai School of Medicine. The cost is usually about $1,200 for a series of five monthly sessions. Or you could use an at-home peel product that uses aluminum oxide crystals that you apply to your face with a manual or battery-powered rotating or vibrating wand. Your skin will appear smooth, though you won't have the same texture changes you get with the collagen-stimulating professional version.

Get longer-lasting results. Many women want to have fresher, younger-looking skin, but they don't want to spend a lot of time on home or professional treatments. One option is to have a peel called the trichloracetic peel. It's performed by a dermatologist or plastic surgeon, and it will improve the appearance of the skin for as long as a year, says James W. Goodnight, MD, director of the Facial Plastic Surgery Center in Teaneck, New Jersey. The procedure takes under an hour.

This is one procedure that you won't want to have done during your lunch break. The skin will burn during the procedure, and it will peel off in large pieces in the days to come. Women who have this treatment usually plan to stay close to home for about a week, until the peeling is complete. It costs between $300 and $600.

Masks leave your face feeling clean and refreshed.

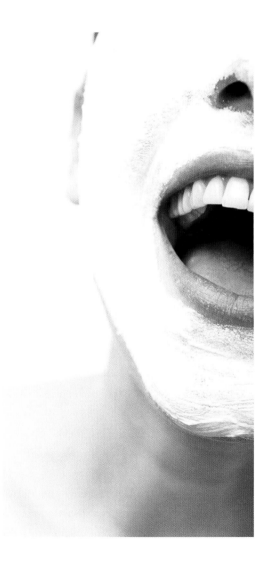

Go for the power cleanse. These exfoliating treatments dislodge oil and dead cells from your skin, leaving it looking healthier and finer textured, and more absorbent of moisturizers. These $65 to $100 an hour sessions use steam to soften pores and dilate blood vessels, which will boost circulation. Your aesthetician will then clean and exfoliate your skin, removing blackheads and whiteheads and applying moisturizer. At home, you can use battery-operated brushes (that work similarly to an electric toothbrush) to massage cleanser into your skin at up to 300 rotations per second, which will also remove makeup, oil, and dead skin cells, though not as extensively as microdermabrasion or a peel.

Step 6: Say Goodbye to Puffy Eyes

Few things can make you look more tired (or older) than puffy eyes. They're usually caused by such things as fatigue, water retention, allergies, or even a reaction to eye makeup. To quickly tighten the skin and help your eyes look younger, here's what doctors advise.

Try grape seed extract. It's found in Caudalie's products, jO2 Firming Lotion, and Napa Valley Grape Seed Spa products. Some people report good results from their personal experience, and preliminary studies suggest that applying grape seed extract to the skin can reduce eye puffiness caused by water retention or poor circulation. As a bonus, it helps smooth the complexion and may protect against the sun's harmful rays. It can be used nightly. Grape seed extract has also been found to help skin wounds heal faster with less scarring.

Reduce puffiness with tea bags. Brew a cup of tea using two tea bags. Set the bags aside until they're cool, then place them on the puffy areas of your eyes for a few minutes. The cool moisture can reduce swelling for up to 24 hours. In addition, tea contains tannins, compounds that reduce eye inflammation, says Dr. Matarasso.

You can get similar effects by placing cool cucumber slices or even cooled spoons on the puffy areas, Dr. Matarasso adds.

Apply products that contain caffeine. Caffeine can help reduce swelling under the eyes.

Balancing Your Emotions

Imagine a time when you felt at peace. Relaxed. Content. Free of worry. Now imagine that you could feel that way every day. Sounds impossible? It's not. You can balance your emotions.

Although psychologists have different views of what constitutes emotional balance, they agree that it involves spending more time at peace than blowing up in anger, writhing with jealousy, or being dragged down by sadness.

"Internally, we all have a central home base," says Terry Murphy, PsyD, a clinical psychologist in private practice in Philadelphia. "It's a state of normal calm and contentment."

No one spends all their time in that peaceful zone, of course. Life is full of conflicts. But a reasonable goal—one that any woman can achieve—is to return to that soothing home base after a setback, such as a clash with a coworker or a disagreement with your husband.

You'll feel better immediately, but that's not the only benefit. You'll also enjoy better health. Negative emotions such as anger and anxiety can weaken the immune system and leave you vulnerable to illness. Stress and tension also increase the risk of high blood pressure, heart disease, and dozens of other serious conditions.

Experts don't suggest that women should never get mad, jealous, or sad. What you can do is minimize the amount of time you spend experiencing these or other negative emotions. In just six steps, you can strengthen your ability to handle any situation with calm and confidence.

Step 1: Take an Emotional Inventory

Before you start working on your emotional skills, it's helpful to know just how balanced you already are. Start with a quiz.

1. **How often do you feel physically healthy, energetic, and well rested?**

   A. Almost every day

   B. About 50 percent of the time

   C. Rarely

2. **How often do you experience the gamut of emotions: sadness, guilt, fear, joy, love, and excitement?**

   A. Every week

   B. Every month

   C. I can't remember the last time I felt some of those emotions

3. **How often do you express your emotions to other people?**

   A. Only when I think it's appropriate

   B. Only when the emotions are strong

   C. All the time

4. **How often do you feel physically or emotionally numb after an activity, such as watching television, exercising, working, browsing the Internet, or reading a book?**

   A. Hardly ever

   B. Once in a while

   C. Every day

5. **When you're sad, what are you most likely to do?**

   A. I look for people to be with

   B. I spend time with others, if it's convenient

   C. I'd rather stay home when I'm sad

6. **How often do you find yourself struggling to do things that were easy in the past, such as balancing the checkbook or completing projects on time?**

   A. Only when stress is very high

   B. Once in a while, but not regularly

   C. Regularly

7. **Do your spouse, family, children, and close friends support you?**

   A. Every day

   B. Only when I really need them

   C. Not enough

8. **How often do you ask friends and family for help?**

   A. Daily or weekly

   B. Monthly

   C. Only when I'm desperate

9. **Do you have hobbies?**

   A. Yes, and I do them regularly

   B. One or two, which I tend to neglect

   C. There's no time for hobbies

Step 2: Identify Your Emotional Strengths and Weaknesses

If you answered the quiz questions honestly, you'll have a pretty good sense of how good a job you're doing staying balanced. If most of your answers were A, congratulations: You're on the right track. If most of the answers were B, you could use a little work—and this chapter will help. If most of your answers were C, you're going to have to try harder to find your emotional center.

Let's take a moment to look at each of the quiz questions to see how they measure emotional health and wellness.

Question 1. Negative emotions frequently result in physical symptoms. It's normal, for example, for people to feel tired or lethargic before they actually feel the underlying emotions, such as anger or rage. When you're feeling physically "off" and there's no good reason for it, it's likely that your emotions are out of balance.

Question 2. Many people don't feel comfortable with certain emotions, such as anger or jealousy. These feelings still have to come out, however. What people often do is transfer their energy to another emotion, such as guilt, says Vivien D. Wolsk, PhD, a clinical psychologist and dean of faculty of the Gestalt Center for Psychotherapy and Training in New York City. Soon guilt will overwhelm you because it's the only emotion you allow yourself to feel.

Question 3. Expressing emotions to others is important. This doesn't mean blowing your temper at the slightest provocation, of course. Nor does it mean you should always say exactly what's on your mind. In healthy human relations, emotions have to be expressed appropriately, says Dr. Murphy. Suppose, for example, that your husband says something that annoys you. If it's a minor issue, the healthy thing would be to respond to it as if it is a minor issue. If you overreact and go into a rage, your emotional balance is a little off, and your relationships are going to suffer.

Question 4. Most people have ways of coping with emotional troughs. A common strategy is to numb negative emotions, such as guilt or anger, by engaging in routine activities—watching television, working extra-long hours, or even exercising long past the point you'd normally quit, says Lisa Firestone, PhD, a clinical psychologist and education and program director at the Glendon Association in Santa Barbara, California. When you're in this defensive state, you push away the people who can help you through rough times.

Question 5. Negative thoughts become more powerful when you're alone. And the more powerful the thoughts become, the less likely you are to seek out human contact. That's why therapists advise people who are feeling blue to spend time with others. Even if you decide not to talk about your problems, the simple human contact will boost your mind and even relieve mild depression.

Question 6. When you're emotionally out of balance, concentration and focus diminish.

A Quick Course in Anger Management

I n the traditional view, women aren't supposed to get mad. Maybe that's why women often cry instead of confronting the people who are pushing their buttons. Why they're nice to people who have insulted them. Or, in some cases, why they blow their tops at the slightest provocation. The pent-up anger just has to come out.

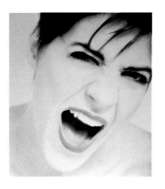

Whether you express your anger or suppress it, there are a number of ways to understand it and keep it at healthful levels.

Use anger as a signal. Rather than push anger away, figure out what it's telling you, says Vivien D. Wolsk, PhD, a clinical psychologist and dean of faculty at the Gestalt Center for Psychotherapy and Training in New York City. Say to yourself, "I'm angry because something's wrong here." It will help you figure out what needs fixing.

Think before you act. Feeling the emotion isn't the same as acting on it. When you're boiling with rage, ask yourself if this is the time and place to express it. You may want to go to a private place to vent, or take a long walk to think things over.

Confront the source. There's nothing wrong with confronting people who have made you angry, says Dr. Wolsk. Wait until you cool off, then explain how their words or actions made you feel. As long as you approach people calmly and with a genuine desire to work things out, they'll usually work with you to find a solution. ■

Tasks that should be easy become increasingly difficult and fatiguing.

Question 7. Women are responsible for a lot these days. They keep the house clean, take care of children, do the shopping. And all this is often on top of working at jobs outside the home. If you aren't getting a lot of support in your life, your emotions—and your health—are going to suffer.

Question 8. "Women expect themselves to be able to handle everything," Dr. Murphy says. "They haven't given themselves permission to ask for help."

Feeling uncomfortable with or overwhelmed by your workload is a red flag. Not only does it mean that your physical and emotional resilience is needlessly being sapped, but it also means that you're not taking responsibility for getting the help you need.

Question 9. Hobbies—such as collecting antiques, bird-watching, or writing short stories—are a great way to incorporate downtime into your life. If you don't have a few hobbies that you enjoy, there's a good chance you're spending too much time working, caring for others, or generally assuming the burdens of the world.

Step 3: **Keep a Journal**

If you completed the quiz above, you have a pretty good sense of your emotional strengths and weaknesses. But that's just the beginning. Inside everyone are vast, subterranean networks of emotions. These emotions guide everything you do—and everything you think and feel. To find and maintain your emotional

When You're Worried All the Time

as many as 6.1 million Americans are in a constant state of anxiety—even when their lives seem to be going just fine. Called generalized anxiety disorder or GAD, the condition is characterized by free-floating worries that may flit from finances, work issues, health, to family problems. And even though people with GAD know their concerns are unfounded or bigger than they should be, they can't seem to control them.

People with GAD have problems concentrating and falling or staying asleep, and feel keyed up and restless or fatigued. They sometimes have physical symptoms, such as shakiness or headaches.

Cognitive behavioral therapy (CBT) is an effec-tive treatment for GAD. This form of therapy teaches you to challenge the thoughts and emotions that are the basis for your irrational worry. It's a time-limited therapy, usually lasting only 10 to 20 weeks, that leaves you with skills for controlling your thoughts so they don't control you. A sense of mastery replaces the sense of helplessness that can lead to fear and panic.

Your therapist may also recommend antidepressants, in particular selective serotonin reuptake inhibitors or SSRIs such as sertraline and fluoxetine. If those don't work, you may be given a prescription for antianxiety medications, which can't be taken long term because of dependence issues. ∎

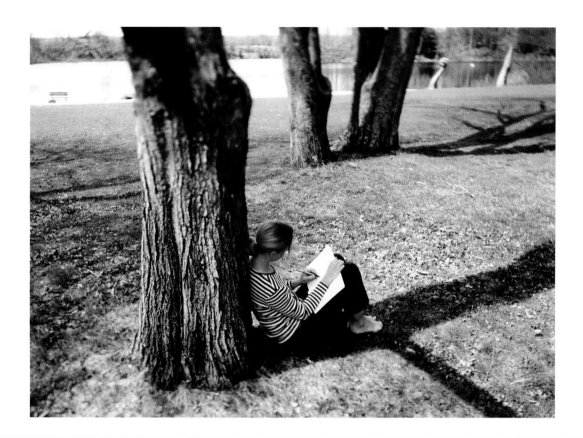

THREE THINGS I TELL EVERY FEMALE PATIENT

LISA FIRESTONE, PhD, *a clinical psychologist and director of research and education for the Glendon Association in Santa Barbara, California, offers this advice for achieving emotional balance.*

1

ACCEPT ALL YOUR EMOTIONS, THE GOOD AND THE BAD. Nobody chooses to feel a certain way, she says. Allow yourself to experience all your feelings—including emotions typically labeled as negative, such as hostility and anger. Accept all your emotions, but know that you choose your behavior in response to them.

2

MOVE BEYOND NEGATIVE THOUGHTS. Everyone is self-critical at times. Pay attention to how you criticize yourself, and expose these thoughts to a more rational evaluation. Write them down or tell them to a friend. It is important to act in your own self-interest, not on negative self-critical thoughts. Taking action in your own self-interest can help combat these thoughts.

3

MAKE A LIST OF THE ACTIVITIES AND PEOPLE THAT BRING YOU JOY. Then make a list of those that bring negative emotions. Look at the lists daily—and do everything you can to embrace the "good" and avoid the "bad." ■

balance, it's essential to understand what's happening deep inside—and keeping a journal is a great place to start.

Studies have shown, for example, that people who write in journals, especially about the traumas in their lives, report feeling better about themselves. Their immune systems also get a boost, which protects them from stress-related illness. An increasing number of psychologists and psychiatrists have begun incorporating journal writing into their practices as a treatment for depression and anxiety disorders. There's also some evidence that keeping a gratitude journal—writing down the things you're grateful for and the positive things that happen each day—can make you feel uplifted, even in times of trouble.

There are no formal rules for keeping a journal. In fact, the opposite is true—your personality and desire for creativity should be your guides. To get started:

Please your personality. Your journal can be leather-bound or made of recycled paper. It might have leopard-print designs or flower petals on the pages. It can be as simple as a spiral notebook. Everyone has different tastes, and this is your chance to indulge them.

Write as much or as little as you like. You don't have to write in a journal every day to achieve emotional balance. Keeping a journal is simply a tool, and it's up to you to decide how it works best for you, says Susan Heitler, PhD, a clinical psychologist and author of the book *From Conflict to Resolution* and the audiotape *Anxiety: Friend or Foe.*

On one day, for example, you might sit down

Getting a Grip on Guilt

guilt is what you feel when you've done something wrong or when you are toying with the idea of doing something wrong. It's what you feel when you call in sick at work to go shopping with a friend or fantasize about having an affair with an attractive man.

Women suffer from guilt to a disproportionate degree, says Karen Clark-Schock, PsyD, a licensed psychologist and board-certified art therapist in private practice in Philadelphia. "I think that it comes from feeling as though they can never do enough."

Women are raised to be caretakers, Dr. Clark-Schock explains. As a result, they focus on the needs of others. And when the other person isn't happy, for whatever reason, women can feel responsible, thinking either that they caused the unhappiness or that they must fix it or solve it—or both.

As with many emotions, guilt can easily take on a life of its own, especially if you don't talk about it. One of the best ways to come to terms with guilt and to shrink it to a manageable size is to discuss your feelings with others, be it a friend, family member, or therapist, advises Dr. Clark-Schock. The guilt that looms so large in your own mind will probably appear pretty small to others. Plus, your friends can share their own guilty secrets, which will put your own in perspective. ■

to write and realize that you don't have a lot to say, maybe only a sentence or two. That's fine. On another day, especially one with a lot of emotional challenges, you might find yourself writing page after page as you think about what happened, what people said, and how you reacted to everything.

Put it on your schedule. While it's best to avoid feeling obligated to write in a journal, it's often helpful to set aside certain times when you're going to write—first thing in the morning, for example, or right after dinner. If you miss an "appointment," fine—but setting a schedule will make it easier to keep at it.

Date the pages. Some journals have the dates already on the pages. If yours doesn't, jot down the dates, including the year, you're writing. When you review your journal entries months or even years later, the dates will provide fascinating insights into what you were thinking or feeling at different stages of your life.

Write anything. Nearly everyone experiences writer's block when they first start keeping a journal, says Dr. Heitler. This might be the time to remind yourself that you're not trying to create literature for the ages but only to explore and understand your innermost feelings.

Still blocked? Dr. Heitler suggests that you close your eyes for a moment and imagine a stressful situation in your life. That's your topic: Describe the situation in as few or as many words as you wish. Once you start, you'll probably find that the words will flow faster than you can write them down.

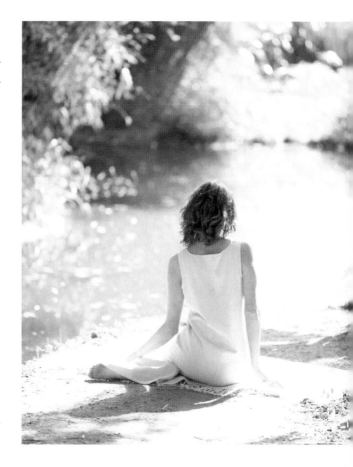

Step 4: Create Pockets of Tranquility throughout the Day

In today's busy world, it's easy to get so caught up in responsibilities that you never set aside quiet times for yourself. Women who don't take time to recharge their physical and emotional batteries will experience ever-escalating amounts of stress and tension.

It may feel like an indulgence to give yourself some daily quiet time, but it's not: It's as important for good health as eating nutritious foods or getting a good night's sleep. Here are some places to start.

Take the time to breathe deeply. According to a proverb, "He who half breathes, half lives." It's extremely common for women to hold their breath briefly when they're under stress—or to breathe shallowly throughout the day. Apart from the fact that shallow breathing doesn't supply the body and brain with the necessary oxygen, doing so also makes it more difficult to experience emotions fully, says Dr. Wolsk.

She advises women to set aside a few minutes each day to do nothing but breathe deeply. Breathe in through your nose, and keep taking in air until your abdomen swells. Hold the breath for just a moment, then slowly exhale through your mouth. This technique, called diaphragmatic breathing, floods the tissues with oxygen and makes it possible to get in touch with your emotional life, she explains.

Find a safe place. When you're overwhelmed with a negative emotion, it helps to have a private room or place to let the emotion out. When you're feeling sad or depressed at home, for example, you might want to retreat to the bathroom and have a long, hot shower. At work, people often sit in an empty office or even their car for a few moments. Giving yourself the time to escape makes it possible to release negative emotions as they accumulate, rather than allow-

New Help for Bipolar Disorder

We all experience emotional ups and down from time to time—feelings of elation followed by sadness. For most of us, these emotional swings are triggered by real-life events: Getting a raise at work or a compliment from a supervisor might be followed by finding out a roof needs repair. We deal with the emotions, then get on with our lives.

For people with bipolar disorder, however, the emotional swings come out of the blue—and the emotions may be so extreme that it's almost impossible for them to function normally without medical help, says Francis Mark Mondimore, MD, associate professor in the department of psychiatry and behavioral science at Johns Hopkins University School of Medicine in Baltimore and author of *Bipolar Disorder: A Guide for Patients and Families*.

People with bipolar disorder—an estimated 2.6 percent of Americans or 5.7 million adults have this condition—may go from being profoundly depressed to being wildly elated, or manic. During the depressive stage, they may lose their appetite and have little interest in their normal activities. When they're manic, they almost seethe with energy. They can't keep up with their own thoughts, they have little need for sleep, and they may have hallucinations.

There's no cure for bipolar disorder and suicide is a high risk for people with this condition, who will need lifelong treatment with drugs and psychotherapy. But with a combination of medications and lifestyle changes—such as avoiding alcohol, getting enough sleep, and exercising regularly—many people with this condition are able to keep it under control, says Dr. Mondimore. ∎

WHAT TO DO IF YOU HAVE ONLY **5 MINUTES**

Set aside at least 5 minutes every day to meditate and get away from the distractions of the world, says Lucy Papillon, PhD, a clinical psychologist, author of *When Hope Can Kill: Reclaiming Your Soul in a Romantic Relationship,* and director of the Center of Light in Beverly Hills, California, and Santa Fe, New Mexico.

Find a quiet place that's free of distractions, she advises. Close your eyes, or maybe look at the flame of a candle. Allow your thoughts to float through your mind, but don't dwell on them. If you practice this regularly, you'll find that you'll be able to disregard self-critical thoughts and self-destructive emotions, no matter where they come from or when they arrive.

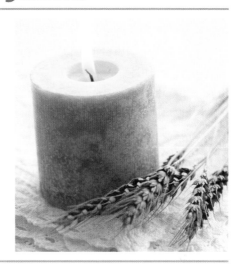

ing them to build and surge throughout the day, says Dr. Wolsk.

Move your body. Any kind of exercise—walking up and down stairs, raking a few leaves, jogging in place—increases your breathing rate and triggers the release of endorphins, chemicals in the brain that help regulate mood. One study at the University of Vermont found that people who rode an exercise bike for 20 minutes at a moderate pace experienced a significant lift in their moods right afterward—and as long as 12 hours later—when compared to a similar group that didn't exercise.

Don't wait until you're stressed to start moving. Women who get aerobic exercise 4 or more times a week will feel physically and emotionally stronger, says Dr. Wolsk.

Give yourself positive messages. Everyone deals with a lot of negativity throughout the day, and it's normal to feel overwhelmed

and frustrated. Over time, however, these negative feelings can begin to take over, which is why it's so important to remind yourself of how strong and special you really are," says Lucy Papillon, PhD, a clinical psychologist, author of *When Hope Can Kill: Reclaiming Your Soul in a Romantic Relationship,* and director of the Center of Light in Beverly Hills, California, and Santa Fe, New Mexico. "It could end up being a self-fulfilling prophecy," she says. "When you're having a tough time, tell yourself, 'This is hard, but I have the strength to get through it,'" she advises.

Step 5: **Plan and Conquer**

Emotional stress and negative emotions come in infinite forms, and they're often unpredictable. But that doesn't mean you can't anticipate them and plan ahead for how you're going to deal with them.

Imagine, for example, that you're blindsided at work—by a difficult coworker, for example, or an unexpected problem with a supervisor. On top of the challenge of working things out, you'll also have to deal with the rush of adrenaline and other stress hormones that are released when the unexpected hits. Multiply this by a few dozen times a day, and it's easy to see why so many women feel embattled and exhausted.

You can't anticipate all the specific problems you're likely to face every day, but you probably have a few emotional hot buttons in your life—things that consistently sap your strength and batter your emotions. If you take a few minutes to plan your coping strategies ahead of time, you'll be less likely to be taken by surprise, and you may be able to circumvent the problems altogether. Whatever the issue is, plan ahead for it by identifying at least three alternative ways to approach it.

When you plan your options, you'll be much more likely to achieve your goals, and you'll also feel stronger and more confident, she explains.

Put the Brakes on Anxiety

anxiety is a normal reaction to threatening situations. For some women, however, the emotion is so intense or frequent that they find it difficult to go about their lives.

Doctors estimate that 40 million Americans, a majority of them women, suffer from anxiety disorders. These can result in panic attacks, a racing heart, nausea, chest pain, dizziness, and other symptoms. The attacks can be so severe that people rush to emergency rooms because they think they're having a heart attack.

A full-fledged anxiety disorder is a serious problem that requires medical attention. In most cases, however, women can control mild to moderate anxiety with a few simple steps.

Prepare yourself. Some things in life, like job interviews or talking to groups of people, are especially likely to provoke anticipation anxiety. One of the best ways to control it is to be as prepared as possible—by rehearsing a presentation ahead of time, for example, or by learning more about the company you're applying to, says Susan Heitler, PhD, a clinical psychologist and author of the book *From Conflict to Resolution* and the audiotape *Anxiety: Friend or Foe*.

Take some deep breaths. It's one of the best ways to reduce shortness of breath, a speeding heart, or other anxiety symptoms, says Brenda Wiederhold, PhD, executive director of the Virtual Reality Medical Center in San Diego.

Stop irrational thoughts. People often feel anxious because of what experts call "catastrophic thinking"—the belief that the worst is about to happen.

When this is happening to you, imagine a red flashing light and mentally yell "Stop!" advises Dr. Wiederhold. At the same time, distract yourself—by counting backward from 100, for example. Your mind will find it difficult to return to the same troublesome thoughts, she explains. ■

Plan your words. Confrontation is a fact of life. Hardly a day goes by when you don't have to deal with uncomfortable situations: a mail-order package that didn't arrive when it was supposed to; a friend who always says something inappropriate; a neighbor who plays loud music late at night. Just thinking about it gets you upset—and the tension keeps building.

Plan ahead of time what you'll say. You'll be less likely to respond in the heat of the moment (which can make a bad situation worse), and you'll also feel more confident about your ability to handle it.

You can't eliminate confrontation, but as long as you plan for it and give yourself choices, you'll always feel you are in charge—and that's an essential part of keeping your emotions in a healthy balance.

Step 6: Practice the Art of Acceptance

Women who achieve a sense of control in their lives are often amazed by how much stronger and confident they feel. Unfortunately, there are thousands of things we all wish we could control—everything from dress size to the behavior of teenagers—but can't. Sometimes you just have to accept that some things are out of your hands.

Allow yourself to feel your emotions. Emotions are going to come and go whether you want them to or not. Instead of pushing uncomfortable emotions away, be honest and allow yourself to feel them. Cry when you're sad. Don't automatically say "fine" when someone asks how you're doing. Admit it when you're depressed or anxious.

"People believe that if they feel an emotion, it will take over," Dr. Firestone says. But being aroused emotionally can last only so long. The sooner you allow yourself to feel an emotion, the sooner it will go on its way.

Be good to yourself. And say it with words. Every morning, look in the mirror and say something positive: "I appreciate you" or "I love you." Saying things out loud helps them become real, says Dr. Wolsk.

Remember the anchors in your life. When things feel like they're spinning out of control, take an inventory of all the things you know are solid and reliable: Your child is safe on the bus; your car will get you to work on time; your computer will turn on and work. When you realize how much in your life is dependable, you'll have more trust in your ability to work through life's problems, says Dr. Murphy.

Healthy Sex at Any Age

One 2010 sex survey published by *Time* magazine garnered worldwide headlines: Women prefer food to sex. Another survey of 1,774 Swedish women reported that our Scandinavian sisters think jogging is just as important as making love. And *Cooking Light* readers ranked drinking enough water higher than having enough sex on a survey on factors important to health and well-being.

That doesn't appear to bode well for women's sexuality, but those are not scientific surveys. Sex therapists, on the other hand, say that most women want to be more in touch with their sexuality.

In her book, *Why Women Have Sex,* researcher Cindy Meston, PhD, of the Sexual Psychophysiology Laboratory at the University of Texas at Austin, reveals that women fall into bed for the same reasons men do: sexual attraction and gratification. They have their own reasons too—a need for love and commitment and the kind of intimacy and bonding that only sex can bring. "For many women, living without an intimate sexual relationship is like living without chocolate or their favorite meal," says Bonnie Saks, MD, clinical professor of psychiatry at the University of South Florida in Tampa. And, presumably, water and jogging.

The real science bears out that a good sex life is important to most women—and more lasting than we might think. More than three-quarters of the 46,000-plus participants in the Women's Health Initiative, the largest-ever study of women's health in the United States, told researchers they were satisfied with their sex lives. And these were women from 50 to 79, mainly postmenopausal women who were likely to be having some problems—low-energy, menopausal discomfort, and side effects of medications—in the bedroom. Tellingly, sexual satisfaction rose with age—as well as with being slim, active, and not smoking—suggesting that a

Drug "Cocktails" Are the Closest Thing to a Cure

It's hard to imagine that until about 30 years ago, no one had ever heard of AIDS. Although scientists first identified the human immunodeficiency virus (HIV, the virus that causes AIDS) in 1959, it wasn't until 1982 that it got its name and was recognized as a disease transmitted through bodily fluids. The first cases in the United States were among gay men, then IV drug users.

Today more than 1.1 million Americans are living with the AIDS virus. Nearly three-quarters of those are men, who contracted the virus via male-to-male sex and drug use. Women make up the rest, with the most likely route of transmission heterosexual sex or injecting drugs with a contaminated syringe. Women who have other sexually transmitted diseases have a higher risk of being infected with the AIDS virus.

HIV can survive in the body for years without causing symptoms. In the early stages, the only way for a woman to know she's been exposed to the virus is to have a blood test.

Scientists have made tremendous progress in understanding the AIDS virus, but there still isn't a cure. However, it's often possible to reduce levels of the virus in the body dramatically by giving people a combination of antiviral drugs. There are many medications to choose from, so when one combination doesn't work, another probably will.

Until doctors find a way to beat the virus, the best strategy by far is prevention. For women who aren't in long-term, committed relationships, this means always using a condom during sex. Sex with a condom isn't as spontaneous as some women would like, but it's among the best ways to stay healthy and infection-free. ■

good sex life can surmount many obstacles and that pleasure and intimacy just never get old. In fact, an Indiana University survey found that 61 percent of women said they liked sex more than they did 20 years ago. One rea-son: "A woman's ability to orgasm gets easier as she ages," says Debby Herbenick, PhD, a research scientist at Indiana University. And in a *Prevention* survey, most women said they'd have sex every day if they could (the big rea-

Dealing with Herpes

When a woman diagnosed with herpes first learns that she's infected with the virus, she'll probably assume two things: that she'll suffer from frequent and pain-ful outbreaks and that her current partner hasn't been faithful.

Neither is necessarily true. Although there isn't a cure for herpes, many women can live most of their lives free of outbreaks. And it's not uncommon for men and women to harbor the virus unknowingly for years or even decades and to be free of symp-toms, says Marian Dunn, PhD, director of the Cen-ter for Human Sexuality at State University of New York Downstate Medical Center in Brooklyn.

The herpes virus often lives silently in the mouth or genitals. When an outbreak starts, a woman may experience itching or burning, pain in the legs or buttocks, or a feeling of pressure in the abdomen. After a few days, she may develop small, painful sores, either on the mouth or on the genitals, depending on the type of herpes she's infected with.

The first outbreak usually lasts for 2 to 3 weeks, but future episodes tend to be less severe. However, the virus is highly contagious during the active phase. A woman who has sex without a condom at that time could very well pass the virus to her partner.

Here are a few ways to ease the discomfort and possibly prevent the outbreaks from occurring.

- The prescription drug acyclovir (Zovirax) can reduce the discomfort of outbreaks and shorten their duration. A prescription drug called fam-ciclovir (Famvir) also treats herpes outbreaks, and may help prevent future attacks. Valcy-clovir (Valtrex) boosts the effectiveness of acyclovir so you need to take less of it. It's usu-ally prescribed if you have six or more out-breaks a year.

- Try aspirin. Taking 125 milligrams of aspirin at the first sign of cold sores (caused by the her-pesvirus) may speed their healing time and will relieve pain.

- Take soothing baths, or gently dab the sores with a warm, moist towel. Applying moist heat is one of the best ways to reduce irritation.

When you become pregnant, tell your doc-tors that you have genital herpes. Although your antibodies should protect your fetus and newborn, there is a small risk that a herpes infection can cause lasting damage to a baby's central nervous system, mental retardation, or death. If you have an active outbreak during labor, your doctor can perform a cesarean sec-tion to prevent the baby from coming into con-tact with the virus. ■

son they don't: too tired, survey respondents admitted).

If fun and pleasure don't hook you, how about these reasons to work on a flagging sex life? Studies have found that sex can ease pain, boost your immunity, lower your risk of cancer, reduce stress, and even cure one of the main reasons menopausal women have pain during sex: vaginal dryness.

Here's a three-step plan that will help keep your passion at healthy and satisfying levels.

Step 1: Get a Healthy Attitude about Sex

It's hard to believe in an age when celebrities parade their sexuality—and sometimes their malfunctioning wardrobe—on stage, but there are still some women who have a tough time being sexual. Some women were raised to think of sex as something "forbidden" or improper. Some feel that it's inappropriate for a woman to express her full range of sexual desires—or even to admit them to herself. These and other emotional barriers may prevent women from fully exploring—and enjoying—their sexuality.

Open your mind to possibilities. Sexuality is a natural part of who you are. You may choose how much or how little sex you have, but the feelings will always be there, says Marian Dunn, PhD, director of the Center for Human Sexuality at State University of New York Downstate Medical Center in Brooklyn.

Millions of Americans—men and women alike—aren't entirely comfortable with their sexuality, she adds. One solution is to browse your favorite bookstore or online catalog. There are literally hundreds (if not thousands) of informative books that explore all aspects of female sexuality. You'll discover many emotional and physical possibilities that you may want to explore for yourself.

THREE THINGS I TELL EVERY FEMALE PATIENT

MICHAEL PLAUT, PhD, *is a psychologist with a specialty in sexual problems and past president of the Society for Sex Therapy and Research. Here's what he advises women who want to explore and renew their sexuality.*

1

COMMUNICATE WITH YOUR PARTNER. Men aren't mind readers. The only way your mate will know what pleases you—and what you don't like—is if you're honest and forthright about your preferences.

2

ALLOW INTIMACY TO HAPPEN. It's easy to get so caught up in life's responsibilities—overdue bills, looming deadlines, problems with the children—that you never really let yourself go. During intimate moments, try to focus entirely on the moment at hand. Deal with the responsibilities later.

3

BE OPEN TO NEW THINGS. The sex that you enjoyed when you were 20 may not be what you enjoy today. Men and women are constantly changing, and there's no reason for sex and intimacy to stay the same. ■

Learn to love your body. Research has shown that body perceptions, positive as well as negative, strongly affect sexual satisfaction. A University of Texas study found that women who liked their bodies had higher levels of sexual desire. And more than 20 percent of women who responded to *Prevention*'s sex survey said that it was dissatisfaction with their looks that held them back in bed.

Few women are completely satisfied with their bodies—but don't let this hold you back. When you're with your partner, focus on the parts of your body that you feel good about, suggests Dr. Saks. Write down five features you really love about the way you look. It might be your soft skin or delicate hands, or the gentle curve of your neck. When you think about the things that please you most, you'll feel more attractive, and feeling attractive will make you more confident and assured.

Conquer old memories. Negative feelings about sex are often caused by early experiences. For some women, it was sexual abuse; for others it was the result of having sex before they were fully ready. They may see sex more as a service than as a means to self-fulfillment, says Dr. Saks.

One way to overcome these feelings is to let your partner know that you want more control in the bedroom. This might mean that you'll be the one to initiate sex, and you'll also take charge of setting the pace. Limit touch to only what is comfortable for you. As you gain a greater sense of control, your enjoyment will also increase, says Dr. Saks.

Set sexual goals. If you want to feel sexier and get closer to your partner, try something new—write it down, and do it. A 2008 study found that people who had positive goals for their sex lives were less likely to have a dip in sexual desire over time than people who had negative goals such as "stop fighting with my partner."

Have morning sex. If being tired is preventing you from having a good sex life, this is the best time to remedy that. "Biochemically speaking, it makes sense to have sex first thing in the morning," says Eva Cwynar, MD, an endocrinologist and assistant clinical professor of medicine at the University of California Los Angeles. "Cortisol is at its peak so you have the energy to do it. Then afterward you release other hormones like oxytocin so you're in a good mood all day." Don't set the alarm: You don't need much time. Research shows that most couples enjoy quickies—sex that only lasts 7 to 13 minutes. And don't wait for the mood to hit you. Have sex whether or not you feel like it. Desire actually increases during intercourse.

Kiss and touch a lot. Building more intimate moments into your daily life keeps sex and intimacy alive and well.

Step 2: Keep Your Body Healthy

It's hardly a coincidence that the line "Not tonight, I have a headache" has become a catchall cliché for avoiding sex. If you don't feel good physically, you aren't going to want to have sex—and you probably won't enjoy it very much when you do.

How do you maintain or improve your "sexual fitness"? By doing the things that promote your health overall.

Eat a healthful diet. Apart from preventing illnesses and improving energy, a diet that's high in essential nutrients and low in fat will make you feel better—and maybe sexier—overall, says Lily A. Arya, MD, associate professor of obstetrics and gynecology at the University of Pennsylvania in Philadelphia.

Stay physically active. A 2009 University of Pittsburgh School of Medicine study of

The Pill versus Libido

When researchers from the Kinsey Institute for Research in Sex, Gender, and Reproduction, located in Bloomington, Indiana, followed 79 women who took birth control pills for a year, they found a life-altering side effect that women and their doctors usually don't mention: lowered libido and less sex.

"There's currently no way to predict which women will experience adverse sexual or emotional side effects or which pills are more likely to cause them. We each have our own individual chemistry," says Stephanie Sanders, PhD, associate director of the institute and associate professor of gender studies at Indiana University, also in Bloomington. "The important message is this: If you like the convenience and reliability of oral contraceptives, you can usually work with your doctor to find a pill that's right for you—if you let her know what it is that's bothering you."

What's going on: The Pill can inhibit testosterone (the male hormone that promotes sexual feelings) and other male hormones and increase sex hormone-binding protein, which attaches itself to testosterone and makes it impossible for it to latch on to and stimulate cells—and your desire.

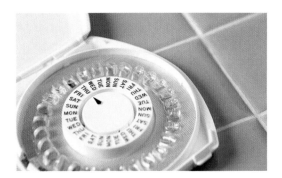

Here's how to preserve your sex life without discontinuing the Pill.

Discuss your symptoms with your doctor. Research shows that health professionals rarely discuss the emotional and sexual side effects of the Pill with their patients. Speak up.

Don't skip a dose. In addition to the obvious—an unplanned pregnancy—missed doses or irregular timing may cause hormonal fluctuations that could dampen your mood and sex drive.

Consider a switch. There are dozens of different birth control pills sold in the United States. If one pill causes side effects, you can try another or switch to a nonhormonal form of contraceptive, such as an intrauterine device (IUD) or a diaphragm. ∎

women ages 41 to 68 found that they enjoyed sex more if they were more physically active. "The better your health, the better your sexuality," says Sheryl Kingsberg, PhD, psychologist and chief of behavioral medicine, University Hospitals Case Medical Center at Case Western Reserve University in School of Medicine in Cleveland. "Exercise relieves stress, increases energy, and puts you in touch with your body. Plus, if you're in better shape and feel great, you'll want to share that with someone else." Aim for 30 minutes most days of the week.

Reduce stress. You may want to try a little yoga, which combines exercise with relaxation. Always end with "corpse pose"—the one in which you lie still and face up. It sounds easy, but it's not, says Ellen Barrett, author of *Sexy Yoga*, because the aim is to quiet your mind. That means no unwanted thoughts (to-do lists, work issues, relationship problems) that can get in the way of intimacy and arousal.

Protect yourself. Nothing dampens ardor faster than the thought of an unwanted pregnancy or sexually transmitted diseases. Your best move: Choose an effective form of contraception and, if you don't have one committed partner, always use a latex condom, whether or not you use other forms of birth control, says Michael Plaut, PhD, associate professor of psychiatry at the University of Maryland School of Medicine in Baltimore and past president of the Society for Sex Therapy and Research. Fortunately, many sexually active couples are heeding this advice; many common STDs are on the decline, including human immunodeficiency virus (HIV), which causes AIDS.

Step 3: Give Nature an Assist

Lack of desire is the most common sexual problem for women. This may be caused by issues in the relationship, but it can also result from physical changes or underlying health problems. Breast-feeding, for example, lowers your body's production of three chemicals you need for a robust sex life—the hormones estrogen and testosterone and the brain chemical dopamine. They're all sublimated for prolactin, the hormone you need for milk production.

Menopause is prime time for libido to vanish, along with your estrogen. For one thing, sex may become painful because of vaginal dryness. Insomnia can make you too tired to make love. Low moods may put sex and other things that once gave you pleasure on the back burner. Or you may be taking a medication or have an undiagnosed physical ailment that affects your sex drive.

Start with lubrication. The vagina naturally produces less lubrication as menopause approaches; women who take low-dose birth control pills or who are breast-feeding also may be too dry for comfort. Don't let this slow you down. Pharmacies stock a variety of water-based lubricants that are safe and comfortable to use, says Dr. Saks. You can also use topical estrogens such as Estrace, though studies show that just having sex regularly can help keep you feeling "juicy."

Look into side effects. A number of medications—including some antidepressants, birth control pills, and drugs for controlling blood pressure—may inhibit sex drive in some women. If you've noticed a dip in your libido, ask your doctor if switching to a different prescription would be helpful, says Dr. Saks.

Ask about hormone tests. If your thyroid gland is underactive, you may have decreased levels of androgens, hormones that fuel the sex drive. Conversely, high levels of prolactin, a female hormone, also can cause libido to diminish. Your doctor can check hormone levels with a simple blood test. If they're lower (or higher) than they should be, you may need medications to restore the proper balance.

Spice it up. Since having sex makes you want to have sex, schedule time to cuddle with your honey whether you're motivated or not. If sex has become perfunctory, do something different, or in some place you've never done it before. Fantasize about sex with your partner, which will help arouse you. Women's prime erogenous zone is the brain.

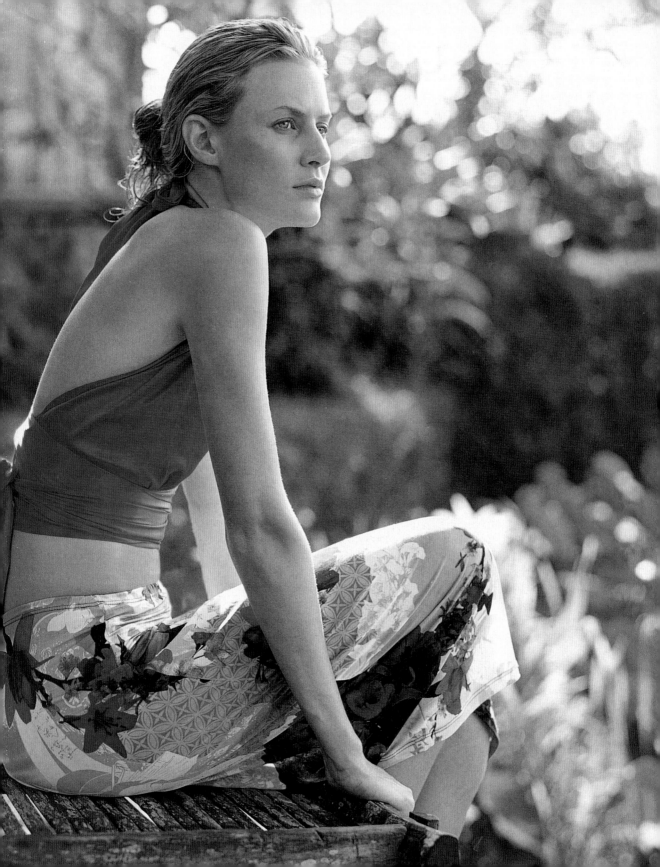

PRIMARY CARE:

ESSENTIAL

PROTECTION

Heart Disease

If you're like most women, breast cancer tops your list of health worries. But heart disease is more likely to claim your life. In fact, it kills 6 times as many women as breast cancer and is the leading cause of death—for both men and women—in the United States.

More than one in two women will die from a stroke, heart attack, or other forms of cardiovascular disease. Yet it's among the most preventable diseases. Studies have shown that women who follow a healthy lifestyle—refraining from smoking, exercising regularly, eating a healthy diet, reducing stress—can slash their risk of heart disease by 82 percent.

Even if you're premenopausal, don't put off taking care of your heart. More than one in five women who have heart attacks are under age 65.

A woman's heart disease risk does increase as she gets older. After menopause, when the body's production of estrogen declines, there's an increase in atherosclerosis—the accumulation of fatty deposits in the arteries that can reduce blood flow and increase the risk of heart-damaging clots. But atherosclerosis actually starts much earlier.

"We see the beginnings of it in teenagers," says Rose Marie Robertson, MD, chief science officer of the American Heart Association and professor of medicine at Vanderbilt University Medical Center in Nashville. "Many women have the sense that they don't need to worry about heart disease until after menopause. But they may be ignoring risk factors that could be treated, such as high blood pressure or high cholesterol, because they don't think they have to worry about them yet."

Here's what the country's leading cardiologists say women should be doing, right now, to protect their hearts.

Lifestyle Strategies

Maintain a healthful weight. For every 8.8 pounds you gain, your risk of heart disease goes up by more than 50 percent, according to a 2010 Danish study that looked at combined data from three studies tracking 81,000 women and men. Women who are overweight are much more likely to develop diabetes, a major risk factor for heart disease. People with diabetes have heart disease death rates 2 to 4 times higher than people without the disease. Obesity also increases cholesterol and blood pressure and puts more strain on the heart.

Your scale, your clothes, and the mirror will tell you if you're overweight. But how your weight is distributed can tell you how it may be affecting your health. Belly fat, for example, may be worse for your heart and other organs than having thunder thighs or saddlebags. The fat that lies deep within your abdomen, called visceral fat, is biologically active, secreting hormones that can raise your cholesterol, increase your desire to overeat, boost your blood sugar, and damage tissues. A recent study found 20 new hormones and other previously unknown chemicals in the fat cells of belly pooches. To be healthy, a woman's waist size should be under 35 inches. Doctors also often use the body mass index (BMI) to determine how close you are to your ideal weight. You'll find a detailed guide to calculating BMI on page 98. For now, just remember that your BMI should fall somewhere between 18.5 and 24.9. If your waistline is larger than 35 inches and if your BMI is above 25, it's time to get serious about losing weight.

If you follow the guidelines in Chapter 6, you'll find that losing weight doesn't have to be an all-consuming chore—and the more you lose, the healthier your heart will be.

Get serious about exercise. Every woman knows that exercise is important for health, but people don't always realize just how damaging a sedentary lifestyle can be, says Lori J. Mosca, MD, PhD, associate professor of medicine and director of preventive cardiology at New York

Angina: Heed this Warning Sign

about 4 million women suffer from angina, a condition that may cause chest pain or other symptoms that occur when narrowed blood vessels prevent the heart from getting all the blood and oxygen that it needs. Women are nearly twice as likely as men to get angina. In a way, angina may be a good thing because it's often a clue that a woman is developing heart disease.

"Often there's not actually a sensation you would call 'pain' with angina, but rather a deep discomfort or tightness under the breastbone that can radiate up to the shoulder or jaw," says Rose Marie Robertson, MD, chief medical officer of the American Heart Association and professor of medicine at Vanderbilt University Medical Center in Nashville. The lack of suffi-

cient blood flow to the heart that causes angina symptoms can also result in fatigue or shortness of breath. It usually comes on when you're doing something physical and subsides when you're at rest. "Hopefully, angina will lead a woman to seek medical attention before things become worse."

If you experience any of the pain or other symptoms associated with angina and they last for more than 5 minutes, call 9-1-1. You could be having a heart attack and need medical attention right away.

Angina doesn't always mean that surgery or angioplasty is needed, Dr. Robertson adds. It can often be treated with medications, although some women may need surgery to improve blood flow to the heart. ∎

Presbyterian Hospital of Columbia University in New York City. Women who are sedentary have about twice the risk of heart disease as those who are physically active. In fact, not getting regular exercise is potentially as harmful as smoking or having high cholesterol.

The American Heart Association recommends getting moderate-to-vigorous aerobic exercise for at least 30 minutes on most days of the week at 50 to 85 percent of your maximum heart rate. Don't think you don't have the time to spare: Although one longer daily walk of 30 minutes is preferable, women who exercise 3 times daily for 10 minutes each time will get measurable cardiovascular benefits, too. You don't need to run marathons. Studies have shown that even modest levels of activity can make a real difference. Women who walk, ride a bike, or exercise at the gym for 30 minutes most days of the week can achieve nearly the same health benefits as those who go all out, says Dr. Robertson.

In addition to helping you lose weight, lower your blood pressure, and improve heart function (the heart, after all, is a muscle), regular moderate exercise can help keep your arteries healthy and flexible. Having arteries that are more elastic keeps blood pressure down and can increase blood flow if you do have blockages. (Want to know how flexible your arteries are? A 2009 study found a correlation between how well people can do the "sit and reach" exercise—in which you sit on the floor with your legs in front of you and reach for your toes—and how elastic their arteries were.)

It doesn't really take much to keep your arteries and heart healthy. You don't even have to do "formal" exercise to protect your heart. "Vacuuming can be exercise if you do it vigorously," says Dr. Robertson. So can gardening, making the beds, or

Good News for Chocolate Lovers

Who says heart-healthy eating has to be dull? Researchers have found that chocolate contains chemical compounds called antioxidants, which prevent harmful oxygen molecules in the body from damaging cholesterol—the process that makes it more likely to stick to artery walls. (It shouldn't be surprising; chocolate comes from the cocoa bean, which is actually a seed.)

Chocolate is so effective, in fact, that it blocks free radicals better than green tea, grape juice, or blueberries, all of which are potent antioxidants. As a bonus, the active compounds in chocolate, called flavonoids, make the blood thinner and may reduce the risk of harmful clots in the arteries. Studies have found it also lowers blood pressure and improves blood sugar levels in diabetics.

Of course, chocolate is high in sugar, calories, and fat. While it may have some benefits, it's not a replacement for fresh vegetables, legumes, or other wholesome foods. But as an everyday treat? Yes—with a caveat.

"The key is moderation," says Carl L. Keen, PhD, professor of nutrition and internal medicine at the University of California Davis. "For the average person who's physically fit, having an occasional cup of cocoa or a bar of chocolate can be part of a healthy diet." ∎

putting away clothes and clutter, especially if you have to take the stairs. "Look for opportunities to exercise throughout the day," she adds. This might involve walking around the perimeter of your office building on your lunch hour, taking stairs instead of elevators, and walking to the corner store instead of hopping in the car and driving. "Taking a dog for a walk is great, too, whether you have a dog or not," Dr. Robertson suggests. Offer to walk your neighbor's pooch.

If you smoke, quit. The risk of heart disease in smokers is 2 to 4 times higher than in non-smokers. As every ex-smoker knows, quitting is hard; it may be the hardest thing you've ever done. But the payoff is dramatic. If you haven't been able to quit smoking on your own, talk to your doctor about starting a stop-smoking program. (For more information on getting cigarettes out of your life, see Chapter 8.) It's also important to avoid secondhand smoke. Studies have been consistent: Exposure to someone else's tobacco smoke can cause a heart attack; even brief exposure may trigger one.

Consider aspirin. Studies have shown that this over-the-counter painkiller thins the blood and reduces the risk of heart-damaging blood clots. But the jury is still out on whether aspirin prevents heart attacks in women the way it does in men. However, taking a baby aspirin (81 mg) daily does reduce the risk of one kind of stroke in women by about 17 percent and will improve survival in women with stable heart disease.

WHAT WORKS FOR ME

LORI J. MOSCA, MD, PHD, *associate professor of medicine and director of preventive cardiology at New York Presbyterian Hospital of Columbia University in New York City, has seen too many women suffering unnecessarily from heart disease. In her own life, she does everything possible to keep her heart and arteries healthy.*

I definitely practice what I preach in terms of heart health. No matter how busy the family gets, we have a couple of priorities. We sit down every night and eat well together—and we exercise together, too.

We always cook meals that are heart healthy. The meals might include salad, soup, and a main course—something like a stir-fry made with garlic, olives, capers, broccoli, and chicken, served over pasta.

One trick I've learned is to do a lot of cooking on Sundays. I make things like soup or pasta sauce and store them in plastic containers. That way, if we're stretched for time during the week, we don't have to cook hamburgers. We can take something out of the freezer, make a quick salad, and have a nutritious meal.

I always find time to exercise. I work out in the mornings before I wake my two boys. As a competitive Ironman triathlete, I do 20 minutes of swimming, 20 minutes of biking, and 30 to 40 minutes on the treadmill. One day a week, I do strength training, and another day I take a stretching class. I also swim with my kids regularly, and I ride a bike with my husband.

Exercise helps me unwind, too. Sometimes I run through the nature center near our home and listen to the frogs and birds. It's so serene. I love the feeling of the sun on my back and the wind through my hair. ∎

WHEN BAD THINGS HAPPEN TO HEALTHY WOMEN

She Woke Up with a Heart Attack, Not the Flu

Nancy Loving woke up early one morning because she was nauseated, light-headed, and achy. She figured it was the flu and tried to get back to sleep. But the symptoms kept getting worse, so she decided to go to the emergency room—and that's what saved her life.

"The next thing I knew, a doctor was leaning over me, telling me I was having a heart attack," says Loving, executive director of WomenHeart: The National Coalition for Women with Heart Disease in Washington, DC. "I was 48 years old and never had any symptoms. I didn't even know that women had heart attacks."

While she was in the hospital, Loving learned that her cholesterol was a frightening 313 mg per deciliter. Obviously, she had suffered from high cholesterol for years, but none of her doctors had ever discussed her choles-

terol or her risk for heart disease—despite the fact that she had been a smoker and that her father and three uncles had all died young of heart attacks.

For 3 years after the heart attack, Loving was terrified of what might happen next. She was, she admits, a "basket case." "The doctors offered no counseling or support groups," she says.

Loving finally took charge of her recovery. She quit her high-powered job as a public relations executive and set up a small agency in her home. She now swims 4 or 5 days a week, and she tries to walk for 30 minutes every day.

"I was a driven, type A workaholic before the heart attack," she says. "Now I'm a lot more careful about how I spend my time, and I try to keep the stress levels down. I take bubble baths, listen to music, and read. I give myself permission to put my health first." ∎

Talk to your doctor about whether aspirin therapy is right for you. Aspirin can cause bleeding.

Nutritional Treatments

Eat 5–9 servings of fruits and vegetables each day. Women who follow this simple advice can dramatically reduce their risk for heart disease.

What makes fruits and vegetables so powerful? They're packed with antioxidants—powerful plant chemicals that block the effects of free radicals,

harmful oxygen molecules in the body that make cholesterol more likely to stick to artery walls. Fruits and vegetables are high in fiber, which helps remove cholesterol from the body. They're also filling, which means that you'll be less likely to fill up on other, less healthy foods, and avoid obesity, a major risk factor for type 2 diabetes, which itself ups your risk of cardiovascular disease. Studies have also found that high intake of produce lowers blood pressure, another top-ranking risk factor for heart attack and stroke.

The American Heart Association recommends

that women eat at least five servings each of fruits and vegetables daily, up to nine depending on their calorie intake. (Most Americans eat three.) "It's so simple, it's unbelievable," says Dr. Mosca. Don't let the numbers scare you. A serving is only about a cup for most fresh or cooked vegetables. For leafy greens such as lettuce and spinach, a serving is 2 cups and for dried fruit, only ½ cup.

Large studies of both women and men have found that people who average eight or more servings of produce a day are 30 percent less likely to have a heart attack or stroke. (Having five lowers risk by 20 percent.) While all vegetables and fruit are good, some are more likely to confer major benefits. Those include green leafy vegetables such as spinach, lettuce, Swiss chard and mustard greens; cruciferous vegetables such as broccoli, cauliflower, cabbage, brussels sprouts, and kale; and citrus fruits such as oranges, lemons, limes, and grapefruit.

Cut back on fat. This includes cooking oils, butter, and lard, as well as fatty foods such as red meats, fast foods, and rich desserts and snacks. The fats in foods—especially saturated fats and trans fatty acids—raise blood cholesterol levels and increase the risk of heart disease.

Women should limit total fat intake to 25 percent of total calories; 20 percent is even better. In addition, do everything you can to restrict your intake of saturated fat—the kind found in red meat, regular milk, and other animal foods—to no more than 7 percent of total calories. Keep trans fats at less than 1 percent.

Study after study has shown that women who limit their consumption of animal foods and fill up on fruits and vegetables can dramatically lower the risk of heart disease, says C. Noel Bairey Merz, MD, director of the Cedars-Sinai Preventive and Rehabilitative Cardiac Center in Los Angeles. In fact, a 2010 study by researchers at the Harvard School of Public Health found that replacing saturated fat in the diet with unsaturated fat reduces the risk of heart disease by 19 percent. The DASH diet, or "dietary approaches to stop hypertension," which emphasizes produce and low-fat foods to lower blood pressure, also reduces heart attack risk by 18 percent.

Follow the Mediterranean example. Even though people in Italy, Greece, and other Mediterranean countries consume more fat than Americans, their rates of heart disease are a fraction of what they are in this country. What are they doing differently?

For one thing, they consume very little saturated fat. They enjoy meat, but they have much smaller portions than Americans do. Much of the fat in their diets comes from olive oil, which contains heart-healthy monounsaturated fats. They also eat large amounts of whole grains, fresh fruits and vegetables, and other plant foods. As a result, the Mediterranean diet is among the healthiest in the world, says Stephen T. Sinatra, MD, a cardiologist at New England Heart Center in Manchester, Connecticut, and assistant clinical professor at the University of Connecticut School of Medicine in Farmington.

Sip a little wine with meals. Or pour a glass of grape juice. They contain chemical compounds called flavonoids, which have been shown to reduce fatty buildups in the arteries and reduce the risk of heart disease. Researchers at the University of Michigan report that even eating grapes can help lower risks of both type 2 diabetes and heart disease. In their animal study, grapes lowered blood pressure, improved heart function, and reduced physical indicators of inflammation in rats that also experienced lower triglycerides and better glucose tolerance, a measure of how the body handles dietary sugars.

Eat more fish. It's among the most powerful strategies for preventing heart disease. One study found that men who ate mackerel, herring, salmon, or other fish several times a week were 34 percent less likely to die from heart disease than those who ate less. The results are assumed to apply to women as well.

Prevention recommends eating fish twice a week. If you don't care for fish, take fish oil supplements. Look for products that contain docosahexaenoic acid, or DHA. The recommended dose is 300 mg daily, more if you already have heart disease. Talk to your doctor about the dose that's right for you. There is also some evidence that taking fish oil with a cholesterol-lowering statin drug reduces risk of a coronary event by as much as 19 percent.

Mind-Body Techniques

Keep stress under control. Studies have shown that women with high levels of stress in their lives may have a higher risk of heart disease, says Dr. Bairey Merz. If you're in a demanding job, you could have a 56 percent

The Couples Connection

marriage is about sharing— everything from tackling the daily chores and caring for the children to making the monthly mortgage payment.

Now there's some evidence that sharing may go further than anyone imagined. If your husband has heart disease, your risk for getting it may also be high.

In one study, researchers surveyed 177 couples in Oklahoma and Washington 2 months after the husband had either had a heart attack or undergone open-heart surgery. They found that even though spouses didn't share the same physical risk factors as their husbands—they were unlikely to have high cholesterol or elevated blood pressure, for example—they often shared unhealthy lifestyle habits, such as smoking or being overweight.

In some cases, the wives had even greater risks than their husbands after the initial hospitalization because they didn't always join their husbands in adopting heart-healthy habits. After the hospitalizations, in fact, the women were twice as likely as the men to continue smoking.

Of course, just as couples may share bad habits, they can also work together as a team to reverse them, says Lynn C. Macken, MSN, RN , coordinator of cardiac and pulmonary rehabilitation at the Regional West Medical Center in Scottsbluff, Nebraska, and one of the study researchers.

"It's not easy to change these kinds of risky behaviors, but when couples work together, it's probably easier to do," Macken says. ■

greater chance of having a heart attack or stroke than a woman with less stress on the job.

You can't eliminate stress, of course, but you can take steps to keep it under control—by exercising, practicing yoga or meditation, or simply taking some deep breaths during the day.

Accept what you can't change. Stress itself doesn't necessarily increase the risk of heart disease, it's how you respond to it, says Dr. Robertson. "Many of the things we get stressed out about just aren't that important. You have to step back and ask yourself, 'Am I going to let this bother me or not?'"

Don't skip the annual vacation. A recent study showed that men who took annual vacations were less likely to die of heart disease than those who kept their noses to the grindstone. The same applies to women. It makes sense because few things reduce stress more quickly than taking a vacation. In addition, vacations are a good way to spend quality time with family and friends, and studies have shown that maintaining social connections is an important strategy for keeping the heart healthy.

Take mini-breaks. To combat job stress, "take a break during the workday, even if it's only 5 minutes," suggests Helen Coons, PhD, clinical associate professor of psychiatry at Drexel University School of Medicine in Philadelphia. "Get up and stretch and remind yourself to breathe deeply. When you're stressed you're more likely to hold your breath, which can make you feel dizzy and panicky. If you have a lunch hour, go for a walk. And if you can't go on a week's vacation, take a long weekend to recharge."

Let go of anger. The same goes for chronic hostility and irritability. If you're always on edge and ready to snap at people or overreact to difficult situations, your heart may be paying the price.

"Studies show that the less angry and hostile you are, the less your blood pressure responds when you're provoked," says Dr. Robertson. "Having a positive, optimistic view of the world is clearly good for you."

WHAT WORKS FOR ME

ALICE H. LICHTENSTEIN, SCD, *nutrition professor at Jean Mayer USDA Human Nutrition Research Center on Aging at Tufts University in Boston and a spokesperson for the American Heart Association, believes that you don't have to make dramatic changes in your eating and exercise habits to keep your heart healthy.*

Make small changes by eating a little less and exercising a little more.

When preparing dinner, and at other times when hunger's likely to strike, I keep clementines, carrots, and raw snow peas on hand. That way, I'm less tempted to eat high-fat, high-calorie fare. I cook with small portions of lean cuts of meat, and I choose fat-free milk, reduced-fat cheese, and fat-free yogurt. And I skip butter and other spreads altogether.

To get more exercise, I make it a point always to use the stairs, and I take them to and from my fifth-floor office several times every workday. ∎

But don't bury momentary irritation or anger. Studies have found that speaking your mind sometimes can cut your body's production of the stress hormone, cortisol, which is linked to obesity and heart disease. Anger isn't always a negative emotion. It can make you feel in control, which can counteract any helplessness or vulnerability you feel, which is also stressful.

Get in touch with your spiritual side. Research has shown that people who are spiritual have a lower risk of heart disease than those who don't practice a religion or cultivate spiritual beliefs.

"Spirituality provides important support in many ways," says Dr. Robertson. "It allows you to take a bad event and put it in a different perspective. It allows you to have less fear and anxiety, and it provides solace. Going to church also performs a very important social function by providing a sense of community."

Medical Options

Many of the things that increase the risk of heart disease, such as smoking, gaining weight, or not getting enough exercise, are easy for women to recognize—and reverse—on their own. But other types of risk factors are "silent"—you won't know you have them unless you work with your doctor.

"The first step in taking action against heart disease is to identify all your risk factors, but many women have nowhere near the awareness that they need," says Dr. Mosca.

Some risk factors you can't change, of course. If you have a family history of heart disease, you can't just drop out of your family. But other risk factors can be controlled—if you know you have them. That's why it's important to discuss your concerns about heart disease with your doctor.

Don't wait for your doctor to bring it up, Dr.

Women's Heart Attack Symptoms: When to See a Doctor

heart attack symptoms are usually the same in both men and women. They include:

- Pain, pressure, fullness, discomfort or squeezing in the center of the chest
- Shortness of breath or difficulty breathing
- Stabbing chest pain
- Pain radiating to shoulders, neck, back, arms or jaw
- Pounding heartbeats or feeling extra heartbeats
- Upper abdominal pain
- Nausea, vomiting, or severe indigestion

- Sweating for no apparent reason
- Dizziness with weakness
- Anxiety or panic

But about a third of women have no chest pain and 71 percent have flu-like symptoms for 2 weeks to a month before having their first bout of chest pain. If you're at risk of heart disease, watch out for these milder symptoms and call your doctor or go to the emergency room if you experience them. If you think you're having a heart attack, call 9-1-1 and say, "I think I'm having a heart attack." Chew an uncoated aspirin immediately to help reduce heart damage. ■

Mosca adds. Many doctors aren't aware that women, including premenopausal women, can have a high risk for heart disease. "Women need to ask questions. Always ask your doctor what your risk factors are and what you can do about them."

Heart disease in women can often be predicted years or even decades before it occurs, adds Dr. Bairey Merz. "But if you don't know you have high cholesterol or high blood pressure, you'll have missed the opportunity to prevent future problems."

Get regular blood pressure checks. High blood pressure has been called a silent disease because it doesn't cause symptoms at first. By the time it does, damage to the arteries has already occurred. It's essential to get your blood pressure checked regularly, because high blood pressure boosts the heart's workload and greatly increases the risk of heart disease and other cardiovascular problems.

You want your blood pressure to be under 120/80. If your blood pressure has climbed to 140/90 or higher, it's essential to take fast action–by exercising, limiting salt intake, losing weight if you need to, or taking medications.

Keep an eye on cholesterol. If you were to do only a few things to protect your heart, maintaining healthful levels of cholesterol would certainly be near the top of the list.

Cholesterol, also known as lipids, enters the bloodstream every time you eat. Over time, the fatty molecules are taken up into artery walls, where they restrict blood flow, promote the development of blood clots, and greatly increase the risk of heart attack and other cardiovascular conditions.

According to the latest guidelines from the American Heart Association, here's what you should strive for.

- Total cholesterol: Keep it under 200 mg per deciliter. Women whose cholesterol is between 200 and 239 mg per deciliter are considered to have borderline high cholesterol; those whose cholesterol is above 240 are putting their hearts at serious risk. Keep in mind that a total cholesterol reading over 200 may not be a bad thing if your HDLs are high (50 or above).

- LDL: It stands for low-density lipoprotein, the "bad" cholesterol. Ideally, your LDL should be below 100 mg per deciliter.

- HDL: Shoot for keeping your high-density lipoprotein, the "good" cholesterol, at 50 mg per deciliter or above. Levels under 40 put you at considerable risk for heart disease. Having low HDL levels are a stronger risk factor for women than men. The best way to raise good cholesterol levels is by exercising briskly 30 minutes a day, which has been shown to boost them by about 5 percent. It can also help you lose weight, another boost for the good cholesterol.

- Triglycerides: Keep them under 150 mg per deciliter. These fats tend to be sensitive to diet. Eating too many simple carbohydrates and sugary foods can send them soaring. Fish oil can bring them down, though in higher dosages.

Many doctors believe that the ratio of total cholesterol to HDL is more accurate than total cholesterol alone as a marker for heart disease. To determine your ratio, divide your total cholesterol reading by your HDL number. The

Framingham Cardiovascular Institute recommends a total cholesterol/HDL ratio below 4.

Keep in mind that these guidelines are variable, depending on other risk factors you may have. If your doctor says your risk for heart disease is low to moderate, for example, it may be acceptable to have an LDL reading of up to 160. If you have multiple risk factors for heart disease, on the other hand, you'll want to keep LDL below 100.

These days, there's no reason for most people to have high cholesterol. Apart from lifestyle changes, such as lowering your intake of saturated fat, there are a number of very effective cholesterol-lowering drugs that can bring the numbers down to a healthy level.

Ask your doctor for a blood protein test. Scientists have identified a number of proteins in the body that can increase (or decrease) your risk for heart disease. One type of protein, called apolipoprotein B (apoB), causes cholesterol and other fatty substances to stick to artery walls. Another protein, apolipoprotein A (apoA-1), scavenges fat and cholesterol from the blood and transports it to the liver for disposal.

In a study of more than 1,000 people who had suffered a heart attack, those with low levels of apoA and high levels of apoB were four times more likely to have a second heart attack than those with a healthier protein balance. If test results indicate you have a low apoA-1 level or a high apoB level, a low-fat diet, regular exercise, and cholesterol-lowering medications can help.

Think twice about hormone replacement therapy (HRT). If you were considering taking it to help protect your heart, don't. Although it was once thought that estrogen replacement would help prevent heart attacks, results from a number of large recent studies found that rather than being protective, HRT actually increased the risk of coronary heart disease and stroke.

Statins: Are They for You?

Statin drugs, which shut off cholesterol production in the liver, lower the risk of death over 4 to 5 years even in people without diagnosed heart disease. Because they also reduce inflammation, they're effective in people with low cholesterol but who have elevated levels of C-reactive protein, an inflammation marker. And they lower death rates in people with diabetes. But should you take a statin if you're healthy? National Cholesterol Education Program guidelines suggest that women with two or more risk factors for heart disease should consider taking one. That's something you'll have to decide with the help of your physician.

While statin drugs have relatively few side effects, there is a small risk of liver and muscle damage, pain, and weakness. If you can't take a statin drug, there's emerging evidence that a Chinese remedy, red yeast rice can lower cholesterol significantly—LDL (bad) cholesterol by 35 mg per deciliter on the average with no side effects. That's as good as a moderate dose of statins.

But like statins, red yeast rice can cause liver damage, so check your liver enzymes twice a year. Caution: A 2010 study found that 4 out of 12 products contained citrinin, a contaminant that causes kidney damage in animals. Talk to your doctor about trying this statin alternative. ∎

14

High Blood Pressure and Stroke

Often called the "silent killer," high blood pressure, or hypertension, doesn't cause any symptoms in the early stages. Even when your numbers reach potentially dangerous levels, you probably won't feel different than you did before.

But even in the absence of symptoms, the force of blood roiling through the arteries will be doing serious damage. Unless high blood pressure is diagnosed and treated early, it can lead to a host of cardiovascular conditions, including stroke and heart disease, says Debra R. Judelson, MD, a clinical cardiologist and medical director of the Women's Heart Institute at the Cardiovascular Medical Group of Southern California in Beverly Hills.

About one in four Americans has high blood pressure, and more than a third of them don't know it. One in every five adult women in the United States has high blood pressure, and more than 60 percent of all deaths from stroke are women. Women often enjoy healthy blood pressure levels until they reach menopause. Then, when their estrogen levels decline, blood pressure starts creeping upward—and the women won't even suspect there's a problem.

Understanding the Numbers

Blood pressure measures the force with which blood travels through blood vessels. The numbers typically start to rise when artery walls thicken, constrict, or lose their elasticity, which makes it harder for blood to push through them. In the majority of cases, the change in blood vessels occurs long before actual changes in blood pressure can be detected. There's usually no known cause; only about 10 percent (or fewer) of cases of high blood pressure can be attributed to specific conditions, such as kidney or blood vessel abnormalities.

You don't want your blood pressure to be too low because that can result in dizziness or fatigue. But for most women, the lower the blood pressure, the healthier they'll be, says Marilyn M. Rymer, MD, medical director of the Brain and Stroke Institute at Saint Luke's Hospital in Kansas City, Missouri, where she is also director of research.

When you get your blood pressure taken, there are two numbers to consider. The first, higher number measures systolic pressure—the pressure that's generated when the heart is pumping blood. The second, lower number measures diastolic pressure—the pressure when your heart rests between beats.

Here's what the readings mean.

■ Ideally, blood pressure should be below 120/80 mg per deciliter.

■ If your systolic pressure is 130 to 139, and the diastolic pressure is 85 to 89, you're heading into risky territory, especially if you have other risk factors for stroke or heart disease, such as obesity or a family history of high blood pressure, or if you're postmenopausal or African American.

■ A reading of 140/90 or higher means that it's time to take action. Even if only one of the numbers is high, you may need medical treatment.

BRINGING THE NUMBER DOWN

Many people require medications to control high blood pressure, but this isn't always necessary.

"With a healthy lifestyle, many women can prevent hypertension from developing—or at least reduce its severity," says Samuel J. Mann, MD, professor of clinical medicine at Weill Cornell Medical College in New York City and author of *Healing Hypertension: A Revolutionary New Approach*.

Here's what doctors advise.

Lifestyle Strategies

♀ **Maintain a healthful weight.** "Excess weight is the biggest risk factor for high blood pressure," says Matthew Gillman, MD, professor and director of the obesity prevention program in the department of population medicine at Harvard Medical School. Studies have shown, in fact, that men or women who lose as little as 10 pounds can send their blood pressure plummeting.

WHAT WORKS FOR ME

DEBRA R. JUDELSON, MD, *is a clinical cardiologist, medical director of the Women's Heart Institute at the Cardiovascular Medical Group of Southern California in Beverly Hills, and former president of the American Medical Women's Association. Here's what she does to make sure that her risks for high blood pressure and stroke are as low as they can possibly be.*

I eat fewer processed foods these days, and I also go for a brisk walk every morning before I shower. This is my thinking time. By the time I'm dressed and ready to leave the house, my day is already planned.

I've also worked to reduce the stress in my life—and not just by using relaxation techniques. I've changed my entire life.

I used to be a type A personality. I was working incredibly hard—always in a hurry. Then, just before I turned 45, I began wondering why I was working so hard. I realized that I was trying to make a lot of money to pay for a fancy house and fancy vacations or other things I really didn't need. But I wasn't necessarily reaching my goal of happiness.

I stopped the 80-hour weeks. I now keep my office time limited. Sometimes I go in at 9 o'clock—it gives me time to spend time with the kids in the morning. I don't rush very much anymore. I have a degree of peace and comfort throughout the day that sustains me. ■

The only way to lose weight is to consume fewer calories than you burn. You can do this by eating smaller servings, consuming fewer high-fat foods (fat contains more calories than protein or carbohydrates), and avoiding snack foods. "Portion size is important, and be aware that manufacturers of processed low-fat foods tend to replace the fat in those foods with sugars, which also contribute to weight gain," he notes. At the same time, you'll need to exercise regularly to burn off the calories you consume. "Concentrate on increased physical activity," Dr. Gillman recommends. (For more information on healthy weight loss, see Chapter 6.)

Keep your body moving. Even if you're at a healthful weight, regular exercise is among the best ways to prevent–or reverse–high blood pressure. Studies have shown, in fact, that men and women who are sedentary are 20 to 50 percent more likely to develop high blood pressure than those who are physically active.

How much exercise do you need? A total of at least 30 minutes a day of gardening, walking, jogging, bicycling, weight lifting, or other types of exercise is probably enough to keep blood pressure in check. (For more information on exercise, see Chapter 5.)

If you smoke, try to quit. Every time you light up, your blood pressure climbs–and it stays elevated for an hour or more afterward. (For information on how to quit smoking, see Chapter 8.)

Nutritional Treatments

Follow the DASH diet. It stands for "dietary approaches to stop hypertension," and it's considered one of the most effective ways to keep blood pressure in a healthful range. The diet calls for having:

- Eight to ten daily servings of fruits and vegetables (each about $\frac{1}{2}$ cup)

- Seven to eight daily servings of whole grains (one slice of bread, or about $\frac{1}{2}$ cup)

- Two to three daily servings of low-fat or fat-free dairy foods (each 1 cup, or $1\frac{1}{2}$ ounces)

- Two or fewer servings of meat (each about 3 ounces)

The DASH diet is so effective that one study found that men and women who followed the eating plan were able to lower their blood pressure as much as they would have had they taken prescription drugs.

For more information on the DASH diet, visit the National Heart, Lung, and Blood Institute's Web site at www.nhlbi.nih.gov.

Cut way back on salt. The government's dietary guidelines call for limiting salt consumption to 2,400 mg daily (1 teaspoon). However, several recent studies suggest that this number may be too high. When men and women without high blood pressure lowered their salt intake by about a third of the recommended limit–to $\frac{2}{3}$ teaspoon, or 1,500 mg–their systolic pressure fell by 7 millimeters; in those with high blood pressure, the drop was $11\frac{1}{2}$ millimeters. People who lowered salt intake and followed the DASH diet had even more improvement.

"We eat huge amounts of salt in this country because of all the processed foods," says Dr. Judelson. When buying soups or other processed foods, look for the words "low sodium" or "sodium free" on the label. Avoid ultra-salty foods such as chips, pickles, and soy sauce, and use the saltshaker sparingly.

If you must use salt, shake on a potassium salt (as opposed to sodium). A 2010 study in the *Archives of Internal Medicine* that looked at potassium intake in 21 countries found that those who had the most potassium in their diets had lower blood pressure. Switching from sodium to potassium salt—and increasing intake of potassium-rich vegetables and low-fat dairy—would reduce systolic pressure by between 1.7 and 3.2 mmHg. In one study, people who just replaced sodium with potassium lived longer and spent less money on medical care than those who stuck with sodium.

Eat fish 2 or 3 times a week. It's rich in omega-3 fatty acids, which have been shown to help lower blood pressure. Fatty fish has the largest amounts of omega-3s. This includes salmon, tuna, and sardines.

If you're not a fish eater, you can get the same beneficial fats by eating flaxseed or walnuts or using oils made with flaxseed, canola, or walnuts.

Imbibe moderately. Moderate drinking (one glass of wine or beer daily for women, two for men) won't affect blood pressure and has been shown in several studies to be good for your heart and arteries. Drinking to excess, however, can cause long-term rises in blood pressure, and more than a drink a day increases the risk of breast cancer. So if you do drink, limit yourself to about 1½ ounces of hard liquor, 5 ounces of wine, or a 12-ounce bottle of beer a day.

Indulge—a little—in chocolate. In 2010, Australian researchers looking at 15 previously published studies reported that the flavonol antioxidants in dark chocolate modestly reduce systolic blood pressure—the top number—in people with hypertension by about 5 mmHg, which is about the same drop you can get with 30 minutes of daily exercise. They estimated it could reduce the risk of a cardiovascular event by about 20 percent over 5 years.

Keep cholesterol in check. It makes the arteries less elastic, and it also leads to accumulations of fatty material, called plaque, on the artery walls—the cause of heart attacks. As the arteries narrow, blood moves through them with greater force.

The best way to control cholesterol is to avoid saturated fats in the diet and increase your consumption of whole grains, legumes, and other fiber-rich foods. (For more information on controlling cholesterol, see Chapter 13.)

Alternative Therapies

Drink hawthorn tea. It dilates blood vessels, which can result in modest drops in blood pressure, says Dr. Judelson.

To make a tea, steep 1 to 2 teaspoons of crushed herb in a cup of boiling water for 10 minutes. You can drink the tea several times daily.

Get in touch with "hidden" emotions. Stress isn't a confirmed risk factor for chronic high blood pressure, though it clearly sends blood pressure soaring in the moment. However, emotions that are held deep inside may boost blood pressure, at least in some women.

"One-quarter to one-third of the hypertension cases I see are related to repressed or, so to

WHEN BAD THINGS HAPPEN TO HEALTHY WOMEN

Job Stress Raised Her Blood Pressure

In retrospect, Brita Hudson-Smith shouldn't have been surprised that her blood pressure rose to 140/90. When she was in her early thirties, she suffered the death of her mother. She had also gained weight, and she had a family history of hypertension. At the time, however, she was shocked to find that her blood pressure was soaring,

"You don't really pay attention to your risks until it happens to you," she says.

Her doctor immediately put her on hypertension medication, but she didn't work very hard at making basic lifestyle changes until she left her high-stress job at a suburban Philadelphia health organization a few years later.

"I started walking every day," she says. "I got involved in my community, and I read books about health and spirituality. I also meditated every day and became a vegetarian. It took time, but my blood pressure went down even further."

But the changes didn't last. When she started a new job the following year, her health routine fell apart. Her blood pressure rose higher than it had ever been. In fact, she wound up in the hospital after a test revealed that her blood pressure had risen to an alarming 170/100.

Hudson-Smith admits that she struggles to find a balance between career demands and healthful living. "I keep saying a mantra to myself: 'I'm not going to let my job keep me from eating right and exercising.'"

She continues to take medication, but she also eases daily stress by visiting friends and doing things she enjoys, like flower arranging and going to the theater. "I know I don't have to do everything, that it's okay to let some things go," she says. "I write little notes to myself about the priorities in my life. I read them whenever I feel things getting crazy." ∎

speak, hidden emotions," says Dr. Mann. "These are people who have had childhood traumas or who cope with emotional stress by not dealing with it. They're the ones who are even-keeled, who never complain, and are actually less likely than most to feel depressed."

People whose hypertension is related to hidden emotions tend to achieve less success with blood pressure-lowering medication. "For some women, shifting attention to what has been hidden away can rapidly lower blood pressure.

Some can heal themselves, and others can benefit from consulting with a psychotherapist."

Meditate. Transcendental meditation—a form in which you meditate with the use of a word called a mantra, such as peace, God, or "om"—lowered blood pressure by as much as 7 points in a group of African American women, some of whom were able to reduce their use of high blood pressure medication as a result. One meta-analysis—a study that looks at a variety of published research on a subject—found that TM, as it's called, results in a 23 percent lower rate of premature death and 30 percent lower rate of cardiovascular disease deaths compared with groups that didn't meditate. For more information about TM, go to the Web site www.tm.org.

Medical Options

Ask your doctor to check your blood pressure twice. Nearly one in four people, including women, suffers from "white-coat hypertension." In other words, their blood pressure is usually normal, but it spikes when they visit the doctor, often because of simple anxiety. They could wind up being treated for hypertension that they don't have.

The opposite can also happen. It's normal for blood pressure to rise and fall periodically. It's possible for a woman to have normal blood pressure in the doctor's office, but soaring blood pressure at home.

"Always make sure that you really have hypertension before getting treated," advises Dr. Mann. The way to do this is to ask your doctor to take more than one blood pressure reading during your visit.

There is some evidence that people who regularly experience white coat hypertension do go on to have sustained high blood pressure, so make sure you and your doctor don't treat it as a benign condition. Buy a blood pressure cuff and periodically check your own pressure at home.

Consider medications. If you aren't able to control your blood pressure with lifestyle changes, your doctor will probably advise you to take pressure-lowering medications. There are many classes of drugs to choose from. Some of the main ones are:

- Diuretics. Also called "water pills," they cause the body to eliminate sodium and water, which causes blood pressure to fall. They're often used with other drugs to control blood pressure and may come paired with another drug in the same pill.

- Beta-blockers. They block the action of a body chemical called epinephrine, thereby slowing the heart rate and causing a drop in blood pressure.

- Calcium channel blockers. These drugs prevent calcium from entering the smooth muscle cells of your heart and arteries, which lowers the force of the heart's contraction. These drugs also relax and open up narrowed blood vessels and reduce heart rate.

- ACE inhibitors. Angiotensin-converting enzyme inhibitors, as their name suggests, help reduce the production of an enzyme that causes the arteries to narrow. They cause the blood vessels to stay dilated, allowing blood to flow with less force, lowering blood pressure.

- Angiotensin II receptor blockers. These drugs block the cell receptors for angiotensin, the enzyme that narrows the arteries, so it fails to constrict them.

- Alpha-blockers. They relax the muscle tone in the vascular walls.

- Alpha-2 receptor agonist. By decreasing the activity of the sympathetic (adrenaline-producing) nervous system, these drugs lower blood pressure and are often used in pregnancy since they have few adverse effects.

■ Central agonists. Though they act differently than alpha- and beta-blockers, these drugs accomplish the same results—lower blood pressure by decreasing the ability of the blood vessels to contract.

■ Vasodilators. They cause the muscles in the walls of the blood vessels to relax and widen, which allows blood to flow through more easily.

Blood pressure drugs are safe for most women, but they can cause a variety of side effects, including dizziness, dehydration, decreased levels of potassium, or sedation. They can even cause blood pressure to drop too low in some cases. Doctors usually resort to medications when lifestyle measures aren't effective, says Dr. Mann.

REDUCE YOUR RISK FOR STROKE

Heart disease and cancer get all the headlines, but stroke is the third leading cause of death in both men and women in the United States. Overall, one in six women will die of stroke, compared with one in 25 who will die from breast cancer. About 25 percent of those who suffer from strokes are younger than 65, and 60 percent are women.

"We've done such a good job of educating women about breast cancer, but stroke is much more common," says Dr. Rymer.

There are two main types of stroke: ischemic strokes, which occur when a blood clot blocks the flow of blood through an artery in the brain, and hemorrhagic strokes, which occur when brain blood vessels leak or burst.

The same strategies that lower blood pressure—

such as cutting back on salt and eating a low-fat diet—also reduce the risk of stroke. It makes sense because high blood pressure damages arteries throughout the body, including those in the brain. Other stroke-preventing strategies include the following.

Home Remedies

Quit smoking immediately. It's bad for blood pressure, and it's even worse for stroke. Studies have shown, in fact, that compared with nonsmokers, smokers have double the risk of having a stroke. If you quit, within 5 years your risk will be the same as that of a nonsmoker.

Take aspirin daily. It reduces the tendency of blood to form clots in the arteries, which can help prevent ischemic strokes (although it can raise your risk of hemorrhagic strokes slightly). Studies have found it lowers women's risk of ischemic stroke by 19 percent. Aspirin is usually advised for those who have already had a stroke or who have a high risk for having one. Even if your risk for stroke is low, you may want to take a daily baby aspirin, which contains 81 mg, says Dr. Rymer. Of course, check with your doctor to make sure daily aspirin is right for you.

Walk every day. Try to exercise every day for 30 minutes to reduce stroke risk.

Nutritional Treatments

Get extra B vitamins. They lower levels of a chemical in the body called homocysteine. "High homocysteine levels may be as risky as high cholesterol," explains Wayne M. Clark,

MD, director of the Oregon Stroke Center at Oregon Health Sciences University in Portland.

Leafy green vegetables and beans are among the best dietary sources of folate and vitamins B_6 and B_{12}. You may want to take supplements as well. Look for a multivitamin that contains 1 mg of folic acid, 25 mg of vitamin B_6, and 250 micrograms of vitamin B_{12}, Dr. Rymer advises.

Eat fish twice a week. Salmon, tuna, trout, mackerel, halibut—have two servings a week of these omega-3-rich fish to lower your risk of both stroke and heart attack.

when to see a doctor

If you experience migraine headaches that are preceded by difficulty talking or partial paralysis on one side of your body, call your doctor right away. These types of migraines mean you may have a slightly higher risk of stroke, says Wayne M. Clark, MD, director of the Oregon Stroke Center at Oregon Health Sciences University in Portland.

If you experience sudden numbness or weakness in the face, arms, or legs, or if you're having trouble speaking, walking, or maintaining your balance, get to an emergency room. You may have experienced a "mini-stroke" or stroke warning called a transient ischemic attack, which could potentially be followed by a full-fledged stroke.

If you notice that your pulse is irregular. This is sometimes caused by atrial fibrillation, an irregular heartbeat that increases the risk that blood clots will travel to the brain.

Limit sodium. Aim for less than a teaspoon of salt a day (1500 mg).

Medical Options

Treat depression. The Framingham Heart Study—one of the longest-running research projects of its kind—found a strong link between depression and stroke. Of 4,120 study participants, the risk for stroke or transient ischemic attack (mini-stroke) was 4.21 times greater among those under 65 who were depressed. Depression rates in women are twice those of men's. If you have depression symptoms—sadness, difficulty concentrating, feelings of hopelessness and pessimism, loss of interest in activities that were once pleasurable, thoughts of suicide—see a counselor who can help you with talk therapy or medication.

Don't go in for a second round. In an international study that followed 6,105 stroke survivors for 4 years, those who took the blood pressure drug perindopril (Aceon) plus the diuretic indapamide had 43 percent fewer second strokes than those who took placebos.

Twenty percent of stroke survivors will have another one within 5 years—and second strokes are often more disabling, or deadly. "Now, we're finally seeing evidence that secondary strokes can be prevented," says Stanley Rockson, MD, a cardiologist at Stanford University and a spokesman for the National Stroke Association. Discuss this with your doctor if you've had a stroke.

Diabetes

ctress Halle Berry, singer Patti LaBelle, author Anne Rice, tennis legend Billie Jean King and talk show hostess Sherri Shepherd have something in common: They all have diabetes. A few decades ago, a diagnosis of diabetes meant a lifelong sentence of dietary austerity, and a vastly increased risk of blindness, nerve damage, and other serious symptoms.

Things have improved dramatically since then. Diabetes is still a serious illness but, as these celebrities prove, it can almost always be controlled—and one type may even be prevented and possibly reversed through a combination of medications and lifestyle changes.

"Diabetes is a very manageable disease—but it does take some work," says Karen E. Friday, MD, an endocrinologist, clinical core director of Tulane Xavier National Center of Excellence in Women's Health, and associate professor of medicine at Tulane University School of Medicine in New Orleans.

Diabetes occurs either when the pancreas doesn't make enough insulin or when the insulin that is produced isn't efficiently used by the body's cells. Insulin is a hormone that transports glucose, the sugar found in foods, into the cells,

where it's the basic energy supply. (When you eat, your body breaks down sugars and starches into glucose.) When insulin is in short supply, the cells don't get all the glucose they need. Instead, the glucose accumulates in the blood. Small amounts of glucose are essential for health, but at high levels it literally becomes toxic. Uncontrolled high blood sugar can lead to kidney failure, blindness, stroke, nerve damage, and heart disease.

There are two main forms of diabetes. Type 1—formerly called juvenile-onset or insulin-dependent diabetes—occurs when the immune system destroys beta cells, insulin-producing cells in the pancreas, an organ located behind the stomach. Like rheumatoid arthritis, in which the body attacks healthy joints as though they were a foreign invader, type 1 diabetes is considered an autoimmune disease. It accounts for 5 to 10 percent of all diagnosed diabetes cases and is thought to be caused by genetic and environmental factors that trigger the immune system to mistakenly target healthy beta cells. People with type 1 diabetes need daily insulin shots or insulin delivered by a pump to manage their blood sugar.

The second form of diabetes, which accounts for 90 to 95 percent of all diabetes cases, is type 2, previously known as non-insulin-dependent or adult-onset diabetes. Those with type 2 have a condition called insulin resistance in which their bodies do not respond efficiently to insulin. Blame this one on lifestyle factors. People who are genetically susceptible and are overweight, eat a lot of processed foods, and don't get regular exercise have the highest risk of developing it. "It's mostly associated with obesity and sedentary lifestyles," says Mitchell A. Lazar, MD, director of Penn Diabetes Center at the University of Pennsylvania School of Medicine in Philadelphia.

Diabetes is now considered epidemic in the United States and it comes hand-in-hand with rising obesity rates. An estimated 25.8 million children and adults have diabetes; 79 million have prediabetes, a precursor to the full-blown disease, and about 7 million people with diabetes have not yet been diagnosed. As many as 25.6 percent of all women over the age of 20 have the disease.

There are some nonlifestyle-risk factors for type 2 diabetes. Those include a family history of the disease, age, and ethnicity: African Americans, Hispanics, and Native Americans are more likely than Caucasians to get type 2 diabetes. Women with a history of gestational diabetes—a type of diabetes that occurs during pregnancy and then disappears—and those who have had a baby with a birth weight exceeding 9 pounds are also at an increased risk for later developing type 2 diabetes.

If you have diabetes, one of the most important things you can do, apart from controlling it, is to keep an eye on your heart health. People with diabetes have a 2 to 4 times higher risk of heart disease, as well as stroke.

Almost before anything else, doctors advise people with diabetes to get their other risk factors under control. These include controlling body weight and blood pressure (be sure to keep it under 120/80 mg/dl), exercis-

Follow the Glycemic Index

the glycemic index or GI is a carb-controlled eating plan used widely in the United Kingdom to help prevent and control diabetes.

The index ranks foods based on their propensity to raise your blood sugar when you eat them. So foods such as white bread, potatoes, snack goods, fruit in heavy syrup, sugared sodas, and candy are considered high GI foods because they send blood sugar soaring. Low GI alternatives such as whole wheat bread, sweet pota-

toes, brown rice, peanuts, fresh fruit, soy or fat-free milk keep your blood sugar on an even keel.

You can think of them as good carbs and bad carbs. You can make them work for you by sticking to a diet that's rich in whole grains, fresh fruit, and vegetables. A 2008 Australian review study found that a low GI diet was linked to lower risk of diabetes and heart disease. Other studies have found links between high GI foods and postmenopausal breast cancer. ■

ing regularly, and maintaining healthy levels of cholesterol.

The National Cholesterol Education Program of the National Institutes of Health recommends that people with diabetes keep low-density lipoprotein (LDL, the "bad" cholesterol) below 100. After this goal is reached, women should then try to get their high-density lipoprotein (HDL, the "good" cholesterol) over 50, and keep their triglycerides under 150.

■ Pregnancy. About one in 20 pregnant women will develop gestational diabetes. Your doctor can screen for gestational diabetes around the sixth month of pregnancy. If you have it, you'll have to be especially vigilant about taking care of yourself later on.

Catch It Early, Treat It Well

The goal of treating type 2 diabetes is straightforward: to keep blood sugar levels as normal as possible with a combination of lifestyle changes, or with lifestyle changes plus medications, including insulin when necessary. Women with type 1 diabetes need to maintain a healthy lifestyle, too, and take insulin. If you have either type of diabetes, your doctor will also instruct you on how to monitor your blood sugar levels at home. Your physician also can check for kidney problems by measuring protein in the urine. This is important because diabetics have a higher risk of kidney disease. You should also go for yearly eye exams to check for early, treatable changes in the eyes.

The sooner diabetes is diagnosed, the better your chances of managing it effectively. Type 1 diabetes, if not well controlled, can lead to life-changing and life-threatening complications, including cataracts, damage to the blood vessels and nerves in the legs and feet, foot ulcers that can necessitate amputation, blindness and an increased risk of heart attack and stroke. An early diagnosis for type 2 diabetes is important because if it continues uncontrolled for years, the high glucose and insulin levels eventually destroy the pancreas so it can't produce a sufficient amount of insulin. Once the pancreas is no longer producing insulin, there may be no going back; you might require medications for the rest of your life. Of particular importance to women of child-bearing age: Nearly half of all women who have diabetes prior to becoming pregnant have a cesarean section that could have been avoided and their babies are twice as likely to die as those born to women without the disease. People with type 2 diabetes also have increased cancer risk.

"But type 2 diabetes may possibly be reversed in some people, up to a point, if they lose weight and exercise," says Katherine D. Sherif, MD, director of the Drexel Center for Women's Health and associate professor in the Division of Internal Medicine at Drexel University College of Medicine in Philadelphia. In some cases, in fact, people are able to quit taking medications once they make these fundamental lifestyle changes. To catch type 2 diabetes in its early stages, when it's most reversible and little damage has been done, you need to know its warning signs. This is especially important for women because they have a higher risk than men for developing heart disease as a result of diabetes. Here's what to look for:

Extreme thirst

Frequent urination

Fatigue

Blurred vision

Frequent or slow-healing infection

Increased appetite

The main symptoms of type 1 diabetes are unexplained weight loss and hunger, sometimes called "starvation in the midst of plenty." You may also have dry, itchy skin and a tingling or lack of feeling in your feet. But if you are at risk for either form of diabetes, see your doctor regularly for checkups, even if you don't have any symptoms.

What puts you at risk? In the case of type 2 diabetes, along with the risk factors mentioned earlier, having a family history, carrying a lot of weight around your midsection, a sedentary lifestyle, and a poor diet up your chance of getting the disease. Other factors include HDL levels of less than 35 mg per deciliter or triglyceride levels greater than 250 mg per deciliter; high blood pressure; and polycystic ovary syndrome (or PCOS, an imbalance of a woman's sex hormones that can cause menstrual cycle irregularities, acne, ovarian cysts, and infertility).

Preventing diabetes, of course, is a lot better than treating it later. Long before people actually develop the disease, the body's cells may become increasingly resistant to insulin, mainly because of poor lifestyle habits.

"If we could get people to restrict calories, exercise, and eat right, in theory we could prevent type 2 diabetes," says Francine Ratner Kaufman, MD, former president of the American Diabetes Association and head of the Center for Diabetes, Endocrinology and Metabolism at Children's Hospital of Los Angeles.

Must-Have Monitoring

If you have diabetes, get these five checks regularly. If your doctor's office has a diabetes educator on staff, he can help teach you how to do these.

- Blood sugar self-monitoring (daily)
- Blood test for glycosylated hemoglobin (at least once a year)
- Foot check for sores or ulcers (performed by your physician at least once a year)
- Eye screening for retinopathy, a condition that can lead to blindness (once a year)
- Lipid panel (total cholesterol, HDL, LDL, and triglycerides) to check heart disease risk (once a year) ■

Lifestyle Strategies

If you don't have diabetes, the following lifestyle tips will help ensure that you never get it. Even if you've already been diagnosed with diabetes, you can use this guide to help control your glucose levels, reduce symptoms, and generally keep the disease at a manageable level.

Control your weight. Even if you didn't inherit a propensity for overweight from your parents and grandparents, the tendency to overindulge and hold on to every last calorie is hardwired into the human genome.

"Our genes aren't that different from those in our caveman ancestors," says Dr. Kaufman. "If a bison came along only once a week, those genes enabled us to survive by storing calories incredibly efficiently. Now, with a convenience store on every corner and fast food everywhere, we're still storing those calories efficiently, but it leads to obesity."

The problem with obesity is that it increases the risk of insulin resistance. This means that it's more difficult for glucose to enter the body's cells. The glucose sits in the blood and starts to poison the blood vessels, nerves, and pancreas. Insulin resistance is more likely to occur when body fat is stored in the abdomen rather than in the hips or buttocks—but any fat accumulation may be a factor. As little as 20 extra pounds of fat can make you insulin resistant.

The best way to lose weight is to follow *Prevention*'s weight-loss guidelines, which are discussed in detail in Chapter 6. But one point is worth mentioning here: Diets that promise dramatic weight loss in a short period of time almost never succeed. Traditional diets, which involve a combination of physical activity and smart eating, may be slower, but they've been proven to work.

"I always try to be realistic when I advise a woman about weight loss. For example, I might say to aim for losing 10 percent of her weight over 6 months," says Dr. Sherif. "If you weigh 180, that means losing 18 pounds—which is just 3 pounds a month." And studies have found that even extremely overweight people were 70 percent less likely to develop diabetes when they lost just 5 percent of their weight, even without exercising.

If the diabetes is at an early stage and your body's cells and insulin levels are close to normal, losing as little as 10 pounds may be enough to keep your blood sugar from getting into the diabetic range, says Dr. Lazar. If you are able to control your blood sugar and keep your blood pressure down, you can significantly reduce your risk of death, stroke, heart failure, and other complications.

A height and weight chart—and your scale—can tell you if you're overweight. But you may also want to check your body mass index, or BMI. We discuss this is more detail in Chapter 6, but here's how it works. To find your BMI, multiply your weight in pounds by 703 and divide that number by your height in inches. Divide that number again by your height in inches, and you have your BMI. A BMI of 25 to 29.9 means that you're overweight. Anything above 30 is considered obese.

To make the calculations easier, check out the online BMI calculator of the National Heart, Lung, and Blood Institute. The Web address is www.nhlbisupport.com/bmi/bmicalc.htm.

Get regular exercise. It's among the best strategies for treating both types of diabetes, and evidence suggests it may also help prevent type 2 diabetes.

"Exercise has two beneficial effects. It alters muscle cells to improve their resistance to insulin, and it also allows sugar to get out of the blood into the skeletal muscle in the absence of insulin," says Dr. Lazar. If you exercise regularly, your cells will be less resistant to insulin and will take in more glucose, which in turn keeps blood sugar levels in a healthful range.

Getting regular exercise will also help you maintain a healthful weight, control your cholesterol, and keep your blood pressure numbers normal. It can dramatically reduce your risk of heart disease, which is important because women with diabetes are 2 to 4 times as likely to die from heart disease as those without diabetes.

For a complete guide to exercise, see Chapter 5. Keep in mind, however, that even if aerobics classes or weight lifting isn't for you, simply walking for as little as 35 minutes a day can reduce your risk of diabetes by an impressive 58 percent, as it did for people in a Finnish study (who didn't all peel off the pounds).Closer to home, the medical professionals in the Nurses' Health Study

The Blues-Blood Sugar Connection

doctors have known for a long time that depression and diabetes seem to go hand in hand. But which comes first: the depression or the diabetes?

Studies are suggesting that, in most cases, depression arrives earlier.

Scientists looked at dates from the medical records of 1,680 people with newly diagnosed type 2 diabetes and compared them with records for the same number of people without the disease. They found that those with diabetes had suffered significantly more bouts of depression prior to their diagnoses. In fact, in those who had been diagnosed with diabetes and depression, the depression came first three-quarters of the time.

"I'm not sure we can say that depression causes diabetes," says lead researcher Gregory A. Nichols, PhD, an investigator at Kaiser Permanente Center for Health Research in Portland, Oregon. It's possible, he says, that both depression and diabetes are linked to a common factor—one that hasn't yet been identified.

If you have a family history of diabetes or if you have other risk factors for the disease, it's worth paying attention to your moods, Dr. Nichols says. "I'd consider depression a possible warning sign. If you notice you're depressed, get it treated, and get your blood sugar checked, too." ∎

reduced their diabetes risk by 30 percent by working up a sweat more than once a week.

Another study found that type 2 diabetes responds well to a one-two punch—doing aerobic exercise some days and resistance training on others controlled blood sugar levels better than either type of exercise alone, say researchers from the Pennington Biomedical Research Center at the Louisiana State University System in Baton Rouge.

Talk to your doctor before starting an exercise routine, particularly if you already have diabetes or if you haven't put on your walking shoes for a while. Your doctor might recommend that you have a stress test, just to make sure that your heart can handle the workouts.

"There's no reason to go from being sedentary to running a marathon," says Dr. Lazar. "Increase your pace gradually. Start by walking ¼ mile, then slowly increase the distance," he advises.

Get regular sleep too. A Yale University study found that people who regularly got less than 6 hours sleep a night were 50 percent more

WHAT WORKS FOR ME

KATHERINE D. SHERIF, MD, *is director of the Drexel Center for Women's Health and associate professor in the Division of Internal Medicine at Drexel University College of Medicine in Philadelphia. She comes from a family of immigrants, and she saw firsthand what happens when people switch to the overabundant Western diet and lifestyle, which puts them at high risk for developing diabetes.*

My father is Egyptian, and our family members who eat the traditional diet of lots of fruits and vegetables and who get regular exercise are very healthy. But those who have sedentary lifestyles and eat a typical Western high-calorie, high-carbohydrate diet have developed diseases like heart disease, stroke, hypertension, diabetes, and high cholesterol. The transformation I've seen in just one or two generations is striking.

I've always tried to eat a healthful diet. For example, I have one of three breakfasts: Sometimes a couple of hard-boiled eggs and fruit, sometimes a cup of plain yogurt with soy protein powder and fresh fruit mixed in, and sometimes high-protein Egyptian beans with vegetables, which are a staple of the Egyptian diet in the countryside. Lunch might be a can of tuna and fruit, and my afternoon snack is typically roasted soybeans or string cheese with fruit. Dinner often consists of tofu and stir-fried vegetables, or a piece of fish or chicken, served with a salad or vegetables.

I also take multivitamins. I get 100 mg of B vitamins, 2,000 mg of vitamin C, 400 IU of vitamin E, and 2,000 mg of fish oil.

It's so hard sometimes to play sports or go to the gym, so I try to walk 10,000 steps daily. One mile is roughly 2,500 steps. I wear a pedometer throughout the day so I can show my patients how I incorporate exercise into my life.

If I park a little farther down the parking lot, I add 500 steps coming into the office and 500 steps going out. On weekends, I walk nine blocks from my house to the Philadelphia Art Museum. That's 2,500 steps there and 2,500 back. The exercise really adds up. ∎

likely to get diabetes than people who slept more. But sleeping too long–more than 8 hours– doubles your risk. "When you sleep too little–or too long because of sleep apnea (a condition in which you stop breathing briefly many times a night)–your nervous system stays on alert," says lead researcher Henry Klar Yaggi, MD, assistant professor of pulmonary medicine at the Yale School of Medicine. An over-alert nervous system interferes with the hormones that regulate blood sugar. Getting too little or too much sleep has also been linked to obesity and high blood pressure, so aim for 7 hours of sleep a night. Trouble sleeping? Avoid caffeine after noon, don't work in your bedroom, keep bedroom temperatures comfortable (not too hot or too cold), skip late-night TV, and invest in room-darkening shades to keep the sun from waking you up too early.

Nutritional Treatments

Eat natural foods. Humans didn't evolve to grab burgers at a drive-thru window or pop barbecue chips or chocolate sandwich cookies while sitting and staring at a TV screen. The ideal diet today is the same one that fueled our ancestors: fiber-rich whole grains, fresh fruits and vegetables, and legumes–and the "good" fats, such as olive and flaxseed oils and the omega-3 fats, says Burton Berkson, MD, PhD, founder of Integrative Medical Centers of New Mexico, and author of *Syndrome X* and *The Alpha Lipoic Acid Breakthrough*.

In the past, people with diabetes were advised to avoid desserts and other sugary foods. Nutritionists still worry about this, but research has shown that the key to controlling diabetes is to eat a balanced diet. Keep your overall diet healthy and have only small portions of cake, candy, cookies, and other sweets very occasionally. (In fact, a study done in Italy found that flavonoid-rich dark chocolate may help the body metabolize sugar, as well as lower cholesterol and blood pressure.)

The optimal diet, according to the American Diabetes Association, includes 10 to 20 percent of daily calories from protein; 30 percent (or less) of total calories from fats with less than 10 percent coming from saturated fats; and the rest from complex carbohydrates, which are mainly found in fruits, vegetables, beans, and grains. If your LDL cholesterol is 100 or more, you need to take extra care to make sure your saturated fat intake is less than 7 percent.

Include more fiber in your diet. A study done at the University of Texas Southwestern Medical Center at Southwestern Medical School in Dallas found that people who increased their fiber intake from 24 to 50 gm daily had dramatic improvements in blood sugar levels. In fact, the high-fiber diet was as effective as some diabetes medications.

Rather than try to calculate the fiber in the foods you eat, simply plan to get a total of 13 daily servings of a mixture of fruits, vegetables, beans, brown rice, and whole grain pastas, cereals, and breads. For optimal glucose control, try to get an equal mix of soluble fiber (found in oranges, grapefruit, prunes, cantaloupe, raisins, lima beans, oat bran, and granola) and insoluble fiber (found in some greens, vegetables, legumes, and whole grains).

Ask for vinaigrette on your salad. In an Arizona State University study, people with type 2 diabetes or insulin resistance had lower blood sugar levels if they had about 2 tablespoons of vinegar before they ate a high carb meal. "Vinegar contains acetic acid, which may inactivate certain starch-digesting enzymes, slowing carbo-

hydrate digestion," says lead researcher Carol Johnston, PhD.

Avoid sugary drinks. There's nothing wrong with having fruit juices or sodas on occasion, but they're brimming with sugar and little else. When you take in a lot of calories from sugar, you'll be less likely to get enough calories from wholesome, nutrient-packed foods, says Dr. Kaufman.

She advises people with diabetes to drink mainly water. When you do have a hankering

Protect Your Oral Health

gum disease may threaten more than your teeth and gums. Scientists now believe that gum disease may be a trigger for the clinical onset of diabetes in individuals already predisposed to the disease. One study, for example, found that women with gum disease were more likely to develop gestational diabetes. Another reported that periodontal disease was an independent predictor of type 2 diabetes in a population of more than 9,000 people. There is also evidence that gum disease can worsen the degree of control of diabetes.

Using data from the Third National Health and Nutrition Examination Survey (NHANES III), researchers found that among overweight adults with the highest insulin resistance levels, one in two also suffered from severe gum disease.

It's possible that gum disease, which is caused by chronic bacterial infections that affect the whole body, may somehow trigger insulin resistance. The process is believed to be a result of inflammatory substances produced in response to the infection. Molecules of these substances prevent insulin from docking on its receptors on the cells' surface. This reduces the uptake of glucose by the cells and results in insulin resistance.

"Oral health is far more important than we previously thought," says Sara G. Grossi, DDS, a faculty member at the Brody School of Medicine at East Carolina University in Greenville, North Carolina. "Gum disease may affect other conditions in the body, such as heart disease, stroke, respiratory diseases, and diabetes. Periodontal disease in people with diabetes constitutes a significant health risk since it could lead to difficulty in controlling blood sugar and therefore worsen diabetic status."

The best way to prevent gum disease is to brush and floss your teeth twice daily, eat a balanced diet rich in antioxidants, and visit your dentist regularly for checkups and teeth cleanings. Your dentist will advise you on the recommended frequency of your visits. ■

for soda or a juice, look for products that are sugar-free and drink them in moderation, no more than one a day, she advises.

Add a pinch of cinnamon. A teaspoon of cinnamon a day may help improve blood sugar control, particularly if you already have diabetes. What's at work? Some researchers suspect it may be the chromium and polyphenol antioxidants in this spice. Chromium plays a role in insulin sensitivity.

In studies at the Nutrient Requirements and Functions Laboratory at the Agricultural Research Service in Beltsville, Maryland, lead scientist Richard A. Anderson, PhD, has tested more than 50 spices and herbs—including cinnamon, allspice, catnip, and turmeric—to see which ones make fat cells more responsive to insulin. The research is important because insulin-resistant cells can't take in enough energy-giving glucose from the blood, which can lead to diabetes. "Cinnamon is the champ," says Dr. Anderson. It contains a substance called methylhydroxy chalcone polymer, or MHCP, which in laboratory studies increased glucose metabolism up to twentyfold.

Dr. Anderson recommends eating ¼ to 1 teaspoon of cinnamon daily, particularly if you have high blood sugar, insulin resistance, or type 1 or type 2 diabetes. He suggests sprinkling cinnamon on your oatmeal and stirring it into foods like yogurt throughout the day to reach the total amount.

"We've heard from people with diabetes who have begun adding cinnamon to their diets," he says. "They say it's the best thing they've tried since sliced bread."

Grab a handful of nuts. Once a diet no-no, nuts are back on the healthy menu where they may contribute to weight loss (they quash your appetite), lower cholesterol, and even lower blood sugar.

Have a cup of coffee. There's increasing evidence that caffeine may reduce the risk of type 2 diabetes. In one 2010 study, coffee-drinking mice specially bred to get diabetes had lower blood sugar and better insulin sensitivity. They also had a number of other beneficial biochemical changes that would reduce their risk of developing diabetes.

Alternative Therapies

Until recently, most physicians dismissed alternative healing techniques for serious conditions such as diabetes. But recent studies have shown that remedies outside of mainstream medicine, such as medicinal herbs and mind-body techniques, may play an important role in keeping diabetes under control.

Let go and relax. Simply taking a deep breath and relaxing your muscles may result in significant dips in blood sugar. A study of 18 people with diabetes found that relaxation exercises were able to reduce blood sugar levels by 9 to 12 percent.

"When you're under stress, the brain secretes hormones that make you more susceptible to all diseases, including diabetes," says

Dr. Berkson. In fact, part of your body's stress response is to raise your blood sugar to give you the energy you'll need to fight or flee the perceived danger.

There are many relaxation techniques to choose from, from meditation to yoga to prayer. One of the easiest is called progressive relaxation. Begin by breathing deeply for a minute or two. Spend the next 10 to 15 minutes progressively relaxing all the muscles in your body, starting at your toes and working upward to your head. In your mind, imagine that the muscles are getting heavy, warm, and loose. By the time you're done, you'll notice that stress and tension have slipped away. If you do this every day, you may find that your blood sugar levels have dropped into a safer zone. (For more relaxation techniques, see Chapter 7.)

Battle depression. Studies have shown that people with diabetes are twice as likely to suffer from depression than nondiabetics. A Harvard study appearing in the November 2010 issue of the *Archives of Internal Medicine* found that the link was especially strong in middle-aged women and that it went both ways: Women with diabetes were more likely to be depressed, and depressed women were at higher risk of diabetes.

Being depressed may even worsen diabetes symptoms, possibly because it keeps you from focusing on the positive lifestyle changes you need to keep blood sugar under control. The researchers also speculated that antidepres-sants may exert some biochemical effect on blood sugar that has not yet been identified. Some antidepressants may also lead to unwanted weight gain, which could also play a role. If you've been feeling depressed or anxious, your doctor may recommend that you talk to a therapist or get a prescription for anti-depressant medications (some are not linked to weight gain). On the home front, really push yourself to get more exercise and to spend time with friends. They're among the best ways to ease depression.

Try milk thistle. It contains a compound called silymarin, which appears to improve insulin resistance and glucose control, says Dr. Berkson. He advises people with diabetes to get 140 to 210 mg of silymarin from standardized milk thistle extract daily. The supplement label will tell you how much silymarin the milk thistle product contains.

Insulin Resistance: The Beginning of Diabetes

Long before people develop diabetes, their bodies begin laying the groundwork. They may have what doctors refer to as insulin resistance, which leads to other problems, including high cholesterol and triglyceride levels, high blood pressure, and accumulations of fat around the middle, a condition called metabolic syndrome. These conditions can increase the risk of diabetes as well as heart disease.

"People who are diabetic may have been

insulin resistant for years," says Dr. Sherif. "One day, the pancreas just can't crank out enough insulin anymore. Blood sugar builds up, which leads to diabetes. And by that time, half of them also have developed coronary artery disease."

Between insulin resistance and diabetes is a condition doctors are now calling prediabetes—elevated blood sugar that's not high enough for a diabetes diagnosis. Sometimes called impaired fasting glucose (IFG) or impaired glucose tolerance (IGT), it's estimated that one in four adults over 20 in the United States has the condition and most will have diabetes within 10 years unless they lose 5 to 7 percent of their body weight.

What causes your body to stop responding to insulin the way it should? In some people it's genetic. But for most people it's excess weight, a couch potato lifestyle, and eating too many refined carbohydrates, which are generally found in snacks and other processed food. The problem with refined carbohydrates, and possibly with refined fats and excess protein, is that they're quickly turned into glucose in the body. The cells get overloaded with glucose, so the body stores it in the form of fat, explains Dr. Berkson.

That fat does more than cling to just the abdomen. It promotes the production of a number of hormones, including one called resistin, which essentially orders cells to ignore instructions from insulin to usher glucose that's circulating in the blood into the cells where it can be used for energy. In other words, it makes the cells resistant to insulin, one hallmark of type 2 diabetes. Although this mechanism is not proven—a 2009 study found that resistin caused insulin resistance in mice—researchers think that resistin may be the link between obesity and type 2 diabetes.

"We're all at risk from insulin resistance, which is caused by poor diets and lifestyles," says Dr. Berkson. "But you can reverse it, and

Does Television Cause Diabetes?

For years, doctors have known that an active lifestyle protects against diabetes and all of its life-threatening complications. But researchers at the Harvard School of Public Health wanted to find out if the reverse was true: Would long stretches of TV watching—the sedentary activity that consumes 40 percent of our leisure time—increase the odds?

They analyzed the viewing habits of nearly 38,000 men, ages 40 to 75, for more than 10 years. After adjusting for age, physical activity levels, alcohol use, and smoking, those who watched TV more than 4 hours a day doubled their odds of getting diabetes, compared with those who watched less than 2 hours weekly. Those who viewed 40 hours a week tripled their risk.

And if TV watching keeps you up late, you may face a second risk: lack of sleep, which is linked to insulin resistance and diabetes. ■

sometimes type 2 diabetes as well, by eating a proper diet, getting regular exercise, and reducing stress," he explains. If you have a family history of diabetes, or if you have high cholesterol, high blood pressure, or abdominal obesity, it may be helpful to see your doctor for an oral glucose tolerance test. "It tells how your body handles sugars after eating," says Dr. Sherif. "If sugar levels don't drop after a couple of hours, it means that your body isn't handling glucose and you're probably insulin resistant."

The test may be helpful for women with a condition called polycystic ovary syndrome, which causes symptoms such as irregular periods, unexpected weight gain, and acne outbreaks. Most women with PCOS are insulin resistant and have a very high risk of developing type 2 diabetes. If they're not treated, many do go on to develop the disease, says Dr. Sherif.

16

Cancer

Almost every week, another cancer myth makes the Internet rounds. You've probably gotten e-mail cancer alerts about deodorant, shampoo, and even electrical appliances. It's enough to make women swear off consumer products forever. Your best bet is to delete those e-mail warnings and empower yourself with facts. Those lists of "carcinogens" looping through cyberspace have no basis in truth.

What does count is how you live. If every woman ate well, exercised, didn't smoke, and safeguarded herself against sexually transmitted diseases, nearly three-quarters of cancer deaths among women would never happen.

"The majority of cancer risk can be attributed to lifestyle," says Therese Bevers, MD, medical director of the Cancer Prevention Center at the University of Texas MD Anderson Cancer Center in Houston. Diet and smoking make up most of the risk pie, she explains, with inherited cancers accounting for between 5 and 10 percent of cases. "But even then, lifestyle or environmental factors may actually trigger it," she says.

Does that mean you'll stay cancer-free if you follow the rules of good health? Not necessarily, says Mitchell L. Gaynor, MD, founder and president of Gaynor Integrative Oncology and clinical assistant professor of medicine at Weill Cornell Medical Center for Complementary and Integrative Medicine, affiliated with New York Presbyterian Hospital-Weill Cornell Medical Center in New York City. But you greatly improve your odds.

Many Diseases, Similar Strategies

Cancer may sound like one disease, but it's actually hundreds of diseases that attack different organs and spring from different causes.

What all cancers share, though, is the uncontrolled growth and spread of abnormal cells—cells that eventually destroy the body if they aren't stopped.

Your immune system is uniquely equipped to recognize and destroy deviant cells before they become cancerous. The liver is your body's detoxification system, ridding you of cancer-causing toxins. If cancer cells begin to form, your immune system produces an army of cells to attack and kill them, then produce antibodies that "remember" the invader so your immune cells will attack quickly next time. But sometimes this arsenal of defenses fails and cancerous cells may slowly begin accumulating. "A tumor is the manifestation of a process that may have taken decades to happen," says Dr. Gaynor.

That's why keeping your body, mind, and spirit in potent fighting shape is the key to preventing cancer and to living with cancer once you have it.

"If you get cancer, the healthier you are, the less likely you'll be to have other medical conditions that might interfere with treatment, and the better you'll be able to get through it," says Marilyn Leitch, MD, a surgical oncologist, professor of surgery at the University of Texas Southwestern Medical Center, and medical director of the University of Texas Southwestern Center for Breast Care in Dallas. "You don't have to die from cancer."

Here's how to lower your general cancer risk, plus ward off the most common women's cancers.

Turning Out the Lights May Help Turn Off Cancer

the hormone melatonin, which is secreted by the pineal gland at night when it's dark, and is curtailed by light, has been lauded as everything from a promising sleep aid to the fountain of youth. But its greatest potential may lie in its potency against breast cancer.

In one study, Steven M. Hill, PhD, professor at Tulane University Health Sciences Center in New Orleans, and the Edmond and Lily Safra Endowed Chair for Breast Cancer Research, gave female rats a preparation to induce breast cancer. Then he treated them with a combination of melatonin and 9-cis-retinoic acid, a derivative of vitamin A. The animals given the treatment developed significantly fewer tumors than those that didn't get the treatment. In addition, the onset of tumors was delayed from 5 to 7 weeks.

The vitamin A derivative is a known cancer fighter, and adding melatonin to the mix appeared to make it even more effective, Dr. Hill explains.

Besides its ability to prevent or delay breast cancer, melatonin may aid in the treatment of existing breast tumors by altering estrogen receptors and by starving tumor cells of the hormone they need for growth. A study by Dr. Hill and his colleagues, published in *Breast Cancer Research* in 2010, also found that melatonin can prevent breast cancer from becoming invasive. While it's too early in the research to recommend melatonin supplements, it's a good idea to encourage the pineal gland to produce as much of this healing hormone as possible by turning out the lights when the sun goes down and going to sleep early—no easy task in today's busy world.

"By getting up at 5:00 every morning and staying up until 11:00 or 12:00 every night, with artificial lights on, you're giving your pineal gland only a short period in which to make melatonin," says Dr. Hill. He suspects, in fact, that melatonin deprivation may explain why some reproductive cancers are on the rise. ■

YOUR CANCER PREVENTION PLAN

Today, you can get a vaccine that can help prevent two kinds of cancers—one against the hepatitis B virus that can cause liver cancer, and one against the human papillomavirus type 16 and 18, which cause cervical cancer. Vaccines that boost the immune system to prevent and treat cancer are one of the hottest areas of medical research today, but it's still in its early stages. Your best bet: do everything you can to lower your risk—starting with dietary changes.

Nutritional Treatments

Eat well. Like so many lifestyle diseases, cancer risk can be reduced by a good diet. The American Cancer Society recommends having five or more servings of fruits and vegetables daily, plus plenty of other plant-based foods, such as whole grain breads, rice, pasta, and beans. Prepare low-fat meals, and limit your consumption of meat, particularly high-fat red meats.

Women who try to overhaul their diets all at once often get frustrated and fail. Dr. Leitch advises making the changes slowly. For example, substitute fruit or vegetables for french fries one day; on another, replace red meat with fish, whole grains, or legumes. "You can't go on a grapefruit diet for the rest of your life, nor would you want to," she says. "But if you have a more comprehensive plan that lets you eat enough to feel satisfied, then you're more likely to stick with it over time."

Stack your odds with cancer-fighting foods. "I think the most exciting advance in the next decade will be predicting who's at risk for cancer, and preventing it largely through nutrition," says Dr. Gaynor. Scientists have found that many foods contain protective antioxidants and phytonutrients, which boost your body's natural defenses against carcinogens. Some of the best include:

- Tomatoes and tomato sauce. They contain lycopene, a plant pigment that blocks the harmful effects of naturally occurring molecules called free radicals. Lycopene has been linked to reductions in lung, breast, colon, cervical, and other cancers.

- Cruciferous vegetables. Cabbage, broccoli, cauliflower, brussels sprouts, and kale contain formidable cancer fighters, including sulforaphane and indole-3-carbinol. In one study, eating 9 ounces each of broccoli and brussels sprouts a day significantly reduced the formation of a carcinogen found in well-done meat, effectively cutting off the cancer process before it starts. Dr. Gaynor recommends having six servings of cruciferous vegetables weekly.

- Mushrooms. They're packed with compounds called polysaccharides, large, chainlike molecules that have both antitumor and immune-stimulating properties. Enoki and maitake mushrooms contain the largest numbers of these molecules.

- Olive oil. It contains anthocyanins, flavonoids, and phenols, which are known cancer combatants. They're not bad for your heart, either.

- Green tea. Population studies have shown that people who drink about 4 cups of green tea daily have a lower risk of cancer than those who don't drink tea, though other human studies have been inconclusive. Why researchers think tea can fight cancer? It contain antioxidant compounds that can prevent the cellular damage that can lead to cancer.

- Garlic. Along with scallions, leeks, and onions, it contains sulfur compounds, which have anticancer properties. Population studies have found that regular garlic consumers have lower risks of cancers of the breast, stomach, colon, esophagus, and pancreas. A few small studies have found that taking a garlic supplement can reduce tumor incidence and may even decrease tumor size when applied to skin cancers.

Lifestyle Strategies

Get physical. Regular exercise can reduce your risk of a variety of cancers, including colon, breast, endometrial, and ovarian cancers. According to the National Cancer Institute, getting moderate intensity physical exercise at least 30 minutes 5 or more days a week, or intense physical activity 20 minutes a day on 3 or more days a week could reduce your risk of colon cancer by 30 to 40 percent. Studies have also found that physically active women have lower risk of breast cancer (up to 80 percent lower). To achieve that, you need 30 to 60 minutes of physical activity a day. Exercise may also lower endometrial cancer risk, in part

Do Low-Calorie Diets Prevent Cancer?

before you sit down to your next big meal or hit the refrigerator for a midnight snack, consider this: Eating much less than you usually do could potentially add years to your life and prevent or delay the development of cancer or other diseases.

For decades, scientists at the National Institute on Aging in Baltimore have been studying two groups of 60 male and 60 female rhesus monkeys that typically live an average of 25 years. Animals in one group are allowed to eat as much as they want, while those in the second group consume about a third fewer calories.

Results suggest a dramatic difference between the groups. Of the 60 well-fed monkeys, six have developed cancer. In the restricted-calorie group, only two have developed cancer. Other animal studies have shown similar effects.

It's possible that calorie restriction significantly slows cell division in the body, which reduces the likelihood of diseases that rely on cell proliferation, such as cancer and endometriosis, says Mark Lane, PhD, head of the Nutritional and Molecular Physiology Unit of the Laboratory of Neurosciences at the National Institute on Aging and principal investigator of the NIA's primate calorie restriction and aging project.

Animals who eat less also have lower incidences of heart disease, cataracts, and ulcers. They live longer, too. "In human terms, you'd see an average increase in life span from age 80 to 100, and the maximum age limit would rise from 120 years to 140 years," Dr. Lane says.

Should you reduce your calorie intake by one-third? Probably not. "That would mean skipping a meal a day every day for the rest of your life. It's just not realistic." ■

because it alters estrogen metabolism—a factor in this kind of cancer—and helps you lose weight. (For a complete guide to fitness, see Chapter 5.)

Live lean. An estimated one out of three cancers is linked to excess weight, poor nutrition, and lack of exercise. But of the three, the strongest evidence is for weight, which contributes to 14 to 20 percent of all cancer deaths. "Excess weight gain has been associated with increased breast cancer risk" among postmenopausal women, Dr. Bevers says. It's also linked to colon, endometrial, esophageal, and kidney cancers, and may play a role in cancers of the gallbladder, pancreas, thyroid, ovary, and cervix, as well as multiple myeloma and Hodgkin's lymphoma.

Though there's not a lot of research on whether losing weight will help reduce your risk, there is some evidence that weight loss can lower levels of hormones known to trigger cancer, such as insulin and estrogen.

Views That Heal

mother Nature's beauty calms frayed nerves and soothes tired eyes. But can its magic have an effect on cancer and other diseases?

Absolutely, says Richard Enoch Kaufman, MD, assistant clinical professor of medicine (immunology) at Yale University School of Medicine. "Even having a hospital window with a view of nature, or having flowers in a room, is healing," he says.

Research suggests that people who are able to experience nature have an increase in immune activity. Nature also activates hormones that promote healing and neuropeptides that ease pain. One study showed that hospital patients who had a view of nature had shorter stays, less need for pain relievers, and fewer complaints during recovery.

Many of the nation's cancer departments have gone beyond providing pleasant views; they actually bring nature inside. At Marin General Hospital in Greenbrae, California, for example, patients about to undergo radiation treatments can look through a wall-length window from the waiting room into a sea of multihued foliage. They can hear the soothing sounds of a stone fountain. Paths and benches are arranged throughout the Healing Garden for those who wish to enter. There is also a walking path.

"The patients are vulnerable. They're usually wearing their gowns and are right in the throes of the most intense part of their treatment," says Leslie D. Davenport, who was founding manager of the hospital's Institute for Health and Healing Humanities Program and established guided imagery programs at five Bay Area hospitals. "The garden gives the feeling of being in a private inner sanctum."

To heighten the connection between nature and healing, the plants and trees in the garden are selected for their cancer-curing properties. One example is yew, a tree that yields a medication (taxol) that's used to treat ovarian and breast cancers.

"One cancer patient took home a cup of water from the fountain and put it in a bowl on her home altar," Davenport recalls. "It somehow represented her path to wellness, out of the artificial, harsh, technological world to a more natural place of healing." ■

A body mass index (BMI) of 25 to 29.9 is considered overweight, and anything over 30 is obese. To calculate your BMI, multiply your weight in pounds by 703. Divide that number by your height in inches. Divide that number again by your height in inches, and you'll have your BMI. A woman who's 5 feet 5 inches tall is overweight if she weighs between 150 and 179 pounds. (For more information on weight control, see Chapter 6.)

Take a stress break. When you experience stress in your life, the body produces higher amounts of stress hormones, which suppress immunity and increase the likelihood of cancer, particularly those triggered by viruses, such as lymphoma. Stress may indirectly promote cancer by encouraging the growth of new blood vessels that nourish tumors, causing them to grow and thrive. A recent study from the MD Anderson Cancer Center in Houston found that stress hormones such as adrenaline can actually prevent cancer cells from dying when they break away from their colony—a normal process for healthy cells called anoikis. Cancer cells that leave their point of origin can spread

WHAT WORKS FOR ME

JULIE R. GRALOW, MD, *is director of Breast Medical Oncology at Seattle Cancer Care Alliance, professor of medical oncology at the University of Washington School of Medicine in Seattle and co-author of* Breast Fitness: An Optimal Exercise and Health Plan for Reducing Your Risk of Breast Cancer. *She is also medical director of Team Survivor Northwest, an exercise and fitness program for women cancer survivors. Here's what she does to reduce her own risk of cancer.*

I try to practice what I preach on cancer prevention, but I'm the first to admit I'm not perfect. I don't smoke, but I do drink a glass or two of wine a week. A little bit is enjoyable, and it relaxes me.

I travel around the world a lot for work, and I try to be reasonable about my diet. I don't eat much meat, but I do eat fish. But I'm always struggling to get enough fruits and vegetables. In hotels, if I'm ordering room service, I have some control. During business meetings, I often order the vegetarian plate. Airport lounges now offer baskets of fruit, so I take some along. It's a little more work to get what you need, but it can be done.

Of course, there are days I look back and am mortified by what I've eaten, so I take a multivitamin with extra calcium just to make sure I'm getting everything I need. I definitely believe in exercise. When I'm staying overnight anywhere, I always carry my running shoes, bathing suit, and exercise clothes and try to fit in exercise, even if it's only at the hotel gym or around the neighborhood. I've actually jogged around the Kremlin and through Shanghai.

At home, I run a couple of times a week, and my husband and I try to plan an event every weekend, such as a bike ride or hiking. We've climbed nearby Mount Rainier and Mount Hood, and occasionally we've biked 50 miles a day. Every August I participate in a sprint triathlon (swimming, biking, running) as part of Team Survivor.

To reduce stress, I make sure to schedule quiet time. I love novels, and I read a couple of nights a week and on weekends. I'm also a big fan of massages, and I try to get them whenever I can, especially when I'm traveling in Asia. ■

throughout the body forming new tumors, a process called metastasis.

"Get in touch with your essence," says Dr. Gaynor. "Make a list of things in your life that serve you and things that don't—and try to get rid of those things not serving you. Play music that you find relaxing. Try yoga, deep breathing, guided imagery—anything that relaxes you." (For a stress-reduction action plan, see Chapter 7.)

Medical Options

Get a complete checkup. If you've never had a formal cancer risk assessment, now's the time to do it, says Dr. Bevers. "Knowing your risk for certain cancers allows you to pay attention to specific risk reduction strategies and screening techniques that are right for you," she says.

Your doctor can perform the assessment, but you can also do it on your own on the Internet. Check www.diseaseriskindex.harvard.edu/update/, the Web site for Harvard's Cancer Center, to learn more about your risk for specific cancers such as breast, ovarian, uterine, and cervical cancers, visit the Web site of the Women's Cancer Network at www.wcn.org, which also provides an online assessment of female-specific cancer risk.

BREAST CANCER

It's true that breast cancer strikes more women than any other kind of cancer. But your overall risk is probably much lower than you think, and there are ways to make it lower still.

About one in eight women will develop breast cancer during her lifetime. Hereditary factors, such as carrying the BRCA1 or BRCA2 breast cancer gene, account for only 5 to 10 percent of all breast cancers. The rest are mainly due to what you eat and how you live.

Here's an anti-breast-cancer plan that will tilt the odds in your favor.

Nutritional Treatments

Have 10 daily servings of fruits and vegetables. In one study, women at high risk for breast cancer increased their daily intake of fruits and vegetables from 5.8 servings to 10 or more servings. After 2 weeks, researchers found that free radical damage to the DNA in the women's white blood cells had dropped by 21.5 percent. Though the most current research, including a 2010 study from the Black Women's Health Study, have not found a significant relationship between produce intake and breast cancer, most experts still believe this is advice worth taking.

When choosing fruits and vegetables, look for those that contain a variety of phytochemicals, says Caroline M. Apovian, MD, director of nutrition and weight management at Boston Medical Center, and associate professor of medicine and pediatrics at Boston University School of Medicine. Some of the best include citrus fruits and berries, cruciferous vegetables (such as broccoli and cabbage), leafy green vegetables, tomatoes, and yellow and orange vegetables. In the Black Women's Health Study, women who ate carrots were less likely to develop estrogen-negative breast cancer (the kind of cancer not caused by estrogen exposure).

Get more fiber in your diet. Dietary fiber helps reduce the amount of estrogen that circulates in the blood, and it reduces estrogen's impact at the cellular level, says Dr. Apovian. Over a woman's lifetime, this can reduce the risk of breast cancer. Fiber also makes the stools bulkier, which can allow the body to excrete estrogen more efficiently.

All plant foods contain fiber. When you plan your menus, be sure to include plenty of fruits, vegetables, whole grains, legumes, and nuts.

Prevention recommends 25 to 35 gm of fiber per day for general good nutrition.

Get "good" fats in your diet. Diets that are high in animal fats and high in foods containing trans fatty acids have been linked to higher breast cancer rates. Replace these with monounsaturated fats, such as those in olive and canola oils, or with omega-3 fatty acids, such as those in fish and flaxseed.

Drink moderately or not at all. Research suggests that woman who have two drinks a day may increase their risk of breast cancer by 25 percent. If your overall breast cancer risk is

Women Blame Stress for Breast Cancer

Science has found strong links between cancer and diet, genes, and lifestyle. But cancer survivors tend to finger something else: stress. Do patients' beliefs—even when not scientifically proven—help them survive?

To find out, Donna Stewart, MD, senior scientist at the Toronto General Research Institute and chairperson of women's health for the University of Toronto's University Health Network, surveyed nearly 400 breast cancer survivors who had been disease-free for at least 2 years. They were asked what they felt was the cause of their cancers, and why the cancers hadn't recurred.

Stress was overwhelmingly named as the leading culprit, cited by 42 percent of the respondents. Known scientific risk factors—such as genetics (26.7 percent), environment (25.5 percent), hormones (23.9 percent), and diet (15 percent)—trailed considerably.

"We know that stress alters immune function, and these women may in fact be partly right that stress contributed to their cancers," says Dr. Stewart. "But the evidence isn't very clear."

When the women were asked why their cancers hadn't returned, 60 percent credited their positive attitude. This was followed by diet (50 percent), healthy lifestyle (40.3 percent), exercise (39.4 percent), stress reduction (27.9 percent), and tamoxifen (3.9 percent).

Dr. Stewart and her colleagues, who have also done surveys with similar results among ovarian cancer survivors, concluded that patients' personal beliefs about the cause of their cancers—even when their opinions were at odds with scientific evidence—were important in helping them cope with and manage the disease and that these beliefs should be worked with and not be discounted by doctors. ∎

average, it's probably safe to have a drink or two on occasion. "One drink a day may be too much for women who already have breast cancer or for those at high risk," says Dr. Apovian.

Lifestyle Strategies

Get up and go. Don't underestimate the power of physical activity to safeguard you against breast cancer. Even a little bit of exercise can help–but the harder you exercise, the greater your protection. Brisk walking or jogging for 3 or more hours a week can lower your breast cancer risk by 30 percent, possibly by altering both body weight and estrogen metabolism.

"I recommend exercising for at least a half an hour, 3 or 4 days a week," says Julie R. Gralow, MD, director of Breast Medical Oncology at Seattle Cancer Care Alliance, a professor of medical oncology at the University of Washington School of Medicine in Seattle, and coauthor of *Breast Fitness: An Optimal Exercise and Health Plan for Reducing Your Risk of Breast Cancer*. She is also medical director of Team Survivor Northwest, an exercise and fitness program for women cancer survivors. "Then augment that with a bike ride or something else on weekends or other days."

Stay slim. One reason exercise is so crucial is that it controls fat, a tissue that produces large amounts of estrogen–and estrogen increases the risk of breast cancer. Fat is even riskier after a woman reaches menopause, when the incidence of breast cancer rises.

"If you're 150 pounds, and then you gain 15 pounds at menopause, your risk increases," says Dr. Gralow.

Medical Options

Avoid estrogen. Hormone replacement therapy is no longer the automatic prescription for menopausal symptoms, particularly if you're at high risk of breast cancer. Exposure to estrogen over a long period of time increases your chances of developing breast cancer. That's why early menstruation and late menopause are risk factors, while being pregnant and nursing are protective. However, using estrogen alone (without progesterone) does decrease your risk, though it ups your chances of getting uterine cancer. It's best to try to deal with menopause symptoms in a more natural way. (See Chapter 29.)

See your doctor regularly. Although headline-grabbing studies have suggested that mammograms may not be as effective as once thought for reducing deaths from breast cancer, leading experts recommend that you should still have an annual breast exam and mammogram, starting at age 40. If you have a high risk for breast cancer, your doctor may recommend starting mammograms earlier. You'll also want to practice monthly self-exams on your breasts throughout your life and see your doctor annually for a clinical breast exam.

Some women, including those with dense breast tissue, may benefit from having a yearly MRI. Women who have a very high risk for breast cancer may be advised to undergo a procedure called ductal lavage, which can detect malignant cells years before a tumor shows up on a mammogram.

Consider chemoprevention. If you have a strong family history of breast cancer or you've had an estrogen-positive cancer yourself, talk to your doctor about taking a SERM–short for selective estrogen receptor modulator. These drugs act like estrogen on some tissues and block it on other tissues. One, tamoxifen, is called an antiestrogen because it blocks the effects of estrogen in the body. It may reduce a woman's risk of developing the disease by almost 50 percent even after she stops taking it. Studies suggest that an osteoporosis drug, raloxifene, may be similarly beneficial. Your doctor may also talk to you about aromatase inhibitors, which decrease the amount of estrogen your body makes. These drugs may lower breast cancer risks in postmenopausal women with a history of breast cancer. All these drugs can have significant side effects and aren't recommended for anyone who is not at high risk.

Explore surgical options. Some women who have a high risk of breast cancer—they have the BRCA1 or BRCA2 genes, for example—sometimes choose to have either one or both breasts removed or their ovaries removed, as they also run a high risk of ovarian cancer. It's important to have genetic tests and counseling before making this decision.

LUNG CANCER

Preventing lung cancer can be summed up in two words: Don't smoke. If we all heeded this advice, lung cancer cases among men and women alike would drop by 80 percent.

Your chances of getting breast cancer are greater, but lung cancer is more likely to kill you if you get it. In fact, it's now the number-one cancer killer of women (felling more women than breast, ovarian, and uterine cancers combined), mainly because more women start to smoke at an earlier age, when their lungs are most vulnerable.

Mutational changes in the lungs start

The Power of Acceptance

I am putting myself in God's hands."

For years, when doctors heard cancer patients say these words, they felt that they were surrendering to almost certain death. Better to display a fighting spirit, it was assumed, than to accept the disease. But what sounds like resignation may actually be an effective coping style.

"We used to think that fatalism meant that someone believed that they were going to die and that there was nothing they could do," explains Ellen G. Levine, PhD, a senior scientist at San Francisco State University where she is co-founder of the Cancer Health Disparities research group. "But for a certain group of women, that may not be so."

Dr. Levine and former graduate student Cory Fitzpatrick, PhD, assessed the coping styles of 120 women with breast cancer. Contrary to the prevailing notion that fatalism means giving up, the researchers found that adopting a fatalist attitude was linked to feelings of control, acceptance, spirituality, and engagement in religious practices. The women also reported a higher quality of life and less depression and anxiety.

"A better way to think of fatalism may be as spiritual acceptance," says Dr. Levine. "The attitude seems to be 'I'm doing everything I can; now it's up to God. I trust there will be spiritual help along the way.'" ∎

immediately, so quitting as soon as possible is the most important thing you can do.

The most common lung cancer in women is adenocarcinoma, which is found in the lung tissue that produces mucus. It's also the most common lung cancer in nonsmokers—and about one in five women who have lung cancer are in that group. In fact, as the death of Dana Reeve brought to light, women nonsmokers are more at risk for developing lung cancer than men who don't smoke, possibly because of their higher risk for certain genetic mutations.

If you've smoked for years, and you've smoked a lot, your risk of lung cancer is naturally greater than if you never smoked. But the risk drops dramatically once you quit and your lungs start repairing the smoke damage. In just 10 years, your risk may be up to half that of a smoker. Even if you wait until middle age to quit smoking, you can reduce your risk considerably.

For tips on giving up the habit, see Chapter 8. Or point your browser to the American Lung Association's free online smoking cessation program at www.lungusa.org/stop-smoking/.

Nutritional Treatments

Eat your way to lung health. The chemical compounds in fruits and vegetables can protect the lungs from cancerous changes. In one study, women who ate more than six daily servings of fruits and vegetables were able to reduce their lung cancer risk by 21 to 32 percent. Animal studies suggest that compounds in vegetables and fruits may affect the expression of genes involved in the processes by which cancer develops or is quashed by the body.

Some of the best choices include cruciferous vegetables (such as cabbage and broccoli), citrus fruits, and vegetables high in carotenoids (such as tomatoes, winter squash, and carrots). Apples and onions are also good choices because they contain a compound called quercetin, which has been shown to reduce lung cancer rates.

A large Japanese population study published in 2010 found that nonsmokers who ate the most soy, including soybeans, tofu, and soy milk, were 57 percent less likely to be diagnosed with lung cancer than nonsmokers who ate the least amount of soy. Other potential lung cancer fighters include:

Vitamin D. A new study launched at Harvard School of Public Health may provide the definitive proof that vitamin D prevents a number of cancers, including lung cancer. Preliminary research suggests that the sunshine vitamin may be a key preventative.

Green tea. A 2010 Taiwanese study of more than 500 people found that one cup of green tea, which is chock full of antioxidant flavonoids, reduces the risk of lung cancer, especially in smokers.

Curry. This Asian spice contains curcumin, a compound that appears to detoxify smoking-related carcinogens in lung tissue.

Lifestyle Strategies

Exercise early or late. Avoid exercise outside in highly polluted areas. Air pollution may be linked to increased risk of lung cancer. If you can't avoid the fumes from urban traffic or industry, at least get your exercise in the early morning or later in the evening, when traffic is lighter.

Check for radon. After smoking, radon is the main cause of lung cancer. This odorless gas is formed during the natural breakdown of radium in rocks and soil, and it gets trapped in basements and other airtight spaces. If you live in a high-radon area, or if you just want to make sure that your house doesn't have elevated levels of this odorless, radioactive gas, look in your phone book for a testing service.

Medical Options

If you ever smoked or still smoke, get tested. One reason lung cancer is so deadly is that the most common diagnostic test, a chest x-ray, isn't sensitive enough to detect tumors when they're small enough to be cured. If you're 60 years or older and you're a smoker or former smoker, talk to your doctor about getting an annual spiral CT (computed tomography) scan, in which a doughnut-shaped machine takes pictures of cross-sections of your body, called "slices." Several studies have shown that these scans can catch early tumors better than chest x-rays, but they may not be covered by health insurance because until recently they haven't been shown to increase lung cancer survival. But in November 2010, a study sponsored by the National Cancer Institute found 20 percent fewer cancer deaths among people with a high risk of lung cancer who got spiral CT scans compared to those who got chest x-rays. The research looked at 53,000 smokers and ex-smokers over six years.

COLORECTAL CANCER

For some reason, people often think that cancers of the colon or rectum (colorectal cancers) are more likely to strike men than women. The opposite is true: slightly more women now die from colorectal cancer each year than do men.

However, this is one type of cancer that can almost always be prevented. "If you get tested and have a reasonable diet, you shouldn't get colorectal cancer," says Ernestine Hambrick, MD, founder of the Stop Colon and Rectal Cancer Foundation in Chicago.

Most colorectal cancers begin as a polyp, a tissue growth inside the colon or rectum. Over many years, they may gradually change to cancer.

"Usually there's adequate time to prevent cancer by removing polyps before they turn cancerous," says Mary Elizabeth Roth, MD, allopathic family medical residence director at Geisinger Medical Center in Wilkes Barre, Pennsylvania. Even a malignant polyp, if caught before the cancer spreads, can be removed almost all the time for full recovery.

"That's why it's so important to assess your risk and get tested regularly," says Dr. Roth.

Medical Options

Have regular tests. Americans have seen TV news anchor Katie Couric and cardiac surgeon Mehmet Oz, MD, undergo colonoscopies on television, and this resulted in an increase in the number of these gold-standard colon cancer screenings done every year. If you're at average risk for colorectal cancer, get a digital rectal exam as part of your annual physical exam along with a fecal occult blood test, starting at age 50. Also starting at age 50, *Prevention* recommends that you undergo a colonoscopy every 10 years or as ordered by your doctor. Research has found that colonoscopy is the most effective method of screening for colon cancer because it allows the doctor to view the entire colon and rectal area and remove any precancerous or cancerous polyps she finds. During the procedure, a slender, flexible lighted tube is inserted through the rectum while you are under anesthesia. If you're not having a colonoscopy, then at least have a flexible sigmoidoscopy every 3 to 5 years. During this test, the doctor gently inserts a soft, bendable tube about the thickness of the index finger into the anus (rectal opening) to examine the rectum and lower colon. It's not as thorough as a colonoscopy and may not give you the most peace of mind.

If you have a high risk of colorectal cancer—because you have a family history of colon cancer, for example, or if you have inflammatory bowel disease—you may be advised to start having the tests at an earlier age, and having them more often. For example, if you have a first-degree relative who had colorectal cancer before the age of 60, you will probably need your first colonoscopy at 40, or 10 years before the youngest case in the immediate family, whichever comes first. You'll then need to repeat it every 5 years. If you have an inherited condition such as familial adenomatous polyposis, screenings should start in childhood.

Talk to your doctor about hormone therapy. If you're postmenopausal and are at high risk for colon cancer, ask your doctor about taking estrogen-plus-progestin hormone therapy. A study done at the Fred Hutchinson Cancer Research Center in Seattle found that women on postmenopausal hormones have a 40 percent lower risk of getting colon cancer than women not taking hormones or those who take estrogen alone. Since HRT may raise your risk of breast cancer and heart attack, work with your doctor to weigh the benefits and disadvantages.

Ask about aspirin. Research has found that people who regularly take aspirin to help prevent blood clotting or other nonsteroidal anti-inflammatory drugs for pain have a lower risk of colorectal cancer and polyps. These drugs have also been found to prevent the growth of polyps in people who have had polyps removed or who had colorectal cancer. Since you can run life-threatening risks such as internal bleeding when taking these drugs, do not take them on a regular basis without checking with your doctor.

Lifestyle Strategies

Slim down to your ideal weight. Being overweight is an established risk factor of colorectal cancer for both men and women. See Chapter 6 for how to lose weight permanently.

Stop smoking. You know that the carcinogens in your cigarette can damage your lungs, but some of those cancer-causing chemicals are also swallowed which can cause colon and other digestive system cancers. See Chapter 8 for advice on how to quit.

Stick to one drink a day, max. Heavy alcohol use is associated with colon cancer, possibly because people who drink a lot have low levels of folic acid.

Get a move on. Regular moderate to vigorous exercise—4 hours of brisk walking a week—may reduce your risk of colorectal cancer by 35 percent. It may also improve your survival rate if you do get the disease, suggests results from the Nurses' Health Study.

Keep regular bowel habits. If you exercise regularly, drink plenty of fluids, and get enough fiber in your diet, your bowel movements will naturally stay regular. This is important because constipation may increase the risk for colon cancer by allowing harmful substances to linger in the intestine, says Dr. Roth.

Nutritional Treatments

Eat loads of fruits and vegetables. Along with their beneficial phytochemicals, they contain fiber. "The best sources of fiber are raw fruits and vegetables," says Dr. Roth. "Fiber literally cleans away potential carcinogens from your intestine."

One study found that people who ate more than six daily servings of fiber-rich fruits and vegetables had a 40 percent lower risk of colorectal cancer than those who only ate two daily servings.

Cut way back on meat. The saturated fat in meats, butter, and other animal foods may cause cellular changes in the intestine that can lead to cancer. Other colon enemies: processed meats like hot dogs or lunch meat.

Eat grilled foods sparingly. Meat that's charred on the grill (or in the broiler) produces cancer-causing compounds that can increase the risk of colon cancer, says Dr. Roth. She recommends grilling only on occasion. When you do grill, don't let the flames touch the meat, which increases the production of cancer-causing compounds.

Get a daily dose of vitamin D. D is an emerging superstar in the fight against cancer. Get it from fortified foods such as low-fat dairy products or in supplement form. It's best to take it with calcium.

Get extra calcium. This essential nutrient is believed to bind to toxic bile acids released from the liver. This is important because bile acids may trigger cancer when they come into contact with the colon wall.

The best dietary sources of calcium include low-fat milk and cheese, fortified cereals or soy milk, and vegetables such as broccoli and turnips. You also may want to take a calcium supplement. Dr. Gaynor recommends taking 1,500 mg daily if you're postmenopausal and you aren't undergoing hormone replacement therapy. Younger women can take 1,000 mg daily.

UTERINE OR ENDOMETRIAL CANCER

A woman's body produces estrogen, which offers significant protection to your heart and bones. But too much estrogen can boost the risk of uterine and other reproductive cancers, which usually strike after menopause. In fact, high exposure to estrogen over many years may be your single biggest risk factor for uterine cancer.

If you started menstruating before age 12, entered menopause after age 50, never gave birth, and have a history of infertility, you've been exposed to relatively large amounts of estrogen over time, and your chances of getting uterine cancer are elevated.

You can't change your menstrual or reproductive history, but there are other ways to reduce your lifelong exposure to estrogen. Here's what doctors recommend.

Lifestyle Strategies

Maintain a healthful weight. Fat tissue does more than hug your thighs and hips. It converts certain hormones into estrogen. Women who are obese are 2 to 5 times more likely to develop endometrial cancer than are slimmer women. (For more information on achieving and maintaining a healthful weight, see Chapter 6.)

Nutritional Treatments

Follow a low-fat diet. Foods that are high in fats, particularly animal fats, can raise your risk of uterine cancer in two ways. Fatty foods lead to weight gain, and fat tissue itself, as we've seen, increases the risk of cancer. High-fat foods also appear to boost the body's production of estrogen.

The Benefits of Healing Retreats

In 1995, Nancy J. Raymon and Donna Farris founded Healing Odyssey, a retreat and follow-up support program for female cancer survivors. Since then, they have witnessed again and again how group support can powerfully transform and extend the lives of women with cancer. More than 700 cancer survivors have experienced a 3-day retreat in California.

Raymon, an oncology clinical nurse specialist and urologic cancer nurse coordinator at the Hoag Cancer Center in Newport Beach, California, decided to demonstrate the effectiveness and long-term benefits of weekend retreats. She surveyed 41 women, mostly breast cancer survivors, who were to participate in a retreat held in a remote location. The retreat included a coping with fear and sexuality workshop, a spirituality session, yoga, meditation, and guided imagery sessions, nature walks, a Saturday-night celebration, and an Empowerment Walk.

The survey looked at physical, psychological, social, and spiritual well-being. Raymon and a colleague evaluated participants before the retreat, directly afterward, 6 weeks later, and again at 6 months.

"We found a statistically significant increase in all four quality-of-life domains following the retreat," says Raymon. What's more, the effects remained strong after 6 months.

Raymon believes that healing retreats are effective because more and more patients are now living long lives with cancer. Many are looking to sharpen their survival skills and maintain long-term physical, psychological, and spiritual health by connecting with others.

"Cancer has become more of a chronic disease, unlike in the past, when most people either died or were cured," says Raymon. "These retreats are designed to help people deal with the challenging emotional and psychological issues of survivorship. It's also building a community of support and learning practical tools for moving forward with life." ∎

Research has shown that women who consume diets low in fat and high in complex carbohydrates have a reduced risk for developing endometrial cancer, says Linda R. Duska, MD, a gynecological oncologist and gynecologic oncology fellowship director at the University of Virginia in Charlottesville.

Get plenty of fiber. Fiber helps rid your body of excess estrogen. You should be getting 25 to 35 grams a day from vegetables, fruit, and whole grains.

Medical Options

Consider birth control pills. Taking oral contraceptives for up to 5 years defends against endometrial cancer, not only while you're using them but for years afterward. Most birth control pills contain progesterone, which helps reduce the body's exposure to estrogen. It's the same reason that pregnancy—which shifts the hormonal balance toward greater levels of progesterone—also safeguards the uterus.

Add progesterone to hormone replacement therapy. There's no question that the use of supplemental estrogen after menopause has given new meaning to the term "golden years." But taking estrogen without balancing it with progesterone may increase the risk for endometrial cancer.

"It's pretty clear that a lot of uterine cancer is preventable with the use of progesterone during estrogen replacement," says Joanna M. Cain, MD, chair of the department of obstet-

rics and gynecology at Women and Infants Hospital and assistant dean for Women's Health Programs at Alpert Medical School at Brown University in Providence, Rhode Island.

Be wary of tamoxifen. Used to prevent breast cancer, it acts like estrogen in the uterus, sometimes encouraging growth of the uterine lining and slightly raising the risk of endometrial cancer. If you're taking tamoxifen, have a yearly gynecologic exam—and be sure to report any abnormal bleeding to your doctor.

Report unusual bleeding to your doctor. A number of conditions, many of them harmless, can cause abnormal menstrual bleeding. With endometrial cancer, however, abnormal bleeding is almost a given. "If you're bleeding abnormally, especially after menopause, contact your doctor," says Dr. Duska.

See your gynecologist. Starting at age 21, visit a gynecologist every year for a pelvic exam and Pap test. If you are under age 21 but are sexually active, you should go earlier.

The Pap test is most effective at detecting cervical cancer (in the lower uterus), but it may detect endometrial cancers as well. Don't rely on it solely, however. Your best bet is to be alert to symptoms and report them immediately. If you have the hereditary form of colon cancer or are at risk for it, your chance of developing uterine cancer is also higher. Get an annual endometrial biopsy—a test that looks for cancerous changes in the tissue lining the uterus—beginning at age 35.

OVARIAN CANCER

"The most significant factor related to ovarian cancer is the number of ovulations that you have over a lifetime," says Dr. Cain. "Things that suppress ovulation–such as birth control pills, having children, breastfeeding, later menstruation, or early menopause–will all decrease your risk."

About 10 percent of ovarian cancers are genetic. If your mother, sister, or daughter has had ovarian cancer or breast cancer, particularly at a young age, or if you've had breast cancer yourself, your chances of getting ovarian cancer are greater.

Whatever your initial risk, following the general anticancer plan that we discussed at the beginning of this chapter will go a long way toward providing lifetime protection. In addition, here are some other strategies you'll want to follow.

Medical Options

Get tested regularly. Have an annual pelvic exam and Pap test starting at age 21, earlier if you are sexually active. The exams are particularly important after age 65, when half of all ovarian cancers show up. Pap tests, which are best at finding cervical cancer, sometimes detect advanced ovarian cancers as well.

If you have a family history of cancer, you may want to visit a genetic counselor to find out if you carry the BRCA1 or BRCA2 gene. These genes raise the risk for both ovarian and breast cancers.

"You'll want to discuss what you're going to do if you have the gene," says Dr. Cain. "Doctors recommend removing the ovaries after a woman is done having children. If someone's not at that point yet, we can test with transvaginal ultra-sound (with a small instrument inserted into the vagina) and a CA-125 screen every 6 months." CA-125 is a blood protein that's sometimes elevated in women with ovarian cancer. These tests are recommended only for women with a higher-than-average risk of ovarian cancer, Dr. Cain adds, because the test can produce too many false positives to be used for regular screening.

Enroll in a clinical trial. "If you carry the BRCA genes, my recommendation is to be involved in a study," says Vicki Seltzer, MD, chairman of obstetrics and gynecology at Long Island Jewish Medical Center and North Shore University Hospital in New Hyde Park, New York, and past president of the American College of Obstetricians and Gynecologists.

Your doctor can tell you how to enroll in a clinical study. Or contact the American Cancer Society at www.cancer.org or (800) ACS-2345.

Report symptoms immediately. "Many women have subtle symptoms, such as mild nausea, a little diarrhea that doesn't get better, or a slight pain in the pelvic region, about 6 months to a year before they're diagnosed with ovarian cancer," says Dr. Cain.

Other symptoms of ovarian cancer include long-term swelling of the abdomen, unusual vaginal bleeding, pelvic pain or pressure, back pain, leg pain, or digestive disorders, such as gas, indigestion, or stomach pain.

Chances are, the symptoms will turn out to be nothing to worry about, but having prompt checkups can ease your mind and also aid your chances of recovery if it turns out to be ovarian cancer.

Take oral contraceptives. Studies have been consistent: Contraceptive use may result in a 50 percent lower relative risk of developing ovarian cancer.

Review reproductive options with your doctor. Having one or more pregnancies is one way to reduce the risk for ovarian cancer, especially if your first baby arrives before you're 30. If you breast-feed for a year or more, you'll improve your odds further.

This doesn't mean that women should rush into having children before they're ready. The goal is to reduce your body's long-term exposure to ovulation, and this can be achieved with the use of birth control pills. Women who take birth control pills for more than 5 years are 60 percent less likely to get ovarian cancer than women who have never used them.

Consider a surgical route. If you have the BRCA genes, you may choose, as many women do, to have your ovaries removed prophylactically, which will reduce your risk of ovarian cancer by 90 percent.

Nutritional Treatments

Avoid processed meat. Hold the lunch meat sandwich and hot dogs: A 2010 Australian study found that women who eat four or more servings of processed meats are at higher risk of ovarian cancer. Fish, on the other hand, may put you at lower risk, the study authors suggest.

Eat a low-fat diet. Researchers tracking 49,000 postmenopausal women found those who had been asked to cut their fat intake nearly in half (to 24 percent of daily calories) were 40 percent less likely to develop ovarian cancer than a group that ate their regular diet.

CERVICAL CANCER

Your mother and grandmother probably worried more about cervical cancer than you do. Thanks to the development of Pap tests, which allow for early detection, deaths from cervical cancer plummeted by nearly three-quarters between 1955 and 1992. With the introduction of vaccines that prevent human papillomavirus—the cause of almost all cervical cancers, anal cancer, vaginal cancer, and some vulvar cancers—this cancer may slip off the radar screen altogether.

But don't let it slip off yours. Your risk may be higher than you think, particularly if you or your partner has been sexually active outside the relationship, or at other times in your lives.

Since the leading cause of cervical cancer is infection with the sexually transmitted HPV, the more sexual partners you and your partner have had, the greater your likelihood of HPV infection.

"All women may be at higher risk for HPV than they believe," says Dr. Seltzer. Even if you've had few sexual partners in your life, your significant other may unwittingly harbor the infection.

So far, there isn't a sure way to prevent HPV. The use of condoms can help, but it's possible for HPV to be transmitted during skin-to-skin contact with an infected area, such as skin of the genital area not covered by the condom, even if symptoms aren't apparent. Doctors are currently working on an experimental vaccine, and within a few years it could be available. "If successful, it will pretty much wipe out cervical cancer," predicts Dr. Duska.

Here are some other important strategies.

Medical Options

Have an annual Pap test. One of the most important things you can do is have a Pap test beginning at age 21 or when you first start having intercourse, whichever comes first. Pap tests can detect the signs of cervical cancer long before it becomes a real threat.

"Cervical cancer is almost completely preventable with regular Pap tests," says Dr. Seltzer. It can also be successfully treated when abnormalities are detected early.

If you don't have any abnormalities, it's safe to have a PAP every 2 years, and every 3 years when you're in your thirties, as long as you've had three clear PAP tests in a row.

It's not uncommon for mild dysplasias (precancerous cell abnormalities) to show up during Pap tests. These abnormalities don't always become cancerous. They may even disappear by themselves. (HPV disappears on its own too in many women, the victim of their immune systems.) If you have a positive test, don't be surprised if your doctor doesn't seem too concerned. He or she might schedule a

Drumming Up Cancer Immunity

group drumming is used as a part of healing rituals around the world. It sounds more like a quaint relic of medicine's unenlightened past than a modern cancer fighter. But drumming circles could soon find their way into oncology's arsenal of potent new weapons.

Barry Bittman, MD, is neurologist and medical director of the Mind-Body Wellness Center in Meadville, Pennsylvania. He and his colleagues have looked at group drumming and its effects on stress levels and immune function.

To enhance camaraderie and lightheartedness, participants in the studies were first asked to pass around, faster and faster, plastic "shaker eggs" filled with sand or gravel until the eggs invariably fell to the floor and the group erupted into laughter. Participants were then asked to drum together in rhythm to their own names, varying the tempo and pace. This was followed by a guided imagery session in which members played their drums as the facilitator told stories.

The researchers found that people who drummed had a reduction in stress levels and an increase in their immune response, including a rise in natural killer cell activity. Natural killer cells are the body's main cancer-fighting cells. Other studies have found that other immune cells are also increased by drumming.

Apart from the physical effects of drumming, it's also a powerful community-building tool, says Dr. Bittman. It allows participants to reveal feelings that may be hard to air verbally. And in studies, Bittman and his colleagues also found that mood improves, particularly among older people under stress.

Dr. Bittman now uses drumming circles with his cancer patients, both to help them de-stress and to give voice to their pain and fears.

"Chemotherapy, radiation, and surgery are certainly valid therapies, but there's also a fourth tool, a whole-person component that provides coping strategies, community, and stress reduction," he says. ∎

follow-up Pap test to keep track of changes.

If the dysplasia is more advanced, your doctor will probably remove the abnormal cells. It's a simple procedure that can be done right in the office, either with the use of liquid nitrogen (cryosurgery) or with a cone biopsy.

Lifestyle Strategies

Don't light up. If you smoke, do everything possible to quit right away. Doctors believe that tobacco smoke creates chemicals that damage DNA in cervical cells. If you smoke, you're twice as likely to get cervical cancer as a nonsmoker.

Nutritional Treatments

Eat your retinoids. Found in a wide variety of fruits and vegetables, retinoids such as vitamin A and beta-carotene appear to slow the growth of epithelial cells in the cervix, which is where most cancerous and precancerous abnormalities occur.

Get folic acid. Women who don't get enough of this B vitamin, which is abundant in fortified grain products, are more likely to get cervical cancer. If you're a smoker, you may need more, so a supplement may be in order. Pick a B-complex vitamin, since the other Bs also may help prevent this cancer.

Serve broccoli. All the cruciferous vegetables (including cauliflower, brussels sprouts, cabbage, and kale) contain indole-3-carbinol, which helps metabolize estrogen in a way that makes it less harmful.

SKIN CANCER

We all like that sun-kissed look, but our love affair with the sun is a prime health hazard. Skin cancer is the most common of all cancers.

"Heredity plays a role, and the more irregular moles you have, the more likely it is that you may develop melanoma," says Diane Berson, MD, assistant clinical professor of dermatology at Weill Cornell Medical College of Cornell University in New York City. "But protecting yourself from the sun is the most important thing you can do."

Fortunately, most skin cancers are highly curable, especially nonmelanomas, such as basal cell and squamous cell carcinomas, which account for the majority of cases.

Malignant melanomas are less common (though on the rise among young women), but they're also less curable. Catching them early is your best shot at making a complete recovery. Prevention is even better. Wearing sunscreen is essential, of course, from the time you're young. Roughly 80 percent of sun exposure occurs before you're 18. *Prevention* recommends wearing a waterproof, sweat-proof sunscreen with at least 30 SPF and full ultraviolet A (UVA) and ultraviolet B (UVB) protection at all times. Apply it 20 minutes before exposure and reapply every 2 hours—more if you've been in the water. You should also avoid the sun as much as possible between 10:00 a.m. and 4:00 p.m. (For a complete guide to skin care, see Chapter 9.) Practicing healthy habits, such as refraining from smoking and eating a low-fat diet, will contribute to the overall health of your skin, including reducing cancer risk and having fewer wrinkles.

And stay away from tanning beds. It's not

true that getting a "base" tan will help protect your skin from the sun and that the UV rays in a tanning bed are more benign than the sun's rays. Experts now think that tanning beds are responsible for the increase in deadly melanoma cancers among women in their twenties.

Dr. Berson recommends that adults have an annual skin exam by a dermatologist. *Prevention* recommends seeing a dermatologist for a head-to-toe skin cancer check at least every 3 years between ages 20 and 40. If you've had skin cancer or are at high risk because of family history, start exams earlier and get them more often.

It's also important to check your skin monthly. When looking at moles, remember the letters A (asymmetry), B (border irregularity), C (changes in color), and D (changes in diameter). If you notice any one of these changes, you could have a higher risk for developing melanoma.

Nonmelanomas often start as pale or pink wax-like, pearly nodules, or as red, scaly patches. Report to your doctor scaling, oozing, or bleeding from bumps or moles. "Skin cancer is the one cancer that shouldn't be missed, because it's visible," says Dr. Berson.

It's also worth drinking a few cups of green tea daily or using skin-care products that contain green tea extract. Green tea is rich in antioxidants, which have been shown to prevent skin cancer in laboratory mice. Some researchers believe green tea is probably just as effective in humans.

The Skin Cancer Foundation also recommends that people who avoid the sun or use protection increase their intake of vitamin D to 1,000 mg daily—not to prevent skin cancer, but to keep up stores of this vitamin that may help protect against other cancers and help your bones absorb calcium. Sunshine is a primary source of vitamin D.

Vaccines That Fight Cancer

It started with melanoma. In the late 1990s, studies found that 55 percent of people with this deadly skin cancer who were given a new, experimental anticancer vaccine survived when only 20 percent would have been expected to beat their diagnosis.

The injectable vaccine, made from the patients' own chemically altered cancer cells, seems to stop the spread of the disease by activating the immune system to attack active cancer cells, explains lead study author David Berd, MD, professor of medicine at Thomas Jefferson University in Philadelphia.

In 2009, University of Pittsburgh researchers began clinical trials of a vaccine that targets pre-cancerous colon polyps and breast and pancreatic tumors, using the body's own antibodies to battle an abnormal protein involved in those cancers.

If the results are positive, it may join three FDA-approved anticancer vaccines (one against human papillomavirus, a cause of cervical cancer; another for hepatitis B, which triggers liver cancer; and the third to treat advanced prostate cancer) as part of standard treatment for cancer.

Other vaccines being studied include those for kidney, breast, ovarian, lung, head and neck, and prostate cancers, as well as leukemia, multiple myeloma, and non-Hodgkin's lymphoma. ■

Osteoporosis

Osteoporosis, a bone-thinning condition that primarily affects women, develops over decades without causing overt symptoms. It doesn't hurt. You won't see any visible signs. But year after year, the bones get progressively weaker. You won't suspect there's a problem until you actually fracture a wrist, hip, or spinal bone—doing something as benign as picking up a shopping bag or even sneezing—or your doctor notices a substantial decrease in your height.

About 10 million Americans have osteoporosis and another 34 million are at risk. Your risk rises with age, especially in the first 5 to 7 years after menopause, when drops in estrogen may result in a 20 percent loss of bone mass. For women 50 years and older, the risk of suffering an osteoporosis-related bone fracture is about 50 percent.

The good news? Even if you have risk factors for osteoporosis—such as family history, a thin or small-framed body, a history of irregular or skipped periods, smoking or drinking excessive amounts of alcohol, not getting enough calcium, being inactive, or having taken steroids or other bone-thinning medications—the odds for preventing it can be very much in your favor.

"Osteoporosis is a disease of heredity and lifestyle," says Bess Dawson-Hughes, MD, direc-

tor of the Bone Metabolism Laboratory at the USDA Human Nutrition Research Center on Aging at Tufts University in Boston. "You can't do much about heredity, but you can prevent much of it with lifestyle modifications."

Nutritional Treatments

You may think of your skeleton as inert, as hard and lifeless as stone. But bone is living tissue and throughout your life bone cells called osteoblasts are continually adding new bone to your skeleton while cells called osteoclasts demolish old bone in order to supply the rest of your body with much-needed calcium.

The prime bone-building years are between childhood and early adulthood, when new bone is added to your skeleton faster than old bone is destroyed. By age 30, your bones are as dense and strong as they'll ever get. After that, bone loss gradually begins to outpace bone construction. Everyone—male or female—needs an adequate level of estrogen to build bone during their youth. Estrogen deficiency in premenopausal women is a significant risk factor for bone loss, and once a woman reaches menopause, declines in the body's estrogen cause bones to lose calcium and break down at an accelerated rate.

"Whether you get enough calcium and build adequate bone mass early in life or not, your body will start reabsorbing bone from your skeleton during your peri- and postmenopausal years, which can lead to osteoporosis," says Ethel Siris, MD, director of the Toni Stabile Center for Osteoporosis at Columbia University Medical Center at New York-Presbyterian Hospital in New York City and president of the National Osteoporosis Foundation. "If you enter menopause with a lower bone mass, obviously you'll be at a disadvantage." The body uses the reabsorbed bone to keep your blood calcium at a healthy level to sustain life.

Get enough calcium and vitamin D. Think of these two essential nutrients as though they were joined together, because your bones won't get enough calcium if you aren't getting the right amount of vitamin D to help them absorb the bone-building mineral. Your needs for both also change over time.

If you're 50 years or younger, you should be getting 1,000 mg of calcium daily through your food, plus a supplement if needed. If you're under 71, you need 600 IU of D daily, which goes up to 800 at 71. If you're older than 50, you need 1,500 mg of calcium daily. That's a lot of calcium, but Mother Nature is generous—many delicious, wholesome foods are brimming with it—and vitamin D, says Robert R. Recker, MD, director of the Osteoporosis Research Center at Creighton University School of Medicine in Omaha, Nebraska. Dairy products are your best bet, followed by calcium- and D-fortified juices, breads, and cereals. You'll also find vitamin D in fatty fish such as salmon, tuna, and mackerel.

How much calcium can you get in your diet? Consider this: Just three daily servings of low-fat or fat-free milk, cheese, or calcium-fortified soy milk or orange juice provide more than 1,000 mg of calcium. When you add the calcium that you get from other foods, such as legumes or salad greens, you'll get the calcium that your bones need to stay healthy—provided you eat all those foods every day. Milk and fortified orange juice supply about 100 IU of vitamin D per cup, but you can get your daily dose of the sunshine vitamin in just 3 ounces of salmon. Other canned fish is also high in D.

Consider supplements. Even women who eat healthful diets most of the time don't always get enough calcium. This is especially true of women who avoid dairy—either because they don't care for the taste or because they find them hard to digest. If you aren't getting enough calcium in your diet, it's fine to make up the difference with supplements, says Dr. Siris.

Siris sometimes advises women to take chewable supplements, such as Tums (an antacid that's calcium-based) or Viactiv soft chews, as a portion of their daily calcium intake. You can also take traditional calcium supplements. Supplements in any form can be overkill, Dr. Siris notes, because your body can absorb only a certain amount of calcium at one time and then excretes the excess. Genetics play a role in determining how much calcium your body can actually use for optimal bone density, she explains. Your body never fully absorbs all the calcium you ingest, but taking calcium in several 500 mg servings or doses throughout the day will optimize absorption.

"You might think you're getting 900 mg of calcium at breakfast if you drink a glass of milk—which has about 300 mg—and take a 600-mg supplement, but in reality you're only absorbing somewhat less," she says.

One more point about supplements: Those that contain calcium carbonate should be taken only with meals, to promote better absorption while those that contain calcium citrate can be taken anytime. Studies suggest that calcium citrate may actually be more effective than the carbonate version.

Be aware of the calcium robbers. Salt, caffeine, and protein play a role in removing calcium from your body. To safeguard your calcium stores, cut back on processed, canned, and fast foods, plus chips, pickles, and other items that are high in salt, says Dr. Dawson-Hughes. The upper daily limit for salt is about 2,400 mg, assuming you consume 2,000 calories daily.

Dr. Dawson-Hughes also advises drinking no more than two cups of coffee a day—although adding milk to coffee will replenish the calcium that's lost due to the caffeine (about 6 mg). It's also helpful to eat moderate amounts of protein. Women age 30 to 50 are advised to get about 10 to 15 percent of their total caloric intake from protein each day.

Lifestyle Strategies

Get a little sun each day. Every time sunshine strikes your skin, the body produces vitamin D, which aids in the absorption of calcium. You also get some vitamin D in fish oil, egg yolks, and fortified milk, but few other foods contain this vital nutrient—so getting a little bit of sun makes good sense.

If you don't get much sun (it only takes 5 to 10 minutes of unprotected exposure daily during the summer) or live in a northern latitude where the sun's rays aren't strong enough in winter to convert the chemicals in your skin to vitamin D, you may want to take a multivitamin that contains it—or take a calcium supplement with vitamin D added.

Get plenty of exercise. Aerobic exercise is good for everyone, but for protecting the bones, you can't beat weight-bearing or resistance exercises, which are essential for increasing or maintaining bone mass.

What's the best exercise? You have plenty to choose from. Felicia Cosman, MD, medical director of the Clinical Research Center at Helen Hayes Hospital in West Haverstraw, New York, advises women to run, walk, ski, or dance. Any activity that gets you on your feet and moving for 30 minutes 5 times a week will keep or modestly increase your bone mass. (For details on starting an exercise program and sticking with it, see Chapter 5.) For additional benefits, add 15 minutes of muscle-strengthening exercises, such as lifting weights. (For more on bone-building exercises, see page 230.)

If you smoke, quit. Cigarettes damage the bones in several ways. Smoking lowers levels of estrogen, which hastens bone loss. In addition, women who smoke may absorb less of the calcium in their diets. (For details on how to quit, see Chapter 8.)

Drink alcohol in moderation. Having more than a drink or two a day will interfere with the bones' ability to absorb calcium. Heavy drinking is even worse because it often results in poor nutritional intake overall, which can increase the risk of osteoporosis and fractures.

Medical Options

As we've seen, the body's levels of estrogen decline at menopause. Combined with the natural bone loss that occurs with age, this can vastly increase your risk for osteoporosis and related bone fractures. Women who have reached menopause need to follow all the bone-protection strategies that they depended on when they were younger—plus some that are unique to this stage of life.

"It's good to have an ongoing dialogue with your physician about your bone status throughout your life," says Dr. Siris. "Simply taking calcium and exercising won't stop osteoporosis. You need to discuss your risk factors and what you can do for protection."

Get a bone test. If you've reached menopause and have one or more risk factors for osteoporosis, you should undergo a test called central DEXA (dual energy x-ray absorptiome-

try), which measures bone density of the hip and spine. If you don't have any risk factors for osteoporosis, you can probably put off the test until you're between the ages of 60 and 65, says Dr. Cosman. *Prevention* recommends that women have a baseline bone density test at the first signs of menopause—or earlier if they have one or more risk factors for osteoporosis. If you're 50 or older, the test may be covered by your health insurance.

If you're still in your thirties and forties, there's no reason to have a bone density test as long as you eat a nutritious diet, get regular exercise, have a healthy lifestyle, and don't have any risk factors for osteoporosis.

Take medications to prevent bone loss. Most women can prevent osteoporosis by maintaining a healthful lifestyle, but if you already have it, your doctor may recommend medications that will prevent further bone loss.

In addition to estrogen, the FDA has approved a number of drugs for the prevention and treatment of osteoporosis. These include the selective estrogen receptor modulator raloxifene (Evista), alendronate (Fosamax), calcitonin (Miacalcin, Fortical), ibandronate (Boniva), zoledronic acid (Reclast), and risedronate (Actonel). Each of these drugs reduces bone loss and also increases bone density; though in 2010 a study found that people who take bisphosphonate drugs (Fosamax, Actonel, Boniva, Reclast, and their generics) could be at high risk of thigh fractures, and the FDA issued a warning about this atypical side effect.

WHEN BAD THINGS HAPPEN TO HEALTHY WOMEN

She Made Up for Lost Time—And Bone

A few years ago Linda Harrigan felt a pain in her hip during aerobics class. It was bad enough to send her to her doctor. Even more shocking was the diagnosis: osteoporosis.

"My reaction was total surprise," she recalls. "I thought, 'This is an old woman's disease.'"

While the reasons for her condition weren't surprising (she had undergone a hysterectomy, which had halted her body's production of bone-building estrogen), she didn't understand why her doctor hadn't recommended supplemental estrogen or extra calcium to offset the bone loss.

"I was angry," Harrigan says. "But I'm also a fighter. I never gave up, and I never stopped to be emotional."

As soon as she got the news, Harrigan went on a bone-strengthening regimen. She began getting 1,800 mg of calcium daily from high-calcium foods and supplements and she launched into an exercise plan that included walking, cycling, lifting weights, and running on a treadmill. Because she has brittle bones, she stays away from pounding activities, such as horseback riding or running on hard surfaces.

Harrigan also decided to begin low-dose estrogen replacement therapy, and she gets a bone-density test every 2 years. Because she has a family history of breast cancer, however, she may discontinue the use of estrogen and begin taking an osteoporosis-stopping drug.

"I've been told that my spine is what you'd find in a 90-year-old, so I worry sometimes that my body will start to crumble and fall apart. But I'm very upbeat about it. I just went for my yearly checkup, and I'm still 5 foot 10 and my posture is excellent. I've been blessed." ■

Ask your doctor about taking estrogen replacement. The Women's Health Initiative hormone trials were stopped early after finding that HRT increased the risk of stroke, blood clots, cognitive problems, and breast cancer. But it ran long enough for researchers to learn that it did help improve bone mineral density and reduce fractures. Still, it's so risky that it's not recommended for osteoporosis prevention.

Strengthen Your Bones with Exercise

If you do have osteoporosis, check with your doctor before starting an exercise plan. Physical activity is good for you, but you'll probably be advised to limit certain activities—such as those that require bending your back forward, or high-impact exercises such as tennis or running. There are two main types of exercises for building and strengthening bones: weight-bearing exercises, in which you move your body against gravity, and strength-training and resistance exercises, which are considerably more strenuous. Here are some of your choices.

Walking

The weight you're bearing is yours, of course. When you walk, your legs are required to bear most of your weight, increasing stress on bones in the legs and hips. Researchers aren't sure why, but the stress felt by bones during exercise stimulates the bone-building cells, osteoblasts, to make new bone.

Walking is easier to do than many types of exercise, and it's an excellent way to retard bone loss as you age. Women who regularly walk throughout their lives have higher bone density than women who are sedentary. They also have a 30 percent lower fracture rate.

Doctors advise taking a 30-minute walk 5 days a week. You don't have to do it all at once. Two 15-minute walks will give the same benefits. To increase the intensity of your workout—and increase the bone benefits—walk faster or choose an uphill route.

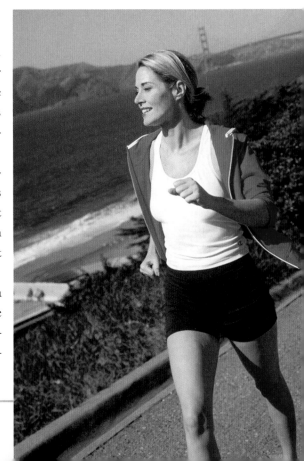

Running

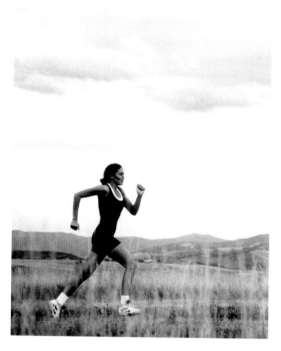

This is a high-impact exercise. It stimulates about 3 times more bone growth than walking according to recent studies. If your bones are already strong, high-impact activities (which include aerobics, dancing, and tennis) are a good choice. If, however, you've already been diagnosed with osteoporosis, ask your doctor if your bones are strong enough for high-impact activities.

Many women incorporate high-impact activities into their regular walks—for example, by breaking into a run for a minute or two, then slowing back to walking speed. To give your body time to adjust to the vigorous exercise, start out by running for just 10 seconds. If it feels comfortable, gradually increase the time. Even a small amount of high-impact activity will prompt significant bone growth.

Gardening

You don't have to belong to a gym to get the bone-boosting benefits of resistance exercises. Activities such as lawn care and gardening require a lot of digging, pulling, and pushing, which can also add bone.

Remember, though, to take it easy. If you haven't done yard work for a while, rest frequently to prevent overexertion and drink plenty of water to prevent dehydration.

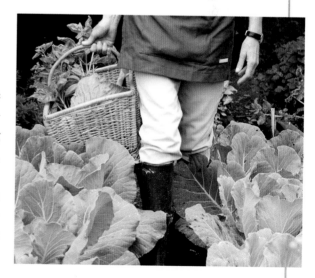

(continued)

Strengthen Your Bones with Exercise

Jumping Jack

If your bones are already strong and healthy, jumping is a good way to increase hip density. In fact, doing this type of exercise for 2 minutes daily can increase bone density in a matter of months.

Jumping jacks are good for beginning jumpers. Find a flat surface, either indoors or out. Avoid slippery spots or extremely hard surfaces, like concrete or tile.

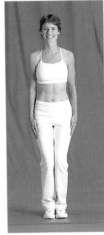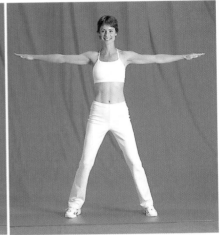

Stand with your feet together and arms at your sides (left). Bend your knees slightly, and jump while simultaneously moving your arms and feet out to the sides. Your feet should be approximately 3 feet apart. Your arms should be parallel to the floor (right). Land on the balls of your feet with your knees slightly bent.

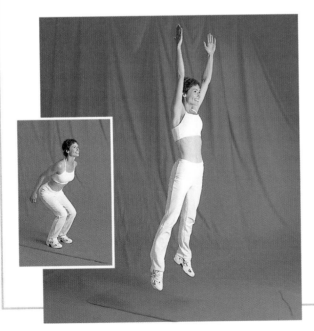

Power Jump

If you've been doing jumping jacks for at least 4 weeks, and you're sure you can jump and land safely, the "power jump" is worth a try.

Stand with your feet hip-width apart and your elbows bent slightly at your sides (far left). Bend your knees 4 to 6 inches, then jump straight up. As you jump, extend your arms up over your head, as if you were reaching toward the ceiling (near left). Land on the balls of your feet, keeping your knees slightly bent.

Seated Reverse Fly

This simple exercise will strengthen your shoulders and back.

Sit in a chair with your feet flat on the floor, hip-width apart. Hold a dumbbell in each hand, with the weights at chest level. Hold them about 12 inches from your body, with your palms facing each other as though you were holding a beach ball. Your elbows should be slightly bent (near right). Bend forward from your hips about 3 to 5 inches.

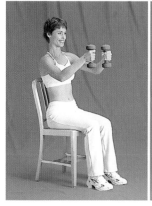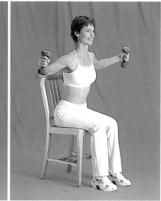

Keeping your back flat and your spine straight, slowly squeeze your shoulder blades together and pull your elbows as far back as possible (far right). Pause, then slowly return to the starting position. Repeat the exercise 8 to 12 times. Rest a moment, then do 8 more.

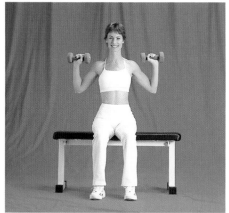

Overhead Press

This offers plenty of lifting and lowering—and lowering weights is what really counts when it comes to stimulating bone growth, according to researchers at California State University Los Angeles.

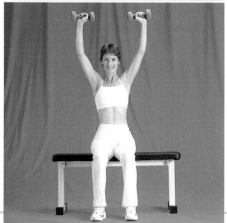

While sitting, hold a weight in each hand (top). Start with the weights at shoulder height; your palms should be facing forward. Raise the weights above your head without bringing them together or locking your elbows (bottom), then bring them back down to your shoulders.

Important: Don't try to lift weights that are too heavy. The weight should be challenging, but not overwhelming. If you find you can easily repeat the exercise more than 12 times, move to a heavier weight. If you can't do 8 repetitions, the weight is too heavy. This advice on weight selection pertains to the military press exercise here, as well as the exercises requiring dumbbells, above and on pages 234 and 235.

(continued)

Strengthen Your Bones with Exercise

Squat

A type of resistance exercise, squats are an excellent way to strengthen the thighs, and new research suggests that the more muscle you have, and the less fat, the higher your bone density will be. Here's how to do them.

Stand with your feet shoulder-width apart (near right). Bend your knees and squat, as though you're sitting; hold your arms in front for balance. Slowly lower your buttocks until your thighs are almost parallel to the ground (far right). Don't let your knees extend beyond your toes. Hold the position for a second, then rise.

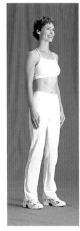
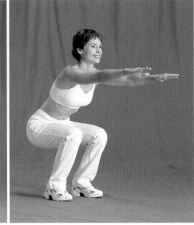

Chest Fly

This exercise improves chest and shoulder strength, as well as your posture.

Lie face-up on an exercise mat, with your knees bent, feet hip-width apart, and toes straight ahead.

Holding a dumbbell in each hand, extend your arms out to the sides, with your palms facing up and your hands at chest level (top). Bend your elbows at about a 45-degree angle.

Keeping your wrists straight and your lower back pressed into the floor, slowly lift both arms up and toward the center of your body in a sweeping arc (bottom). Make sure not to lift the dumbbells directly over your head, and don't straighten your arms.

Stop just before the weights touch in midair over your chest. Pause, then slowly lower the weights. Repeat the exercise 8 to 12 times. Rest a moment, then do them again.

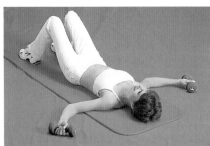
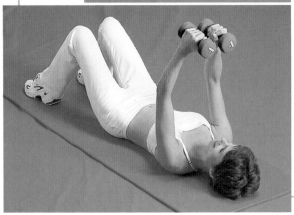

Wrist Flexion

Osteoporosis is responsible for 250,000 wrist fractures each year. This easy exercise will strengthen the wrists and protect against carpal tunnel pain, sprains, and other injuries.

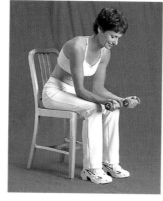
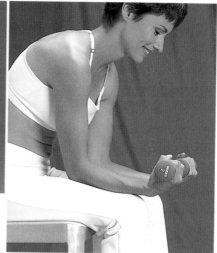

Sit in a chair, your feet hip-width apart. Holding a dumbbell in each hand, place your forearms on top of your thighs so your palms are facing up (left). Your hands will hang over your knees.

Slowly bend your wrists, curling the dumbbells up toward your arms (right). Your wrists and hands should be the only things moving. Bring your hands up as high as is comfortable. Hold, then slowly lower. Repeat the exercise 8 to 12 times. Rest, then repeat the exercise.

Wrist Extension

Like wrist flexions, this exercise will both strengthen and protect your wrists.

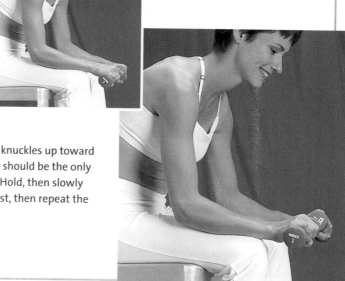

Sit in a chair with your feet hip-width apart. Holding a dumbbell in each hand, place your forearms on top of your thighs so that your palms are facing down (near right). Your hands will hang over your knees.

Slowly lift the dumbbells, bringing your knuckles up toward your arms (far right). Your wrists and hands should be the only things moving. Go as far as is comfortable. Hold, then slowly lower. Repeat the exercise 8 to 12 times. Rest, then repeat the exercise.

Alzheimer's Disease

Occasional forgetfulness is a disconcerting sign of middle age. Maybe you misplace the car keys now and then or find yourself searching for a word that's just beyond reach. Deep down, you may worry that these flashes of forgetfulness are the beginnings of Alzheimer's disease.

The worry is understandable. About one in ten Americans over age 65, and almost half of those over 85, suffer from this debilitating brain condition. Sixty-five percent are women, largely because women live longer than men. Dementia rates double every 5 years after the age of 65. Medications can ease some of the symptoms for a time, but there's no cure, and scientists still aren't sure of the underlying causes. Researchers have found that people with Alzheimer's have abnormal tangles of fibers in and around nerve cells in the brain, which interrupt their normal connections and result in mental and physical deterioration. But it isn't clear what triggers these changes, though it's likely that genetics, environment, and lifestyle each play a role. One recent study found that a gene variant on the X chromosome is related to Alzheimer's development; since women have two X chromosomes (men have only one), they are more at risk. Many memory problems, of course, are entirely normal, although research shows that you can minimize the lapses with a little help. (For more information on memory problems, see page 456.) Even if you have a greater risk for developing Alzheimer's disease—because it runs in your family, for example, or you've had a serious head injury in the past—you may be able to reduce that risk.

Most neurological problems take decades to develop. The earlier you start strengthening and protecting your brain, the better your chances of staying healthy throughout your life, says Dharma Singh Khalsa, MD, president and medical director of the Alzheimer's Research and Prevention Foundation in Tucson.

"The brain is not a computer," says Dr. Khalsa. "It's flesh and blood like any other organ—and it depends on the same things to keep it healthy."

Nutritional Treatments

Reduce the fat in your diet. Ideally, fewer than 20 percent of your total calories should come from fat, especially if you have a family history of Alzheimer's disease. "Fat plugs up arteries in the brain and reduces blood flow," says Dr. Khalsa. A high-fat diet also increases damage from free radicals, harmful oxygen molecules that damage tissues in the brain and other parts of the body.

Eat more fish. People who eat fish once a week are 60 percent less likely to develop Alzheimer's than those who rarely or never eat fish, according to a study done by researchers at Rush University Medical Center in Chicago who believe it's a result of the omega-3 fatty acids in seafood, which are vital to brain health.

Consider an over-the-counter supplement. A soy-based product available in pharmacies and health food stores, phosphatidylserine (PS), is permitted by the FDA to claim that it "may reduce the risk of dementia in the elderly," though that is based on very preliminary evidence. One study showed that people who took PS had an improvement in their ability to remember names. Dr. Khalsa advises taking 100 to 300 mg of PS daily.

Home Remedies

Get and stay slim. It's one of the only ways to avoid diabetes, hypertension, and cardiovascular disease, which are all risk factors for Alzheimer's disease.

Stop smoking. Heavy smoking at midlife can nearly double your risk of Alzheimer's, possibly because smoking encourages inflammation, which seems to be a trigger for the disease, says a 2010 study from the University of California San Francisco. (See Chapter 8 for ways to quit.)

Take ibuprofen. Because brain inflammation appears to play a role in the development of Alzheimer's disease, taking ibuprofen (such as Motrin or Advil) may delay its onset. Because ibuprofen may cause side effects, including bleeding, be sure to talk to your doctor before using it as part of an Alzheimer's prevention plan, Dr. Hershey says.

Stay physically active. In a 5-year study of people ages 65 and older, Canadian researchers found that those who exercised vigorously at least 3 days a week were up to 50 percent less likely to develop Alzheimer's disease and 40 percent less likely to suffer other symptoms of mental decline than their sedentary counterparts.

Even those who did only light activity such as easy walking had a much lower risk, says lead researcher Danielle Laurin of Laval University in Quebec. "We need more research, but exercise may work by improving blood flow to the brain (hence providing more nutrients), which keeps brain cells healthy and alive."

A 2010 study from the Mayo Clinic found that people between the ages of 70 and 90 who exercised moderately but regularly were almost 40 percent less likely to have mild cognitive impairment (MCI) than people who didn't. People who exercise late in life were also 32 percent less likely to have memory problems.

Exercise your brain. "Reading the paper and discussing it, doing crossword puzzles, or taking up a hobby–such as art, music, or learning a foreign language–increases the connections between brain cells and decreases your chance of getting Alzheimer's," says Dr. Khalsa.

Treat your depression. A 2008 French study found that Alzheimer's disease risks are gender-specific. More men were likely to have cognitive

Why Early Diagnosis Is Vital

families often wait 3 to 4 years, dutifully fishing car keys out of sugar bowls and nodding at the same tale repeated over and over in a single conversation, before they seek professional help for a loved one exhibiting early signs of dementia. Those 3 to 4 years could cost dearly. Here's why.

There are three stages of dementia, but prior to stage 1 is the phase called mild cognitive impairment, which is characterized by mild memory and thinking problems that don't interfere with everyday tasks. Not everyone who has MCI gets Alzheimer's or another form of dementia, but many do. Symptoms may include forgetting recent events or conversations, difficulty solving problems, and taking longer to perform difficult mental activities. In stage 1, the patient begins to exhibit language problems (forgetting the names of familiar objects), misplacing things, getting lost on familiar routes, flat mood, difficulty with tasks that were once easy such as balancing a checkbook, as well as, depression, irritability, and anxiety. At this point, a person can still live on her own, but this early phase lasts only 2 to 4 years. Most families mistakenly attribute these behaviors to normal aging. A doctor's opinion is frequently not sought until stage 2, which is often marked by more troublesome behaviors such as agitation, paranoia, or aggression, and by more serious cognitive and physical slippage such as difficulty reading and writing, loss of ability to recognize danger, or forgetting events in your own life, including who you are. Obviously, people at this stage need more care. By the time someone reaches stage 3, they often require around-the-clock care. They can no longer understand language, recognize family members, or do simple things, such as feeding themselves, bathing, and dressing.

An early diagnosis of Alzheimer's—while still in stage 1—can help to slow the progression of the symptoms by as much as a year or more with medications such as Razadyne, Aricept, and Exelon, says Steven Potkin, MD, director of neuropsychiatric research at the University of California Irvine Medical Center.

New evidence suggests that if you miss that window of opportunity, the new drugs may not work as well. In one study, patients with mild to moderately severe Alzheimer's who received Exelon improved after 6 months; expectedly, those given a placebo didn't.

"But then the researchers gave the placebo group Exelon, and checked in with both groups over the next year and a half," says Dr. Potkin. "Much to their surprise, while the original placebo group improved with Exelon, they never did as well as the people who had been given the drug from the beginning."

There is treatment for moderate to severe Alzheimer's—a medication called Namenda (memantine) delays progression of some symptoms, allowing patients to continue to care for themselves, including using the bathroom independently, at least for several months. It works by regulating glutamate, a brain chemical that can lead to brain cell death in large amounts. Aricept is also approved for use in late-stage Alzheimer's. ∎

impairment as the result of stroke; for women, it was depression. To protect your brain, seek psychological counseling or talk to your doctor about drug treatment for depression.

Alternative Therapies

Take a break from stress. "Chronic stress raises levels of the hormone cortisol, which is toxic to the memory center of the brain," says Dr. Khalsa. Cortisol decreases the brain's ability to use glucose, blocks the effects of neurotransmitters, and actually injures and kills brain cells. He advises managing stress by meditating, stretching, or sitting quietly for a few minutes.

Other Causes of Dementia

Alzheimer's disease is the most common cause of dementia, but it's not the only one. Others include:

Strokes. By cutting off the oxygen supply to the brain, a stroke can cause sometimes massive brain cell death that triggers what's called vascular dementia, the second most common cause of dementia and one that's preventable.

Dementia with Lewy bodies. This form of dementia is marked by spherical structures that develop inside nerve cells, where they damage brain tissue.

Pick's disease. Caused by the atrophy of the brain's temporal and frontal lobes, Pick's is similar to Alzheimer's and usually affects people between the ages of 40 and 60.

Parkinson's disease. A degenerative disorder of the nervous system, Parkinson's results in the loss of dopamine-producing brain cells and can cause dementia in addition to its typical symptoms, such as tremors and balance problems. Other motor neuron diseases such as multiple sclerosis may also increase dementia risk.

Endocrine disorders. Addison's disease, which results from adrenal cortex damage, and Cushing's disease, caused by a tumor or excess growth of the pituitary gland, are also associated with dementia.

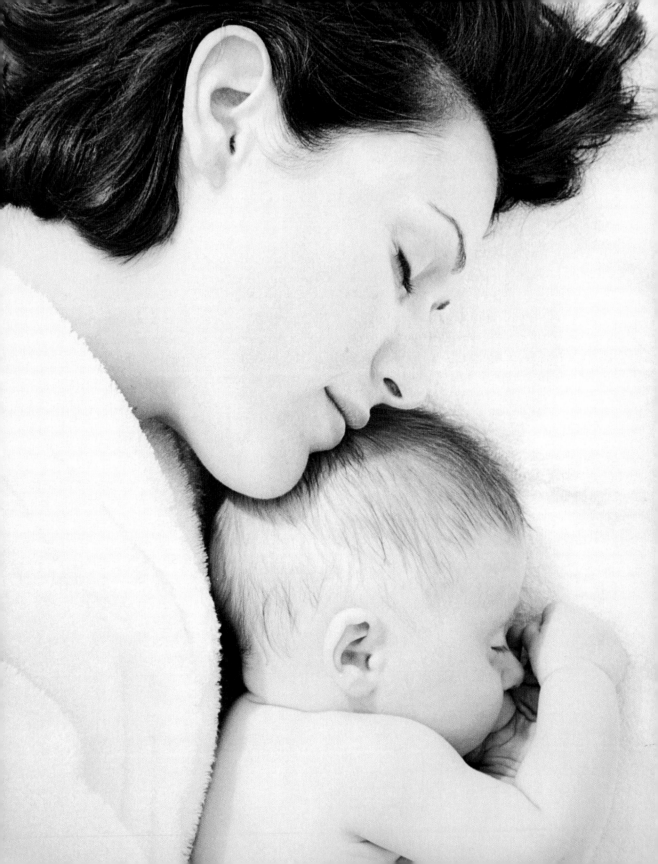

PART
FOUR

HORMONAL

WELLNESS:

THE BEST-EVER

LIFE-STAGE

STRATEGIES

19

PMS and Menstrual Discomforts

You probably know what happens every month during your reproductive years. Nature goes about its work of trying to populate the earth. So once a month, a single egg (usually) passes from an ovary to a fallopian tube, where it lies in wait for sperm. While the egg waits, the ovary releases estrogen and, a bit later, progesterone, in order to create a nourishing and protective nest in the lining of the uterus.

Should the egg remain unfertilized, the uterine lining begins its monthly regenerative ritual by trickling out blood thanks to vessel-constricting substances called prostaglandins. The chemicals stimulate contractions that release the uterine lining, and trigger cramps that may start as early as a week before the period begins and continue until menstruation is done.

Because prostaglandins have inflammatory and pain-causing effects, many women also experience a touch of nausea, bloating, headaches, diarrhea, or breast tenderness. And, for some reason, moods can swing wildly during this time, prompting a diagnosable condition called premenstrual syndrome or PMS.

Perhaps the only woman who has been able to put a positive spin on the often joked about and sometimes dreaded time of the month is comic Roseanne Barr, who once said, "Women complain about PMS, but I think of it as the only time of the month when I can be myself."

What's Normal and What's Not

The cramps, fluid retention, and occasional moodiness that many women experience before and during their periods are nothing more than signs that their reproductive systems are following their normal, healthy patterns, says Ronald Young, MD, director of the division of gynecology at Baylor College of Medicine in Houston.

But there may be other changes that aren't so healthy. Severe menstrual pain, called dysmenorrhea, for example, warrants a checkup with your gynecologist or family doctor because it could be a sign of endometriosis, uterine fibroids, or pelvic inflammatory disease.

Emotional changes can be just as telling. A little moodiness is one thing, but the onset of menstruation shouldn't leave you feeling morose or out of control. Estimates vary, but as many as 85 percent of women have at least one symptom of PMS, including swollen or tender breasts, acne, anxiety, depression, irritability, fatigue, food cravings and memory problems. Anywhere from 3 to

8 percent have a premenstrual dysphoric disorder (PMDD), a serious condition characterized by severe symptoms of depression, irritability, and tension before menstruation. Those symptoms usually interfere with a woman's daily life and may affect her relationships. No one knows what causes either condition, though genetics and lifestyle may each play a role.

In fact, more than 150 physical and emotional changes have been linked to the menstrual cycle. When women are otherwise healthy, menstrual-related changes in their physical or emotional well-being are often caused by lifestyle factors, such as stress, nutritional deficiencies, or a lack of sleep, says George J. Kallins, MD, coauthor of *Five Steps to a PMS-Free Life*.

Because the menstrual cycle can trigger such a wide range of signs and symptoms, there is no cure-all. However, doctors have identified more than 300 treatment options for menstrual or pre-menstrual discomfort, though many come with no supporting evidence of their effectiveness. However, it's worth being optimistic because you're sure to find some simple remedies that will work for you.

Home Remedies

Sometimes even small changes can have profound effects on the way you feel. Women have always treated PMS and menstrual discomfort with home remedies—simple, time-tested strategies that can make a difference. Here are some things you may want to try.

Take ibuprofen right away. Ibuprofen blocks the body's production of pain-causing

prostaglandins—and it's much less likely than other pain medications to cause side effects.

If you start taking ibuprofen at the first sign of symptoms, you'll have protective levels of the medication in the bloodstream, which will prevent the discomfort from getting worse later on, says Melvin V. Gerbie, MD, retired head of the gynecology section and professor of clinical gynecology at Northwestern University Feinberg School of Medicine in Chicago. He

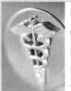

when to see a doctor

If you're experiencing so much discomfort before or during your period that you can't function normally. Make an appointment to see your doctor. Mild menstrual discomfort may be normal, but if it's interfering with your life, there's probably an underlying problem that needs to be addressed, says Melvin V. Gerbie, MD, retired head of the gynecology section and professor of clinical gynecology at Northwestern University Feinberg School of Medicine in Chicago.

If you've been having depression, anxiety, or irritability for more than 3 months, or if the feelings aren't limited to the 7 to 10 days before your period. You could be confusing clinical depression with PMS. Make an appointment to see a psychologist or psychiatrist, or discuss it with your current health care provider. Depression is also a risk factor for PMS and PMDD.

If you're having cramps as well as irregular or heavy bleeding, or if the blood is coming out in clots. You could have physical problems that require professional consultation.

advises taking 400 mg of ibuprofen four times daily. Start taking it 2 days before your period, and keep taking it until the time in your cycle when the cramps usually stop–usually about the second day after menstruation begins.

Water down bloating. Fluid retention caused by high hormone levels can cause uncomfortable swelling in the abdomen, breasts, and ankles. It sounds paradoxical to drink a lot of water when you feel like a sponge, but water acts as a diuretic and removes excess fluid from the body, says Dr. Kallins. He advises drinking at least eight full glasses of water daily before and during your period. (If that doesn't work, talk to your doctor about diuretics.)

Avoid cigarette smoke. Research has shown that even secondhand smoke can make premenstrual discomfort worse. In one study, Chinese researchers looked at 165 female nonsmokers, all newlyweds. None of the women had a history of menstrual discomfort. In the months after marriage (and their exposure to secondhand smoke by household members), there was a significant increase in premenstrual lower-back pain and abdominal discomfort.

Have an orgasm. In one survey of more than 2,600 women, 9 percent told doctors that giving themselves an orgasm through masturbation helped ease menstrual cramps.

Nutritional Treatments

Estrogen regulates the body's metabolism of a variety of nutrients, and it also affects the body's ability to absorb them. New evidence suggests that levels of calcium, vitamin D, iron, and other key nutrients may rise and fall in synchrony with estrogen fluctuations. Some researchers believe that short-term nutritional deficiencies are responsible for some of the premenstrual symptoms that have perplexed doctors for decades.

Many major studies have shown that supplementing the diet with calcium or vitamin B_6 can relieve menstrual or premenstrual symptoms in women who usually don't get adequate amounts of these nutrients.

Supplements can only do so much, of course. Every woman should eat a healthful diet and maintain adequate levels of vitamins and minerals throughout the month, not just before and during the menstrual period.

"Don't think about getting enough fresh fruits and vegetables and avoiding processed foods only when your symptoms hit," says James G. Penland, PhD, a research psychologist and PMS researcher at the USDA Human Nutrition Research Center at Grand Forks, North Dakota. As extra insurance against PMS discomfort, however, it's fine to use supplements containing no more than the daily recommended intakes.

Load up with calcium and vitamin D. These bone-building nutrients are also extra protection against PMS symptoms. In the long-running Nurses' Health Study, women who got the most D and calcium in their diets–from fortified foods such as low-fat or fat-free milk–had the lowest risk for menstrual problems. In fact, women who had four or more servings of low- or fat-free milk daily were protected from the

WHEN BAD THINGS HAPPEN TO HEALTHY WOMEN

Her Monthly Discomfort Led to a New Life

When Charis Lindrooth was a school-teacher in Kutztown, Pennsylvania, she found that any stress and disappointments that she felt during the month would climax in the days before her menstrual period.

"I'd feel fine the rest of the month, and then, a few days before my period, I'd habitually dwell on everything so much that I'd make myself physically sick," says Lindrooth. "When depression set in really hard, it sent me off on a crazy sugar binge."

She finally mustered the discipline to quit eating sweets, and it made a remarkable difference in how she felt. She also consulted an herbalist, who gave her herbs for her moodi-ness and for her digestive problems.

"I also started on chamomile and lemon balm tea, which really helped resolve my anxiety," she says. "After taking these herbs for a month, it felt like suddenly something was really healed inside me."

Lindrooth was so inspired by the changes that she decided to study nutrition and body work. Eventually she left her job as a teacher and went on to become a chiropractor, and she's getting ready to complete a degree in herbal medicine.

"I sometimes tell people that the call to my vocation came through my uterus," she laughs. ■

---

monthly "curse" significantly better than those who had only one or none. Get 1,200 mg of calcium and 600 IU of D from fortified dairy or orange juice. If you are lactose intolerant, use an enzyme such as Lactaid to help you digest dairy products. Other studies support the use of supplements: In one, women who took 300 mg of calcium carbonate four times a day significantly reduced their mood swings, pain, bloating, depression, back pain, and food cravings.

Get enough magnesium and vitamin B_6. "One of the reasons that these two nutrients are so highly recommended for PMS is that they help assure a healthy supply of the mood-regulating brain chemicals serotonin and dopa-mine," says Dr. Kallins. Research suggests that these chemicals, called neurotransmitters, also play a role in easing or preventing physical symptoms, including bloating, headaches, acne, and cramps. Some studies suggest that women with PMS have low levels of magnesium.

You can get a lot of magnesium and vitamin B_6 from figs, raisins, corn, and bananas. To be on the safe side, Dr. Kallins advises women to supplement their diets with 350 mg of magnesium and 100 mg of vitamin B_6. The B vitamins work together, which means that supplemental B_6 won't be helpful unless you also have adequate amounts of the other B vitamins. So it's a good idea to take a multivitamin or a B-complex supplement, he says.

Ease breast pain with a nutritional combo. If your breasts get tender as your period approaches, you might want to try a remedy suggested by Mary Jane Minkin, MD, clinical professor of obstetrics and gynecology at Yale University School of Medicine and coauthor of *What Every Woman Needs to Know about Menopause.*

Talk to your doctor about taking 1,000 mg of evening primrose oil, 400 to 800 IU of vitamin E, and 100 mg of vitamin B$_6$ daily. This supplement combination reduces the pain and inflammation that are triggered by surges in prostaglandins during the menstrual cycle, she explains.

Focus on the "top four" proteins. Many of the foods that Americans depend on for protein—mainly meat and dairy foods—are also high in fat, which has been linked to menstrual cramps. Better sources of protein include fish, soy foods, egg whites, and legumes, says Dr. Kallins.

These foods provide more than just protein, he adds. Soy foods and legumes are rich in phytoestrogens, plant-based chemicals similar to the estrogen that women produce naturally. Fish is rich in omega-3 fatty acids, which may help regulate mood, and egg whites provide an abundance of good quality protein with virtually no fat.

Reduce salt intake. If you find you're taking on more water than the *Titanic,* giving you that unpleasant bloated feeling, abandon the salt-

THREE THINGS I TELL EVERY FEMALE PATIENT

GEORGE J. KALLINS, MD, *coauthor of* Five Steps to a PMS-Free Life, *offers the following tips for controlling PMS and menstrual discomfort.*

1 **DON'T TAKE ANTIDEPRESSANTS UNLESS YOU'VE TRIED CALCIUM FIRST.** Scientific studies have shown that calcium supplements—about 1,200 mg daily—can reverse menstrual-related mood swings, depression, and anger. The mineral also reduces the discomfort of cramps and headaches.

EXERCISE OFTEN. "I see in my patients that those who exercise regularly experience less menstrual symptoms than those who don't," says Dr. Kallins. Natural chemicals called endorphins are released during exercise. Known as "feel good" chemicals, endorphins can help ease cramps, breast tenderness, and other types of menstrual discomfort.

2 For the best endorphin "rush," Dr. Kallins advises women to focus on aerobic exercises, such as fast walking, bicycling, or swimming. Try to exercise for 20 to 30 minutes at least 4 times a week.

LIMIT INDULGENCES. Women who eat a lot of sweets or fast food, or who consume caffeine or alcohol regularly, tend to have more menstrual and premenstrual discomfort than those who eat a healthier diet. "Don't think of it as depriving yourself," Dr. Kallins advises. "Think of it as a gift you're giving yourself to feel more balanced on every level." ■ **3**

shaker and reduce your intake of sodium-heavy foods such as crackers and chips (which you shouldn't eat for many reasons). Sodium causes your body to retain fluid.

Pass on coffee and alcohol. Reducing stimulants can help decrease fluid retention, bloating, and irritability. It can also reduce breast pain, particularly if you have fibrocystic breasts, a condition affecting about half of all women and marked by lumps and bumps in the breast that can get tender just before your period. The lumps are caused by fibrocystic tissue in the breast, says Elizabeth A. Poynor, MD, PhD, a gynecological oncologist and pelvic surgeon in private practice in New York City. As you age, the cells in your breast glands overgrow and form fibrous tissue that blocks ducts and prevents fluid from draining.

Don't give in to cravings for sugary food. Many women crave candy, baked goods, and other sweet foods before and during their periods. Indulging in these foods causes a rapid rise in blood sugar, which in turn can cause your energy and mood to crash. Highly processed carbohydrates, such as bagels, potato chips, and sodas, aren't much better because they supply a lot of calories and not a lot in the way of important nutrients. If you fill up on "empty" calories, you may find that you're not getting enough important nutrients to prevent menstrual discomfort.

It won't hurt to give in to cravings on occasion if your diet consists mainly of fresh fruits and vegetables, whole grains, and other nutritious foods. The fiber in a plant-based diet is especially helpful because it helps remove excess estrogen from the body, which will go a long way toward reducing menstrual and premenstrual discomfort, says Dr. Kallins.

Take advantage of healing oils. As you know, chemicals called prostaglandins are responsible for some of the pain and discomfort that occur before and during your period. But there are actually several types of prostaglandins, including some that inhibit pain and inflammation. Flaxseed, black currant, and hemp oils, available in health food stores, stimulate the body's production of "good" prostaglandins. Adding these oils to your diet may inhibit cramps, bloating, and breast tenderness. These oils aren't used for cooking, but you can add them to salads, shakes, or other foods. Try to get a total of 3 teaspoons of one or more of these oils daily all month.

Alternative Therapies

Most women experience some degree of premenstrual stress. As it turns out, stress is not only a symptom of PMS but also a cause of it.

When we experience stress, the adrenal glands make cortisol, a stress hormone, out of our progesterone. This results in low levels of progesterone, and low progesterone is thought to be a primary cause of menstrual cramps and PMS symptoms.

To reduce your risk of suffering from stress-related PMS, try to develop and practice stress reduction strategies every day.

Each woman has a different approach to reducing stress. Some of the most helpful are meditation, taking hot, lavender-scented baths, and getting at least 8 hours of sleep every night. Other helpful strategies include the following:

Press away symptoms. For centuries, Asian healers have practiced reflexology, a technique in which one "adjusts" the body's internal organs by pressing certain points on the feet, hands, and ears. In one study, women with PMS underwent foot, hand, and ear reflexology sessions in which practitioners manipulated the trigger points that correspond to the uterus and ovaries; other women in the study were given "sham" treatments at inappropriate trigger points. The women who received the real treatment had a significant reduction in symptoms, says Terry Oleson, PhD, director of the department of behavioral medicine at the California Graduate Institute in Los Angeles.

To find a professional reflexologist in your area, go to the Reflexology Association of America's Web site at www.reflexology-usa.org.

Practice relaxation therapies. An easy way to relax and let go of tension is to tense and then relax each muscle in your body. The technique, known as progressive relaxation, is simple. While you're lying down, contract the muscles in your feet. Hold the tension for a moment, then relax. Then move up to the calves . . . the knees . . . the thighs . . . and onward up to your head. It takes about 15 to 20 minutes to work through the whole body. At the end of each session, you'll find that your levels of physical and emotional tension will be substantially reduced.

Go into the light. Several studies have found that exposure to bright light before and during your period may help ease depression and some physical symptoms of PMDD. This is the same kind of cool white light treatment used for seasonal affective disorder, a form of depression caused by lack of light exposure during the winter months. How it works: Light enters through the retina, where it affects your neuroendocrine system via your pineal gland and hypothalamus, including increasing serotonin levels, which can ease depression.

Combine exercise with meditation. Women who exercise tend to have less PMS or menstrual discomfort than those who are sedentary. To get even more benefits from exercise, Dr. Kallins recommends making it mindful. In other words, focus all your thoughts on your body—the stretching of your muscles, the slap of your feet on the mat or pavement, the breath going in and out of your lungs—and not on the things that are troubling you.

The idea, he explains, is to use your movements to put yourself into a kind of mild trance. When your mind is relaxed, you'll be more in touch with your body and feelings—and that's the first step to managing them more effectively.

Use aromatherapy. One study of 67 women found that those who had a 15-minute tummy massage daily with an oil infused with a combination of lavender, rose, and clary sage had a third more pain relief than those who had a massage without the scented oil. On the second day of the massages, the aromatherapy group's cramps had decreased 12 percent while the other women reported a 5 percent improvement. You can make your own aromatherapy oil by adding 6 drops of lavender oil, 3 drops of rose, and 3 drops of clary sage oils to 4 teaspoons of almond oil.

Use vitex supplements. The fruit of the chaste tree, vitex is a popular folk remedy for PMS—and one study suggests that it may work. In a German study, women suffering from PMS were given 20 mg of dried vitex extract daily. After taking the supplements for three menstrual cycles, more than half of the women reported a dramatic reduction in headaches, irritability, and other symptoms of PMS. A review study published in 2010 found that of all purported herbal remedies for PMS, Vitex was consistently better than a placebo in reducing PMS symptoms.

Vitex is available in health food stores and some pharmacies. Try taking two 500-mg tablets twice daily for a few months to see if it helps. (The seeds, also called the berries, are the most effective part.) If it does, you'll have to keep taking it; in the study, women who took vitex and then gave it up had a return of symptoms within 3 months.

Medical Options

Most women can control menstrual or premenstrual discomfort with changes in lifestyle or diet, but some can't. Since there are other causes of severe pain, consultation with a knowledgeable physician is imperative before you start a medication for pain. If your

---

WHEN BAD THINGS HAPPEN TO HEALTHY WOMEN

A Meat-Free Diet Banished Menstrual Pain

Barbara Swanson is an energetic and healthy woman, but for a long time she had such unbearable menstrual cramps that she routinely missed 2 days of work a month.

"When my period hit, I couldn't do anything but lie uncomfortably on the couch in front of the television," says Swanson, an administrative assistant in Washington, DC. "I had to take a lot of over-the-counter pain pills, which only seemed to make me sleepy."

In 1997, Swanson received a postcard calling for women to participate in a Georgetown University study that was looking at the link between vegan (meat- and dairy-free) diets and pain-free periods. She volunteered, and several cooking classes, a restocked pantry, and two menstrual cycles later, her cramps were markedly reduced, she could function at work, and she was up off the couch and jogging.

Swanson has stuck with the vegan diet ever since. "I have some great cookbooks that I use for making simple dinners," she says. For desserts, she enjoys soy ice cream and soy yogurt, and she has even found vegan versions of fast foods, like faux burgers and hot dogs.

She was also pleased to get an additional bonus from the vegan diet: Soon after giving up meat and dairy, she lost 5 pounds and the weight never came back. ∎

symptoms aren't getting better, here are some medical options that might make the difference.

Take high-dose ibuprofen. Available by prescription, ibuprofen tablets that contain 800 mg appear to be more effective than taking 4 over-the-counter pills containing 200 mg each. "It's a mystery why, but it seems to make a difference," says Dr. Gerbie.

Try birth control pills for 6 to 12 months. "For some women, the Pill ends all the discomfort because it stops the hormone fluctuations that occur with ovulation," says Dr. Gerbie, "and it stops the lining of the uterus from building up so much." In many cases, taking the Pill for 6 months to a year will balance the hormones and relieve symptoms for good.

Dr. Gerbie cautions you to let your doctor know if you're using the Pill only for menstrual or premenstrual discomfort, and not for birth control, because you'll need a different dosage.

Consider selective serotonin reuptake inhibitor (SSRI) antidepressants. Usually given for PMDD, SSRIs can reduce physical and emotional symptoms of the disorder when taken either during the luteal phase of the menstrual cycle (the day after ovulation through to the end of your period) or continuously, though they seem to be more effective when taken continuously. Studies have found that in women with PMDD, serotonin levels tend to be low.

Rub away breast pain. Rub your breasts with an OTC painkilling gel or lotion such as diclofenac. A study of 108 women with breast pain found that those who got diclofenac 3 times a day for 6 months saw significant relief from their breast pain compared to women given a placebo.

Contraception

Contraceptives are incredibly effective. When used correctly and consistently, all of the leading contraceptives have been shown to prevent pregnancy more than 99 percent of the time.

So why is it that almost half of unintended pregnancies occur in those who use birth control?

In most cases, it's because people are using birth control that's not right for them or not using the method correctly, says Mitchell Creinin, MD, professor of obstetrics, gynecology, and reproductive sciences at the University of Pittsburgh School of Medicine, where he is also director of the division of gynecologic specialties and senior investigator at Magee-Womens Research Institute.

There are many different types of contraception, from barrier methods, which block sperm from reaching the uterus, to the Pill, which prevents ovulation, to patches, shots, and implants, which work in a variety of ways. By knowing what's out there and choosing products or practices that suit your personality and lifestyle, you'll be able to get maximal protection without sacrificing comfort.

Don't let doctors or other health care advisors limit your options in advance, says Dr. Creinin.

"Your doctor doesn't pay your bills, take care of your kids, deal with your in-laws, or have a relationship with your husband or partner," he adds.

Don't put too much weight on hearsay, either. Just because your sister or mother or most of the women in your book club prefer a certain method does not mean it's the right one for you. With so many options to choose from, don't accept anything less.

The Right Match for Every Woman

Start by asking yourself if you need protection only from unwanted pregnancy or if you also need protection from sexually transmitted diseases (STDs), says Erica Gollub, DrPH, assistant professor of epidemiology at the Robert Stempel College of Public Health and Social Work at Florida International University in Miami.

Some STDs cause infertility, some increase the risk of uterine cancer, and still others can threaten your life. "You have to recognize that they're out there, and if you have any doubt in your mind that your partner has undisclosed relationships, your safest bet is clearly the male or female condom."

If condoms aren't for you, other "barrier" methods of birth control, such as a diaphragm combined with spermicide, might be good alternatives. On the other hand, Dr. Gollub notes, birth control pills or other methods of hormonal contraception, along with intrauterine contraceptives, may increase your risk for STDs because they alter the cervical mucus.

If you are in a mutually monogamous relationship and can use hormonal methods of birth control, you'll have to educate yourself about the pros and cons. The leading contraceptive method among women in their reproductive years is the oral contraceptive, usually just called the Pill. It is an effective method of birth control that offers some protection against ovarian cancer but may increase your risk of breast, liver, and cervical cancer, or lead to serious side effects if you're over 35 and smoke. Another factor to consider when you're making your choices: whether you're planning to get pregnant in the future, and how soon you'll want it to happen. Fertility will usually return immediately upon stopping use of the Pill or a barrier method; even an intrauterine contraceptive or implant can be removed and assure a relatively quick return of fertility. However, Depo-Provera, an injection method of contraception given every 3 months, may delay pregnancy for 10 months after it's discontinued.

Your Guide to Contraceptive Options

As you review your options, here are some other questions to ask yourself.

- What's my comfort level with this method?
- Does this method take away from or add to the pleasure of sex?
- What are the short-term and long-term costs?
- What are the side effects?

BARRIER METHODS

Barrier methods are among the oldest and safest form of birth control. A barrier contraceptive's mission is to prevent a sperm from ever meeting up with an egg. They include the diaphragm, cervical cap, cervical shield, sponge, and male and female condoms. The chemicals in spermicidal foams, jellies, and films eradicate sperm the way antibacterials kill germs, offering a second line of defense against unwanted pregnancy.

One of the first modern variations on the condom theme was the female condom, which was approved in 1993 by the FDA for preventing both pregnancy and disease.

"Women like the female condom because it makes them feel in control," says Dr. Gollub. You place the closed end—an inner ring—up in the vagina as far as it will go, then guide your partner's penis into the outer ring. When used correctly, it can prevent pregnancy as effectively as the male condom, and it may be even more effective in preventing disease since it covers more of the female genitalia.

There's also another version of the cervical cap, a thimble-shaped cone that is placed in the vagina and held in place against the cervix with suction. The cervical shield is a softer and smoother silicone cap with a one-way valve that creates suction, allowing it to fit against the cervix. It comes in one size, so you don't need your doctor to fit you, as is the case with the cervical cap and diaphragm. You need to leave both devices in for 6 to 8 hours after sex to prevent pregnancy, and remove them within 48 hours.

The contraceptive sponge is a soft, disk-shaped device with a loop that allows you to remove it. Made of polyurethane foam, it contains a spermicide for an extra measure of protection. Before you have sex, you wet the sponge and place it inside the vagina. It's effective for up to 24 hours and needs to be left inside for at least 6 hours after sex.

The diaphragm is a shallow latex cup that is inserted before sex and must remain inside for 6 to 8 hours afterward.

The male condom is a thin sheath made of latex, polyurethane, or natural lambskin that is placed over an erect penis, effectively stopping pregnancy at the source. Condoms work best when used with a spermicide. They come in lubricated versions, which makes intercourse more comfortable, and non-lubricated. Only the latex is super-effective at preventing the spread of STDs.

The failure rates of barrier contraceptives when used consistently and correctly is only about 3 percent, but in the real world—where they may not be used every time a couple has sex or may not be inserted correctly—the rate is closer to 14 to 20 percent. Condoms can break or fall off, diaphragms be forgotten in a bureau drawer, and caps dislodged. They work best if you're highly motivated and disciplined.

Here's some expert advice on using barrier contraception.

Get the proper fit. Diaphragms and cervical caps come in different sizes. If yours feels uncomfortable or loose, ask your doctor for a refit, says Dr. Gollub. Always assume you will need a different size after childbirth, abortion, or gaining or losing 10 pounds, which changes the size of your cervix.

Select safe lubricants. Many barrier methods are designed to be used with spermicides or lubricants. Lubricants can increase pleasure and although they do act against sperm, they aren't as effective as spermicides, which typically contain a sperm-killing ingredient called nonoxynol-9. Using commercial lubricants and spermicides can also decrease the odds that a condom will break.

Though bedroom fun may sometimes involve household products such as whipped cream, they're not a substitute for spermicidal lubricants. In fact, whipped cream, petroleum jelly, or cooking or rubbing oils can cause condoms to break down and provide no spermicidal effects.

Get ready ahead of time. If you find that fussing with a contraceptive disrupts the moment, remember that a diaphragm can be inserted 6 hours ahead of time. The female condom can be inserted up to 8 hours in advance, and the cervical cap can be inserted 2 to 3 days before a romantic encounter.

Remember to remove them. More than a few women have left diaphragms or caps in place long past their allotted time, which can result in bladder or even blood infections. It may be worth writing a note to yourself and putting it on the bathroom mirror or somewhere else you'll be sure to see it, suggests Dr. Gollub.

ORAL CONTRACEPTIVES

The Pill has been in use for more than 40 years, and it's safer than it ever was. That's in part because the dose of hormones in the Pill has been reduced and years of clinical experience have identified those who are at high risk of adverse side effects and should not use it. Doctors have found that birth control pills even offer some health benefits that are unrelated to contraception.

There are two basic forms of oral contraceptives: the combination pill and the single-hormone mini-pill. Combination pills contain synthetic estrogen and progestin, which are hormones similar to those produced in a woman's ovaries. Taken daily, these pills prevent your ovaries from releasing an egg every month and alter the lining of the uterus and cervical uterus to prevent conception. Combination pills are available as monophasic pills, which provide estrogen and progestin at the same doses throughout the course of the pill pack, which you take for 3 weeks of your cycle (with placebo pills for the fourth week). There are also triphasic pills, which vary the amount of hormones over the course of the month, and extended cycle pills, such as Seasonale, which you take every day for 12 weeks (followed by a placebo) and which cuts your periods to three or four a year.

Mini-pills contain progestin only. They do not consistently stop ovulation so you always need a backup such as a condom or diaphragm. They do, however, thicken the mucus over the cervix to prevent sperm from entering the uterus. They also stop the uterine lining from growing, which

when to see a doctor

If you're taking the Pill or other hormone-based contraceptives and you experience chest pain, blurred vision, or leg pain, Call your doctor immediately. The symptoms could be caused by inflammation, a blood clot, or even a stroke, says Mitchell Creinin, MD, professor of obstetrics, gynecology, and reproductive sciences at the University of Pittsburgh School of Medicine, where he is also director of the division of gynecologic specialties and senior investigator at Magee-Womens Research Institute.

Women who take the Pill have a slightly increased risk of developing these conditions compared with women who don't use hormonal contraception, although the actual risk is still very small.

If you're developing acne or have unpredictable bleeding. These are common side effects of contraceptive hormones, and changing the dosage (or the medication) will probably resolve the problem.

If an intrauterine device becomes visible. The device has fallen out of position, and you'll want to get it repositioned immediately to prevent damage to the uterus or intestine. Avoid sexual intercourse or use an alternative method (like condoms) until you can talk to your health care provider about other contraceptive options.

makes it more difficult for the egg to get implanted. These pills are usually used by women who are concerned about the possible health risks—such as heart disease, stroke, or breast cancer—of estrogen-based pills. They're often prescribed for women over 35 who can't take estrogen or are at risk of blood clots.

Aside from being highly effective at preventing pregnancy (generally 99 percent when used correctly) women taking birth control pills may have a reduced risk of colon, endometrial, and uterine cancers. The estrogen in the Pill also protects against the bone-thinning disease called osteoporosis.

Because combination pills prevent ovulation, they can relieve or prevent menstrual pain, ovarian cysts, or fibroids. They can also prevent the hot flashes, headaches, irregular bleeding, vaginal dryness, and other symptoms that may occur in the years preceding menopause.

Birth control pills are very effective—but only if you remember to use them. Here are few ways to keep with the program.

Pack your pills. Carry extras in a pill pack just in case you forget your morning dose. You can keep the pills in your purse, wallet, or backpack, where you'll always have easy access to them.

Take them on a strict schedule. Progestin-only pills prevent pregnancy by thickening the cervical mucus. This effect lasts only for 24 hours, so it's important to take the pills at the same time every day. If you doubt your ability to stick to a regular schedule, you may want to choose another type of contraception.

LONG-ACTING HORMONAL METHODS

For many women, the nicest thing about long-acting hormonal methods of birth control is not having to worry. Nobody will find your pills, your partner won't feel an IUD string or the rim of a diaphragm, there's no messy spermicide, and you're less likely to "forget" to use them, says Robert Hatcher, MD, MPH, professor of gynecology and obstetrics at Emory University School of Medicine in Atlanta and senior author of *Contraception Technology*. They include:

- Depo-Provera. This injectable dose of progestin needs to be refreshed every three months. Like the Pill, it stops your ovaries from releasing an egg and alters your uterus and cervix to discourage conception. The shot shouldn't be used for more than 2 years in a row because it can increase bone loss; it's also been linked to weight gain in some women. If you have trouble fitting a monthly doctor's visit into your schedule, ask your doctor for a 6- to 12-month supply of injections, which you can administer to yourself at home, says Dr. Creinin.

- The Patch. Like the nicotine patch, this patch is worn on the body (the lower abdomen, buttocks, outer arm, or lower body) where it releases estrogen and progestin into the bloodstream. You use a new patch every week for 3 weeks, then skip a week to allow your period to come.

- Vaginal ring. This thin, flexible ring releases estrogen and progestin. Called NuvaRing, it's inserted into the vagina by squeezing it between your thumb and index finger and worn for 3 weeks, with one week off.

■ Implantable rod. This matchstick-size flexible rod is inserted under the skin of your upper arm, where it releases progestin. It's effective for up to 3 years.

INTRAUTERINE DEVICES

There's a good reason that many women appreciate an intrauterine contraceptive, also called an IUD. Once it's inserted, it can be left alone for 5 to 10 years.

There are two kinds of IUDs available in the United States, copper and hormonal. Both kinds are small, T-shaped devices with a plastic string attached, and are inserted into the uterus by your doctor.

The copper IUD releases small amounts of copper into the uterus, where it keeps the fertilized egg from implanting. It also immobilizes sperm on its way to the fallopian tubes.

Hormonal IUDs contain levonorgestrel (Mirena), which mimics the effects of progesterone and can stay in place for up to 5 years.

"The hormone is released locally in the uterus," says Dr. Creinin. "The amount of hormone that gets into the rest of your body is only about 10 percent of the amount that comes from taking birth control pills. This means that there's less potential for side effects."

Less than one out of 100 women will get pregnant with an IUD, making it one of the most effective forms of birth control available. It's also one of the cheapest: It can cost about $500 to have a copper IUD inserted. Your ability to become pregnant returns immediately after it's removed.

However, you can experience heavier than normal menstrual bleeding and worse menstrual cramps with the copper IU, and irregular periods in the first 3 to 6 months with the hormonal device. Serious problems are rare.

OTHER CONTRACEPTION OPTIONS

Tubal sterilization, a permanent procedure, is best for women who know that they don't want to have any (or any more) children. For surgical ligation, a small incision is made in the abdomen. The surgeon then seals the fallopian tubes, thereby creating a permanent roadblock on the egg-uterus highway. Essure is the first nonsurgical method of sterilization. A tiny springlike device is threaded through your vagina and uterus into your fallopian tubes. Scar tissue will grow on the spring and block your tubes, preventing egg and sperm from joining. It takes as long as 3 months or more for sufficient scar tissue to develop to block your tubes, so you'll have to use an alternate form of birth control until your doctor makes sure your tubes are actually blocked.

Even if you already have children, don't discount the possibility that you may want to have more later on, especially if you happen to divorce and then remarry. Long-term, reversible methods, such as an intrauterine contraceptive, or a vasectomy for the spouse of a woman in a mutually monogamous relationship, might be better for you, says Dr. Creinin.

Some women depend on the "withdrawal method" for birth control. It is the most unreliable method of birth control short of not doing anything. However, family-planning clinics sometimes teach women what are called fertility awareness methods based on observing menstrual cycle patterns and abstaining from sex before and during ovulation. The more data you take using this method (such as body temperature, the appearance of cervical mucus, self-cervical examinations, and urine tests), the more effective it becomes, says Dr. Gollub. There are at-home fertility tests that can make these methods better than guessing.

"It's a valuable educational tool for every woman to learn," she says. "It can also be quite moving to be so aware of your body's changes throughout the month."

However, anywhere from 2 to 20 out of 100 women will become pregnant using these methods.

EMERGENCY CONTRACEPTION

Emergency contraception is not designed to be your regular contraception. It comes in pill form (the morning-after pill) or as a copper IUD, which can be inserted up to 5 days after intercourse to prevent pregnancy.

As with some other contraceptives, ECPs either prevent ovulation or alter the uterine lining to prevent the implantation of an egg. You can think of them as very strong, fast-acting birth control pills.

To be effective, the pills have to be taken according to strict guidelines. You'll need to take your first dose within 72 hours (or sooner) of unprotected sex, followed by another dose 12 hours later. The pills are unlikely to cause serious side effects, but some women may experience nausea, vomiting, abdominal cramps, headache, breast tenderness, or dizziness.

Here are some additional emergency strategies to keep in mind.

Get checked for infection. If you had unplanned sex outside of a mutually monogamous relationship, you might be at risk for an STD. The symptoms don't always show up right away (or at all). The only way you'll know you're infected is to have your doctor give you an exam.

Go to the source. If you want immediate information about emergency contraception, visit www.not-2-late.com, a Web site provided by the Office of Population Research at Princeton University. You'll find a lot of information about emergency contraceptives, along with lists of health care providers who prescribe them.

Get emergency pills in advance. The effectiveness of ECPs drops off every minute after unprotected sex, and then decreases very rapidly after 72 hours. Since your physician may not be able to see you immediately or the pharmacy may be closed, you may want to get the pills in advance and keep them in a safe place.

21

Pregnancy

You can play classical music to your growing belly, be scrupulous about eating foods that will help your child grow and be healthy, and choose the right colors and décor for the nursery to stimulate your newborn's brain development. As baby-centric as pregnancy makes you, don't forget yourself.

You're doing more than supporting a developing baby over 9 or 10 months. You're also growing as a woman and a mother-to-be, says Deborah Issokson, PsyD, a psychologist and teacher specializing in reproductive mental health at the Boston University Nurse-Midwifery Education Program. Dr. Issokson is also the author of the postpartum chapter in the book *Our Bodies, Ourselves: A New Edition for a New Era.* "The most important advice I can give is not to rush through 40 weeks trying to get everything ready for the baby," she says. "Focus instead on your personal development. Pregnancy is an incredibly reflective time when your sense of being a woman, a wife or partner, and even an employee is evolving to a new level. Make the time and space for that natural shift, and you'll feel emotionally your best before, during, and after pregnancy. Emotional well-being can also translate into physical well-being."

Get the Best Support

Whether you are having a first child or your fourth, getting good prenatal education is one of the smartest parenting decisions you'll make. Birth classes allow you to gain vital new information. Plus, you'll have the chance to talk about the experience with other pregnant women. The more you learn about the physical and emotional changes that other women undergo during pregnancy, the better prepared you'll be to cope with your own.

Birthing educators offer private instruction, classes in hospitals (usually six 1-hour sessions or a 1-day class), and weekend-long retreats, says Sally Riley, CBE, founder and codirector of the Academy of Certified Birth Educators, based in Olathe, Kansas.

Start with a broad-based class that will prepare you, physically and emotionally, for anything that might come up. The class should offer instruction on a variety of relaxation and comfort measures and breathing techniques, as well as discussions and role playing to help you and your partner focus on various scenarios.

Look for the same spirit of flexibility and objectivity in choosing your primary pregnancy caregiver—the person who conducts prenatal exams and attends your birth. Whether you choose an obstetrician, a family practitioner, or a nurse-midwife, try to sense whether her aim is to mold you into a good patient—or a smart mother.

Many women prefer to work with nurse-midwives because they tend to put a strong focus on empowerment and education. Women who work with nurse-midwives generally need significantly less medical intervention, including cesarean sections and labor induction, says Marion McCartney, CNM, a practicing nurse-midwife and author of *The Midwife's Pregnancy and Childbirth Book: Having Your Baby Your Way.* Nurse-midwives have access to the same general technology for prenatal evaluation and labor as doctors, but the Centers for Disease Control and Prevention reports that there is a lower rate of infant mortality when nurse-midwives attend labors compared with those attended by obstetricians. A 2008 review of 11 studies looking at midwife-assisted births found that women who received midwife care were less likely to need episiotomies or pain medication, and less likely to lose their babies before 24 weeks gestation, and that their babies were likely to have a much shorter stay in the hospital. The authors' conclusion: "Most women should be offered midwife-led models of care and women should be encouraged to ask for this option" unless there are substantial medical risks.

To get the best possible care, visit your prenatal caretaker every month up until your 32nd week. After 32 weeks, see her twice a month, then once a week after your 36th week.

Concerns for Older Moms and Higher-Risk Pregnancies

Halle Berry, Emma Thompson, Madonna, Marcia Cross, Kelly Preston—the list of celebrity moms over 35 (and many over 40) grows daily. With high-tech fertility treatments, women have gotten pregnant in their fifties and sixties. About 14 percent of all births in the United States today are to mothers 35 and older, and for the most part the pregnancies are uneventful. "Even women in their early fifties today are expected to have routine and normal pregnancies," says Ronald J. Wapner, MD, a high-risk obstetrician and director of the division of maternal fetal medicine at the Columbia University Medical Center in New York.

However, women who are over age 35 do have a slightly increased risk for fetal chromosome abnormalities. There's also a higher risk if they've had children with a birth defect or a chromosome abnormality such as Down syndrome, says Dr. Wapner. For example, your risk of having a child with any kind of chromosomal problem is 1 in 500 if you're between the ages of 15 and 24. At 35, that risk grows to 1 in 178. It grows dramatically after 40 to 1 in 63 at 40, and 1 in 18 at 45.

If you fit this profile, see a specialist in genetics to assess specific risks before you conceive. You'll also want to consider additional screenings once you get pregnant, such as the chorionic villus sampling (CVS) test in your 11th to 13th weeks, or an amniocentesis procedure in your fourth month. There is a very small risk of miscarriage from these tests, though, so weigh the benefits and risks accordingly. You may also choose a first trimester screen, which combines a maternal blood test with an ultrasound of the fetus to check for specific chromosomal abnormalities, including Down syndrome. It has a combined accuracy rate of 85 percent. However, a positive test doesn't mean your baby actually has any of these abnormalities; it simply means that you have a 1 in 100 to 1 in 300 chance of having a baby with these conditions. Most women also have what's called triple or quad screen blood tests in the 15th and 21st week in the second trimester to detect chromosomal abnormalities and neural tube defects, which create gaps in the protective spinal column that can affect brain development and cause spinal cord damage. The triple test can detect about 70 percent of fetuses with Down syndrome and the quad screen about 10 percent more. Either is about 80 to 95 percent accurate in picking neural tube problems.

Here are some additional issues older women may face.

- Diabetes. The body produces anti-insulin hormones during pregnancy, which can result in a temporary condition called gestational diabetes. It can also aggravate preexisting diabetes. Women who are 40 years or older have a 7 percent chance of developing gestational diabetes,

compared with 1.7 percent for a woman in her twenties. To avoid complications that can be caused by uncontrolled blood sugar—such as an oversize baby—be sure to get dietary advice from a nutritionist or a perinatal specialist.

- High blood pressure. If you have hypertension, it's important to get it under control before you conceive, says Dr. Wapner. Since your heart will be pumping more blood when you're pregnant, you may develop high blood pressure for the first time. You'll need extra rest to avoid a serious complication called preeclampsia, which can rob a fetus of blood flow.

- Placental problems. Women in their late thirties are almost twice as likely and women in their forties almost 3 times as likely as younger women to develop placenta previa, in which the placenta covers part or all of the uterine opening. This can cause severe bleeding during pregnancy and may necessitate a cesarean birth.

- Premature or low-birth-weight babies. Both are common among older moms because they're more likely to be carrying twins or triplets. There are also preterm births because of maternal illness, like high blood pressure. Uncontrolled blood pressure or unhealthy lifestyle factors can also increase the risk of premature or low-birth-weight babies.

- Repeated miscarriage or stillbirth. Losing a baby may be your body's way of coping with genetic abnormalities. As a woman gets older, miscarriages occur more frequently because there are more genetic abnormalities in pregnancy. It may also be a sign of irregularly shaped reproductive organs, a hormone imbalance, or an immune system disorder. Women over age 40 are 2 to 3 times more likely than younger women to have stillbirth, the death of a fetus after the 20th week of pregnancy.

A Healthy Pregnancy

Regardless of your age when you conceive, the following advice will help ensure a safe and healthy pregnancy.

Take folic acid supplements. All women who are thinking about getting pregnant should take a minimum of 400 micrograms of folic acid daily. Folic acid helps prevent spinal cord defects.

Stay fit before and during pregnancy. Regular exercise can keep blood sugar under control, and women who are fit generally have lower blood pressure. In addition, getting in shape will improve your stamina to push out a baby. Check with your doctor first, but if you aren't currently exercising, you might want to begin by walking. Start at an easy pace–so you don't break a sweat–for 10 to 15 minutes at a time the first week. Add a few minutes each week as you feel comfortable, gradually working up to an hour most days, if possible. Stop walking and contact your caregiver immediately if you become short of breath or have uterine cramping. And make sure to drink plenty of water before, during, and after exercise to prevent dehydration and overheating.

Gain a healthy amount of weight. If you're starting out at a good weight, you should gain 25 to 37 pounds over the course of your pregnancy. If you were underweight, you can put on 28 to 40 pounds, and only 15 to 25 if you were overweight. Being too thin or overweight can complicate pregnancy, especially if you have gestational diabetes or high blood pressure.

Don't smoke, and avoid alcohol. Smoking and drinking can raise the risk of miscarriage, birth defects, and low-birth-weight babies. Ideally, women should avoid alcohol and tobacco even before they conceive, says Dr. Wapner.

Eat wholesome foods. Every pregnant woman needs to do her best to get a nutritional diet. It should include lots of fruits and vegetables, whole grains, and other healthful foods. You'll certainly want to avoid excessive amounts of sweets or highly refined (and nutritionally "empty") foods.

Be choosy about fish. Though the omega-3 fatty acids in fish are good for you and your baby, the mercury and other pollutants in fish aren't. The U.S. Food and Drug Administration and the Environmental Protection Agency recommend avoiding certain mercury-laden fish (shark, swordfish, king mackerel, tilefish), and eating up to 12 ounces a week of lower-mercury fish and shellfish such as shrimp, canned light tuna, salmon, Pollock, and catfish. Limit albacore tuna to one 6-ounce serving a week.

Get enough rest. Women who are at risk for preeclampsia or other health problems will usually be advised by their doctors to curtail their working hours. But regardless of risks, listen to your body, and be prepared to slow down when you're feeling fatigued.

WHEN BAD THINGS HAPPEN TO HEALTHY WOMEN

Difficult Pregnancy Led to Lifestyle Improvements

Marla Hardee Milling knew that her pregnancies—one when she was 35, the other at 37—wouldn't be easy. She had received 52 radiation treatments for Hodgkin's disease when she was in her early twenties, and she knew that women in their mid- to late thirties were well past their childbearing prime.

In addition, Milling, a freelance writer in Asheville, North Carolina, discovered during her first pregnancy that she was a carrier of the group B strep bacterium, which could potentially infect her unborn children.

During her second pregnancy, gestational diabetes proved to be yet another challenge. Milling accepted the fact that she would require extensive prenatal testing. And she also knew that she would have to make some sweeping lifestyle changes—such as giving up her favorite sweets. "I became more aware of my body," she says. She walked more, ate a lot more fresh vegetables, and reflected on her physical and emotional changes in the journal she kept.

"All of the little things that were different— even things like fatigue and nausea—made me aware of the miracle that there was a child inside of me," she says. "Besides, a few uncomfortable symptoms were nothing compared to the challenge of a life-threatening illness."

She used her age as an asset as well. "Being an older mother, I was emotionally prepared. I was so mentally and spiritually ready to have children, it was actually the best I ever felt in my life, despite the so-called problems." ∎

Don't change the kitty litter box. It can be a source of toxoplasmosis, an infection that can cause birth defects.

Consider pregnancy yoga. Many yoga centers now offer yoga classes for pregnant women. One 2005 study found that women who practiced yoga while pregnant were less likely to have preterm births and their rates of pregnancy-induced hypertension and fetal growth retardation were also lower. And women who do yoga along with mindfulness meditation get a bonus: They sleep better, according to a 2010 study in *Biological Research for Nursing.*

Feeling Well on Every Level

Between the time your future child is conceived and the time you deliver, your uterus will expand to 1,000 times its prepregnancy size. Your body will be producing 25 percent more progesterone and 100 percent more estrogen. These tremendous physical changes can result in nausea, backache, headaches, digestive difficulties, and fatigue—not to mention potentially overwhelming emotional ups and downs.

Women who mentally prepare themselves for motherhood generally feel better physically as well as emotionally, Dr. Issokson says.

"Women need to stay connected with their bodies and natural rhythms, with their partners, and with other women who want to talk about the birth and mothering experience. Things like journal writing, yoga, swimming, gardening, good self-care, connecting with other women, and talking about what they envision for themselves as mothers are all activities that reflect where women are spiritually and physically when they are pregnant. If they ignore the reflective and spiritual aspects of pregnancy, then women often end up feeling disconnected from themselves—and they feel disconnected from their bodies as birth approaches."

To get in harmony with your mind and body during this important time, here are a few worthwhile strategies.

Allow yourself to feel ambivalence. "I don't think there's any way to go through a life-altering event such as childbearing without some internal conflict, even in the most planned and wanted pregnancy," Dr. Issokson says. It's normal and healthy for women to acknowledge their anticipated losses—like how much they're going to miss sleeping late on Sundays, or giving up a degree of sexual intimacy or the loss of freedom and spontaneity that comes with a child-free life. Admitting and coming to terms with these and other losses and changes will help a woman accept the entire experience of having a baby—the difficulties along with the joy.

Give yourself time to bond. When you're pregnant, set aside time to bond, not only with your spouse but also with your baby-to-be. Try a "story time and music box" ritual every night. Here's how it works.

You and your husband take turns reading. It can be anything from children's books to baseball scores, as long as you are addressing your future child. Afterward, play a music box on your stomach. As the fetus matures, it will respond with a flurry of activity when it recognizes these sounds. Later, as soon as your baby emerges from the womb, playing the music box will orient and comfort your just-born child.

Reduce nausea naturally. One study found that 90 percent of pregnant women had less nausea when they took ginger. Fresh ginger tastes great when it's added to stir-fries, soups, and spicy baked goods, and it's entirely safe during pregnancy.

Because nausea usually increases when the stomach is empty, it's important for women to eat frequent, small meals during pregnancy, says Mary Lake Polan, MD, PhD, professor and chairperson of the department of gynecology and obstetrics at Stanford University School of Medicine. Take your prenatal vitamin with food or before bed to make sure it stays down and eat a small meal when you get up in the morning to go to the bathroom.

Don't lose sleep because of back pain. "During pregnancy, the tissues that support the spine and pelvis naturally get soft in order to allow the pelvis to open for delivery. This, along with the extra strain from her changing center of gravity, strains a pregnant woman's back," says James Cable, MD, an occupational and sports injury physician with the Texas Back Institute in Plano.

He advises pregnant women to sleep on their side with the knees slightly bent. Put one pillow between your legs and another beneath your abdomen for extra support.

Know when to consider therapy. "Mental health services should be a routine part of everyone's prenatal care," says Dr. Issokson. "Pregnancy and birth trigger a lot of issues for women. Some issues are old ones that have never been resolved or that have crept back up, and some issues are new. While not everyone needs therapy, a few sessions with a counselor or therapist can create a wonderful opportunity for women to sort through these issues. For a woman who has a history of depression or anxiety, trauma, violence, or eating disorders, a prenatal session with a therapist can help her evaluate her risk factors for postpartum difficulties, like postpartum depression." Therapists can help with many different issues: the previous loss of a child, anxiety about birth, or the sense of vulnerability that so many women experience. If you suffer depression after giving birth (postpartum depression), working with a therapist is among the smartest things you can do.

Increase communication with your partner. "Discuss what you both think parenthood will ultimately be like and what your fantasies are. Along with these ideal expectations, understand what you both perceive as your roles and responsibilities," suggests Dr. Issokson.

You might, for example, discuss who will be responsible for getting up in the middle of the night when the child cries. Or you might discuss the types of discipline you believe in or who will take days off from work when it's time to visit the pediatrician.

If your relationship has problems, this is the time to seek couples therapy and commit to getting your relationship as a couple in good working order, adds Dr. Issokson. "Don't fall for any fantasies that a baby will make your marriage better. Babies add stress to every relationship. The stronger, healthier, and more communicative a relationship is, the better it is able to handle the stress of new parenthood."

22

Childbirth

The personal touches that were planned for bringing Maureen Angelino's child into the world created the confidence, comfort, and sense of sacredness that she hoped for.

In Allentown, Pennsylvania, her husband and the midwives collaborated like old friends—offering loving massages, assisting her into the whirlpool, or just standing by to change the CD. And when the baby was ready, the warmth of her husband's hands was the first sensation that his son experienced outside the womb. The honor of snipping the umbilical cord went to his 4-year-old brother.

Marla Hardee Milling, who lives in Asheville, North Carolina, needed an entirely different birth plan. Potentially lifesaving procedures were arranged to protect both mother and baby from complications. Medical interventions abounded.

Two different women, two different birth plans. Obviously, no two births are exactly alike. Every woman creates in her mind the ideal situation and circumstances for giving birth. Things can always change, of course, sometimes at the last minute. Planning for childbirth is important, but so is maintaining a spirit of flexibility.

Conceiving a Birth Plan

To increase your chances of having the kind of childbirth experience you want, there are many considerations: the setting you prefer—hospital, birthing center, your own bedroom; who you want around you—doctors, nurses, midwives, family, doula; the procedures you do or don't want, says Marion McCartney, CNM, a practicing nurse-midwife and author of *The Midwife's Pregnancy and Childbirth Book: Having Your Baby Your Way.*

Creating a birth plan will help you think through the decisions that will one day come together to create the optimal scenario. It's a way of clarifying your expectations and ensuring that everyone is working together to fulfill your needs.

To create a birth plan that will help make your childbirth dreams come true, here are some points to keep in mind.

Get information from a variety of sources. Read about the kinds of births that are offered in hospitals, at birthing centers, or at home. Learn about the pros and cons of different medical interventions, from "natural" vaginal births to cesarean sections. Ask the mothers you know to tell you their birth stories. At www.childbirth.org, you can fill out your ideal birth plan (with prompts) so you have a written document that covers all the bases. Always discuss your birth plan with your midwife or physician during your pregnancy, and be realistic about their response. If your caregiver is reluctant to accommodate your plan, you need to find out why and either revise the plan or look for a person who is comfortable with your wishes.

Look into cesarean section rates. There are many situations when surgical delivery, known as cesarean birth, or C-section, is essential. But if a hospital or clinic has a C-section rate that approaches 25 percent as opposed to the more reasonable rate of 5 to 10 percent, it may be a sign of overuse of medical interventions, says Mindy Smith, MD, associate professor in the department of family medicine at Michigan State University in Lansing and coauthor of *20 Common Problems in Women's Healthcare.* (The C-section rate is on the rise in the United States; it was 4.5 percent in 1965 and is around 31 percent today.)

Understand the pros and cons of medications. Epidural anesthesia is highly effective at relieving discomfort in your pelvic area and can be key to helping you have a positive birth experience. It allows you to stay awake and alert and participate in giving birth and helps reduce exhaustion and irritability. The procedure has some drawbacks—your blood pressure can drop suddenly, you may develop a headache caused by spinal fluid leakage; and you may find pushing more difficult, necessitating the use of forceps, vacuum extraction, labor-inducing Pitocin, or even C-section. Drugs such as Pitocin that induce labor can decrease the anxiety of waiting, but they may increase your need for pain medication, which carries some risk to the unborn child.

Many women want to avoid the use of drugs during childbirth, and that's fine. Just be sure to plan ahead. If you want to utilize acupressure to manage pain or nipple stimulation to increase uterine contractions, consider making them part of your birth plan.

Decide about episiotomy. A surgical incision in the area between the vagina and anus, episiotomy is often performed to make more

when to see a doctor

When contractions settle into some sort of a pattern, it's time to call your doctor or midwife. Labor is about to begin, says Mary Lake Polan, MD, PhD, professor and chairperson of the department of gynecology and obstetrics at Stanford University School of Medicine.

When contractions noticeably increase in strength and occur about every 4 to 5 minutes for 60 seconds at time, and this pattern has continued for 30 to 60 minutes. You may be entering the final phase of labor, and you'll need professional assistance.

When your water breaks. It's time to get to the hospital or birthing center, or, if you're giving birth at home, to have the assistance of your doctor or midwife.

WHEN BAD THINGS HAPPEN TO HEALTHY WOMEN

Hiring a Birth Coach Avoided Repeat Delivery Stress

During her first pregnancy, Nancy Battis was immediately hooked up to machines. An electronic monitor was threaded into the uterus and attached to the baby's scalp. She was tethered to an IV and told to stay on her back, where she remained for hours.

It wasn't the kind of childbirth she imagined. A marketing and sales VP in St. Louis, Missouri, Battis had wanted a more comfortable, intimate birth. She felt that she needed someone there to talk her through the experience, and she had hoped for an environment that made her feel as though she was having a healthy, natural delivery. Instead, it felt more like she was having a serious medical procedure.

The next time she got pregnant, Battis hired a professional labor coach and birth advocate known as a doula. She also crafted a detailed birth plan. There was to be no IV or internal birth monitor to restrict her movements. She arranged to have a whirlpool ready, and the doula made sure there was a birthing ball in the room, which Battis practiced using before the birth. "It was almost like she predicted my every need," Battis says.

"It's not that the labor wasn't hard," she adds. "But all of us—my doula, my husband, and the medical staff—got through the hard times together. My doula kept us beautifully focused."

To locate a doula in your area, visit the Doulas of North America (DONA) Web site at www.dona.org, e-mail the organization at Referrals@dona.org, or call (888) 788-DONA. ∎

room for the baby to pass. Some doctors perform episiotomies routinely. They feel that even though the incision may take several months to heal, it's a safer option than risking tissue tears, which sometimes occur during childbirth.

Other doctors, however, maintain that natural tears heal as easily as surgical incisions and are less likely to extend into the rectum. They also cite statistics that indicate that about 20 percent of first-time moms can make it through childbirth without tearing. This soars to 80 percent for subsequent births.

If you're adamant about not having an episiotomy, there are a number of nonsurgical options, such as using a warm compress to soften the tissue prior to delivery or receiving a daily perineal (the area between the vagina and the anus) massage during the last 6 weeks of pregnancy. Perineal massage works best for first-time mothers, who are more likely to tear. Nurse-midwives are trained in the technique and can show you (or your spouse) how to do it at home.

To cover all bases, women sometimes indicate in their birth plans that they want to try nonsurgical measures first, but they'll opt for the incision if there's too much distress to them or their babies.

Discuss the birth plan with your doctor or midwife. Plan on doing this around the sixth or seventh month of pregnancy.

Create an easy-to-read outline. It's not uncommon for women to create birth plans that fill an entire journal. But when it's time for the birth, the doctor or midwife isn't going to have time to read all your thoughts. To make things easy, condense the birth plan into a one- or two-page outline that can be read at a glance. Make duplicates so that everyone who will be present will have a copy.

Be prepared for the unexpected. Despite all your plans, your childbirth experience can take some unanticipated turns, so it's important to be flexible.

Advice from a Birth Coach

The early part of your labor, called the latent stage, typically lasts between 6 and 18 hours. You might experience painful, irregular contractions or nonpainful, regular ones. The latent phase doesn't result in cervical dilatation, but it can hurt, keep you awake, and seemingly go on forever. At this time, you want your labor coach to be nearby, and you may feel better if you stay busy around the house, says Mary Lake Polan, MD, PhD, professor and chairperson of the department of gynecology and obstetrics at Stanford University School of Medicine.

Following the latent stage, you'll have approximately 4 to 8 hours of active labor. That's when the contractions increase in intensity and the baby makes its way down into the birth canal.

Once you are fully dilated, expect to deliver in less than 6 hours—or in as little as 30 minutes, Dr. Polan says.

"Labor takes a lot of support physically and emotionally," says Sally Riley, CBE, cofounder and codirector of the Academy of Certified Birth Educators, based in Olathe, Kansas. Here's what birth coaches advise.

Fill your mind with positive images. Try to clear your mind of worry and all the clutter that you normally carry around. Try to visualize the baby coming through, and imagine how healthy the baby is, Dr. Smith advises.

Ask about birth balls. These air-filled physical therapy balls are often used to help women feel more comfortable and to gain control, from the earliest stage of labor to the actual delivery. Getting on your hands and knees and leaning over the ball helps reduce back pressure, and sitting on the ball opens the pelvis for babies who are having a more difficult time getting through, says Riley.

Water down discomfort. Laboring in a tub of water can significantly reduce your pain. Immersion supports the mother's weight, reduces the opposition to gravity, and reduces pressure on the abdomen. It also relaxes the pelvic floor muscles. In addition, laboring in water can increase the rate of dilation. If a tub isn't available, Riley says, you can use the shower while sitting on a birth ball.

Create a soothing environment. Take full advantage of relaxation aids, such as aromatherapy mists in a scent you find relaxing, your favorite music, soothing "hot pads" made from rice-filled socks gently warmed in a microwave, or your comfiest nightgown.

CHAPTER

23

Infertility

Women naturally have a drop in fertility starting around age 30, when there's a reduction in the quantity and quality of eggs. Research has shown that one out of seven women between ages 30 and 34 will have trouble conceiving. Between ages 35 and 39, the odds change to one in five, and by the time a woman reaches 40 to 45, they're one in four. But age isn't the only factor. About 10 percent of women (6.1 million) ages 15 to 44 have difficulty getting or staying pregnant.

The most common cause of female infertility is some kind of ovulation disorder—failure to produce eggs or to produce healthy eggs. Blocked fallopian tubes (caused by endometriosis or pelvic inflammatory disease), structural abnormalities of the reproductive organs, or uterine fibroids are other common causes. And about a third of all infertility problems can be traced back to the man.

While "infertile" has come to mean a delay or difficulty getting pregnant, it rarely means a woman is unable to conceive, says Ken Gelman, MD, a reproductive endocrinologist and president of Infertility and Reproductive Medicine of South Broward in Cooper City, Florida. Two-thirds of couples who are treated for infertility go on to have babies. Lifestyle factors play a sur-

prisingly large role in a woman's ability to get pregnant. Losing or gaining weight, quitting smoking, giving up alcohol, and practicing stress reduction techniques can increase the chances of conception. When self-care isn't enough, medication or surgery can often make the difference.

For more difficult cases, assisted reproduction wonders such as in vitro fertilization and artificial insemination can make parents out of people who at one time would have been considered sterile. Since 1981, assisted reproductive technologies have made possible the births of more than three million babies worldwide. (The first one, Louise Brown, was born in England in 1978.)

How aggressively a woman chooses to treat infertility depends largely on how much cost—in terms of time, money, risk, and emotion—she is willing to invest. Regardless of the medical options, every woman who is trying to get pregnant needs to maintain a diet and lifestyle that will push the odds in her favor.

Lifestyle Strategies

 Hit a hormone-safe weight. Fat cells in the body stimulate an overabundance

269

of estrogen, which inhibits ovulation. Not enough fat, on the other hand, inhibits estrogen. "Fertility is not supported by extremes at either end of the weight spectrum," says Dr. Gelman. "A body mass index (BMI) between 20 and 27 seems to be the best range to foster fertility." To calculate your BMI–and to take steps to achieve the appropriate weight–see Chapter 6.

Exercise moderately. Women who exercise especially vigorously–by running marathons, for example–may experience delays or disruptions in ovulation. "Limit yourself to 45 minutes of daily workouts, such as strength training, walking, biking, or aerobics," says Dr. Gelman.

Keep your environment pure. Limit your exposure as much as possible to photography chemicals, pesticides, solvents, dust from treated wood, or heavy metals such as mercury or lead. Environmental toxins have been linked to infertility in women and sperm abnormalities in men. If you or your spouse has to work with these or other toxins, wear a respirator or breathing mask and protective gloves and clothing, and always ensure that there's adequate ventilation.

Don't smoke, and avoid secondhand smoke. It reduces the production of eggs as well as sperm.

Drink lightly. One study has shown that among women who consumed alcohol while trying to conceive, the probability of conception dropped more than 50 percent when compared with women who abstained from alcohol.

Giving up alcohol is a good way to promote fertility. If you continue to drink, limit yourself

THREE THINGS I TELL EVERY FEMALE PATIENT

ALICE DOMAR, PhD, *executive director of the Domar Center for Mind/Body Health, director of Mind/Body Services at Boston IVF, and assistant professor of obstetrics, gynecology and reproductive biology at Harvard Medical School gives this special advice to women who are trying to get pregnant.*

1 TRY TO RELAX DEEPLY FOR AT LEAST 20 MINUTES A DAY. Some of the most restorative techniques are prayer, guided-meditation tapes, and deep abdominal breathing.

2 SET PARAMETERS BEFORE YOU START TREATMENT. Infertility treatments are expensive and time-consuming, and sometimes risky to the health of the woman and the baby. Couples should set specific time (and cost) limits based on how far they want to go to achieve pregnancy. Knowing these limits in advance will help reduce long-term stress.

3 RALLY SUPPORT. Infertile couples often feel isolated and alone. Ask your doctor at the fertility center to recommend a local support group. Or go to the Web site of the National Fertility Association, www.resolve.org, for information about group meetings in your area or to join an online support group. ■

to three drinks a week, says Dr. Gelman. On specific days when you're trying to conceive, avoid alcohol altogether, he adds.

Switch to decaffeinated coffee or tea. Studies have shown that beverages with caffeine can cause delays in conceiving, and they may increase the risk of early miscarriage.

Nutritional Treatments

Take prenatal supplements. They contain a number of conception-supporting nutrients, including magnesium, B vitamins, and vitamins C and E. In fact, the chemical name for vitamin E, tocopherol, means "to bring forth offspring."

Supplement manufacturers don't make specific prenatal formulations for men, but there are a few key nutrients that can help boost a man's fertility. They include zinc (30 mg daily), copper (3 mg daily), L-carnitine (2 to 3 grams daily), and vitamin C (1,000 mg daily).

Men who want to be parents shouldn't take more than the recommended daily amount of 30 IU of vitamin E, Dr. Gelman adds. It may lower sperm counts when it's combined with vitamin C. It's always best to check with your doctor before taking any new supplements.

Eat natural foods. To support overall health and fertility, not only do you need the full spectrum of required daily nutrients, but you also need good digestion to absorb them, says Mercedes Cameron, MD, a family practitioner in Grand Junction, Colorado.

She advises women who are trying to conceive

when to see a doctor

Young couples who have not achieved pregnancy within a year of unprotected sex should see a reproductive specialist. There's a good chance that one of you has a physical problem that's going to make getting pregnant a challenge, says Ken Gelman, MD, a reproductive endocrinologist and president of Infertility and Reproductive Medicine of South Broward in Cooper City, Florida. If you're over 35, seek help if you've been trying to conceive for more than 6 months.

If your periods are painful or irregular, or if the bleeding is unusually light or heavy. These are common symptoms of endometriosis, uterine fibroids, pelvic inflammatory disease, or polycystic ovary syndrome, all of which can lead to infertility.

to eat three to six daily servings of digestion-friendly whole grains, such as brown rice, oats, and barley, and nine daily servings of fresh fruits and vegetables. Make sure that you get 70 grams of protein daily. The protein can come from beans, nuts, eggs, lean meats, or cheeses. Buy organic foods whenever possible; it will reduce your exposure to hormone-disrupting chemicals that may be used by industrial farms, she says.

Mind-Body Techniques

Women who are facing infertility often feel anxious, depressed, and discouraged. Apart from disrupting their peace of mind, these and other negative emotions can also disrupt the way the body functions.

"Emotional distress can impair ovulation or cause the fallopian tubes and uterus to contract to the point where an egg is prevented from implanting," says Alice Domar, PhD, executive director of the Domar Center for Mind/Body Health, director of Mind/Body Services at Boston IVF, and assistant professor of obstetrics, gynecology and reproductive biology at Harvard Medical School.

Studies have shown that women with a history of depression run nearly twice the risk of having trouble conceiving. While at Harvard, Dr. Domar and her colleagues developed a behavior-oriented fertility treatment program in which women grappling with infertility learned stress management techniques, dealt with esteem issues, and practiced positive thinking. On average, about 44 percent of the women in the program got pregnant.

In a 2009 study, Domar and her colleagues found that women who participated in a stress management program prior to or during their second IVF cycle had a 160 percent greater pregnancy rate than women who weren't in the program. Some of the most important things women can do include:

Try visualization. A woman might be angry because she had a miscarriage. She might resent her husband for failing to understand her despair, and she'll probably be angry at the doctors who can't "fix" the problem. The more frustration she feels, the more likely she is to have trouble conceiving, Dr. Domar says.

Women need to release their negative emotions—not by venting, but by filling their minds with positive thoughts and images.

Here's an example of how it works. Take a few minutes every day to imagine that a magic carpet has arrived to take you away from your troubles.

Multiple Births Equal Multiple Diapers

Women who undergo assistive reproduction procedures, such as in vitro fertilization and gamete intrafallopian transfer, which involves the injection of one or more eggs mixed with sperm directly into the fallopian tubes, will have multiple births about 38 percent of the time. Among those who use ovulation-inducing drugs, 20 percent of the children are twins or triplets or other multiples.

Fertility specialists advise women that multiple births have higher risks of birth defects or delivery complications, especially in older moms. Then there's the sheer workload. Women who are considering fertility treatments should ask themselves if they have the energy and tolerance that's required, say, for the more than 1,000 monthly diaper changes required by a set of triplet newborns. That comes to three new diapers (one for each of three little bottoms) every 2 hours for an entire month.

A recent study also found that women who have ART are 5 times more likely to give birth to a full-term healthy baby if they have a single embryo implanted as opposed to two or more. In part, that's because multiple births tend to be high risk for premature delivery and low birth weight, both of which are linked to mortality. ∎

WHEN BAD THINGS HAPPEN TO HEALTHY WOMEN

She Shed Negative Thoughts—And Conceived Twins

Valerie Gattozzi Mei and her husband, Richard, desperately wanted children. For 6 years, Mei worked with reproductive specialists. She endured tests, surgeries, and side effects from medications, but nothing helped.

"Each year that went by, the desperation and depression became more unbearable," she recalls. "Summers on the beach, which used to be my favorite getaway, became nothing but a torturous reminder that I had no children to watch play in the sand."

Since she had already exhausted most of the medical options, Mei tried a different approach: changing her state of mind.

She enrolled in a 10-week program at the Mind/Body Medical Institute for Women at Harvard Medical Center and Beth Israel Deaconess Medical Center in Boston, where she worked with trained professionals to develop a more positive attitude and reduce her feelings of anger and depression.

In addition, Mei and her husband decided to stop trying to conceive for an entire summer. Rather than feeling the constant pressure, they put all of their energy into enjoying their new boat on the shore.

At the end of a lovely summer, Mei felt ready to pursue one round of in vitro fertilization. "Before I learned how to manage my feelings, the whole idea of in vitro fertilization scared me horribly, so I never considered it," she says.

One month later, she learned that she was pregnant with twins.

Today Mei is the busy mother of 14-year-old Emily Rena and Olivia Lorraine. She continues to use tools she learned during her long struggle to get pregnant. "I now know that it's pointless to get yourself in a tizzy over nothing," she says. "When I catch myself doing it, I remind myself to stop, think, breathe, relax, and go easier on myself." ∎

As you sail through the clouds, mentally place the day's disappointments inside a stone, then gleefully hurl the stone away from you.

This type of imaginative thinking, called visualization, Dr. Domar says, is an excellent way to cope with anger and anxiety and to replace the emotions with feelings of strength and power.

Permit yourself to lie low. Women who are infertile may find it difficult to be near children—or around people who are always asking if they're making "progress." You can't isolate yourself forever, but you shouldn't feel obligated to maintain a busy social life at times when you'd rather be alone, says Dr. Domar.

Confront destructive ideas. Women who are trying without success to get pregnant often link their self-worth to their ability to have children. Put these feelings behind you, the doctor advises. They distort reality and needlessly cause frustration or fear. Try writing down your thoughts in a diary or talking to a supportive friend or family member. If these techniques don't help, consider talking to your doctor about counseling.

Go to church. In a 2010 study, Domar and her colleagues found a strong correlation between fertility distress and symptoms of depression in women undergoing infertility treatment. But those who held strong spiritual beliefs or were part of a spiritual community had less distress and depression.

Medical Options

When you have trouble getting pregnant, the first order of business is for your partner to see a urologist or fertility specialist, who will probably do a semen analysis to rule out a low sperm count or sperm abnormalities. You'll want to visit your gynecologist or a fertility specialist, who will ask about your menstrual history and perform a complete physical exam.

Both of you may need further evaluation of your reproductive organs to rule out blocked tubes or scar tissue in the woman.

Infertility often occurs when a woman is ovulating irregularly or not at all. These cases are often easy to correct because for more than half of couples, the use of drugs leads to pregnancy after 6 months if there are no other problems.

Assisted reproduction technologies, such as in vitro fertilization, manipulate eggs and sperm outside the womb to improve the chances of pregnancy. IVF is the most effective, used often when a woman's fallopian tubes are blocked or when a man produces too little sperm. A woman takes a drug that causes her ovaries to produce many eggs. When they're mature, they're removed and placed in a petri dish with the man's sperm. Once there are healthy embryos (after 3 to 5 days), they are placed either in the woman's uterus or in her fallopian tube. These procedures sometimes involve donor eggs, donor sperm, a surrogate (who usually donates her egg), or a gestational carrier (who carries the infertile woman's biological embryo to term). According to the Centers for Disease Control and Prevention, 39 percent of women younger than 35 who used assisted reproductive technologies gave birth. In women over age 40, the success rate was 11 percent.

Women are usually advised to progress from the easiest treatment options to the most aggressive, giving each treatment at least three menstrual cycles to take effect. After six menstrual cycles, it's probably time to move on to another approach.

"It may be important to move more quickly through your options if you feel that your proverbial reproductive clock is ticking," says Dr. Gelman. "Some couples in their forties want to bypass medications and elaborate testing and go straight to in vitro fertilization. It's always an individual choice."

There are some risks, including birth defects: a CDC study found that assisted reproduction technology (ART) babies are 2 to 4 times more likely to have certain birth defects, such as heart and digestive system problems, or cleft lips or palate. The risk is low and may have more to do with the age of the parents than the technology itself. For more information about infertility, visit the Web site of the National Infertility Association (RESOLVE) at www.resolve.org.

CHAPTER
24

Polycystic Ovary Syndrome

The most common endocrine disorder among women of childbearing years, polycystic ovary syndrome (PCOS) is trouble on many levels. A condition of scrambled hormones and, in at least some women, multiple ovarian cysts, it's a leading cause of infertility, and can predispose a woman to obesity, high levels of inflammation, heart disease, diabetes, uterine cancer, and fatty liver disease. It also has social and emotional ramifications.

Women with PCOS may develop unwanted hair growth on the face, torso, chest, and/or buttocks, and thinning of the hair on the head. They may develop acne as adults. All women produce a small amount of male hormones called androgens, but women with PCOS produce relatively high amounts. The extra male hormones can alter levels of other hormones in the body. It may cause irregular menstrual cycles and stop ovulation. Because of this, the body continues producing estrogen but stops producing progesterone.

Many women with PCOS don't know they have it. All they know is that they're unhappy with the appearance of their bodies—and they often don't suspect that there's an underlying physical

reason, says Walter Futterweit, MD, clinical professor of medicine in the Division of Endocrinology, Diabetes, and Bone Disease at Mount Sinai School of Medicine in New York City and president of the Androgen Excess and Polycystic Ovary Syndrome Society. In young women, PCOS is the leading cause of infertility. It may not be discovered until a woman is unable to conceive.

when to see a doctor

If you have a history of skipped menstrual periods that are followed by serious acne outbreaks, make an appointment to see an endocrinologist. This is a classic symptom of polycystic ovary syndrome (PCOS), says Walter Futterweit, MD, clinical professor of medicine in the Division of Endocrinology, Diabetes, and Bone Disease at Mount Sinai School of Medicine in New York City and president of the Androgen Excess and Polycystic Ovary Syndrome Society..

If you have hair growth on the face or body and thinning hair on the head. In women this usually means that the balance of hormones has been disrupted, and you could have PCOS.

Luckily, most women with PCOS can control the symptoms with a combination of medications and home care.

Lifestyle Strategies

Exercise regularly and keep an eye on your weight. About 50 to 60 percent of women with PCOS are overweight or obese. In overweight women, the main male hormone, testosterone, is converted in the fat tissue to female hormones. An effective way to restore hormones to their proper levels is to maintain a healthful weight. Losing even five percent of your body weight can help. Talk to your doctor about appropriate exercise and diet plans. As

you lose fat tissue, your estrogen levels will naturally decline.

Nutritional Treatments

Control insulin levels. The majority of women with PCOS develop a condition called insulin resistance. Insulin is the hormone that carries glucose (blood sugar) into cells where it's needed. If the cells become resistant to insulin, the body produces more of it—and this in turn stimulates the production of more testosterone by the ovaries.

There are a number of ways to overcome insulin resistance. In addition to helping to control weight, exercising regularly—it can be walk-

THREE THINGS I TELL EVERY FEMALE PATIENT

WALTER FUTTERWEIT, MD, *clinical professor of medicine in the Division of Endocrinology, Diabetes, and Bone Disease at Mount Sinai School of Medicine in New York City and president of the Androgen Excess and Polycystic Ovary Syndrome Society, advises women with polycystic ovary syndrome (PCOS) to follow these recommendations.*

1 REARRANGE THE FOOD GUIDE PYRAMID. The standard for healthy eating, the food guide pyramid recommends getting the bulk of calories from complex carbohydrates, such as whole grains. Women with PCOS, however, should get about 40 percent of calories from lean protein, such as lamb, fish, or legumes. About 30 percent of calories should come

from vegetables, and only about 30 percent should come from complex carbohydrates. Some women have even more success when only about 10 to 20 percent of calories come from carbohydrates.

2 GET SERIOUS ABOUT LOSING WEIGHT. Many women with PCOS are obese. The good news is that losing as little as 7 to 8 percent of the weight is often enough to lower excess hormone levels.

3 SEE AN EXPERT. PCOS CAN BE COMPLICATED TO CONTROL. Your family doctor can help, but women with PCOS really need to be under the care of an endocrinologist, an expert on the body's hormones. ∎

WHEN BAD THINGS HAPPEN TO HEALTHY WOMEN

She Was Eating All the Wrong Foods

Christine Gray DeZarn had kept her weight at 140 pounds throughout her adult life, so she was understandably alarmed when it suddenly jumped to 200 when she was 27. She responded the way a lot of women do: She went on an ultra-low calorie diet. But even when she was getting a skimpy 800 calories daily, she continued to gain weight.

"The doctor I was seeing was convinced I was cheating on my diet, but I was practically starving," she remembers.

At about the same time, she began getting acne along her jaw. She also discovered hair growing on her face and stomach, and when she and her husband tried to have their first child, they had no success after 6 years and 11 trials of expensive assisted reproduction treatments.

DeZarn first heard about polycystic ovary syndrome (PCOS) via an online infertility support group. "I read everything I could get my hands on about metabolism, and how blood sugar and hormones are affected by the different foods you eat. I found out what a mistake I had made by following a low-fat, high-carbohydrate diet. It doesn't work for people with insulin resistance. I was actually triggering my condition by eating a lot of processed grains and cutting back on protein."

As soon as DeZarn eliminated sugar, pasta, rice, and other high-carbohydrate foods from her diet, the pounds started to naturally drop off. She lost 30 pounds in 3 months, and 50 pounds within the first year. "Within 2 years, I was down to 132 pounds, which is better than where I started," she adds.

As a busy travel industry trainer and sales manager, and founder of the Polycystic Ovarian Syndrome Association, DeZarn has to maintain her eating plan while staying in hotels and eating on airplanes and in restaurants. She always eats the same breakfast: scrambled eggs and fresh fruit. Most restaurants serve grilled chicken Caesar salad, and it's also easy to find her favorite snack—celery with blue cheese dressing.

Today, DeZarn continues to follow a strict diet because it controls her weight and other symptoms of PCOS. "I will eat this way for the rest of my life because it works," she says. ∎

ing, bicycling, hiking, or even working in the yard for 20 to 30 minutes most days of the week—will help the body's insulin become more efficient, says Dr. Futterweit. You also may be told to follow a low-glycemic (low-carbohydrate) diet. (For more information on low-glycemic eating, see Chapter 15.)

Curb your sugar cravings. Sugar increases your insulin levels, which causes weight gain and aggravates hormone imbalances, says Lila A. Wallis, MD, clinical professor of medicine at Weill Cornell Medical College of Cornell University in New York City and founder of the National Council on Women's Health. Replace sugary treats with foods like grains, fruits, and vegetables. Without those sweets taunting your hormone levels, you'll feel healthier and more energetic.

Eat small amounts at a time. "If you are in the habit of eating two or three heavy meals a day, switch to five to six light meals," Dr. Futterweit advises. Each meal should contain between 250 and 300 calories. That's about all that insulin-resistant cells can handle at one time, he explains.

Enjoy protein or low-carbohydrate snacks. For women with PCOS, foods that are high in carbohydrates may cause surges in insulin. Better snack choices include protein (such as plain yogurt, string cheese, or nuts and seeds), or low-starch vegetables, such as cucumber or broccoli.

Drink water, but avoid fruit juices. Juices are generally too sweet for women with PCOS. The ideal beverage is water. It's also fine to drink unsweetened almond milk or fat-free or low-fat milk.

Medical Options

Lower insulin with medications. Doctors often prescribe metformin (Glucophage), an insulin-regulating drug that's commonly used to treat diabetes. Women who take it can often normalize their menstrual cycles. They also may see a reversal in weight gain or unwanted hair growth, says Dr. Futterweit. It can also slow the progression of prediabetes to full-blown type 2 diabetes.

Consider the Pill. Oral contraceptives may be used to restore a normal menstrual cycle and help reduce hair growth and acne. Antiandrogen (male hormones) pills such as spironolactone (Aldactone), which block the effects of testosterone, can also be helpful in conjunction with the Pill. This drug is often prescribed for excess hair as well.

Use topical anti-hair-growth drugs. Lotions containing eflornithine hydrochloride (Vaniqa) can block the enzyme needed for hair growth. It takes up to 2 months to work and doesn't eliminate existing hair.

Try laser therapy. A laser can prevent excess hair from growing, though it may take several sessions, which can be expensive.

See a dermatologist. This skin specialist can treat your acne and recommend over-the-counter or prescribe antiacne medications.

Get fertility help. If you're having trouble conceiving, your doctor may prescribe a medication to induce ovulation such as clomiphene citrate (Clomid, Serophene). Combining it with metformin may increase your chances of getting pregnant. If those don't work, you may try injections of gonadotropins to help promote ovulation. Sometimes surgical intervention is needed: A procedure called laparoscopic ovarian drilling, a minimally invasive surgery, involves using electrical or laser energy to burn holes in follicles on the surface of the ovaries, which can reduce androgen levels.

For more information on polycystic ovary syndrome, see the Web site of the Polycystic Ovarian Syndrome Association at www.pcosupport.org.

25

Fibroids

Years ago, having a fibroid tumor often meant hysterectomy. Today we know that these benign growths of the uterine muscle called leiomyomas can be left alone if they're not causing symptoms.

As many as one in five women in their child-bearing years have fibroids; African American women are at least twice as likely to have fibroids as other women. And more than 30 percent of women between 40 and 60 may have them too. You can have one fibroid or a whole cluster. Most fibroids are between the size of a pea and a tennis ball, although they can potentially grow much larger. It's not known what causes fibroids, but their growth seems to depend on estrogen, so as long as you're menstruating, your fibroid may steadily get larger.

It's not uncommon for women with fibroids to be unaware of them. They're sometimes discovered during routine exams, when a gynecologist feels them while pressing on the abdomen, but they can be so small you'd need a microscope to spot them. The diagnosis is usually confirmed by ultrasound or MRI.

If you do have symptoms, you may experience a dull ache in the abdomen, pelvis, or back, a feeling of fullness, gas, constipation, pain with intercourse, or pelvic cramping and pain with your periods. Fibroids may also cause abnormal menstrual bleeding, including bleeding between periods and bleeding during your period that lasts longer than normal. In rare cases, fibroids can cause pregnancy complications, including premature birth and cesarean sections when the fibroids block the birth canal. You can also have severe pain, anemia, or urinary tract infections.

In many cases, however, they cause no symptoms at all—and doctors advise women simply to get used to the idea that there are harmless guests inside the pelvis.

If you are having symptoms, your doctor may just advise you to wait: Since fibroid growth is stimulated by estrogen, once you reach menopause and estrogen levels decline, the symptoms will usually disappear, says Samuel L. Jacobs, MD, a reproductive endocrinologist and associate professor of obstetrics and gynecology at the University of Medicine and Dentistry-Robert Wood Johnson Medical School in Camden, New Jersey.

In the meantime, you may want to take a few steps to manage fibroids naturally.

Home Remedies

Manage your weight. Excess body fat leads to excess estrogen, which can increase the size of fibroids. The best way to maintain a healthful weight is to eat a diet rich in vegetables, fruits, whole grains, low-fat dairy, and lean protein, and to get regular exercise. A combination of weight training and aerobic activities—such as running, bicycling, or fast walking—decreases fat tissue and adds muscle, which can help lower excess levels of estrogen in the body. (For a complete guide to maintaining a healthful weight, see Chapter 6.)

Ease the ache. Applying heat to the abdomen will often relieve discomfort, especially when you're having your period. Mercedes Cameron, MD, a family practitioner in Grand Junction, Colorado, advises using a castor oil pack.

Pour 4 ounces of castor oil on a thick piece of cotton cloth. Fold the cloth in half and put it on your abdomen. Cover it with plastic wrap and a thin towel, then put a heating pad or hot-water bottle on top. Leave the pack on your tummy for up to an hour a day, and repeat the treatment daily, says Dr. Cameron.

Nutritional Treatments

Eat less meat. "The estrogenic additives used in the beef industry can disrupt your hormone levels enough to signal fibroids to grow," says Dr. Jacobs.

In one study, Italian researchers compared the diets of 2,400 women. They found that women with fibroids ate more beef, ham, and other red meats than those without fibroids. A plant-based diet is beneficial because fruits and vegetables contain natural plant compounds called isoflavones, which help prevent estrogen from fueling fibroid growth, Dr. Jacobs says.

Consume more dairy. African American women in the US Black Women's Health Study

THREE THINGS I TELL EVERY FEMALE PATIENT

LYNN BORGATTA, MD, *director of clinical research at Boston University School of Medicine and past research coordinator for Planned Parenthood Federation of America, offers this advice to women with fibroids.*

1 **DON'T BE FRIGHTENED.** Fibroids are tumors, but they're benign and won't increase your risk for cancer. They're almost always harmless, and the symptoms (if there are any) will probably be easy to manage, possibly with medications that shrink fibroids, among other options.

2 **BE CONSERVATIVE.** If you need relief from fibroid symptoms and you're planning to have children, talk to your doctor about medication before considering surgical procedures like myomectomy or uterine embolization.

3 **TALK TO YOUR DOCTOR ABOUT HYSTERECTOMY OPTIONS.** If you need a hysterectomy, let your doctor know that you don't want the ovaries and cervix removed along with the uterus unless it's absolutely necessary. A supracervical hysterectomy is less traumatic and healthier in the long run. ∎

who ate the most calcium-rich dairy products had a lower risk of developing uterine fibroids. While consuming more dairy products may help every woman, the researchers speculate that it's the low dairy intake among African American populations that may contribute to the higher risk for fibroids among black women.

Stick to low glycemic foods. In the same study that found a link between dairy and fibroids, researchers also unearthed another clue: African American women whose diets were higher in foods that raised blood sugar—high-glycemic foods such as refined carbohydrates—were more likely to get fibroids, particularly women over 35.

Don't overdo alcohol. In a 2009 *British Journal of Nutrition* study, researchers found a link between alcohol consumption and increased risk of fibroids in a group of Japanese women. Alcohol is known to raise levels of estrogen in the body.

Medical Options

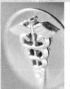 Fibroids need to be treated when they're causing heavy or abnormal menstrual bleeding, chronic pain, bowel or urinary obstructions, or other symptoms, says Lynn Borgatta, MD, director of clinical research at Boston University School of Medicine and past research coordinator for Planned Parenthood Federation of America. You'll also need treatment if you're trying to conceive and the fibroids are interfering with pregnancy.

The treatment options include:

■ Gonadotropin-releasing hormone (GnRH) agonists (Lupron/Lupron Depot). These are medica-

when to see a doctor

If your periods are heavier than usual, or you're having irregular bleeding. See your gynecologist. This is often the first symptom of fibroids, says Lynn Borgatta, MD, director of clinical research at Boston University School of Medicine and past research coordinator for Planned Parenthood Federation of America .

If you're having trouble urinating or moving your bowels. It can mean that fibroids are getting large enough to exert pressure on the bladder or intestine.

If you've been diagnosed with fibroids, whether or not they're causing symptoms. You'll need to have them monitored regularly—3 months after the diagnosis and every 6 months thereafter.

tions that shrink fibroids temporarily. Their main use is to shrink fibroids prior to surgery. The drawback to these medications is that they may cause menopause-like symptoms, such as hot flashes and vaginal dryness. Over time, they can also raise cholesterol levels and increase the risk of osteoporosis, so they are usually not used longer than 6 months.

■ Myomectomy. This means removing fibroids surgically. Small fibroids can be cauterized (destroyed) with a laser or electrical needle; larger fibroids are cut away from the uterine wall. Depending on the location of the fibroids, surgery may be done through the abdomen or through the vagina. The surgery is usually successful, although there's a small chance that a hysterectomy will be needed to finish the surgery. There is also a 30 percent chance that the fibroids will

Acupuncture Saved Her from a Hysterectomy

After an emergency room visit for abdominal pain, Sharon Sanders, a cookbook writer in Allentown, Pennsylvania, discovered that she had a fibroid the size of a 16-week pregnancy. The fibroid had grown so fast and was causing so much discomfort that her gynecologist recommended a hysterectomy.

Saunders wasn't convinced that surgery was her best option, especially because she knew that fibroids often shrink with the onset of menopause. At 48, she was hoping to find a treatment that would tide her over for a few years.

After reading an article about the use of acupuncture for treating fibroids, she decided to give it a try. She made an appointment with a practitioner of traditional Chinese medicine, who recommended weekly acupuncture treatments along with medicinal herbs. After 4 months, she checked back with her gynecologist, who reported that the fibroid had shrunk by a third.

"I got to keep my uterus, and the pain went away entirely," says Sanders, who says estrogen depletion during menopause "took care of the fibroid." ■

return. Fertility is usually preserved, but pregnancy can sometimes be complicated.

■ Hysteroscopic resection. If your fibroids are growing inside the uterine cavity, your doctor may schedule this outpatient procedure in which a small camera and instruments are inserted through the cervix and into the uterus to remove the fibroids.

■ Hysterectomy. This means removing the uterus. Once the uterus is removed, the fibroids are also gone and won't come back. The problem with hysterectomy is that it's major surgery and there may be a long recovery time. Also, women who have this procedure won't be able to have children afterward. A supracervical hysterectomy is limited to removal of the uterus only, leaving the ovaries and cervix intact.

■ Uterine artery embolization. This is a surgical procedure in which the blood vessels that supply

the fibroids are destroyed with a bombardment of plastic particles. The advantage of this procedure is that it's less stressful than other forms of surgery and it's unlikely to interfere with a woman's ability to conceive. It's a relatively new procedure, however, and experts aren't sure how effective it will prove to be over time.

"When medical interventions are necessary, ask your doctor about all your options. The right treatment will be different for everyone," says Dr. Borgatta. There are a lot of considerations to keep in mind, including the severity of symptoms, whether you'll want to get pregnant in the future, and how close you are to menopause. The size of the fibroids and where they're growing can also affect your treatment options as well as your risks," Dr. Borgatta adds.

26

Endometriosis

Your uterus acts as a nest for fertilized eggs, so it's lined with soft, spongy tissue called the endometrium. Normally, an egg is released each month, and if it isn't fertilized, the endometrium swells, breaks down, and sloughs off, exiting the body as menstrual fluid.

Sometimes, however, things go awry. The cells that make up the endometrium grow outside the uterus on nearby organs, such as the fallopian tubes or ovaries. The cells also sometimes implant themselves on the outside of the uterus. They can even spread to the lungs, digestive tract, or other parts of the body. This disease is called endometriosis, and it can result in painful and potentially serious symptoms.

Because endometrial cells are sensitive to the hormonal changes of the menstrual cycle, the symptoms often flare during the menstrual period. Women may experience severe, even incapacitating pain, fatigue, and many other symptoms. Endometriosis also can result in gastrointestinal symptoms, painful sex, or, during periods, painful urination. More than 30 percent of women with endometriosis also face infertility.

Endometriosis sometimes can be controlled with the use of birth control pills or other hormone-altering medications. Surgery to remove the tissue is another treatment that can help. But for about one in three women, the renegade tissue will eventually come back, says Carolyn R. Kaplan, MD, a reproductive endocrinologist, director of In Vitro Fertilization at Georgia Reproductive Specialists, and an assistant clinical professor of obstetrics and gynecology at Emory University School of Medicine, both in Atlanta.

Doctors aren't sure what causes endometriosis. Evidence suggests that the cells get "scattered" around the pelvis when menstrual blood doesn't effectively make its way out of the body. The immune system should recognize and destroy these errant cells, but for some reason it doesn't, says Dr. Kaplan, so the cells implant themselves wherever they end up. Another theory is that endometrial tissue travels to other parts of the body via the bloodstream or lymph system. There may be a genetic component as well.

There are a number of treatment options for endometriosis. A good starting place is for women to strengthen their immune systems and do everything possible to keep their hormones in the proper balance, says Deborah A. Metzger, MD, PhD, associate clinical professor of reproductive endocrinology and obstetrics and gynecology at Stanford University and medical director of Helena Women's Health in San Jose, California.

Some women with endometriosis will require medical treatment, either to remove the tissue or to manage the monthly flare-ups. In many cases, however, women can control the discomfort with home care.

Home Remedies

Take NSAIDs. Painkillers such as ibuprofen, naproxen, or prescription painkillers can help ease cramps.

Treat yourself to heat. Applying warmth to the lower abdomen is a very effective way to soothe the uterus, says Toni Bark, MD, founder and medical director of the Center for Disease Prevention and Reversal in Evanston, Illinois. Taking warm baths or applying a hot-water bottle or a heating pad is the easiest approach. For longer-lasting heat, your doctor may advise you to use a patch that releases heat for long periods of time, such as ThermaCare therapeutic heat wraps, available in drugstores.

Exercise regularly. Walking, swimming, and other forms of exercise increase circulation, which helps the body remove excess estrogen from the blood. Exercise also stimulates endorphins, natural chemicals that help reduce pain.

Avoid pollutants. The hormones in a woman's body are exquisitely balanced, but modern society has thrown a wrench into the works. Humans have introduced more than 70,000 industrial chemicals into the environment, and some of them suppress immunity and disrupt

THREE THINGS I TELL EVERY FEMALE PATIENT

TONI BARK, MD, *founder and medical director of the Center for Disease Prevention and Reversal in Evanston, Illinois, has seen great success when women with endometriosis do the following:*

1
TAKE 1 TABLESPOON OF GROUND FLAX-SEED DAILY. Flax contains an oil that reduces painful inflammation. It's also high in fiber, which can help remove excess estrogen. "I recommend having it for breakfast every morning," says Dr. Bark. "You can mix it with sunflower seeds, fruit, and almond milk."

2
USE EVENING PRIMROSE OIL. Available as a supplement, evening primrose oil reduces inflammation and often relieves pain within a month, says Dr. Bark. The recommended dose is 500 mg twice daily.

3
TAKE A MULTI SUPPLEMENT THAT CONTAINS B VITAMINS AND VITAMIN E. Vitamin E carries oxygen to tissues and helps reduce scar formation in women with endometriosis. The B vitamins are particularly important because they help balance the body's hormones, says Dr. Bark. ∎

the natural balance of hormones, says Dr. Metzger.

Dioxin, for example, a manufacturing waste chemical that's widespread in the environment, might have profound effects on a woman's hormones. In one 13-year study, female rhesus monkeys were exposed to dioxin and 79 percent developed endometriosis. These studies were in monkeys, not humans, but something similar may occur in humans, says Dr. Metzger.

An important place to start, according to the Endometriosis Association, is to avoid food that may have high amounts of dioxin in it (see below). Products that have been bleached with chlorine may contain dioxin and other chemical contaminants. Although a survey by the Endometriosis Association did not show a connection between tampon use and endometriosis incidence, some women like to use non-chlorine-bleached tampons and sanitary napkins.

Some people may find it's also helpful to use dioxin-free bathroom tissues (available in health catalogs and stores), cosmetics, and other products whenever possible. Opt for cloth towels and cloth napkins instead of paper.

Avoid plastic products made with bisphenol-A, another endocrine disrupter. A 2010 animal study found that prenatal exposure to the chemical caused an endometriosis-like condition in mice.

Nutritional Treatments

 Eat organically. Commercial livestock typically is injected with growth hor-

mones and antibiotics—and women who eat meat may suffer the effects. "In my opinion, an immediate way to protect your hormone balance and immune system is to make sure that you don't eat meat and dairy products that aren't certified as organic," says Dr. Bark. One study found that eating red meat and ham were linked to endometriosis. Red meat in particular can contain levels of environmental hormone disrupters such as dioxins and the fat content may raise estrogen levels.

Filter your drinking water. Use water purifiers that filter out lead, mercury, chlorine,

when to see a doctor

If you have abdominal pain that increases with your period, around ovulation, or with intercourse. There's a good chance that you have endometriosis, and it may get worse without prompt treatment, says Carolyn R. Kaplan, MD, a reproductive endocrinologist, director of In Vitro Fertilization at Georgia Reproductive Specialists, and an assistant clinical professor of obstetrics and gynecology at Emory University School of Medicine, both in Atlanta.

If you're having trouble getting pregnant. Endometriosis is a common cause of infertility, says Dr. Kaplan. It may cause scarring around the tubes and ovaries that could lead to infertility. If other women in your family have had endometriosis, you have a higher risk of getting it as well, she adds.

WHEN BAD THINGS HAPPEN TO HEALTHY WOMEN

Natural Treatments Gave Her Control

Menstrual periods are rarely as regular as the textbooks would have you believe, but for Karen Susag, they were unusually erratic from the beginning.

"My periods varied greatly. Sometimes I would only get a period every 6 months, and when I did, I'd be immobilized with pain. There also were times that I would end up at the emergency room," says Susag, a development director at a nonprofit organization in the San Francisco Bay area.

At one point, the pain was so severe and frequent that she missed an entire semester of college. That's when a doctor finally recognized that her symptoms were caused by endometriosis.

In the next 10 years, she had surgery 6 times for endometriosis and to remove scar tissue. She also tried a variety of hormone medications, which invariably brought on headaches, nausea, and fatigue.

On the advice of a practitioner specializing in immunotherapy, Susag eliminated dairy, sugar, yeast, alcohol, and caffeine from her diet. In addition to immunotherapy, she underwent acupuncture and took Chinese herbs under the supervision of an Oriental medicine doctor. And she did everything possible to reduce the stress in her life.

"I have a whole different way of approaching things," she says. "I listen to my body, and know when I'm pushing myself too hard. If I work late, then I take the morning off."

The treatments worked, reducing her pain and fatigue. "The hardest thing about having endometriosis is knowing that it's a chronic problem. But I've discovered that if you keep your life in better balance, you can keep it in check." ∎

---

and other hormone-disrupting contaminants, advises Dr. Bark. Check the labels for the specific substances that each type of filter will remove.

Consume omega-3s. A 12-year study of nearly 120,000 nurses ages 25 to 42 who had not been diagnosed with endometriosis at the start of the study, found that those who had the most omega-3 fatty acids in their diets were less likely to develop the disease. And if you already have endometriosis, omega-3s, with their ability to tamp down the effects of pain-causing chemicals in the body, may offer some relief.

Avoid trans fats. The same nurses study found that consumption of these manmade fats—added to improve the shelf life of foods, often snack foods—was associated with a greater risk of endometriosis.

Eat lots of vegetables and fruit. They're loaded with antioxidants, which can help prevent the cellular damage caused by wayward molecules called free radicals, the product of both normal metabolism and environmental forces, from pollutants to cigarette smoke to sun exposure. Studies have found evidence of free radical damage in the peritoneal fluid and blood of women with endometriosis, which could increase the growth of endometrial cells and their adhesion to body tissues. In one Mexican study, women with endometriosis had lower intakes of vitamins A, C, and E, as well as zinc and copper, but were able to bring them up to higher levels by changing their diets.

Alternative Therapies

Relax as much as you can. Stress management helps to improve immune function and may also decrease pain, says Dr. Bark.

Every woman has her own ways of coping with stress, including meditation, yoga, and relaxation exercises. Or try more creative approaches: Take an art class; do volunteer work; get more engaged with your hobbies. Women who nurture their creative sides will naturally experience less stress, Dr. Bark explains.

Medical Options

Consider drug therapy. Gonadotropin-releasing hormone (GnRH) agonists and antagonists, such as leuprolide (Lupron) and nafarelin (Synarel), turn off the signal to ovulate, leading to a reversible "medical menopause," Dr. Kaplan says. This causes estrogen levels to drop. Menstrual periods stop, and over time the errant endometrial cells will shrink. These drugs can cause menopausal symptoms such as hot flashes, vaginal dryness, mood changes, and calcium loss from the bones. Normally women stay on these drugs for no more than 6 months to a year because of the bone loss. You may be prescribed estrogen-progesterone birth control pills to prevent the disease from worsening. They work by stopping the menstrual cycle and creating a "pseudopregnancy."

Look into IUDs. Intrauterine devices (IUDs) were once discouraged for women with endometriosis or other pelvic problems, but Mirena, which releases a synthetic hormone called levonorgestrel into the uterus, appears to suppress endometrial growth, says Dr. Kaplan.

A Finnish study looked at 56 women who were considering hysterectomies to relieve excessive uterine bleeding. Half of them were asked to use the Mirena IUD to see if it helped. Two-thirds of the women experienced enough relief that they decided to cancel the surgery.

Talk about surgery. If you're in severe pain and other treatments don't work, you may be a candidate for minimally invasive surgery to remove or destroy endometrial-related tissue and adhesions (scar tissue). A hysterectomy usually eliminates endometrial symptoms, but you may need to take hormone replacement after your ovaries are removed. If you're trying to get pregnant, surgery may be your best chance to restore your fertility.

Pelvic Inflammatory Disease

If you suspect that you may have contracted a sexually transmitted disease (STD)—symptoms include a foul-smelling discharge, painful urination, and a dull ache in the lower abdomen; pelvic pain; or fever and chills—don't wait to see if it will go away. Call your doctor right away.

You have to act quickly if there's even a hint that you have an STD. That's because untreated STDs can lead to pelvic inflammatory disease (PID), a broad term that refers to infections of the upper genital tract, usually involving the fallopian tubes, sometimes the ovaries, and even the lining of the uterus. As with many infections, intensive treatment with antibiotics is necessary to destroy the bacteria that are making you sick. Delays in treatment, on the other hand, can allow the harmful organisms to rage out of control, potentially damaging your reproductive organs beyond repair. Unfortunately, women don't always see a doctor at the first sign of symptoms. A quarter of PID cases require hospitalization and the use of intravenous antibiotics; in rare cases emergency surgery is needed to drain infectious fluid from the abdomen or repair organ damage. Because the infection can scar and block the fallopian tubes, PID may

result in infertility. Blocked tubes can also put a woman at higher risk for ectopic pregnancy, a dangerous condition in which a fertilized egg grows in the fallopian tube instead of in the uterus.

More than 750,000 American women get PID every year, and in excess of 75,000 become infertile as a result.

The vast majority of cases can be prevented by taking precautions against sexually transmitted diseases by using condoms, says Samuel Jacobs, MD, a reproductive endocrinologist and associate professor of obstetrics and gynecology at the University of Medicine and Dentistry-Robert Wood Johnson Medical School in Camden, New Jersey.

Unwelcome Infections

The organism that results in PID is usually chlamydia or, less commonly, gonorrhea (or both). These STDs are especially prevalent among sexually active women with multiple partners.

If you've had unprotected sex and suspect that you may have been exposed to an STD, get tested right away. One reason that STDs are so dangerous is that one in five people infected with chlamydia or gonorrhea has no symptoms. Women can carry the disease for weeks, months, or even years before the infection spreads or results in full-blown PID, but a woman's reproductive organs can be damaged in the meantime. Sexually active women in the childbearing years are most at risk, as are women under 25 because the cervixes of younger women and teens are not fully matured and are more susceptible to infection.

PID isn't always caused by sexually transmitted diseases. Some women may develop infections after childbirth, abortions, or other types of pelvic surgeries. These types of infections are rare, however. In most cases—99.9 percent—STDs are to blame, says Dr. Jacobs.

Regardless of the cause, STDs can be successfully treated with antibiotics. While completing the antibiotic treatment, you can also relieve much of the discomfort with home care.

Home Remedies

Allow yourself some downtime. Your body has taken a beating, and you need time to recover. Drink a lot of fluid, eat lightly, and get some rest.

Avoid sex until the antibiotic treatment is complete—usually after 2 weeks. Otherwise, you could pass the infection to your partner. When you do resume sexual activity, be certain that your partner has been tested and treated for STDs. You don't want to be exposed to the same harmful organisms that made you sick in the first place.

Steam away infection. Sitting in a hot environment—a steamy shower, for example, or a

THREE THINGS I TELL EVERY FEMALE PATIENT

SAMUEL L. JACOBS, MD, *a reproductive endocrinologist and associate professor of obstetrics and gynecology at the University of Medicine and Dentistry-Robert Wood Johnson Medical School in Camden, New Jersey, gives the following advice for preventing pelvic inflammatory disease (PID). Women who get PID once have a 15 percent risk of infertility; two infections, 30 percent; and a woman who gets PID a third time has a 50 percent risk.*

1 **USE PROTECTION.** If you and your sexual partner aren't mutually monogamous, or if you haven't both been tested for sexually transmitted diseases, use latex condoms, even if you're on another form of birth control, says Dr. Jacobs.

2 **INTRAUTERINE CONTRACEPTIVES AREN'T FOR EVERYONE.** "Although intrauterine contraceptives are an excellent form of birth control, they're not appropriate for women with a history of multiple partners, STDs, or pelvic inflammatory disease," says Dr. Jacobs.

3 **DON'T DOUCHE.** It pushes bacteria up into the reproductive tract, which can increase the risk for PID, says Dr. Jacobs. ∎

deep bath—increases body temperature, which boosts the activity of the immune system and creates an unfavorable environment for harmful germs. The moist heat will also reduce discomfort in the abdomen and back.

when to see a doctor

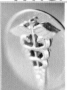

If you have a foul-smelling vaginal discharge, along with a dull ache in the lower abdomen or back, or fever and chills accompanying either of the above, see your doctor right away. These are early signs of PID, says Samuel L. Jacobs, MD, a reproductive endocrinologist and associate professor of obstetrics and gynecology at the University of Medicine and Dentistry-Robert Wood Johnson Medical School in Camden, New Jersey.

If you develop symptoms after having unprotected sex. You could have chlamydia, gonorrhea, or another sexually transmitted disease, which can increase your risk for PID.

If you have flulike symptoms or a heavy vaginal discharge or bleeding, along with pelvic pain, go to the emergency room. If you have PID, the infection may have reached a serious stage. It's not uncommon for PID to be misdiagnosed as endometriosis, so you may want to ask the doctor about getting your white blood cell count checked and having a pelvic ultrasound, advises Dr. Jacobs. These tests will help differentiate between the two conditions.

Don't be hard on yourself. Because of the link between PID and sexually transmitted diseases, women often feel guilty, embarrassed, or ashamed. Put the feelings behind you. It's fine to acknowledge that you may have made some mistakes, but it's more important to look forward to the future.

"Stress, anxiety, and negative thoughts will only make the amount of pain and dysfunction worse," says Emmett Miller, MD, founder and medical director of the Center for Healing and Wellness in Los Altos, California, and author of *Deep Healing: The Essence of Mind/Body Medicine.* "Tell yourself, 'Okay, I got it, and I'm going to take steps to prevent getting it again.' After that, let it go," he advises.

Alternative Therapies

Use live-culture supplements. Antibiotics kill beneficial bacteria in the body along with the bad. To replenish "good" bacteria, take probiotic supplements, which contain live cultures of acidophilus and bifidus. Probiotics improve digestion, assist the immune system, and help prevent yeast infections in women who are taking antibiotics, says Toni Bark, MD, founder and medical director of the Center for Disease Prevention and Reversal in Evanston, Illinois.

Dr. Bark advises taking 1 teaspoon of probiotic powder 3 times daily for as long as you're taking antibiotics. Continue taking the probiotic for an additional 3 weeks.

Look for probiotics that are kept in the refrigerated section of health food stores, she adds. They contain the highest concentration of beneficial bacteria.

Savor spicy stir-fries. The spices ginger, turmeric, and cayenne contain chemical compounds that reduce inflammation, pain, and congestion in the abdomen. Garlic is also helpful because it has powerful antibacterial effects, says Dr. Bark.

Put your mind to work. Some studies have shown that guided imagery, or visualization exercises, in which you form clear mental images of the healing powers of your body, can increase immunoglobulins and possibly help infections heal more quickly.

Here's how it works. Twice a day, find a quiet place and relax by taking slow, deep breaths, says Dr. Miller. Create a mental image of your reproductive organs, but with a slight blur over them; the blur represents the infection. Form a picture in your mind of thousands of white blood cells pouring into your organs. As they work, they'll flush out inflammation and clear away the blur, revealing healthy tissue underneath.

Medical Options

Get prescribed antibiotics immediately. If you're treated for an STD early enough, a single course of oral antibiotics will cure it for good. PID requires long-term therapy with multiple antibiotics, says Dr. Jacobs, because the infection can be caused by more than one bacteria.

Finish the prescription. Often a woman with PID who takes antibiotics starts feeling better within 2 days. But the antibiotics aren't done working. You'll need to finish the full prescription—1 to 2 weeks' worth—to eliminate all the bacteria from your body. Women who quit antibiotics too soon may see the infection come right back, says Dr. Jacobs.

Stay in touch with your doctor. You'll want to make an appointment for 2 to 3 days after you begin treatment with antibiotics to ensure that the drugs are working. Make another appointment for when the treatment is done. Your doctor will make sure that the infection is gone and that you don't need an additional round of antibiotics, Dr. Jacobs says.

28

Perimenopause

Most women experience at least a few baffling patterns as they begin the 4- to 10-year transition to perimenopause. It usually begins in the forties (but can start as early as the late thirties), and can bring a grab bag of symptoms, including depression and anxiety, unpredictable emotions, irregular periods, hot flashes, insomnia, exhaustion, forgetfulness, and migraines. And you thought your regular periods were fun!

It may be small comfort that this is all normal. But fluctuating hormones don't make you any less healthy, confirms Nanette Santoro, MD, director of the division of reproductive medicine at Montefiore Medical Center/Albert Einstein College of Medicine.

The good news is that there's a lot you can do—from diet and lifestyle changes to medications—to manage these womanly delights and reduce your symptoms dramatically. Here's what you can expect and how to successfully navigate this next phase of life with your health and happiness intact.

The "Mystery" Pause

Neither research nor experts can say which symptoms you'll experience and whether they'll continue from month to month. "One of the hallmarks of perimenopause is its unpredictability," says Joann Pinkerton, MD, medical director of the Midlife Health Center at the University of Virginia. That's why experts don't recommend testing your hormone levels to determine if you're perimenopausal. Wildly fluctuating hormones often mean that the test cannot accurately predict where you are in this phase. Instead, pay close attention to your menstrual cycles and note your symptoms. Here are some of the most common.

Yikes! Periods. As hormone levels and ovulation become more erratic, your cycle may shorten by a day or two and then by several days, and your flow may go from light to super heavy and clotty; you may also experience severe cramping. When you don't ovulate, the endometrium, which sheds during menstruation, tends to overgrow, causing the excessive blood. Eventually, you'll have fewer and fewer periods, though they may still be heavy.

Hot flashes. Though scientists don't know the exact cause, they suspect a drop in estrogen may disrupt your body's thermostat, resulting in a hot flash. About 75 to 80 percent of women experience these, which can last from a few seconds to 10 minutes and be as mild as a flushed face or so intense as to cause perspiration, heart palpitations—and an overwhelming desire to strip down to your scivvies. If you smoke, are overweight, or are African American, your risk of getting them increases. Hot flashes accompanied by intense sweating can also occur during sleep. These are called night sweats and may interfere with your shut-eye a little—or a lot.

Mood swings. Some experts believe unpredictable emotions are the earliest signs of perimenopause, and they may begin even before you notice changes in your cycle. Nearly 40 percent of women have mood swings associated with hormonal changes—from feelings of rage to intense PMS moodiness, anxiety, or despair, says Michelle Warren, MD, medical director of the Center for Menopause, Hormonal Disorders, and Women's Health at Columbia University Medical Center. One study found that the risk of depression doubles when women enter perimenopause. If you've previously suffered from PMS or postpartum depression, you may be even more prone.

Mental fuzziness. A new study published in *Neurology* found that 60 percent of perimenopausal women experience short-term memory loss, do not learn as well, and have a hard time concentrating. The effect is temporary, however. Cognitive function improved back to previous levels during postmenopause, say researchers.

AWOL libido. Sexual desire may change, it may even seem to disappear, but studies show that for many women a good sex drive before perimenopause will continue after.

Vaginal dryness. Low estrogen levels cause the tissue in your vaginal area to lose lubrication and elasticity, which can make intercourse painful. It may also leave you more vulnerable to urinary or vaginal infections.

Peri-Prep: Three Keys

Adopting healthy habits now may not only help ease current problems, but will maximize your overall health as you head into the future. Just think: in the next galaxy (menopause) you're going to be free of periods, pads, birth control, pregnancies, and hormonal roller coasters. You'll want to enjoy every minute of it! With these three keys, you'll not only weather the coming changes, but launch yourself into a phase of freedom you haven't experienced since girlhood.

Eat smart. Cholesterol increases around this time, as does your risk of heart disease and osteoporosis. This is a great time to reduce saturated fat in your diet and concentrate on a high-fiber diet rich in fruits, vegetables, and whole grains. Include more calcium-rich foods and a calcium supplement that also supplies vitamin D, which helps your body absorb calcium and protect against bone loss. Avoid excessive alcohol and caffeine, which can trigger hot flashes. Also key: cutting calories. After menopause, metabolism slows, and shifting hormones cause extra weight to settle in your midsection. Since you lose muscle mass as you age, you'll need fewer calories to maintain a healthy weight.

Move more. Regular activity helps prevent weight gain, reduces heavy bleeding and cramping, and improves mood and sleep. Talk about a major perimenopausal payoff! Alternate between strength-training (to maintain muscle mass) and vigorous aerobic exercise (to burn calories and strengthen cardio). Aim for at least 30 minutes most days of the week.

Relieve stress. Practiced regularly, stress management techniques can offer relief and a sense of control when you're dealing with significant life and body changes. Scientists believe emotional stress exacerbates many of the symptoms of perimenopause, like hot flashes, depression, and anxiety. Now's the time to embrace practices such as yoga, meditation, guided imagery, and deep breathing. For example, slow, deep abdominal breathing in for 5 seconds, then out for 5, done 15 minutes twice a day, can decrease the intensity of hot flashes by 39 percent, research shows.

Home Remedies

Watch your thermostat. Note—and avoid—your triggers, such as heat, spicy foods, alcohol, and caffeine. Don't order hot buffalo wings unless you're willing to suffer the consequences. The spices used in Cajun, Mexican, and Eastern cuisines can trigger hot flashes. In the kitchen, you may want to cut back on salsa, curry concoctions, hot-pepper sauce, and black pepper.

External heat sources can fire up your flashes, too: You may find yourself recruiting a family member to take things out of the oven. If a hot hair dryer sets you off, use the cool-air setting.

Dress the part. Wear layers, so you can peel off one at a time when you start feeling steamy.

You may want to leave turtlenecks, heavy fabrics, or body-clothes in the closet for a while. Try wearing a thin camisole of wicking fabric under your dress clothes, and if night sweats are a problem, look for lightweight, wicking pajamas specifically designed for hot mamas.

Keep good bedtime habits. Turn off the TV, keep the bedroom cool and dark, and drink calming teas. Progressive relaxation techniques may help, too. Start with your toes; tighten them for 5 seconds and release. Move your way up to your calves, thighs, abdomen, and so on, tightening each for 5 seconds and releasing, until you reach your eyes (scrunch and relax).

Protect your sleep schedule. If your natural sleep cycle is disrupted, you may try to compensate by snoozing late on weekends—but that can make it even harder to get back on track. Go to bed and wake up around the same time every day as much as possible. A regular sleep/wake cycle helps minimize hormonal fluctuations, too. (A quick nap in the afternoon is okay, but sleeping more than 15 minutes may make it harder to fall asleep at night.)

Create night breezes. Keep a fan near your bed. One with a remote control is ideal: With a control within reach, there's no need for you to jump out of bed each time you need to cool off. An inconspicuous fan near your desk at work also allows you to respond quickly to daytime flashes.

For juice. Declines in estrogen affect the amount of blood flow to the pelvic area, as well as mucus production in the vagina. You may find you need extra lubrication, often for the first time, during sex. Vaginal lubricants such as K-Y Jelly or Astroglide will help prepare mucous membranes for intercourse. Look for a product that's water-soluble and designed for the vagina.

If your vagina always feels dry, you can use an over-the-counter vaginal moisturizer such as Replens or K-Y Long Lasting Vaginal Moisturizer every day. These are longer-lasting creams that act directly on the tissue to relieve vaginal dryness, itching, and irritation.

For fun. It's not uncommon for women to blame their hormones for a decline in libido, when problems in the relationship itself are an equally if not more important factor, note women's' health experts. If physical discomfort or arousal is a problem, you need to discuss what will make you comfortable and raring to go again. If you and your partner have grown apart emotionally, make an effort to invest more time in order to recapture the fun and intimacy that you shared earlier in the relationship. Don't be afraid to seek professional counseling, as well.

Medical Options

The Women's Health Initiative study in 2002 found that long-term use of hormone therapy increased risk of breast cancer and did not protect against heart disease, but scientists say that short-term use (a few years, if needed) is safe. Unless you're at high risk of developing breast cancer or blood clots, you may be a candidate for a low dose of hormones for the shortest time possible, says Jan Shifren, MD, director of the Vincent Menopause Program at Massachusetts General Hospital.

Try an oral contraceptive. Low-dose birth control pills are often effective in regulating periods, reducing hot flashes, and relieving vaginal dryness.

If you have irregular periods, but can't—or choose not to—use oral contraceptives, cyclic progesterin therapy may regulate periods. Some women with heavy bleeding during perimenopause may find relief from a progestin-containing intrauterine devise (IUD).

THREE THINGS I TELL EVERY FEMALE PATIENT

MONA SHANGOLD, MD, *director of the Center for Women's Health and Sports Gynecology in Philadelphia, offers this special advice for women approaching perimenopause.*

1 **EXERCISE REGULARLY.** All women should get 20 minutes of aerobic exercise daily, combined with strength training 2 to 3 days a week.

2 **MAINTAIN A HEALTHFUL WEIGHT.** You'll have more energy and will be healthier overall than if you allow those extra pounds to accumulate.

3 **USE EXERCISE TO CONTROL MOODINESS.** Whether mood changes are caused by sleep deprivation, night sweats, or changes in brain chemicals associated with aging, they can often be prevented with exercise. ■

Other Rx approaches. For intense hot flashes that don't respond to natural remedies, some doctors may prescribe medications "off-label"–that is, blood pressure medications, antidepressants or blood pressure drugs that studies have shown can lessen the severity or duration of flashes–depending on your personal history, of course.

Endometrial ablation. A procedure in which the uterine lining is destroyed using a laser, electrical energy or heat is another option to relieve heavy perimenopausal bleeding.

Switch your contraceptive. If you are already using oral contraceptives at perimenopause, your remedy for a flatlined libido may be as simple as switching to a different progestin formula, says Mary Jane Minkin, MD, clinical professor of obstetrics and gynecology at Yale University School of Medicine and coauthor of *What Every Woman Needs to Know about Menopause.* Certain progestins have androgenic effects that boost sex drive; others can depress libido.

Ask your doctor about products that contain androgenic progestins, such as levonorgestrel (Mirena), norethindrone (Aygestin), or ethynodiol (Demulen). Nonandrogenic formulations have norgestimate (Ortho-Cyclen) or desogestrel (Apri) as the key ingredient, Dr. Minkin says.

Apply as needed. Applying estrogen cream, available by prescription, to the vaginal area will help improve tone and comfort. Some products are inserted outside of the vagina; others are designed to treat vaginal dryness and sensitivity and come in the form of a ring, which is inserted in front of the cervix

Have your thyroid tested. Low levels of thyroid hormones can drain your energy and lead to depression, while an overactive thyroid can produce feelings of anxiety and panic. Make sure that you are getting your thyroid levels screened every year.

Since thyroid hormones and estrogen affect one another, it's likely that you'll need to have your thyroid medication adjusted at perimenopause, especially if you're undergoing HRT, says Steven Petak, MD, associate professor at the Texas Institute for Reproductive Medicine and Endocrinology in Houston and clinical assistant professor at the University of Texas Medical School at Houston.

when to see a doctor

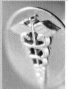

If you have abnormally heavy bleeding or spotting between periods, make an appointment to see your doctor. These symptoms are often normal at the time of perimenopause, but they can also be caused by endometriosis, fibroids, or even cancer.

If you experience hot flashes, vaginal dryness, or other perimenopausal symptoms prior to age 40. About one in 100 women between the ages of 15 and 40 will experience premature ovarian failure, also known as "early menopause." You may need medical treatment to protect your bones and maintain fertility.

29

Menopause

"Going through menopause" is the phrase women use to describe it: the transition between regular menstruation and the end of periods. Formerly—and cryptically—referred to as "the Change," usually in whispers, and restricted to the company of female relatives, no matter what you call it, menopause is actually reached when a full year has past since your last period. Most women will have experienced some of the symptoms of the Big M in varying degrees during the 1- to 3-year period that precedes it, called perimenopause. The average age of a woman having her last period is around 51. But some women reach menopause in their forties, and some have it later in their fifties. The facts about this finale of our reproductive cycles haven't changed. What have changed are the ways we think about, talk about, and understand it medically—as well as the options for the best ways to deal with its symptoms and the health issues accompanying it.

Your hormone levels have been fluctuating throughout perimenopause. Now, at menopause, you have less than half of the estrogen of your reproductive years, and the progesterone that once was released from the ovaries is nearly phased out. Although these changes have an impact on your health, they're completely natural, not a medical illness. It may help to think of menopause as a phase, like puberty: Some of its symptoms can seem strange at first, and it makes you deal with new aspects of your body, but it's a normal part of life.

"Menopause is a natural transition," confirms Margery Gass, MD, consultant at the Center for Specialized Women's Health, Cleveland Clinic.

The reason the ovaries stop putting out massive quantities of estrogen and progesterone is that the hormones are no longer needed for reproductive functions. Progesterone's main purpose is to service the uterus either to stimulate a monthly period or to nurture a growing baby, so if there aren't any more eggs, it's logical for progesterone levels to diminish.

After menopause, estrogen and other sex hormones continue to affect parts of the body that aren't involved with reproduction. That's why the ovaries and adrenal glands continue to produce maintenance levels of sex hormones between 10 and 50 percent of the amounts that were produced in the reproductive years.

Menopause can also be brought on by certain medical conditions, treatments, or surgery. A hysterectomy that removes your uterus, but not your ovaries, usually doesn't cause menopause. Although you no longer have periods, your ovaries still release eggs and produce hormones. An operation that removes your ovaries in addition to your uterus (total hysterectomy and oophorectomy), however, does bring about menopause immediately. Chemotherapy and radiation therapy can also induce menopause. And it may result from a condition called primary ovarian insufficiency, in which ovaries fail to produce normal levels of hormones. This can be caused by genetic factors, autoimmune disease, or unknown factors.

Women can experience a variety of symptoms at menopause, because estrogen is used by many parts of the body, and because our bodies are all different. Some changes are caused in part by aging as well, not just drops in hormone levels. Here's help in sorting it all out.

The Signs

It's over, period. During perimenopause, your periods may have become shorter or longer than usual, and the bleeding may have been heavier or lighter. Now it's been an entire year. They're gone! Imagine what you'll do with the money no longer spent on tampons and pads. And if you do suffer some of the less-than-thrilling symptoms that follow, it helps to remember back to decades of monthly cramps, painkillers, heating pads, surprise spotting, and birth control hassles.

Hot flashes. You've probably experienced some in the years preceding menopause. Thought to be related to fluctuating estrogen levels, these are the sudden feelings of intense heat in the upper part of your body. Your face and neck may become flushed; heavy sweating and the chills can follow. Hot flashes vary greatly from woman to woman. They can be very mild and fleeting, or sudden, drenching, and strong enough to wake you from sleep (night sweats). They can also be accompanied by heart palpitations. Most last between 30 seconds and 10 minutes, and can generally continue a few years beyond menopause. Luckily, inventive creatures that we are, women (and the healing professions) have developed a variety of coping techniques.

Sleep disturbances. It's not uncommon for women to experience troubles getting a good night's sleep during midlife. Some of this is probably related to the menopausal changes you're going through, although experts say that the pressures and stresses we're juggling at this point in life shouldn't be discounted. You may simply find it more difficult to fall or stay asleep. Night sweats are the biggest sleep wreckers for many women.

Vaginal dryness. Changing estrogen levels can cause genital tissues to become drier and thinner, making sexual intercourse uncomfortable. They may also contribute to more frequent vaginal or urinary infections.

Mood swings. Whether you experienced PMS with your monthly cycles in the past or not, you may undergo heightened emotional reactions to everyday ups and downs during menopause. Unfortunately, it's not as easy to acknowledge the hormonal changes responsible when there's no outward reminder (namely, your period) to connect to these strong emotional responses. Research shows that nearly 40 percent of women experience mood swings associated with menopause—from anger to intense moodiness, anxiety, or despair.

Urinary incontinence. Some women experience urine "escapes" during exercise, sneezing, coughing, laughing, or running. But for many women, this kind of leaking can begin earlier than menopause, in large part a result of pregnancies and childbirth. Good news: Simple pelvic floor exercises (Kegels), which can be performed anytime, anywhere, provide significant improvement for many women.

Cognitive glitches. The car keys, that appointment, why you walked into the dining room, even someone's name: Marked forgetfulness can be frightening, but it's also common. Over half of menopausal women report short-term memory loss, difficulty learning new things, and a hard time concentrating. Happily, the effect seems to be temporary. Research shows that you'll return to your usual sharp self.

Waist expansion. Before menopause, many women store fat in their hips and thighs (which is better for pregnancy). Now, the combo of dropped estrogen levels and increase in testosterone causes extra weight to settle into your midsection. The stress of hormonal fluctuations can also cause the body to secrete more cortisol, and high levels of that hormone stimulate the storage of fat around the belly. At the same time, metabolism continues to slow (as it has by about 5 percent per decade), so you're going to need fewer calories to maintain the same weight.

Contrary hair. If you haven't already taken the tweezers to the unwelcome hairs that began appearing on your chin in the last decade as your perimenopausal hormones did the hokey pokey, you will probably need to now. When female estrogen declines and male androgen remains (where it had always been, by the way, during baby-making years), hair can pop up in areas that are androgen-sensitive, like the chin and upper lip. This shift can also have the opposite effect, causing thinning hair in places where you'd rather not lose it, like the top of your head.

Libido dive. Night sweats, sleep loss, and normal hormonal shifts can negatively impact your sex drive. Studies show that for many women, a good sex drive before menopause will return. (Some women even see an increase in desire during this time: New research suggests that social and psychological factors play a bigger part in sex drive than hormonal changes, and that sexual activity during menopause differs greatly between individuals.)

The Real Meno-Perils

Unlike the irksome signs of menopause that grab our attention, several chronic health problems can start at menopause yet remain undetected. The "squeaky wheel" hot flashes, memory hiccups, and AWOL sex drive are hard to ignore, and we can find solace—and coping tips—among our girlfriends of a certain age. But it's the changes we can't see or feel at menopause that are the health equivalent of the Big Bad Wolf . . . except that you can't hear him at the door. These silent threats need to be acknowledged and sent packing (or, at the very least, managed). Now.

Heart disease. When estrogen levels decline, your risk of cardiovascular disease increases. Heart disease is a leading cause of death in woman as well as men, but traditionally has not received as much attention, especially when it is critically needed—at this time of your life.

Osteoporosis. Following menopause, you can lose bone density rapidly, increasing the risk of brittle, weak bones, and the danger of fractures. Postmenopausal women are especially prone to fractures of the hip, wrist, and spine.

Weight gain and body composition change. Many women gain weight at menopause and may also start to carry more excess in their midsection. This, in turn, can increase physical inactivity, high blood pressure, high cholesterol, and diabetes, all risk factors that can lead to heart attack and stroke. Excess weight also plays a role in some cancers, as well as arthritis.

Hormone Therapy: Then and Now

Just a decade ago, Hormone Replacement Therapy (HRT), was considered the best treatment option not only for a variety of relatively harmless yet nasty symptoms that rock the boat of the majority of menopausal women, but also for the serious health threats. HRT was thought to help prevent risks that increase dramatically after menopause, such as heart disease and stroke, cancer, and osteoporosis. And it did offer relief for many women who experienced symptoms that made life difficult, if not downright miserable. But beginning in 2002, findings from large clinical trials showed a very different story—to the shock of many doctors and the millions of women currently using or having been prescribed hormone therapy in the past. Findings emerged from the Women's Health Initiative, a major research program, suggesting that the widely believed protective benefits of HRT were just not there, and worse, that long-term use of hormone therapy could increase some of those serious risks.

Both the estrogen-plus-progestin combination therapy and the estrogen-alone trials of the WHI were halted early because of this evidence of failure to prevent heart disease. And to researchers' further dismay, unexpected threats emerged from the data: The same standard combination estrogen-progesterin therapy appeared to boost risks for strokes, blood clots, and breast cancer. (It was later found that these risks diminished somewhat after stopping therapy.) Combination hormone therapy also seemed to double the risk of dementia and memory loss, other concerns of postmenopausal women, rather than cut risks. It should be noted that one reassuring confirmation of the WHI study was that combination hormone therapy was found effective in reducing risks of colon cancer and bone fractures, as had been believed.

In addition, estrogen-alone therapy (typically prescribed for women who'd had hysterectomies), was also found to increase risks for stroke and deep vein thrombosis and showed no reduction of coronary heart disease risk. It, too, failed to show any benefit against memory loss. (One benefit noted: Estrogen alone did reduce the risk of bone fractures, as did combination therapy.)

In the years since the shocking 2002 WHI data, follow-up analyses have clarified some results and have also created many new questions to be answered.

For example, follow-up research looking at cardio factors suggests that the health consequences of combination hormone therapy may vary by the age of the women involved (younger seems safer) and by the time between menopause and the start of therapy (starting hormone therapy right at menopause rather than 10 years later, for example).

They also found that the increased risk of heart disease from hormone therapy in older women was primarily in those who also had hot flashes and night sweats. Since participants who had those symptoms were also more likely to have risk factors for coronary heart disease, such as high blood pressure or high blood cholesterol, it isn't clear whether those contributed to the higher risks seen during hormone therapy.

The increased risk of stroke seen during the original research was confirmed, however, and did not seem related to age or time since menopause.

And the increased risk of breast cancer observed—even in those women taking combination therapy within 10 years of menopause—was confirmed.

Meanwhile, ongoing studies are being designed and conducted in the hopes of sorting out the future of hormone therapy.

Jacques Rossouw, MD, chief of the WHI Branch at the National Heart, Lung, and Blood Institute, and lead author of "Postmenopausal Hormone Therapy and Risk of Cardiovascular Disease by Age and Years Since Menopause," published in the *Journal of the American Medical Association* in April 2007, noted that these findings may reassure younger women considering hormone therapy for short-term relief of symptoms. But they don't change the current recommendations that hormone therapy should not be used at any age for prevention of cardiovascular disease.

Current Hormone Options

As you might expect, the 2002 WHI findings brought about a dramatic change in treatment practices. The number of women with prescriptions for the higher-dose hormone therapy fell by half between 2001 and 2004. Data showed that trend continuing with a more gradual decline in high-dose prescriptions between 2004 and 2009. During that period, evidence indicated that a lower dose of hormones could treat menopausal symptoms just as effectively as larger doses previously prescribed—with lower risks of breast cancer and cardiovascular disease.

Accordingly, many experts now believe that the lower-dose formulations and skin patches may be a safer way to deliver hormone therapy. The patches, in particular, may reduce the amount of hormones reaching vulnerable organs. However, if you have high cholesterol, high blood pressure or other risk factors for heart disease, many doctors believe you should avoid hormone therapy completely.

Despite this follow-up evidence regarding the relative safety of lower-dose MHT, a recent study by Stanford University School of Medicine found that as of 2009, physicians' practices weren't keeping up with the newest research. It indicated that although the use of lower-dose therapy did increase between 2001 and 2009, it was not nearly enough to suggest that physicians were fully incorporating the new evidence into everyday practice. For example, despite the fact that as many as two-thirds of women with menopausal symptoms find relief with low-dose therapy, researchers found that less than one-third of the women on hormone therapy were prescribed a low dose.

"We're disappointed," said Randall Stafford, MD, PhD, associate professor of medicine at Stanford Prevention Research Center, "because the switch to low-dose therapy was not sizeable." Study authors are unsure why clinical practice has not caught up with research findings. They note that older women who have been satisfied with high-dose hormone therapy for years may not be aware that breast cancer and heart disease risks increase with age—or may be unwilling to change to low doses. Per-

haps their doctors, who've long seen the immediate benefits of higher doses, are also reluctant to change. For women who have had a total hysterectomy (removal of ovaries as well as uterus) low-dose estrogen-only hormone therapy may be an option for easing menopausal symptoms. This carries fewer risks than combination hormone therapy, and should be discussed with your doctor so your entire medical history will be considered.

As research continues regarding various hormone therapies, you and your doctor will have additional evidence to incorporate into your decision process. One example: A recent, large study found that postmenopausal women taking estrogen alone had nearly double the rate of developing asthma compared to women who had never used any form of hormone therapy. And among estrogen-only users, those who had never smoked and those who had had some form of allergy previously were at an even higher risk of developing asthma. This is despite the fact that the incidence of asthma tends to fall after menopause. (Study authors note that previous research has suggested that female hormones may have a role in the development and severity of asthma.) This confirms the importance of remaining up-to-date on current findings, as well as working with your doctor to consider the impact of your menopausal symptoms against the larger picture of your own medical history.

When you discuss your symptoms, risk factors, and medical treatment options (including alternative/complementary therapies), ask about your personal risk-benefit equation. If your doctor agrees that hormone therapy could help, ask about a short-term, low-dose regimen. And as always, don't hesitate to get a second or third opinion.

While important questions remain and additional research is conducted to better identify and understand the health implications of hormone use for menopausal women, experts generally agree on the following guidelines to protect yourself at menopause and beyond:

■ Do not take estrogen alone or with progestin to prevent heart disease.

■ Do not take hormone therapy to prevent memory loss or dementia.

■ Work with your doctor to reduce risks of heart disease and strokes through preventive measures, like lifestyle changes and medications to reduce cholesterol and high blood pressure.

■ Ask your doctor about nonhormonal treatments that are safe and effective in preventing osteoporosis and bone fractures.

■ If you're considering hormone therapy for relief of symptoms such as hot flashes, insomnia, and other annoying symptoms, discuss the impact of short-term, low-dose hormone treatment.

■ Review your health regularly with your doctor: Your risks for heart disease, stroke, osteoporosis, and other conditions may change as you age. Also, new treatments that are safe and effective may become available.

■ Keep your doctor in the loop about any complementary and alternative options you use to ease symptoms.

Your Checkup

It's a fact that your risks of various serious conditions increase in your postmenopausal years. But another thing that comes with age is wisdom—and an appreciation of the importance of your health. Consider menopause your bugle call to grab life by the tail and make the most of it. Pick up the phone and schedule these appointments to take care of yourself. Your doctor will help you determine how often these tests should be performed based on your medical history and test results.

■ Keep abreast. Regular mammograms become even more important for women over 50. Also, continue with your regular breast self-exams and your doctor's yearly clinical breast exams.

■ Check your blood pressure. Do this at least every 2 years—more often if it's elevated.

■ Know your lipoprotein profile. Your blood levels of LDL, HDL, and total cholesterol and triglycerides should be checked at least every 5 years, more often if they are elevated.

■ Test your fasting blood glucose (blood sugar) level. This determines if you have or are likely to develop diabetes. Women who are overweight or have other risk factors for diabetes need blood sugar levels checked more frequently.

■ Get an electrocardiogram. EKGs or ECGs record your heart's electrical activity baseline if you haven't already done so.

■ Monitor your weight—and waist. Know your Body Mass Index (BMI), a measure of your weight relative to your height, and your waist circumference, a measure of your abdominal fat. They're important factors in your overall health and will tell you if you need to lose weight.

■ Measure your bone density. A DEXA scan is an x-ray that determines bone thickness and strength, and will show if you are at risk of or have developed osteoporosis, the bone-thinning disease that can lead to fractures.

■ Continue Pap tests. Done annually when you were menstruating, a Pap test checks for cancerous cervical cells. Ask your doctor how often you need it now (generally every 1 to 3 years after menopause).

■ Get a colonoscopy. This painless exam examines the inside of your colon for cancerous changes. This should be scheduled every 10 years beginning at 50, or more often if previous tests have found problems or if you have a family history of colon cancer.

■ Stop smoking. Good smoking-cessation treatments, including prescription medications, and programs can help you stop lighting up and lower your risks of serious health complications.

Maximum Lifestyle Therapies

Regardless of any decision you make about hormone therapy, there are essential measures that can make you feel and look as good as possible as possibly better than ever before in your life. They also happen to be the same actions proven to protect you against major health threats.

Get Moving

Exercise can help manage many of the uncomfortable symptoms of menopause—as well as its related health risks, such as heart disease, stroke, cancer, and osteoporosis. A 3-year German study of early postmenopausal women found that those who did an hour of aerobic and strength-training exercises 4 days a week had fewer migraines, mood swings, and bouts with insomnia than their sedentary peers. They also maintained bone mass, lost 2 percent body fat and an inch off their waists, and reduced cholesterol by 5 percent. Nonexercisers saw these numbers go up, while losing up to 8 percent of their bone mass. Exercise compensates nicely for declining levels of estrogen, says study author Wolfgang Kemmler, PhD. Both help maintain muscle, bone, and metabolism.

YOUR EXERCISE RX

Aerobic Workouts

In addition to its proven benefits for your heart, lungs, stamina, and weight control, the mood-elevating, tension-relieving effects of aerobic exercise help reduce the depression and anxiety that often accompanies menopause. It also promotes the loss of abdominal fat, the place most women more readily and dangerously gain weight during menopause. In addition, some research studies have shown that the increased estrogen levels that follow a woman's exercise session coincide with an overall decrease in the severity of hot flashes.

Strengthening Exercises

Weight-bearing exercise that stimulates bone, especially of the hips, legs, and spine, to retain minerals that keep them dense and strong, can prevent the onset and progression of osteoporosis. Weight-bearing activities include walking, strength training (with weights, resistance bands), yoga, and many kinds of household work, like gardening.

A Balanced, Consistent Routine

Aim for some moderate activity for at least 30 minutes daily, or at least most days of the week, every week.

New to It? Try Walking

Experts agree: Walking's benefits are stellar. Regular walking has been shown specifically to prevent menopausal weight gain and headaches, and also boosts overall mental and physical well-being. It costs little or nothing, can be done anywhere, anytime, and even promotes social ties.

Donald E. Waite, DO, MPH, professor emeritus of the Department of Family Medicine at Michigan State University in East Lansing, suggests walking in shopping malls if bad weather is an obstacle or if you don't have access to a safe neighborhood or level terrain.

Natural Symptom Relief

As fewer women opt for HRT, the interest in nonhormonal remedies has exploded. Luckily, there are many options, and research has increased in the effort to find safer, more effective ways to ease the menopausal transition from "peri" to "post."

HOT FLASH HELP

Take notes. By keeping a what/where/how diary of your hot stuff moments, you can understand what's triggering them, and that will give you options to reduce the flare-ups. Judi Chervenak, MD, associate clinical professor of gynecology

What Exercise Can Do for You

- Control your weight
- Condition your heart, lungs, muscles, and joints
- Slim your middle
- Fight hot flashes, vaginal, and bladder atrophy
- Boost mental health and memory
- Reduce stress, anxiety, irritability, and depression
- Prevent osteoporosis and fractures
- Promote better sleep
- Improve digestion
- Prevent arthritis
- Prevent the onset of and help manage diabetes
- Improve your balance
- Make you feel sexy

and women's health at Montefiore Medical Center/Albert Einstein College of Medicine in New York City, says that after one of her patients kept a diary, she realized the stress of going to confession at church was giving her hot flashes. "Knowing the cause allowed her to use relaxation breathing before going to church, and that helped her avoid future hot flashes in that situation," explains Dr Chervenak.

Avoid food triggers. Red wine, caffeine, chocolate, and spicy foods such as wasabi and curry dishes can trigger hot flashes in some women. If you find that those foods turn up the heat, you'll probably want to avoid them in the future. Of course, that doesn't mean you have to take them off the menu completely, but you do have to keep in mind that eating them means you're more likely to have a hot flash. "I know that when I have red wine, I'll have a hot flash, but sometimes I really want red wine," notes Dr. Chervenak. If you want to indulge in something that you know will turn up your thermostat, try making it a treat you enjoy only at home, or plan ahead and wear light clothes or a cardigan that you can take off when you're at a restaurant or a party and you feel a hot flash coming on.

Ease stress. The temperature control areas of the brain are located near estrogen receptors, so doctors think that when the fight or flight hormones (epinephrine and norepinephrine) are released during stress, they may trigger the estrogen receptors and cause a hot flash, Dr. Chervenak says. Avoiding stress or learning how to better deal with it—whether that means saying no to some responsibilities, planning to relax on vacation rather than complete projects around the house, or scheduling regular massages—will go a long way in helping you avoid hot flashes. Find out what particular stress relievers work for you. Some swear by yoga, for example.

According to Japanese researchers who studied 15 women, those who indulged in 20-minute massages with aromatherapy twice a week and gave themselves a massage with scented oil 3 times a week suffered from fewer hot flashes and slept better after one month.

Drink it and think it. If you think you're about to have a hot flash, try dampening it by sipping a cold drink. Or imagine a cool mountain, water, rain, air, wind, snow, trees, leaves, or forests whatever image makes you get that Peppermint Patty sensation when you feel an imminent ignition. A new Baylor University study found that hypnotic relaxation therapy works dramatically to relieve hot flashes. "The areas of the brain activated by imagery may be identical to those activated by actual perceived events," explains study author Dr Gary Elkins, professor of psychology and neuroscience at Baylor.

Breathe with your belly. Experts think that deep breathing may offer relief from hot flashes. "Relaxation breathing is invaluable," Dr. Chervenak says, and research supports her. When 33 women who experienced frequent hot flashes were taught belly breathing, muscle relaxation, or a placebo, the women who practiced belly breathing saw a 50 percent drop in the frequency of their hot flashes, while the other women saw no change in the number of hot flashes they experienced.

The key is to breathe abdominally by pushing out your stomach muscles and filling your belly with air as you take a deep breath in through your nose for 5 seconds. Then exhale through your mouth for 5 seconds as you pull in your stomach muscles. Try doing the technique for several minutes a couple of times a day or when you feel a flash coming on.

Stick 'em with acupuncture. The Chinese medicine that involves sticking very thin needles into the skin to rebalance the body's energy seems to lower the frequency of hot flashes among some women. When researchers compared legitimate acupuncture procedures with fake acupuncture procedures, the authentic procedures lowered the intensity of hot flashes that occurred at night by 28 percent. Another study found that acupuncture significantly improved feelings of well-being and quality of sleep while reducing the frequency and severity of hot flashes.

Cool off with soy. Soy contains plant estrogens that seem to even out the estrogen roller coaster that causes hot flashes, says Mary Jane Minkin, MD, clinical professor of obstetrics and gynecology at Yale University School of Medicine and coauthor of *What Every Woman Needs to Know about Menopause*. She recommends getting two servings of soy a day. Try soymilk, tofu, tempeh, or edamame (edible soybeans).

Although many women find relief from eating soy, few studies have found a connection between soy and hot flashes. However, one study by researchers at Johns Hopkins School of Medicine showed promise. Among the 35 women who participated in the study, half received 160 mg of soy isoflavones a day and half received a placebo. After 3 months, those who got the soy supplement had almost a third fewer hot flashes.

Doctors don't recommend aiming for high doses of soy, however. Keep your servings to two a day because of concern that too much soy can increase the risk for breast cancer and hypothyroidism.

Use black cohosh to quell the heat waves. Dr. Minkin recommends taking 20 mg of black cohosh twice a day for menopause symptoms. In a German study of 304 women, half took 40 mg of Remifemin and the other half took a placebo for 12 weeks. The black cohosh worked as well as estrogen therapy in reducing hot flashes and night sweats.

Dr. Minkin recommends buying the German brand Remifemin because herbal products are regulated in Germany but not in the United States. Other supplements that have been studied and found by a watchdog group to have accurate label claims are Jarrow Formulas Black Cohosh, Sundown Naturals Black Cohosh and Swanson Health Products Premium Brand Black Cohosh.

Reset your thermostat with flaxseed. Flaxseed is a phytoestrogen that seems to help relieve hot flashes, Dr. Minkin says. You don't need a lot, just about a tablespoon of ground flaxseed sprinkled onto your cereal, stirred into your yogurt, added to your salad, or baked into bread and muffins will do. Choose ground instead of whole because whole flaxseeds will pass through your body without being digested.

Tamp external temps. Even a small rise in your body's temperature can trigger a hot flash, so dress in light clothes, use a fan or air conditioner, open a window when it's cool outside, or turn down the thermostat at home.

Exercise every day. You won't get rid of hot flashes by moving more, but women who get vigorous activity regularly seem to experience less discomfort than women who don't. Doctors recommend getting at least 30 minutes of exercise a day most days of the week.

Remake the bed. You can find nightgowns and pajamas, even sheets and mattress pads, made from materials that wick away the moisture your body produces at night from hot flashes, preventing you from awakening at night with a soaked nightshirt.

Crush out cigarettes. If you smoke, now is the time to quit. Women who smoke experience more hot flashes, so quitting will help you manage your inner burn while also lowering your risk of heart disease, stroke and cancer.

LACKLUSTER LIBIDO

Midlife is a time for some women when hot and bothered takes on a new definition: the hots aren't fun and you just can't be bothered. More than likely, this didn't happen overnight, and isn't simply a matter of hormones, although changes associated with menopause play an important role. Some experts begin by questioning the term "libido" as a label for women's sex drive, since their sexual desire is more complicated than men's. "Women are much more complex, and to minimize libido to being an on/off switch isn't giving enough validation to woman's symptoms," says Dr. Chervenak. Whatever you call it, diminished sexual interest affects millions of postmenopausal women. Here are some of the causes—as well as solutions.

Menopausal hormone changes. Nearly 40 percent of women report a drop in sexual interest during perimenopause and menopause. In the 2 to 8 years leading up to menopause, your reproductive hormone levels (estrogen and progesterone) begin to drop. But they don't just taper off. They tend to resemble a roller coaster ride, going down, then up, then down again, which can play havoc with your sexual self. Now, at menopause, levels have dropped and left you at the bottom of the ride.

Since estrogen keeps the vagina well lubricated, when your estrogen levels drop, you lose that natural lubrication. Your vaginal walls thin and lose elasticity. In addition, blood supply decreases to the vagina, which makes your vagina drier—so intercourse may become painful. Factor in hot flashes and night sweats causing you to lose sleep, and you're bound to be irritable and moody. "Sleep deprivation is a major factor in decreased sex drive," says Donnica L. Moore, MD, founder of a women's health information Web site called DrDonnica.com and president of Sapphire Women's Health Group, a multimedia health education and communications firm.

Doctors also believe that another natural hormone, testosterone, made by the ovaries and adrenal glands in women, can be key to libido. But at menopause, your testosterone levels have dropped by about 50 percent, and that, along with hormone changes related to menopause, pack a double whammy to your ooh la la.

Partner problems. You're not the only one experiencing hormone-related libido changes. As men age, they lose testosterone, too, which leads to a lower sex drive and problems with erection and ejaculation. If your partner isn't being as amorous, you may lose interest in sex as well. Even if your partner is ready and willing, resentments and arguments over everything from who's doing the dishes to a growing stack of bills may keep you from wanting to jump into bed with him. Or, like many couples, he may not be pleasing you in bed because you haven't been an open communicator about what you want.

Hysterectomy or oophorectomy. Having your uterus surgically removed (hysterectomy) can sometimes reduce blood flow to the vagina and clitoris, making it difficult to become aroused and have an orgasm. Having your ovaries removed (oophorectomy) makes you go into menopause rapidly. Your ovaries are the biggest producer of estrogen, so when they're taken out you'll experience all the side effects of lost estrogen, including vaginal thinning, dryness, and a lack of elasticity. At the same time, oophorectomy causes testosterone levels to fall, which lowers your libido, as well.

Chronic or acute illness. Hormones aren't the only factor in your changing sex drive. The odds of diabetes, hypothyroidism, heart disease, high blood pressure, and depression increase as you age. If your body is dealing with an illness, that takes a toll on sex drive. Getting your blood sugar and blood pressure under control, eating a heart-healthy diet, exercising, and taking medications prescribed by your doctor will help you regain your energy and, with it, your interest.

Body image. Normal menopausal changes may make that woman in the mirror begin to look like a stranger. You may see hair growing in new places, and disappearing—and increasingly graying—in places where it had always been abundant, like on your head. It's not uncommon to gain weight as your metabolism slows, especially around the middle. Tack on the redness (although temporary) of hot flashes on your neck and upper chest, and it may be hard to feel like your old sexy self.

BRING YOUR SEXY BACK

Seek the real problem. A recent study has found that social and psychological issues—not changing hormones—have the biggest influence on women's sexual behavior at menopause. Women's sexual experiences at menopause were found to vary greatly depending on individual differences and what else was going on in their lives. So although much research has shed a negative light on menopause's influence on sexual activity in the past, this study found that some women experienced an increase in their sexual desire at menopause.

Cool it. Hot flashes and sleeping problems are a major factor in low libido. In a study of 341 women ages 45 to 55, researchers noticed that women who had low libido also had night sweats, interrupted sleep, and depression. If you're waking up night after night drenched with sweat, exhaustion and frustration can bump sex from your to-do list. Finding relief from hot flashes can restore your sleep and help you regain your sex life. Now may be the time to try new things in the bedroom like special sweat wicking pajamas and a remote control fan stationed by your side of the bed. (That's one remote your partner may gladly concede.)

Go through the motions. A drop in estrogen causes your vagina to lose elasticity and actually shrink slightly, so sex may be painful. And if it doesn't feel good, you may understandably try to avoid it. But that's exactly what you shouldn't do, says Jennifer Wu, MD, an ob/gyn at Lenox Hill Hospital in New York City. "The worst thing a woman can do is decide sex is painful and put it off for a month to avoid the pain," she says. Having sex regularly–once or twice a week–will help stretch out your vagina and make it pleasurable again.

Move your whole body. Not only will exercise improve your mood, help you burn calories, make you feel good about the way you look, and lower your risk of heart disease, diabetes, and cancer, research has shown that it can also make sex better. In a study of women ages 45 to 55, their fitness levels directly correlated with sexual satisfaction. When you exercise, you also increase blood flow to your vagina, making you feel aroused. Experts recommend getting at least 30 minutes of exercise every day.

Target these muscles. Kegel exercises, typically used to reduce urinary incontinence, can also improve blood flow and elasticity to the vagina and get your pelvic floor muscles in prime shape for heightened orgasms. You do the exercise by pretending you're stopping the flow of urine by squeezing the muscles around your vagina. Contract the muscles for a few seconds and then release, repeating several times a day.

Add juice. If pain from vaginal dryness is putting sex at the bottom of your to-do list, pick up a personal lubricant, such as Astroglide or K-Y Personal Lubricant Jelly, at the drugstore. It will help relieve pain during intercourse. This is such a help that sales of personal lubricants have been rising over the last several years; the average customer is a 52-year-old woman who buys 3 or 4 times a year. Another option: an over-the-counter vaginal moisturizer such as Replens or K-Y Long Lasting Vaginal Moisturizer. These are longer lasting creams that help relieve vaginal dryness, itching, and irritation.

Limit booze. Alcohol may be a social lubricant, meaning it may help you go to bed with your partner more easily than if you hadn't been drinking, but too much alcohol decreases your body's responsiveness and can make it hard to have an orgasm. It's also not a good idea to try to keep up with the number of drinks your partner is having. Even when a man and a woman are the same size, one drink has the same effect on her that two drinks have on him. Another reason to avoid more than two drinks in one evening: It's just not good for your health, period.

Work on your relationship. Your brain is still the most important part of your sex drive, so it's going to be difficult to restart your engine if you're raving mad at your partner on a regular basis. In that case, you need to have an honest talk with him about your relationship. If you need more help, get expert help: Iron out the kinks with a therapist or marriage counselor.

If you and your partner are still love-y but the thrill-y is gone, make your relationship a priority. Give it more attention. Schedule dates. Try something new or different, like salsa dancing, a hike together, or a picnic lunch. Or if you've stopped going somewhere or doing something together that you once loved, bring it back. You may have such a good time that you'll start feeling desire kick back in.

Try something new. It's too easy to get bored always having sex in the missionary position in your bed. Get playful in a new room in your house, the table instead of the bed, in your backyard, or on vacation. Or simply try being more affectionate in public. It may get your juices flowing for later. Don't forget the power of shared massage. Skin-on-skin contact will stimulate your sex hormone oxytocin and increase your sexual desire.

Honor your geography. One of the biggest sex myths is that women are supposed to have an orgasm through intercourse, but the truth is most women don't. Women need stimulation of their clitoris to reach orgasm, and most don't get it through intercourse. If not having an orgasm has made you want to give up sex altogether, stop trying to achieve one through intercourse and start telling your partner what you need to feel satisfied.

Look up. Don't forget that the brain is a vital sexual organ. Even if you're having physical problems that are affecting your sex life, nourishing a positive attitude about sex and your relationship can go a long way.

Check your medicine chest. Some prescription medicines can affect your libido negatively. Antidepressants that fall in the class of selective serotonin reuptake inhibitors (SSRIs) such as Prozac or Zoloft can make it hard for women to have orgasms. They lower dopamine levels in the brain, which makes it harder to become aroused enough to have an orgasm. If this is a problem for you, discuss the possibility of switching to another type of antidepressant with your doctor. Also, blood pressure medications, such as diuretics and beta-blockers, have been found to create sexual problems for men, and experts think women may experience the same side effects.

Diet and Supplements

Eating a healthy, well-balanced diet can help you reduce the discomforts and risks associated with menopause. A diet low in saturated fat and cholesterol, for example, may reduce your risk of heart disease by lowering LDL ("bad") cholesterol and triglycerides (fats in the blood), lowering blood pressure, and helping you maintain a healthy weight. Some evidence suggests that eating soy-based foods such as tofu might help reduce certain symptoms of menopause, including hot flashes.

Adding plenty of calcium and vitamin D to your diet should help you avoid bone loss. High-fiber foods may also help lower your risk of high cholesterol and heart disease. Here are some specific recommendations regarding menopausal well-being.

Calcium. Declining estrogen levels put you at greater risk for osteoporosis, the bone-weakening disease. The National Institutes of Health and the North American Menopause Society (NAMS) recommend that postmenopausal women who do not take hormone ther-

Your Herb Guide

black Cohosh (*Cimicifuga racemosa*). This is traditionally known as the menopause herb. It's been shown to be effective at reducing the severity of hot flashes, memory loss, depression, and mood swings, and to improve the thickness and elasticity of vaginal tissues. Even The American College of Obstetricians and Gynecologists (ACOG) in Washington, DC, agrees that black cohosh may be an alternative for women who choose not to take HRT.

How much to take. Dried root: two 500-mg tablets or capsules. Dry standardized extract: Follow package instructions for each dose equivalent to 1.5 mg of 27-deoxyacteine. Tincture 1:5: 1 teaspoon. Tincture 1:1: 20 drops.

How often. Three times a day.

How long. Take for at least 3 months to determine if it's working for you. It can be taken as long as you need it.

Cautions. Occasionally causes mild digestive complaints when first taken. Do not use black cohosh in combination with HRT. Women with estrogen-dependent cancer, including breast, cervical, uterine, and ovarian, should definitely consult their physician before taking it.

Chasteberry (*Vitex agnus-castus*). Chasteberry is probably better known as an herb for smooth-ing out the hormonal ups and downs of the menstrual cycle and PMS. In Europe, however, it is widely used at menopause.

How much to take. Fruit: two 500-mg tablets. Dry standardized extract: Follow package instructions for each dose equivalent to 250 mg of 4:1 chasteberry extract. Tincture 1:5: 60 drops. Tincture 1:1: 12 drops.

How often. Two times a day

How long. Take the herb for at least 3 months to determine if it's working for you; it can take several months to have the full effect.

Despite taking black cohosh or chasteberry, some women may still have hot flashes, insomnia, mood swings, or even heart palpitations. It's appropriate to take another step, which is to choose an herb that specifically targets a breakthrough symptom. If a specific symptom is bothering you, here are some suggestions that may offer relief.

Sage (for hot flashes). Add common garden-variety sage (the cooking herb) to your program if hot flashes and night sweats persist. It's traditionally used to dry up secretions, including excessive perspiration.

How much to take. As a tea: 1/2 teaspoon of dried leaf in 1 cup of boiling water. Tincture 1:1: 20 drops.

apy get 1,500 mg of elemental calcium per day through diet and supplements to keep bones strong. Your body can only absorb about 500 mg of calcium at one time, however, so if you take more, try to divide it into doses. Foods rich in calcium include low-fat dairy, green leafy vegetables, black strap molasses, almonds, and dried beans. Since it can be difficult to get enough calcium through your diet, you may need to take a supplement. It is important to read the label to see how much elemental calcium a supplement contains (how much

How often. Three times a day.

How long. Sage works right away, so use it as needed.

Valerian (for insomnia). Interrupted sleep patterns are very common at menopause. Some women have a hard time falling asleep, wake up frequently, or have difficulty falling back to sleep once awakened. *Prevention*'s favorite all-purpose herbal sleep remedy is valerian, which has been shown to help you drift into a deep sleep and stay there.

How much to take. Tincture 1:5: 1 teaspoon in water or juice.

How often. A half hour before bed.

How long. Valerian works immediately. It can be used for as long as is required to improve sleep patterns.

Cautions. Do not drive after taking valerian because it causes drowsiness. Valerian should not be used while taking sleep medications or tranquilizers.

Saint-John's-wort (for depression/mood swings). If the blues or mood swings persist, try Saint-John's-wort. It's helpful for treating mild to moderate depression.

How much to take. Dried herb: two 500-mg tablets.

Dry standardized extract. One 300-mg tablet standardized to 0.3 percent hypericin. Tincture 1:5: 1 teaspoon. Tincture 1:1: 20 drops.

How often. Three times a day.

How long. You must use this herb continually for 4 to 8 weeks for it to take effect. It can be used long-term.

Cautions. Do not use Saint-John's-wort with prescription antidepressants. It can cause sensitivity to the sun, so use the strongest sunblock available and reapply it often. If your depression worsens, see your health care provider.

Hawthorn (for heart palpitations). Some women experience fluttering or racing sensations of the heart, or palpitations. Although benign, they can be alarming the first time you experience them. (Check with your health care practitioner to be sure it's nothing more serious.) A classic European women's herb, hawthorn, has been used for centuries. It acts on the nervous system to calm palpitations.

How much to take. Tincture 1:1: 20 drops in water or juice, or follow label directions.

How often. Three times a day.

How long. Hawthorn is safe to use long-term.

Caution. If you're using any kind of cardiac medication, consult your physician before taking hawthorn. ∎

calcium your body can actually use). There are several kinds of calcium supplements. Calcium citrate seems to be more easily absorbed by the body, but it has less elemental calcium than calcium carbonate. Calcium carbonate, however, requires an acid environment to be absorbed, so is best taken with a glass of orange juice. Again, no matter which form of calcium you take, it's better to divide your doses throughout the day so that you are not taking more than 500 mg at a time.

Vitamin D. Your body needs vitamin D to absorb calcium. Levels of vitamin D can decline as you age, so ask your doctor whether you need a supplement. Sources of this vitamin include sunlight, fatty fish, and low-fat dairy fortified with vitamin D. The recommended dietary intake for vitamin D is currently 600 IU per day for women between 19 and 70 years of age and 800 IU for those older than age 70.

Omega-3 fatty acids (fish oil). Omega 3 fatty acids help reduce LDL ("bad") cholesterol and decrease the risk of heart disease. Women who are at greater risk of heart disease after menopause may want to ask their doctor whether they should take a fish oil supplement as well as increase the amount of fish they eat.

More good news: A recent study from the Fred Hutchinson Cancer Research Center in Seattle was the first to demonstrate a link between the use of fish oil supplements and reduced rates of the most common kind of breast cancer. Omega-3 fatty acids also appear to ease hot flashes for some women, and new research indicates that it may ease the types of depression sometimes seen in menopausal women.

Alcohol. If you drink, it's a good idea to assess alcohol's benefit/risk impact on your postmenopausal health and consider how much is enough. Important questions remain unanswered about what role alcohol plays in breast cancer risk, including which women who drink are at greatest risk, and by what means it might trigger breast cancer. Since there is consistent evidence that moderate alcohol consumption may protect against heart disease, another postmenopausal concern, this reinforces the importance of discussing your family history–particularly regarding heart disease and breast cancer–with your doctor. The American Institute for Cancer Research says that if women choose to drink, they should limit their consumption to one alcoholic beverage per day.

"Our data show that women who report having just several drinks a week don't have an increased breast cancer risk, and that the risk begins somewhere between that and two drinks per day," says Dr. Arthur Klatsky, MD, senior consultant in cardiology at the Division of Research at the Kaiser Permanente Medical Center in Oakland, California. "Good research supports the theory that alcohol may increase breast cancer risk via an effect on estrogen, but results are not entirely consistent, and highlight the difficulty in establishing a risk threshold, adds Dr. Klatsky.

Some experts feel that until more is known, for those who have an established risk like a family history of breast cancer, the safest course would be to avoid alcohol.

Herbal Remedies

The use of herbs is a time-honored approach to strengthening the body and treating disease. Herbs, however, can trigger side effects and can interact with other herbs, supplements, or medications. For these reasons, you should take herbs with care, under the supervision of a health care practitioner. Treatments used to relieve menopause symptoms vary in their effectiveness from woman to woman. As with prescription medication taken to relieve menopause symptoms, some women may find relief with complementary therapies while others may not.

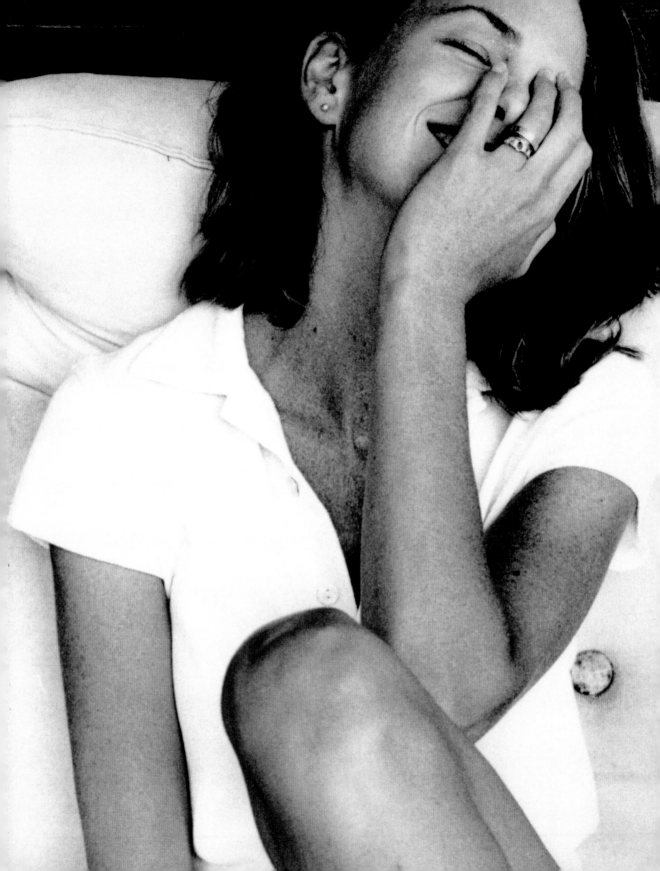

P A R T
F I V E

DOCTORS'

BEST

SYMPTOM

SOLVERS

abdominal fat

How big an issue is belly fat for women? One YouTube video shows a comedy troupe practicing the art of "poo chi," in which the instructor uses her own belly pooch to make a shelf. A ball of dough that rises into a loaf, then into her smiling lips, got almost a million hits and hundreds of appreciative comments. Clearly, it strikes a nerve, if not always a funny bone.

Belly fat is a major issue, and not just because it keeps you out of a bikini or ruins the sleek look of that little black dress. Studies have linked the propensity to accumulate fat around the midsection—which is encouraged by everything from overeating to changing hormones at menopause—to increased risk of heart disease, diabetes, and breast cancer.

But it's not as tough as you might think to slim your waist and protect your health. The good news—you don't need to do a thousand crunches a day. In fact, crunches will only tone the muscles underneath the fat, not make it go away. Leading weight-loss and fitness experts agree that an overall healthy living plan that includes some lifestyle changes along with simple exercises and everyday activities such as walking, gardening, and playing tennis, can lead to a leaner waistline, because they help decrease overall body fat.

"If a woman takes in more calories than she's expending, she will gain weight and store fat in certain areas of her body, such as the abdomen," explains Ellen Glickman, PhD, professor of exercise physiology and coordinator of the exercise science program at Kent State University in Ohio.

"Women are genetically predisposed to store fat in the abdominal area because it's nature's way of protecting the childbearing area of our bodies," she explains. "Extra calories get stored as fat around the abdomen and hips to protect a baby against trauma."

When it comes to abdominal fat, genetics may dictate that women have an uphill climb, but that doesn't mean it's not worth the effort. A firm tummy not only looks great, but keeping weight off your midsection prevents fat inside the abdomen from releasing fatty acids into the liver and sending excessive amounts of cholesterol and insulin into the bloodstream, which contribute to the development of disease.

"Women with large bellies also complain of back pain," says Dr. Glickman. "Back pain is often caused by weak abdominal muscles, so strengthening these muscles helps your back support your body and takes pressure off the back. Where there's less pressure, there's less pain and discomfort."

Here are some strategies to make your belly bulge less noticeable or lose it entirely.

Immediate Solutions
home remedies

Drink up. For premenstrual bloating, drink lots of water. This will help flush away excess fluid, not increase it. Avoid carbonated drinks and those with lots of sugar, which can blow your belly up like a balloon.

Skip the chips. Salt makes you retain water,

especially before your period. Processed and canned foods tend to be high in sodium.

Get some java "to go." If you're feeling overdue for a bathroom session, studies show that a cup or two of coffee can get things moving.

Stand up straight. Imagine a string with one end attached to the top of your head and the other tied to the ceiling. Pretend it's tugging you upright. Your belly will instantly look flatter.

Don't slump. Sitting in a slump accentuates your stomach. To improve your posture, check your chair. If the seat is too high to let your feet touch the floor without making you slump, use a footstool about 4 inches high, or place a pillow at the small of your back to help move you forward in your chair.

Shape up underneath. Body shapers—high-waisted spandex waist slimmers and panties—can take off an inch or more. The more spandex (Lycra) they contain, the more control you'll get.

Wear black. "Wearing black makes women of all shapes and sizes look thinner and taller,"

notes Dr. Glickman. If you're older, black can be harsh on aging skin, so pair dark clothes with lighter accessories such as sweaters and scarves.

Keep your outfits monochromatic. Wear the same color top, skirt or pants, and shoes for an elongating effect.

Choose belly-slimming fabrics. Rayons, silks, knits, and nonclingy matte jerseys generally work best. And pick flat fronts instead of pleated pants, which make you look less bulgy, taller, and better proportioned.

Accessorize. Choose eye-catching earrings and necklaces or colorful scarves. They'll draw attention away from your belly and toward your face.

Long-Term Solutions

home remedies

Aim for at least 30 minutes of exercise most days of the week. To do that, set a specific time to work out, and stick to it. "Women are increasingly taking on more roles, and they

Stay Calm and Trim Your Middle

Stubborn flab called stress fat can pad a woman's midsection when levels of the stress hormone cortisol are high—even if she's thin. When researchers checked how well 59 premenopausal women adapted to laboratory stress tests, they found that those with bigger bellies performed more poorly on the tests—and secreted significantly more cortisol—than those without tummy bulges. In addition, although overweight women with belly fat gradually adapted to stress (their cortisol levels dropped), lean women with bellies didn't (their cortisol levels stayed high).

Researchers suspect that large amounts of cortisol can increase visceral fat, a particularly dangerous type of fat that's associated with increased risk of diabetes and heart disease.

To help balance levels of cortisol, practice this quick stress reducer. Find a quiet, comfortable place to sit. Next, take several slow, deep breaths to help clear your mind. Continue breathing deeply and repeat the word "one" to yourself as you exhale. (If you get distracted, just bring your focus back to the word "one.") Practice this for 5 to 10 minutes once or twice a day. ∎

tend to put themselves last," notes Dr. Glickman. "We put our jobs, children, and house before our own health and wellness. We claim to have less and less time to be physically active and do daily exercise.

"Most women in this country expend a lot of time and effort counting fat grams and calories," she points out. "But what they need to realize is that exercise combined with a reduction in calorie intake is the best way to a flat tummy because you reduce your overall body fat while maintaining lean muscle tissue."

Start at the top. "When you do upper-body weight-lifting or resistance exercises, your lower body, especially the abdomen, will work to stabilize the body," says Dr. Glickman.

Another bonus: Building upper-body muscles, such as those in your arms and shoulders, can make your waistline look smaller. Dr. Glickman recommends starting out slowly, then working your way up to at least 3 sets of 12 repetitions.

Sign up for a few Pilates classes. Dancers have used this series of stretching-type exercises—done on the floor and on special equipment—for decades. Now hundreds of others, including many celebrities, attribute their tight abs to this low-impact form of exercise. Check your local gyms and YMCAs for classes near you.

Give kickboxing a whirl. Aerobic kickboxing is more than just a great fat-burning cardiovascular workout. All those arm thrusts and high kicks firm the abs, too. To learn kickboxing, pick up a videotape from a library or video store. Or contact a local gym, hospital, or community center and ask about classes.

Do a clean sweep. Does the sidewalk or garage need sweeping? Grab a broom (not the push type) and get to it. The back-and-forth motion is a great ab toner. And don't forget the dustpan: Bending over works the abs, too, mostly when you exhale.

(continued on page 326)

WHAT WORKS FOR ME

ELLEN GLICKMAN, PHD, *professor of exercise physiology and coordinator of the exercise science program at Kent State University in Ohio, talks about how she stays in shape.*

"I find sit-ups extremely boring and obnoxious. That's why I refuse to do them. People say, 'Your stomach is so flat.' But I haven't done any sit-ups.

"My approach is to combine an aerobic exercise program with an anaerobic one. For the aerobic workout, I jog 4 miles every day. For the anaerobic exercise, I lift weights 3 times a week, focusing on my upper body. I do lateral pulldowns and a lot of triceps work. The tummy gets flat naturally because while doing the upper-body workout, the abdominal muscles are contracting to stabilize the body, and they become more toned.

"I'm conscious of my calorie intake in the sense that I make a mental note of how many calories I take in each day. I read labels, and I eat basically the same foods, so I've memorized how many calories each food has. For example, I eat bananas all the time, and I know that each one has about 100 calories. I also eat low-fat, high-complex-carbohydrate meals such as pasta dishes or broiled salmon." ■

Shoot for Strength

Strong, flat abs don't just look great. They also improve your posture and protect your back. Try these exercises recommended by *Prevention* to trim and tone your belly. (*Note:* If you experience back pain while doing any of these exercises, stop and check with your doctor before continuing.)

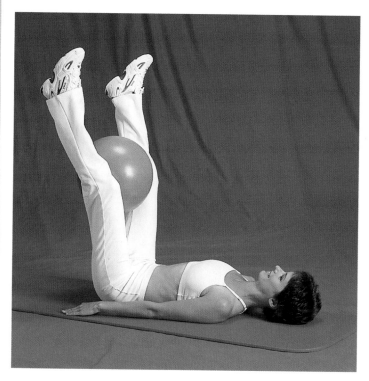

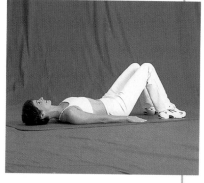

Pelvic Tilt

Lie on the floor with your arms at your sides, knees bent, and feet flat on the floor. Press your lower back to the floor so that your pelvis tilts upward. Straighten your legs by slowly sliding your heels along the floor, and stop when you can no longer hold a full tilt position; hold for a count of six. Next, move one leg at a time back to the starting position, maintaining the pelvic tilt throughout. Hold the starting position for six counts, then relax.

Leg Raise

Lie on the floor and raise your legs straight up. Place an exercise ball between your knees, then do a slight pelvic tilt from the hips. Squeeze the exercise ball for 1 second, then relax.

(continued)

Shoot for
Strength

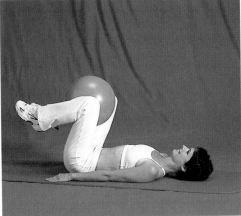

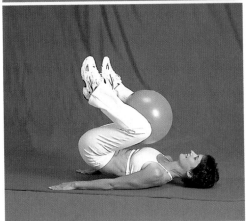

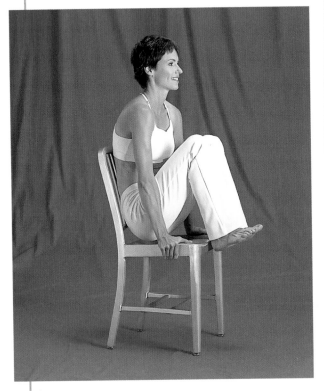

Seated Body Lift

Sit erect in a firm, armless chair and place your hands on the sides of the chair in front of your hips. Tighten your abs and support yourself with your hands as you slowly pull your knees up toward your chest. Keep your lower back against the chair back. Hold and then slowly lower. (This move is performed more easily without shoes.)

Hip Raise

Lie on the floor and place an exercise ball between your bent knees (top). Lift your hips off the floor, and bring your knees toward your chest (bottom). Squeeze the ball for 1 second, then relax.

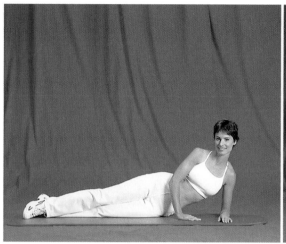 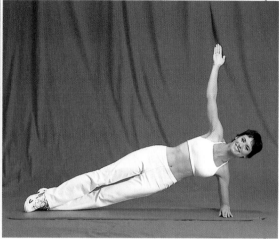

Side Body Lift

Lie on your left side, supporting your upper body on your left elbow, forearm, and hand. Your elbow should be directly under your shoulder (left). Slowly lift the rest of your body off the floor so that only your forearm and feet are on the floor (right). (Use the other arm for balance. For an advanced move, hold that arm straight up in the air.) For maximum effect, keep your body as straight as possible. Hold for as long as is comfortable or until you can no longer maintain good form, then slowly lower and relax. Repeat on the other side.

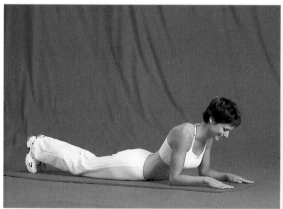 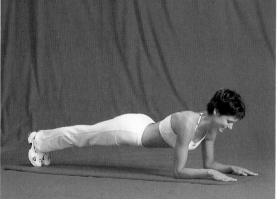

Front Body Lift

Lie facedown on the floor, supporting your upper body on your elbows, forearms, and hands (left). Slowly lift the rest of your body off the floor until you're balanced on your toes (right). Keep your body straight, hold for as long as is comfortable, then slowly lower and relax.

Be Posture Perfect

The following exercises will strengthen your shoulders, chest, and back so you can stand tall and minimize the appearance of your belly.

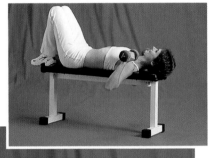

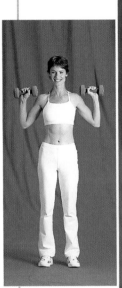

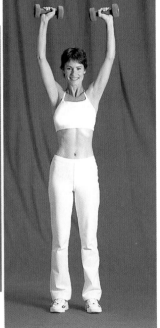

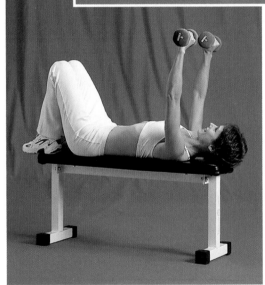

Shoulder Press

To target your shoulder muscles, stand erect with your feet firmly on the floor, holding a dumbbell in each hand at shoulder height, palms facing forward (left). Slowly press both dumbbells straight up until your arms are fully extended (right). Don't arch your back. Hold, then lower the weights.

Bench Press

This exercise works your chest muscles. First, lie on the floor or an exercise bench with your knees bent and your feet flat on the floor or the bench. Hold two dumbbells or a barbell at chest height with your hands slightly more than shoulder-width apart (top). Slowly press the weights straight up until your arms are fully extended and your elbows almost locked (bottom). Hold, then lower the weight.

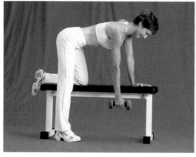

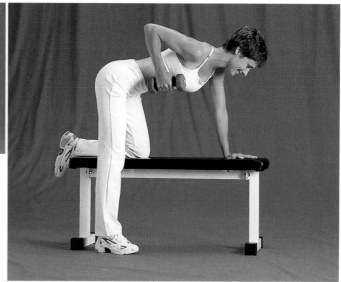

One-Arm Row

This is a great way to strengthen the muscles of your middle and upper back. Put your left knee and left hand on a bench or a chair, keeping your back flat. Hold a weight in your right hand with your right arm straight and the weight hanging toward the floor, parallel to the bench (left). Raise the weight, keeping it close to your body, until it's even with your waist; your elbow should be pointed toward the ceiling (right). (The movement is like starting a power lawn mower, only slower and smoother.) Hold, then slowly lower the weight. Switch sides.

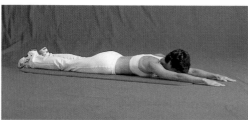

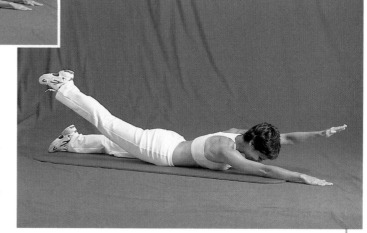

Back Strengthener

Lie facedown with your legs extended straight behind you, toes pointed and arms extended straight over your head. Keep your chin up off the floor at a comfortable level (above). Slowly raise your left arm and your right leg at the same time until they are both a few inches off the floor (right). Hold, then slowly lower them back to the starting position.

Get out and garden. Gardening involves bending, lifting, pulling, pushing, and digging. The spinal twisting and abdominal contractions you do while digging are a particularly good ab workout.

Go for a walk. According to the Nurses' Health Study, women who walked regularly were 16 percent less likely to gain inches at the waist than those who didn't. "Walking is an outstanding exercise for overall weight reduction for women of all body shapes, all ages, and all weight ranges," says Dr. Glickman. "It's the safest form of exercise, with a very low risk of injury. Research shows that it helps to maintain the integrity of bone, which will reduce the chances of developing osteoporosis."

Try tennis. As you play a few sets of backhand and forehand, you'll feel it around your middle. Each time you turn to make a stroke, you strengthen the oblique muscles on either side of your abdomen.

Go for a swim. A vigorous crawl stroke can tighten abs. Since you must breathe in and out forcefully as you swim, your abdominal muscles contract constantly. The reaching forward and pulling back in the butterfly stroke also tones the abs.

Play a few holes. Swinging a golf club shapes up the oblique muscles on the sides of your abs. Playing 9 or 18 holes is a real workout. (For an aerobic workout, skip the cart.)

Don't smoke, and skip the alcohol. Both increase levels of the stress hormone cortisol, which in turn can increase abdominal fat.

Consider yoga. Not only can this exercise help you stretch and sculpt your muscles, it's relaxing, so it can help tamp down your body's production of the stress hormone cortisol, which loads fat on your middle.

Eat more fiber. Not only is fiber great for overall weight loss (it fills you up so you don't eat as much), but it also prevents constipation,

THREE THINGS I TELL EVERY FEMALE PATIENT

ELLEN GLICKMAN, PHD, *professor of exercise physiology and coordinator of the exercise science program at Kent State University in Ohio, offers this special advice for keeping in shape.*

1 DO SOMETHING AEROBIC EVERY DAY. Walking is great because it will help you lose overall body fat, including abdominal fat.

DO SOMETHING ANAEROBIC 3 TIMES A WEEK. Weight lifting is really helpful. "I emphasize upper-body workouts that include lat-

eral pulldowns and triceps pullbacks because they not only help flatten the tummy; they also strengthen the part of the body that's used a lot," says Dr. Glickman. "As we get older, **2** the activities that we're engaged in most often—such as getting out of a bathtub, getting off the commode, getting out of a car—rely on upper-body strength."

ENJOY WHAT YOU'RE DOING. If you do, you'll be more likely to stick to your exercise program. ■ **3**

which can cause a tummy bulge. To stay regular, aim for 20 to 35 grams of fiber a day by eating more whole grains, fruits, and vegetables, or try a fiber supplement such as Metamucil.

Have a MUFA. Monounsaturated fats—the kinds in nuts, seeds, olives, oils, avocado, and dark chocolate, as part of a healthy Mediterranean-style diet recommended by *Prevention*, has been shown to help reduce belly fat. The study, done at the Yale-Griffin Prevention Research Center and commissioned by *Prevention* magazine, found that women who followed this eating plan for 28 days lost an average of 8.4 pounds, but even more important, sheared 2 inches off their waists and reduced belly fat by 33 percent, as measured by a cross-sectional MRI. They also saw their cholesterol drop by an average of 21 points and their fasting insulin decline—bringing home the fact that belly fat is more than just a cosmetic issue.

"This diet study is exceptional because few have used MRI to look at the effects of a particular diet on abdominal fat," says David L. Katz, MD, director of the Yale-Griffin Prevention Research Center. "It shows the plan not only significantly reduces visceral fat but also lowers cholesterol, blood pressure, inflammation, and insulin resistance."

Stop smoking. Though many smokers claim that cigarettes keep them thin, the truth is that smokers have more belly fat than nonsmokers. See Chapter 8 for ways to quit.

anemia

Every time you take a breath, oxygen is picked up by hemoglobin, an iron-rich protein in red blood cells, and carried to tissues throughout the body. Without enough hemoglobin or red blood cells, your cells and tissues can't get all the oxygen they need. This condition, called anemia, can result in weakness, fatigue, headaches, heart palpitations, difficulty concentrating, and other symptoms.

Anemia rarely causes serious health problems for women, but doctors take it seriously because something is causing hemoglobin or red blood cells to decline. There are about 400 different kinds of anemia, most of them uncommon. Heavy menstrual bleeding or a deficiency of iron in the diet is often to blame. There could also be internal bleeding—resulting from ulcers, for example, or some forms of cancer, says Barbara Goff, MD, associate professor of obstetrics and gynecology at the University of Washington School of Medicine in Seattle. Even hemorrhoids can result in anemia if they bleed profusely.

Vegetarians sometimes get anemia because the iron in plant foods isn't as easy for the body to absorb as the iron found in meats. Pregnancy also affects iron levels, which is why women are often advised to take iron-containing prenatal supplements when they're expecting.

Most cases of anemia are caused by insufficient iron in the diet, but a deficiency of vitamin

B_{12} also can result in a decrease in red blood cells that may lead to anemia. This nutrient is found only in animal foods, so strict vegetarians and vegans may not get enough. Pernicious anemia, which often affects elderly adults, is caused by the lack of a stomach protein that's needed to transport vitamin B_{12} from the stomach to the small intestine, and the inability to produce the stomach protein leads to inadequate absorption of vitamin B_{12}. People with disorders such as celiac disease (an inability to process gluten in foods) and inflammatory bowel diseases, such as Crohn's disease, have malabsorption problems that may make it difficult for them to absorb iron from foods. If you exercise intensely–you jog or cycle, particularly competitively–you may also run the risk of iron depletion that can lead to anemia.

Anemia always needs to be checked out by a doctor–but once you have the green light from your doctor, there are a variety of home-care options that can offer effective treatment.

For Immediate Relief

home remedies

Increase your iron intake. The Institute of Medicine recently revised the guidelines for iron intake. Women between the ages of 19 and 50 are advised to get 18 mg of iron daily; during pregnancy, your doctor will increase the amount to 27 mg. Women 51 years and older need only about 8 mg of iron daily.

Eat lean red meats. They help prevent–or reverse–anemia in two ways: They're rich in dietary iron, and the form of iron they contain, called heme iron, is easy for the body to absorb.

Enjoy iron-rich greens. Spinach, chard, turnip greens, and spirulina (seaweed) are good sources of iron. The one problem with these foods is that they contain a type of iron called nonheme iron, which is somewhat harder for the body to absorb than the heme iron found in meats.

Put beans on the menu. Pintos, navy beans, and lentils are good sources of iron. Half a cup of navy beans, for example, provides about 2.3 mg of iron; $\frac{1}{2}$ cup of lentils provides about 3.3 mg.

when to see a doctor

If you have heavy menstrual periods and you're also suffering from constant fatigue, see your doctor right away. The odds are very good that you have iron deficiency anemia, says Scott A. Fields, MD, vice chairman of family medicine at Oregon Health Sciences University in Portland. You'll probably need to get extra iron in your diet, and your doctor will want to ensure that the bleeding is normal and that there isn't an underlying problem.

If your energy is low and you're a strict vegetarian. You could have low levels of vitamin B_{12}, which is found only in animal foods. If you avoid eggs and dairy foods as well as meats, you may need to take B_{12} supplements. The Daily Value is 6 micrograms.

If your stools appear black or tarry. Bleeding from the gastrointestinal tract is a common cause of anemia, and it always needs to be investigated by a physician.

Drink orange juice with meals. Or finish off your meals with a few slices of orange or grapefruit. Citrus fruits are very high in vitamin C, which enhances iron absorption. This is especially important when you're eating plant foods that contain difficult-to-absorb nonheme iron.

Save the tea and coffee for later. Tannins in tea and coffee reduce the body's absorption of iron. It's fine to enjoy these beverages as long as you have them a few hours after meals. Red wine also has iron-blocking tannins. However, these foods are usually not a problem for those who get plenty of iron in their diets.

Take advantage of breakfast cereals. If you find that you're eating less meat in order to reduce the amount of fat in your diet, you'll have to make an effort to find other sources of iron in the diet. Fortified breakfast cereals, which contain added iron, are good choices. A cup of regular instant oats, for example, provides only about 1.6 mg of iron. A cup of fortified oats, on the other hand, may provide more than 8 mg.

Take multi supplements. Multi supplements will help your body keep pace with the normal iron losses that take place during menstruation, according to *Prevention*. Premenopausal women should take a multi containing 100 percent of the Daily Value of iron. Most over-50 vitamins don't contain iron because of the potential for increased risk of heart attack from iron excess.

THREE THINGS I TELL EVERY FEMALE PATIENT

SCOTT A. FIELDS, MD, *is vice chairman of family medicine at Oregon Health Sciences University in Portland. He sees a lot of women who suffer from anemia, and he always offers this advice.*

DON'T TREAT IT ON YOUR OWN. Many women know the signs of anemia, such as fatigue around their menstrual periods, and they assume that getting extra iron is all they need to do. Iron will certainly improve your levels of red blood cells, but it won't correct the underlying problem, says Dr. Fields. It's essential that you see your doctor, who will run laboratory tests to determine what's causing your symptoms.

TELL YOUR DOCTOR IF IRON SUPPLEMENTS ARE CAUSING SIDE EFFECTS. Many women with anemia quit taking iron supplements because they can't handle the diarrhea, nausea, or other disagreeable digestive symptoms that sometimes occur when taking them. "We may try different types of supplements that you'll be able to digest more easily," says Dr. Fields. "Or we might be able to manage your symptoms with dietary management."

BE PATIENT. "It usually takes weeks or months for supplemental iron—either from foods or supplements—to correct anemia," says Dr. Fields. "In the meantime, rest when you feel tired and take comfort in the fact that we've found an explanation for your symptoms." ■

Don't take iron supplements without checking with your doctor first.

Ask your doctor about the Pill. Some women lose so much blood during menstruation that they're almost always anemic. Your doctor may recommend that you go on the Pill. It will normalize your periods and help prevent excessive blood loss, says Dr. Goff.

Report strange cravings. It doesn't happen very often, but women will sometimes develop powerful, nearly overwhelming cravings for unsavory substances, such as dirt, clay, laundry starch, or even cigarette ashes. This condition, known as pica, is often a sign of iron deficiency anemia.

Doctors aren't sure if iron deficiency causes pica or if pica causes iron deficiency anemia because women eat so much of the nonnutritious substances that they don't get enough wholesome foods in the diet.

In either case, be sure to report unusual cravings to your doctor. If you're suffering from pica, taking supplemental iron will often cause the cravings to disappear, sometimes in as little as 24 hours.

Check out restless legs. If you're awakened at night by a strong urge to move your legs, you may have Restless Leg Syndrome or you could have iron-deficiency anemia. Have your doctor check your iron levels before putting you on medicine for restless legs.

arthritis

Arthritis, an autoimmune disease that can cause pain and disfigurement, used to be considered a disease of old age, but we now know it can happen to people of all ages. Even children can get rheumatoid arthritis. Although osteoarthritis—the wear-and-tear version caused by using your joints in the course of daily living—increases with age, if you've led an active life, those pings and twinges and shooting pains you're experiencing are probably arthritis, even if you're on the sunny side of 50.

An estimated 50 million Americans have some form of arthritis, according to the Centers for Disease Control and Prevention, and it is the most common cause of disability in the United States. The CDC predicts that by 2030, that number will rise to 67 million, owing in part to the epidemic of obesity in the United States (overweight is a leading cause of the disease).

The term arthritis (literally, "joint inflammation") refers to a group of more than 100 diseases and conditions that can cause pain, stiffness, and swelling in the joints. If not diagnosed and treated, arthritis can cause irreversible joint damage. With treatment, however, women with arthritis can minimize the discomfort and avoid permanent damage.

Osteoarthritis is far and away the most common form of the disease. The pressure of gravity and the wear and tear of everyday life cause some kinds of osteoarthritis, which was once called degenerative joint disease. Genetic predisposition also plays a role. The resulting damage to the joints and surrounding tissues leads to pain, tenderness, swelling, and disability.

Osteoarthritis primarily affects the cartilage, the slippery tissue that covers the ends of both bones in a joint. Healthy cartilage is thick enough to let the bones glide smoothly over each other and absorb energy from the shock of physical movement. In osteoarthritis, the cartilage breaks down, wears away, and becomes thin, so the bones rub together and cause pain, swelling, and stiffness. Over time, the joint can lose its normal shape. Small, bony growths called bone spurs can form on the edges of the joint, and bits of cartilage can break off and float inside the joint space, causing more pain and damage.

In its early stages, osteoarthritis may cause swelling, but its onset is subtle and gradual, usually involving only one or two joints, such as the knee, hip, and hand. Pain is the earliest symptom.

For Women, Osteoarthritis Is Most Common

Osteoarthritis affects more than 27 million people, says the CDC. It is the most common type of arthritis to affect women, mostly after age 45. The risk increases with age, especially if there's a family history of the disease.

"Often a woman's mother, grandmother, or aunt had osteoarthritis," says Jeffrey R. Lisse, MD, medical director of the Osteoporosis Program and chief of adult rheumatology at the

when to see a doctor

If you have severe pain or disability that interferes with normal activities, contact your physician right away. Many remedies take at least 8 weeks to start working, so it's best to get an early, accurate diagnosis.

Arizona Arthritis Center, and professor of medicine at the University of Arizona College of Medicine in Tucson. "We now know that there's a genetic component to it. It tends to run in families."

A woman in her fifties, for example, can begin to feel pain and stiffness in her knee, then recall a sports injury or accident when she was a young adult. Being overweight can also cause damage. Obese adults tend to wear out their joints more quickly than do those at a healthy weight.

Fortunately, having arthritis doesn't have to mean the beginning of the end of playing golf, cooking gourmet meals from scratch, or doing anything else you love. Here's how you can ease the pain if you already have arthritis, and possibly lower your risk of developing it if you don't.

For Immediate Relief

home remedies

Broil a salmon for dinner. The omega-3 fatty acids in fish oil may ease arthritis pain by providing anti-inflammatory building blocks. "Fish oil has a mild anti-inflammatory effect by decreasing prostaglandins, which cause inflammation," says Dr. Lisse. Good food sources of omega-3s include salmon, tuna, sardines, and

(continued on page 336)

Warm Up to Water Walking

When you have arthritis, warm-water exercise can encourage stiff joints to become more flexible and can relax tight muscles. The buoyancy of the water supports the joints.

A warm-up is essential to prevent pain and injury for all exercisers, but especially for people with arthritis. *Prevention* recommends starting with the following set of full-body range-of-motion exercises, done in a pool to increase flexibility. Do these before and after the water-walking routine described on page 335.

The warm-up: Walk into the water to chest height. (The body part you're working on should be underwater. You'll need to go deeper or crouch down to get your shoulders underwater when doing the first exercise.) Do all of these moves slowly, and never stretch to the point of pain or discomfort. Do at least 3 repetitions of each, but depending on your individual needs and condition, you can do as many as 10 reps of any move to help loosen a stiff joint. Repeat the entire set of exercises to cool down after your water-walking workout.

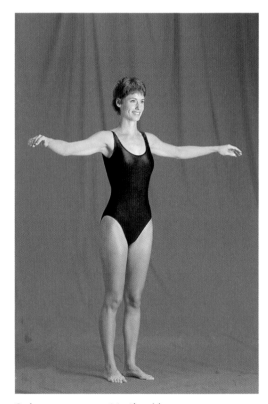

Swing your arms out to the sides.

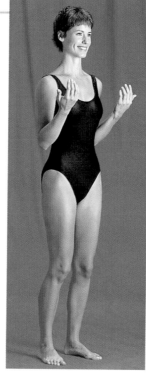

Bend your elbows.

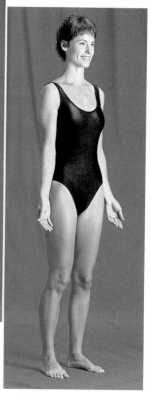

Straighten your elbows.

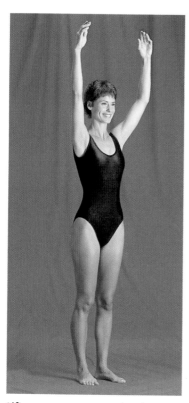

Lift your arms over your head.

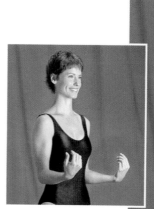

Bend your wrists.

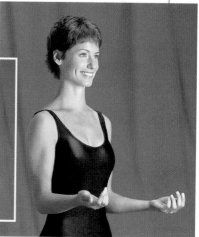

Straighten your wrists.

(continued)

Warm Up to
Water Walking

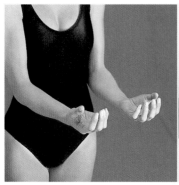

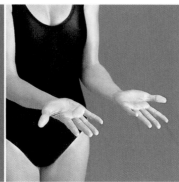

Hold each hand in a loose fist
with fingers bent.

Straighten your fingers.

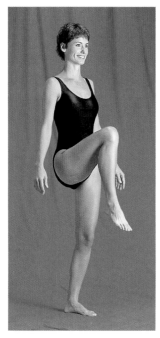

Take high steps, lifting your
raised knee toward your chest.

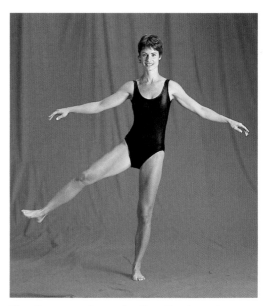

Standing on one leg, swing the other leg out
to the side; then switch sides.

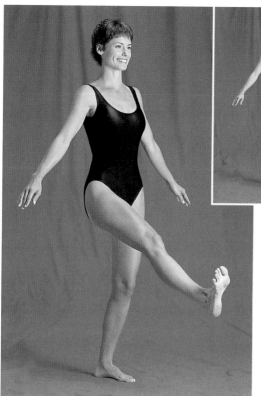

Flex each ankle.

Extend each ankle.

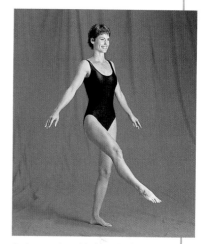

Swing each ankle in a circle.

The exercise: After completing the warm-up routine, you're ready to exercise. Standing in water that's between hip and waist deep, start walking and swinging your arms. Start slowly, then pick up speed and work up to a comfortable, brisk pace. Start with 5 minutes, then gradually increase the time until you feel it could be rated as moderate, which the Arthritis Foundation describes as anywhere from "still light but starting to work" or "still comfortable but harder" to "getting to be somewhat hard." Do the workout 3 to 5 times a week. For more information, check at a YMCA for water-walking classes designed for people with arthritis.

mackerel. *Prevention* suggests eating a 3-ounce serving of fish 2 or 3 times a week. Fish oil is also available in supplements. Three grams, or 3,000 mg, a day of EPA and DHA (omega-3 fatty acids found in fish oil) is the suggested dose. You can get rid of the fishy taste by storing the bottle of capsules in the freezer or choosing a brand with an enteric coating, which prevents them from being digested until they reach your small intestine.

Eat your vegetables. Research has shown that people with high intakes of vitamin C and beta-carotene had a reduced risk of knee pain and disease progression. To be sure that you get enough of these nutrients (as well as other plant-based protective compounds, such as lutein and lycopene), eat lots of carrots, sweet potatoes, broccoli, spinach, tomato sauce and tomato juice, oranges, kiwifruit, and strawberries. The fiber and phytochemicals in vegetables may also contribute to less inflammation. Studies have found that high intakes of veggies and fruit reduce levels of C-reactive protein (a marker of inflammation) in the blood, in some cases by as much as a third. Inflammation not only causes arthritis pain but is implicated in heart disease and some forms of cancer too.

Walk away pain. "Walking is great exercise for women with arthritis because it helps keep muscles warm and flexible, which eases pain," says Dr. Lisse. "Start slowly, then build up to walk-

THREE THINGS I TELL EVERY FEMALE PATIENT

JEFFREY R. LISSE, MD, *medical director of the osteoporosis program and medical director of the Osteoporosis Program and chief of adult rheumatology at the Arizona Arthritis Center in Tucson, offers this special advice.*

USE A CREAM. "I have some luck with capsaicin cream with my patients," says Dr. Lisse. Capsaicin is a substance found in hot peppers, and in this topical analgesic cream, it acts on nerve endings to ease arthritis pain. The cream doesn't work instantly, so repeated applications are key. It produces a burning feeling when you first apply it, but this side effect diminishes over time. Follow label directions carefully, and thoroughly wash your hands after each application to avoid stinging if you accidentally contact your eyes or other sensitive areas later. Capsaicin cream is available at drugstores.

EXERCISE. "It's important to exercise daily to keep the joints and muscles flexible and moving. If you stay physically active, you'll see an improvement in symptoms."

KEEP YOUR WEIGHT DOWN. "Obese women have more problems with arthritis because extra weight puts pressure on the joints. Keeping weight within the normal range may lower the risk of developing osteoarthritis," says Dr. Lisse. "For the woman who already has arthritis, keeping her weight in check will reduce the pressure, which eases pain. If you're overweight and can't lose on your own, talk to your doctor. He can put you in touch with a dietitian who can design a weight-loss program tailored to your tastes and needs." ■

ing for at least 30 minutes 3 to 5 days a week."

Concerned that you might do more harm than good? In several studies involving people with osteoarthritis of the knee, none has shown any harm from 30 to 45 minutes of moderately brisk walking on a good walking surface while wearing well-designed shoes. If walking does cause pain, try walking more slowly, or use some type of shoe insert or orthotic. Take a good look at your walking shoes: It may be time for a new pair. If the pain continues, stop the brisk walking and contact your physician.

Adjust your surroundings. Some advice from the experts at *Arthritis Today*: Arrange your work area so you're about 20 to 26 inches from your computer, the top of which should be even with the top of your head so you're not giving yourself a pain in the neck. Use a document holder positioned at eye level and a hands-free telephone headset to reduce neck strain. Keep your arms at your sides, elbows at right angles, and wrists relaxed, preferably on a wrist wrest, while you type.

Have some pepper. Capsaicin, the chemical that makes hot peppers hot, can be applied topically as a counterirritant to reduce arthritis pain. Don't do it yourself, though; capsaicin creams are available in every drug store. Alternatively, use a salicylate-based cream.

Long-Term Solutions

home remedies

Apply heat. "For chronic arthritis pain, place a heating pad on the painful site for 10 to 15 minutes 3 times a day," says Dr. Lisse. "Heat can be very soothing for sore, stiff muscles and joints. It relaxes them so they move more freely."

Try SAM-e. There's evidence that this chemical, which occurs naturally in the body, can reduce inflammation and pain in osteoarthritis. It may do so by boosting levels of an amino acid, adenosine triphosphate (ATP), and supporting cartilage production. The Arthritis Foundation recommends 600 mg to 1,200 mg daily for osteoarthritis.

Consider glucosamine and chondroitin. Early studies that found this combination of natural chemicals could reduce joint deterioration and pain in arthritis have not been borne out in subsequent research, except for a subgroup of people with arthritis. In 2010, researchers with the National Institutes of Health Glucosamine/Chondroitin Arthritis Intervention Trial (GAIT) reported that among more than 1500 people with knee arthritis, the supplements were more effective combined than taken singly. However, they worked no better than a placebo or a prescription arthritis drug (celecoxib) in people with mild pain. But people with moderate to severe pain did have significant pain relief, even more than with the prescription drug. Dosages used in the trial were 1,500 mg of glucosamine and 1,200 mg of chondroitin.

medical options

Talk to your doctor about drugs. You have many choices. Frontline drugs for osteoarthritis are often NSAIDS—nonsteroidal anti-inflammatory medications that include aspirin, ibuprofen, and COX-2 inhibitors. They all carry a risk of side effects, most notably, gastrointestinal bleeding and stomach upset. COX-2 inhibitors such as celecoxib appear to be safer for the stomach, but they also haven't been on the market as long as the other two. Also available is a nonacetylated salicylate–basically an aspirin developed to have fewer side effects–that will ease your pain but not protect you from stroke as regular aspirin does. Your doctor may recommend acetaminophen, which will give you pain relief but not reduce inflammation. If you have severe pain that isn't relieved by any of these medications, your doctor may talk to you about pain relievers that contain opioids, such as codeine or hydrocodone, that come in pill form and patches. Warning: These drugs can become habit forming.

For more information. Contact the Arthritis Foundation at 1330 West Peachtree Street, Atlanta, GA 30309, 800-283-7800, or visit them online at www.arthritis.org; or the National Institute of Arthritis and Musculoskeletal and Skin Diseases at 1 AMS Circle, Bethesda, MD 20892-2350, or at www.nih.gov/niams.

asthma

Contrary to what many people may believe, feeling rotten doesn't have to be part of living with asthma.

"The American Lung Association did a study of 1,300 families and found that people with asthma think that waking up in the middle of the night with symptoms, getting out of breath, not participating in sports, and going to the ER and being hospitalized are absolutely normal. But this is not normal," says Linda B. Ford, MD, past president of the American Lung Association and an allergist in Papillion, Nebraska. People with asthma who find themselves having "events" or curtailing their normal activities need to be more aggressive about getting the appropriate treatment, she says.

For one thing, studies have shown that allergy shots, or immunotherapy, may prevent asthma, and regular injections can also help after you've been diagnosed.

For others, a host of medications–either inhaled or taken in pill form, or a combination–can keep asthma under control. "With proper diagnosis, treatment, education, and close monitoring, the vast majority of people with asthma can lead normal lives," says William Berger, MD, clinical professor in the division of allergy and immunology at the University of California Irvine and author of *Allergies and Asthma for Dummies.* "The key is to take control of the disease and not let it control you."

Asthma causes what doctors call twitchy lungs, which overreact to stimuli that are harmless to many people. Anxiety, animal dander, dust mites, and even your monthly menstrual cycle can trigger asthma episodes or worsen existing symptoms. When asthma flares, the muscles around your bronchial tubes squeeze tightly, causing the airways to narrow. Then the inflamed bronchial tubes swell even more and produce thick mucus.

Although the exact cause is not known, if you have episodes of wheezing and coughing, you probably inherited the propensity to have asthma from a parent. Then, with repeated exposures to your environment, sensitivity develops and symptoms begin. Doctors also know that childhood allergies increase the risk of developing asthma and that children of women who smoked during pregnancy are also more likely have it. "One study showed that 50 percent of babies delivered to mothers who smoked went on to develop asthma. That increased risk was only from the exposure the baby received in utero," says Dr. Ford.

Here are some strategies that can help you calm your twitchy lungs and breathe easier.

For Immediate Relief

home remedies

Know the signals. Most asthma attacks start slowly, and you can often stop an episode in its tracks by using medication. Anyone with asthma should learn the warning signs, which include wheezing, faster than normal breathing, an itchy or sore throat, tightness in your chest, shortness of breath, coughing, or a drop in your peak flow rate, measured by a device called a peak flow meter. When you blow into this device, a mechanism that moves a small pointer along a scale measures how well your lungs are able to expel air, which is called the peak flow rate. At the first sign of an attack, the best advice for most people is to take their medication and rest.

Relax and breathe. During a mild attack, "sit down and take a few sips of a warm beverage," Dr. Ford advises. Concentrate on breathing slowly. If those steps don't work, use your reliever inhaler. You and your doctor should have previously decided on an "asthma action plan" for attacks, so follow it now. "If you don't have one, ask your doctor for one." The asthma action plan should include self-assessment either with peak flow monitoring or symptom monitoring and self-management prescribed by your doctor, which should include what to do if you have acute asthma symptoms and when to call the doctor or 911.

Long-Term Solutions

medical options

Have an allergy test. To change your asthma, you must change your environment. "In asthma, prevention and avoidance is really the key," says Monica Kraft, MD, director of the Duke Asthma, Allergy and Airway Center at Duke University in North Carolina.

"One of the worst mistakes that people make is not finding out what their triggers are, so they arbitrarily get rid of the cat, or whatever. The answer is to be tested for allergies," adds Ira M. Finegold, MD, chief of the division of allergy and immunology at St. Luke's-Roosevelt Hospital Center in New York City.

home remedies

Reduce your exposure. Know your asthma triggers and avoid them. If you discover that you are allergic to your cat, for example, and you can't bear to get rid of the animal, keep her outdoors or in the basement. At the very least, keep her out of your bedroom. To reduce dander, wash your pet at least 2 or 3 times a month with a shampoo recommended by your veterinarian. Stirring up those colorful leaves during autumn raking can expose you to *Alternaria alternata*, one of the most common autumn molds in the United States, and put you at risk for severe asthma attacks and allergic reactions. If you must rake, take your medication first. Better yet, have a relative or friend take over the chore or hire someone to do it. Avoid leaf blowers—even those used by lawn-care companies—because they spit mold into the air at full force. Chlorine and pool chemicals at the gym or swim club may foil your attempts to exercise by triggering an episode.

Check the medicine cabinet. Some medicines—such as the beta-blockers propranolol (Inderal) and metoprolol (Lopressor) used to treat heart disease, high blood pressure, and migraines—can worsen asthma.

In addition, 10 to 20 percent of all people who experience asthma are sensitive to common over-the-counter painkillers such as aspirin and ibuprofen, and acetaminophen can also trigger asthma attacks. Make doubly sure that any doctor who prescribes medication for you knows that you have asthma.

Lose weight. In a study involving more than 67,000 middle-aged women, those who had the highest BMI (Body Mass Index) had double the risk of developing asthma as those with the least. In another study confirming this finding, the

THREE THINGS I TELL EVERY FEMALE PATIENT

RAN ANBAR, MD, *professor of pediatrics and director of pediatric pulmonary medicine at the State University of New York Upstate Medical Center in Syracuse, offers this special advice.*

TAKE YOUR MIND TO A RELAXING PLACE. Imagine yourself somewhere that's delightful, peaceful, and especially meaningful to you, such as a quiet beach. Do you smell the fresh ocean spray? Can you hear the roar of the surf as it crashes against the sand and feel the warm water on your skin? "The more senses you imagine using, the more relaxing it is," Dr. Anbar says.

CREATE A HYPNOTIC SUGGESTION. Each time you mentally travel to your special spot, touch one thumb with the forefinger of the same hand. Remind yourself that whenever you touch your fingers in this way, you'll be able to relax and breathe more easily. You can use this suggestion as you use your rescue medicine, or try using self-hypnosis first, then see if you still need to use your medication, Dr. Anbar says. "The average adult needs more practice than the average kid. Kids are incredibly imaginative."

FIND A PRO. Dr. Anbar recommends that beginners work with a hypnotist certified by the American Society of Clinical Hypnosis, a professional group that requires significant training for certification. ■

researchers reported that weight did not appear to up a man's risk. They speculated that obesity-related asthma may be generated by a release of excess estrogen in women's fat cells.

Breathe easy with a cup of joe. According to one large study, men and women with asthma who drank 2 to 3 cups of coffee each day reported 25 percent fewer attacks than those who didn't go for java. Caffeine, a chemical cousin of the antiasthma drug theophylline, relaxes the smooth muscles of the bronchial tubes and keeps airways open.

Exercise later in the day. Researchers at the Long Island Jewish Medical Center, following almost 5,000 people over 5 years, found that the lungs are 20 percent more powerful at 5 p.m. than they are at noon. If you have exercise-induced asthma, always keep your quick-relief medications (such as an albuterol inhaler) on hand in case you have an attack.

Become a no-smoking zone. Smoke—even from a fireplace—can irritate your lungs. If you smoke, quit, then encourage those around you to quit. If you live with a smoker, insist that he smoke outside to avoid triggering an asthma attack. While you're at it, avoid sources of perfumes, cleaning fluids, candles, and other airway irritants.

Use your peak flow meter. This simple tube-like device measures the amount of air you can blow out. You should check it in the morning, at night, and after you use your short-acting inhaler such as albuterol (Proventil), metaproterenol (Ventolin), or pirbuterol (Maxair). "National guidelines on asthma recommend that if your airflow falls below 80 percent of your peak flow, you may need to take an additional dose of a short-acting inhaler and call your doctor," says Sally Wenzel, MD, professor of medicine in pulmonary, allergy and critical care medicine and director of the asthma and allergic disease programs at the University of Pittsburgh. Airflow below 50 percent of your peak flow may necessitate a trip to the ER.

mind-body techniques

Help yourself with hypnosis. People with asthma and others with chronic diseases can calm their symptoms with self-hypnosis, says Ran Anbar, MD, associate professor of pediatrics and director of pediatric pulmonary medicine at the State University of New York Upstate Medical University in Syracuse.

In a study done by Dr. Anbar and his colleagues, 82 percent of patients taught self-hypnosis techniques reported improvement or resolution of a variety of symptoms, including asthma, anxiety (an asthma trigger), chest pain, shortness of breath, and hyperventilation. One young girl with severe asthma was able to wean herself off rescue medicine, which she had been using 5 times a day, and dramatically cut back on the oral steroid medications she had been taking for 8 years.

"I want patients to know they have the power themselves, and they can tap into it," he says.

medical options

Take care of monthly problems. Some women notice that their asthma worsens just before and during their periods.

"Check your peak flow readings and see if lower levels are tied to your cycle," advises Harold S. Nelson, MD, an immunologist and professor of medicine at the National Jewish Medical and Research Center in Denver. "If you notice changes, talk to your doctor about changing your maintenance medicines."

Be prepared for emergencies. People who have food allergies as well as asthma are especially susceptible to a life-threatening allergic reaction called anaphylaxis.

"We tell all patients who have both food allergies and asthma to carry Benadryl (an antihistamine) and an EpiPen (a form of lifesaving epinephrine) with them at all times, even if they've never had an anaphylactic event," says Hugh A. Sampson, MD, chief of the division of allergy and immunology in the Department of Pediatrics at Mount Sinai School of Medicine in New York City and former president of the American Academy of Allergy, Asthma and Immunology. And don't forget your rescue inhaler either.

For more information. Contact the American Lung Association at www.lungusa.org or the American Academy of Allergy, Asthma and Immunology at www.aaaai.org.

back problems

The next time you're walking down the street or shopping at the mall, take a look around you—four out of five people you see will experience back troubles at some time in their lives.

"Back pain can come on suddenly and drop you to your knees, or it can be a chronic, long-term condition," says Stephen Hochschuler, MD, clinical instructor at the University of Texas Health and Science Center in Dallas, founder and chairman of the Texas Back Institute in Plano, and author of *Treat Your Back without Surgery*.

It's not surprising that back problems are as common as they are. The back is subjected to enormous amounts of stress. Whether you're sitting, standing, bending over, lifting bags and boxes, or simply turning to look behind you, the muscles, ligaments, and bones in the spine feel the strain. The lower back, called the lumbar region, is especially vulnerable because it supports a tremendous amount of weight. That's why it's the most injury-prone area of the entire spine, says Dr. Hochschuler.

Men and women suffer from back pain equally, but women have some special risks. After menopause, when a woman's estrogen levels decline, the bones begin to lose calcium at an accelerated rate. This makes them thinner and weaker than they should be. This condition, called osteoporosis, increases the risk of spinal fractures. Osteoporosis affects both men and women, but women with osteoporosis greatly outnumber men.

Another problem is the design of the spine itself. The bones of the spine, called vertebrae, are separated by shock-absorbing disks that are somewhat similar in structure to jelly doughnuts: They have a tough outer coating surrounding a soft center. Over the years, the disks lose moisture and flexibility. They literally shrink and lose some of their ability to absorb shocks or impacts. In some cases, the disks actually rupture, or herniate: The soft material in the center leaks out and puts pressure on tissues in the spine, including the spinal nerves.

when to see a doctor

If you've hurt your back and the pain hasn't improved after 3 days, make an appointment to see your doctor. You may have suffered nerve or tissue damage that won't improve without medical treatment, says Deborah Saint-Phard, MD, associate professor of physical medicine and rehabilitation and founder and director of the University of Colorado's Women's Sports Medicine program, in Denver.

If the pain is excruciating and nothing you do seems to help. You may need prescription drugs to reduce pain, muscle spasms, or inflammation.

If you've lost bowel or bladder function, or if you're having numbness, tingling, or a loss of muscle strength. You could have suffered nerve damage that may require surgery or other medical treatments.

"As women start getting into their thirties and forties, the early signs of degenerative disk disease can begin," says Deborah Saint-Phard, MD, associate professor of physical medicine and rehabilitation and founder and director of the University of Colorado's Women's Sports Medicine program, in Denver. As women get older, their risk of developing osteoporosis rises and the bones themselves become increasingly susceptible to damage. "Even if there's very little stress put on the back, compression fractures are common in women with osteoporosis," says Dr. Saint-Phard, a former Olympic athlete.

For men and women, extra weight is among the main risk factors for back problems. Even if you're only a few pounds over your ideal weight, those extra pounds are supported by the back. Year after year, they put unnecessary stress on the spine. Even if your disks hold up and your bones remain strong, the muscles and ligaments in the back will feel the strain.

Keeping your back strong requires a combination of strategies, including getting enough calcium in your diet, watching your weight, and keeping the muscles and ligaments strong and flexible.

Even if you do everything right, there's a good chance you'll eventually suffer a bout of back pain. Most back problems are self-limiting, which means they'll get better on their own. In the meantime, of course, the pain can be excruciating. Here are a few ways to ease the discomfort of minor backaches and strains quickly, along with some long-term strategies for keeping your back strong and healthy.

For Immediate Relief

Ice the pain. "Right after you hurt your back, the first thing you should do is apply ice to the area," says Dr. Hochschuler. "Ice will constrict the blood vessels, which reduces blood flow and decreases swelling."

Ice works best within the first 48 hours after an injury, Dr. Hochschuler adds. If you don't have an ice pack at home, you can wrap a washcloth or dishtowel around some ice cubes. Apply the pack for only 5 to 10 minutes at a time. Or fill a few paper cups with water and freeze them. Peel back the paper and apply the ice directly to the sore spots, in a circular motion, for no more than 5 to 10 minutes at a time.

Follow ice with heat. When you've hurt your back, most of the swelling occurs within the first 2 days, which is why applying ice is the best initial treatment. After 2 days, however, you want to increase blood flow to the area, which will help the damaged tissues heal.

"Put a heating pad on the area for 20 minutes at a time, using a lower setting in order to avoid a burn," says Dr. Hochschuler. Another option is to lounge in a hot bath several times a day. "Standing in a hot shower will also help relieve the pain," says Dr. Saint-Phard.

Take anti-inflammatory drugs. Over-the-counter pain relievers are among the best treatments for back injuries because they inhibit the body's production of prostaglandins, chemicals that excite nerve endings and cause pain. Aspirin, ibuprofen, naproxen, and acetaminophen all can be helpful, says Dr. Hochschuler.

Get some rest—immediately. Back pain is your body's way of telling you that you've done something wrong. Don't ignore the message: Stop whatever you've been doing and give your back a chance to recover.

If you hurt your back playing golf, stop playing and take a break in the clubhouse. If you've been working in the yard, put down the rake and take the rest of the day off. Staying active when the muscles and ligaments are irritated will only increase the damage and the risk of long-term damage.

"Even if the pain is severe enough to warrant bed rest, limit it to 2 days," Dr. Hochschuler adds. "Staying inactive for longer than 2 days will cause the back muscles to weaken and become stiff and inflexible."

Walk it off. "If you can tolerate it, go for a short walk," says Dr. Hochschuler. Walking is a

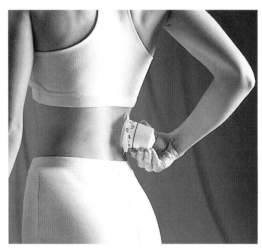

Icing an injury reduces bloodflow and inflammation, which reduces pain as well as the risk of long-term damage.

gentle aerobic activity that gets the blood moving and stretches out stiff muscles. "It can also relieve some of the tension that could be contributing to your back pain."

Try water walking. "If walking on hard surfaces is too painful, try walking in a pool if you have access," says Dr. Hochschuler. "It's less painful because the water creates an environment of near weightlessness. Start out slowly, and as it becomes easier, walk faster."

Long-Term Solutions

home remedies

Change positions often. It's not unusual for back problems to persist for weeks or even months. One of the best ways to relieve stiffness

and prevent future problems is to change positions frequently. This is especially important if you spend a lot of time sitting, which puts a tremendous amount of stress on the lower spine, says Dr. Saint-Phard.

"Every 20 minutes, take a break and change your position," she advises. If you tend to get so focused on your work that you lose track of time, set an alarm or the beeper on your watch. When you hear the alarm, get up and walk around. Do some stretching exercises. Or simply stand up for a while. The change in position will prevent muscles and ligaments in the spine from locking into position.

Lift with your knees, not with your back. "It's of paramount importance that women use their knees and hips to bend down and pick up

---

THREE THINGS I TELL EVERY FEMALE PATIENT

DEBORAH SAINT-PHARD, MD, *associate professor of physical medicine and rehabilitation and founder and director of the University of Colorado Women's Sports Medicine program, in Denver and a former Olympic shot-putter, advises her back patients to do the following:*

1

CHANGE POSITIONS OFTEN. Whether you've recently hurt your back or simply want to avoid problems later, don't spend too much time in any one position. It's especially important not to sit for extended periods because it increases pressure on the spine.

2

BE CONSCIOUS OF HOW YOU MOVE. "Little stresses accumulate to cause back problems," says Dr. Saint-Phard. "Bend your knees when lifting objects, even if you're just picking up a feather. Just because you don't feel pain doesn't mean that you're not creating abnormal stress on the back."

3

FIND EXERCISES THAT WORK FOR YOU. Regular exercise is among the best ways to manage and prevent serious back problems, but there isn't a one-size-fits-all exercise plan. "What works to relieve back pain for one woman may cause it in another," says Dr. Saint-Phard. "If you try a new exercise and have a backache the next day, move on to something else." ∎

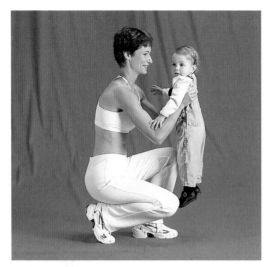

When lifting, always bend your knees and not your back. It's among the best ways to prevent back pain.

kids or groceries," says Dr. Saint-Phard. Whether you're picking up something light, like a piece of paper, or something heavy, like a large carton, bend your knees and get in a squatting position. "The back should remain fairly erect while the knees bend, as opposed to bending forward at the waist."

Bend your knees when you sleep. One reason that people often wake up with stiff backs is that they sleep on their stomachs. This causes the back to arch, which puts a lot of pressure on the muscles and ligaments.

"If you have back pain at night or in the morning, it's a good idea to sleep with the knees bent," says Dr. Saint-Phard. "Lie on your side and put a pillow between your legs. If you're lying on your back, place the pillow beneath the legs."

Try not to twist. "The spine does not like to be bent or twisted, especially when you're lifting

things, says Dr. Saint-Phard. Remind yourself to keep your spine straight whenever possible, she advises.

Plan before you move. A lot of back injuries occur when people are doing simple, everyday activities but doing them the wrong way. When you're vacuuming or making the bed, for example, do you bend forward at the waist? If so, you're putting a lot of unnecessary pressure on the back.

"Use your leg, hip, and butt muscles to move the vacuum cleaner," Dr. Saint-Phard advises. When you're making the bed or unloading the dishwasher, bend your knees or even kneel down. Your goal should always be to keep your back as straight as possible.

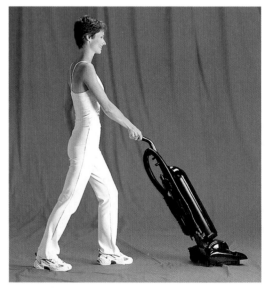

It's always better to bend your knees than to bend your back. Bending your knees slightly and using the hip, leg, and butt muscles can dramatically reduce strain on the lower back.

(continued on page 352)

Strengthen
Your Back Muscles

People who stay in shape don't necessarily have a lower risk for back pain, but they do tend to recover more quickly from back attacks than those who are sedentary and out of shape, says Stephen Hochschuler, MD, clinical instructor at the University of Tex as Health Science Center in Dallas, founder and chairman of the Texas Back Institute in Plano, and author of *Treat Your Back without Surgery.*

One of the best exercises for your back is also the simplest. It's called opposite arm and leg lift, and it strengthens the abdominal muscles as well as those in the back. It protects the spine and also improves your posture.

When doing the exercise, try to complete eight to 12 lifts with each arm and leg. Rest a moment, then repeat the series again. Doing the exercise 2 or 3 times a week will keep your muscles strong and limber.

Opposite Arm and Leg Lift

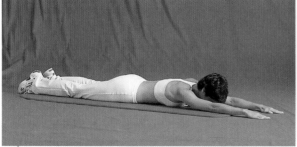

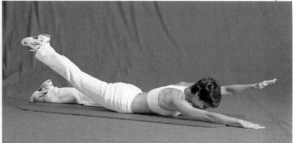

Lie facedown with your legs extended straight behind you, toes pointed and your arms extended straight over your head. Keep your chin up off the floor at a comfortable level.

Slowly raise your left arm and your right leg at the same time until they are both a few inches off the floor. Hold, then slowly lower them back to the starting position. Repeat on the other side.

The Best Exercises for Preventing Back Pain

You need to strengthen your abdominal and back muscles in order to support and protect the spine. It's also important to stretch the hamstrings (the muscles in the back of the thighs) and hips. The following exercises will go a long way toward keeping your back strong and pain-free.

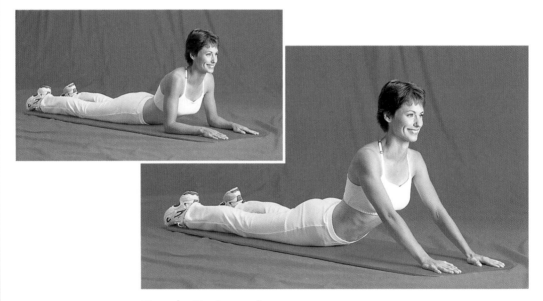

Back Extension

Lie on your stomach. Keeping your hips on the floor, prop yourself up on your fore-arms and raise your chest (left). Hold the stretch for a few seconds, then raise your upper body as far as you can by straightening your elbows and arching your back (right). Go as far as you comfortably can, hold the position for 10 seconds, then relax.

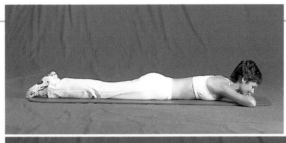

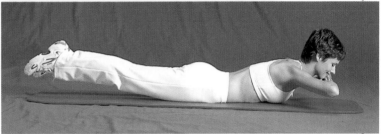

Chest Lift

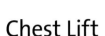

Lie on your stomach with your hands under your chin (top). Lift your head and feet about 1 to 2 inches off the floor; don't arch your back too much (bottom). Hold the position for a few seconds, then lower yourself.

Bridge Lift

Lie on your back with your knees bent and your arms at your sides (top). Slowly lift your pelvis and buttocks off the floor (bottom), hold for about 5 seconds, then lower yourself.

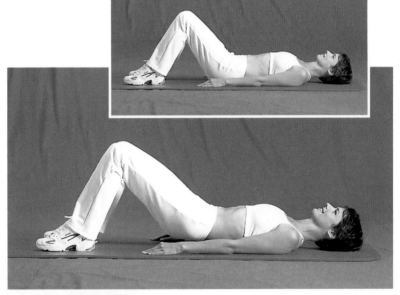

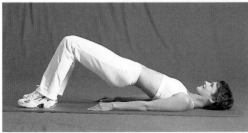

As you get stronger, try to lift your torso until there's a straight line between your knees and shoulders.

(continued)

The Best Exercises for Preventing Back Pain

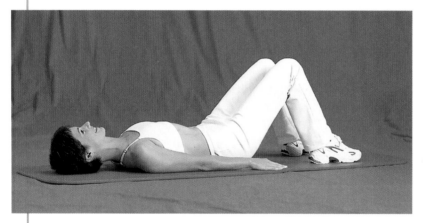

Pelvic Tuck

Lie on your back with your knees bent. Tighten the abdominal muscles and tilt the pelvis upward until the small of your back presses against the floor. Hold for 5 seconds, then relax.

Mini-Crunch

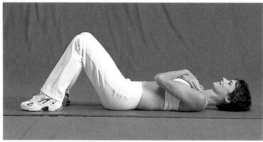 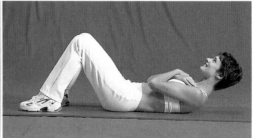

Lie on your back with your knees bent and your arms crossed on your chest (left). Slowly lift your head and shoulders until your shoulder blades come off the floor; don't bend your neck (right). Hold the position for a few seconds, then lower yourself.

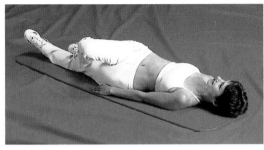
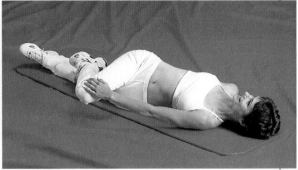

Hip Stretch

Lie on your back with your legs straight. Bend your right leg so it crosses over the left, keeping your foot near your left knee (left). Using your left hand, gently press your right knee toward the floor until you feel a stretch in your right hip and buttocks (right). Hold the stretch for 10 to 30 seconds, then relax. Repeat the exercise with the left leg.

Hamstring Stretch

Lie flat on your back with your legs bent and both feet on the floor. Loop a towel or rope under the arch of your left foot. While keeping a slight bend at the knee, straighten and raise your left leg off the floor and gently pull your leg toward your chest as far as is comfortable. Hold for 10 to 30 seconds, then relax. Repeat on the other leg.

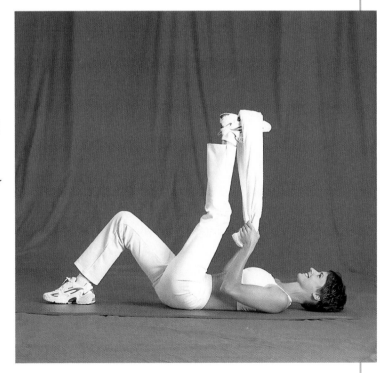

Try to relax. Anxiety and stress cause your muscles to tighten, and tight muscles often lead to back pain. If you already have back problems, emotional stress invariably makes the pain worse. That's why back specialists advise their patients to do everything they can to reduce the tension in their lives.

One technique that often helps is progressive relaxation, says Dr. Hochschuler. It's very easy to do. While you're sitting or lying down, focus on your muscles one at a time. Start with the muscles in your toes; tighten them for a few seconds, then relax. When you're done with your feet, move upward to your legs, hips, back, and chest. It takes 10 to 20 minutes to tense and relax all the muscle groups. When you're done, you'll find that a lot of the tension and stress in your body and your mind will have melted away.

alternative therapies

See a chiropractor. Studies have found that chiropractic manipulation is a cost-effective—and possibly more effective—treatment for back pain than regular medical care.

Get needled. When researchers at the University of Maryland and Peninsula Medical School in the United Kingdom analyzed dozens of studies from around the world, they found that acupuncture—a Chinese medical procedure in which tiny needles are inserted into the skin at specific spots—significantly relieved symptoms of chronic low back pain when compared to sham treatments given as a control.

Bend and stretch. A 2009 study of male and female veterans being treated at Veteran's Administration hospitals found that those with chronic low-back pain who took 8 weeks of yoga classes had a significant reduction in their pain, less depression, improvements in mood and energy, and ranked their quality of life higher than before they took the classes.

medical options

Ask your doctor about TENS. If you've had long-term back pain, your doctor may recommend a procedure called TENS, short for transcutaneous electrical nerve stimulation. Acupuncture-like needles are inserted into the soft tissues and muscles surrounding the bones. A small electrical current passes through the needles, which interrupts pain signals.

Researchers at the University of Texas Southwestern Medical Center in Dallas found that back patients treated with TENS required smaller amounts of painkillers. They also slept better and reported feeling better overall.

For more information. Visit the Web site of the National Institute of Neurological Disorders and Stroke at www.ninds.nih.gov.

blemishes, pimples, and breakouts

You thought you'd put acne behind you, back when you packed away your last prom dress, but there it is again and you're in the prime of your life. Even women in their thirties, forties, and beyond can suffer from occasional breakouts. Acne can run in families and it can flare up because of hormone changes you experience at puberty, during the menstrual cycle, and at menopause.

Even women who never had acne when they were young may have flare-ups in later years—either in conjunction with the menstrual cycle or with the onset of menopause, says Leslie Baumann, MD, director of the Baumann Cosmetic and Research Institute in Miami. Treatments for acne have gotten increasingly sophisticated in the past few decades. You can't prevent the occasional pimple from popping up, but with a combination of medications and home remedies, it's usually easy to keep acne flare-ups under control.

For Immediate Relief

home remedies

Use benzoyl peroxide. A topical antiseptic, it kills the bacteria that cause the inflammation, swelling, and discomfort of acne. Available OTC in cream gel or lotion form, benzoyl peroxide (in products such as Clearasil) may be the only treatment that you need.

After washing your face, spread a thin layer over the affected areas. Individual dosages and product formulations vary, so follow your doctor's advice. Generally, it should be used once a day at first; as your skin gets used to it, gradually increase to 6 or 8 times daily or as needed during outbreaks.

Try salicylic acid. Another OTC remedy, salicylic acid (which is similar to the active ingredient in aspirin), reduces inflammation and loosens the bonds between dead cells, allowing them to shed more easily.

Clean your skin thoroughly, then apply a thin layer of salicylic acid (such as Stridex) to the acne pimple areas. This medication may cause drying of your skin. Dosage varies for each individual and product, so it's best to follow your doctor's instructions. Usually, you start with one application a day and gradually increase to three applications a day as needed.

alternative therapies

Apply a clay paste. Clay has been used for centuries for deep cleaning oily complexions and removing impurities from the skin. To prepare a poultice for blemishes, combine ½ teaspoon of cosmetic clay (available at health food stores and some cosmetics counters and from online stores) with ½ teaspoon of water. You may need to prepare more of the mixture if you have a larger area to treat or if you want to use it as a facial mask. Mix well, then apply a thin layer over the entire face for deep cleaning, or just on the blemishes, and let the clay dry. If the area you're treating is small, you can leave the poultice on for several hours or overnight, then wash it off. Masks need to be rinsed off thoroughly immediately after the clay dries. Repeat the poultice treatments as needed once daily. Use the clay mask only once a week to avoid overdrying your skin.

when to see a doctor

If your acne is accompanied by menstrual irregularities, thinning hair, weight gain, or visible facial hair, call your doctor. You might need blood tests to check for excess androgens, male hormones that can cause acne outbreaks, says Teresa Soriano, MD, associate health sciences clinical professor of dermatology at University of California at Los Angeles School of Medicine.

If you have acnelike bumps on your face, especially on the mid-face (forehead, nose, cheeks, and chin) and facial redness and you can see broken blood vessels resembling threads through the skin. You could have a condition known as rosacea, sometimes called adult acne. Rosacea may require treatment with antibiotics or other medications.

If the acne doesn't get better with home care. Your doctor may recommend medications, including birth control pills, oral antibiotics, and other drugs to get the outbreaks under control.

Use tea tree oil. Studies have found that ointments containing 5 percent tea tree oil are as effective as benzoyl peroxide in treating acne.

Try zinc. This anti-inflammatory mineral may help improve acne. Studies have been conflicting, but in many zinc in a 30 mg dose may be helpful. Make sure you take it with food to avoid stomach discomfort, a side effect of zinc.

medical options

Ask your dermatologist about facial peels. Unlike the mild salicylic acid that's used in home preparations, your dermatologist may recommend treating acne with a highly concentrated form containing 20 to 30 percent salicylic acid. It removes the surface layer of skin and can improve or eliminate acne within 2 to 4 days, says Dr. Baumann.

Try tretinoin. Available by prescription, it's a derivative of vitamin A. It reduces oil production in the skin, taking away the fuel that triggers acne. Applied once daily, tretinoin (Renova) will help eliminate pimples that are already present and may help prevent others from forming.

Ask about these drugs. Adapalene (Differin) is a drug that decreases the formation of pimples, while azelaic (Azelex) helps stop or slow down the growth of acne-caused bacteria and reduces inflammation.

Consider isotretinoin if acne is severe. This is among the most powerful acne remedies, and it's used only for severe inflammatory acne and when simpler (and safer) treatments don't work. Isotretinoin (Accutane) is very effective, but it may cause adverse effects such as itching, headaches, photosensitivity, or hair loss, which may persist in some women. More serious possible side effects include elevations of blood fats, abnormal liver enzymes, inflammatory bowel disease, and hearing impairment. The most significant potential adverse effect is that it can cause birth defects if taken during pregnancy. Your doctor will prescribe this medication only if you're absolutely sure that you won't get pregnant while using it.

For Long-Term Relief

mind-body techniques

Keep stress under control. Emotional stress doesn't cause acne, but it can trigger outbreaks in some women by changing hormone levels and increasing oil gland secretion. If you notice that your complexion tends to get worse during emotionally difficult times, take it as a sign that it's time to unwind—by exercising more, working less, and practicing relaxation techniques such as meditation, deep breathing, or yoga.

breast pain and tenderness

Cramps, mood changes, and food cravings are just a few of the signs that a menstrual period is pending. Many women also experience breast pain. The pain usually starts midway though the menstrual cycle, may get progressively worse until the onset of the period, then dissipates. For some women, it can be severe enough to interfere with normal activities.

"Cyclic breast changes occur in response to fluctuating levels of the hormones estrogen and progesterone during the menstrual cycle," says Eric Whitacre, MD, director of the Breast Center of Southern Arizona in Tucson and president of the American Society of Breast Surgeons. "The breasts may swell and become tender or painful, which may be due to hormonal changes."

Breast pain, called mastalgia, can have many other causes and affects women of all ages. But because it is generally linked to the menstrual cycle, it's much more common in younger women. In fact, hormones are to blame for two-thirds of cases of breast pain among women, and it's most common when you're in your thirties and forties. However, any woman may experience pain because of breast tissue changes.

These changes, referred to as fibrocystic conditions, may cause occasional fluid retention in the breasts. The fluid exerts pressure on breast tissues, which in turn may cause pain, says Dr. Whitacre. In addition, some women develop tiny fluid-filled sacs, called cysts, in the milk glands. These cysts are harmless, but they can make the breasts tender for a few days. More than half of women have lumpy breasts that are tender right before their periods.

If you're breast-feeding, you may also have painful breasts. The hormone prolactin, involved in milk production, may be to blame, but you may also develop an infection caused when bacteria on the skin of your breast breaks through a crack or break in the skin near your nipple and infects fatty tissue. Nonlactating women may also experience inflamed milk ducts near the nipple that can cause pain, lumps, redness, discharge, and retraction of the nipple.

Some drugs, including some diuretics and digitalis medications, also have breast pain as a potential side effect.

when to see a doctor

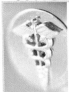

If you've just started experiencing breast pain, regardless of the time of month, make an appointment to see your doctor. It might be a result of normal menstrual changes, or it could be related to medications you're taking, such as birth control or supplemental estrogen or other hormones, says Eric Whitacre, MD, director of the Breast Center of Southern Arizona and president of the American Society of Breast Surgeons.

If there's a lump in or near the breast or in the underarm area; a spontaneous nipple discharge, especially if it's bloody; persistent changes in the breast skin, such as puckering or indentations (called dimpling), redness or scaliness of the breast skin or nipple; pain in the nipple or the nipple turning inward; or a "funny" feeling, such as itching or tingling in the skin of the breast or the nipple. These are potential symptoms of breast cancer, and your doctor will probably advise you to have a mammogram or sonogram, says Dr. Whitacre.

Any type of lump or discomfort in the breasts should be brought to the attention of your doctor right away. In most cases, however, you won't have anything to worry about—and it may be possible to relieve the discomfort with a few simple strategies.

For Immediate Relief

home remedies

Wear an exercise bra. It will give the breasts extra support. This is one of the best ways to reduce tenderness and pain. You can wear the bra any time it helps you with the discomfort, even while you sleep.

Take an analgesic. Aspirin and ibuprofen can provide fast-acting relief from monthly breast pain. They inhibit the body's production of prostaglandins, chemicals that cause pain and swelling.

For Long-Term Prevention

home remedies

Consume less caffeine. Found in coffee, tea, caffeinated sodas, chocolate, and some over-the-counter medications, caffeine stimulates breast tissue, which may cause an increase in monthly pain, says Dr. Whitacre.

Go fish. Or walnuts or another food high in omega-3 fatty acids. They help reduce inflammation and pain related to fibrocystic breasts.

Try vitamin E. There's some evidence that vitamin E may reduce breast pain associated with the menstrual cycle as well as the discomforts of fibrocystic breast conditions. "We're not really sure why it works, but it's worth trying," says Dr. Whitacre. Stick to 400 IU daily and see if it helps.

Give evening primrose oil a shot. Found in OTC supplements, it's rich in gamma linolenic acid, which can inhibit the action of prostaglandins. It can also reduce painful inflammation. The research is inconclusive about its effectiveness in treating the discomforts of fibrocystic breast conditions. Although doctors aren't sure how it works, evening primrose oil supplements have been shown beneficial as a treatment for mastalgia associated with the menstrual cycle.

"At our clinic, we advise women to start with a minimum of 1,500 mg of evening primrose oil per day," says Dr. Whitacre. If that dose doesn't help, you can increase the amount to 3,000 mg daily. "Sometimes you have to start out high, then gradually taper off. We've found that you have to take it for 2 or 3 months to see if it will be beneficial." It's advisable to take 1,000 to 2,000 mg of fish oil daily along with the evening primrose oil in order to provide a balance of omega-6s and omega-3s.

Skip the salt and pass on fat. Sodium can increase breast swelling that can lead to breast pain. Keep fat down too—one small study found that eating a low-fat diet (less than 20 percent of calories) for 6 months helped reduce breast swelling and tenderness.

Keep a food diary. Breast pain is sometimes caused by foods or beverages in the diet. If you keep track of what you're eating and drinking, you may find that pain occurs or gets worse only when you eat certain foods.

"One of my patients was consuming large amounts of soy," says Dr. Whitacre. "Soy contains plant estrogens, and estrogen is implicated in breast pain."

cataracts

magine looking at the world through smudgy glasses, or trying to see the countryside through a windshield that's never been washed. You can probably see fairly well, but things simply aren't as clear as they should be.

"A significant number of people with cataracts don't know they have a problem until they are told during a routine eye exam," says Robert Abel Jr., MD, an ophthalmologist on staff at Christiana Health Care System in Delaware and author of *The Eye Care Revolution*.

Cataracts occur when proteins clump together in the normally clear lenses of the eyes. They can cause blindness in some cases, but more often they make vision a little blurry or decrease your ability to see in dim light.

"It may be possible to keep recently formed cataracts stable and less likely to cause problems," says Dr. Abel.

For Immediate Relief

home remedies

Drink plenty of water. The lenses of the eyes don't have their own blood supply. They depend on a tiny trickle of fluid, called aqueous humor, to get the nourishment they need. "You can't believe how much better people will see when they drink enough water," says Dr. Abel. At a minimum, drink six full glasses of water daily, he advises.

Eat blueberries. They contain chemical compounds called anthocyanosides, which strengthen blood vessels in the eyes and also prevent damage from free radicals, harmful oxygen molecules that often damage tissues in the eyes.

"Periodically go outside and look at the stars," Dr. Abel advises. When you've been eating ½ cup of blueberries daily (or drinking bilberry tea, which has the same active compounds), within 3 days the stars should appear sharper and more distinct.

Give up cigarettes. The smoke unleashes enormous numbers of free radicals. If you're not ready to quit, at least take a vitamin C and B-complex vitamin supplement: It will help protect eye tissues from toxins in smoke, says Dr. Abel.

medical options

Consider eye surgery. Operations to remove cataracts are extremely satisfying for doctors as well as patients because they're quick, safe, and nearly pain free, says John D. Hunkeler, MD, clinical professor of ophthalmology at the University of Kansas School of Medicine in Kansas City.

The surgery is done as an outpatient procedure. More than 95 percent of those who have cataracts removed will have significant improvements in their vision.

For Long-Term Prevention

home remedies

Put on your sunglasses. Researchers at Johns Hopkins School of Medicine in Baltimore found that the risk of cataracts was 57 percent higher in people who had the most sun exposure compared with those who had the least.

"Every time you go out without adequate protection, you're increasing your risk," says Sheila K. West, PhD, professor of preventive ophthalmology at Johns Hopkins University. Plastic lenses are slightly better than glass at blocking the sun's cataract-causing rays, she adds.

Eat brightly colored vegetables. Broccoli, carrots, sweet potatoes, and other fruits and vegetables with vivid hues are loaded with carotenoids, specifically lutein and zeaxanthin, pigments that filter the harmful high-energy blue wavelengths of light and act as antioxidants, preventing the damaging effects of free radicals. One study of more than 50,000 women ages 45 to 67 found that eating five servings of spinach a

when to see a doctor

If you're experiencing changes in vision that are affecting your daily life, get your eyes examined by an ophthalmologist. You could be developing cataracts or another type of eye disease.

If your vision has abruptly gotten worse. There could be a vascular problem that's affecting circulation to the eyes.

week reduced cataract formation by 39 percent.

Don't forget the asparagus. Along with onions, eggs, and lean red meats, asparagus is rich in cysteine, an amino acid that's converted in the body to glutathione. Glutathione is a pow- erful antioxidant that protects the eyes from free radical damage.

For more information on cataracts. Visit the Web site of the National Eye Institute at www.nei.nih.gov.

colds

There's a good reason that colds are called "common." Doctors estimate that men, women, and children alike get one billion colds every year (as many as two to six annually). On any given day, nearly one in four young women is reaching for the tissue box, swabbing her eyes, and counting the days until the miserable infection runs its course.

So far, there isn't a cure for the common cold, and there isn't a lot you can do to prevent them. Vaccines don't help because colds are caused by more than 200 viruses, each of which constantly changes and adapts to whatever medical science throws at it. In addition, cold viruses are every- where—on your hands, in the air, and on door- knobs, washcloths, and toothbrushes.

Colds are rarely serious, of course, and most people start feeling better within a week. But if you act quickly, you may be able to reduce much of the discomfort and even shorten the duration of the illness. Here's what experts advise.

For Immediate Relief

home remedies

Use nasal irrigation. This remedy from the 6,000-year-old Indian Ayurvedic medical tradi- tion really works, say researchers at the Univer- sity of Wisconsin School of Medicine and Public Health. Using a teapot-like pot called a neti pot, you rinse your naval cavities with a saline solu- tion (or you could use a saline spray). In the University of Wisconsin studies, patients with colds and sinus problems reduced their symp- toms, felt better, and used less medication. To make a spray, mix $1/8$ to $1/4$ teaspoon of salt in 8 ounces of water. Suck the solution into a nasal aspirator and give a quick spray. The solution is entirely safe, so you can repeat the spray as often as necessary to get relief.

Take advantage of chicken soup. It's a tra- ditional cold remedy, and there's some evidence that it helps. Apart from the fact that the heat and steam will make you feel better, the onions and garlic in chicken soup contain antiviral com- pounds that will help eliminate the virus, says Mary L. Hardy, MD, codirector of the Integrative Medicine and Wellness Program at the Venice Family Clinic and medical director of the Simms/ Mann Center for Integrative Oncology program at the University of California at Los Angeles.

Add some hot spices. To make chicken soup even more effective, season it with cayenne or chile peppers, suggests Dr. Hardy. Both spices contain a fiery compound called capsaicin, which will quickly clear mucus from the nose and sinuses.

Take plenty of fluids. When you're sick, the body requires extra water to replace fluids that are "burned off" by fever, and also to flush the body of accumulated toxins. Drinking a lot of water, juice, or tea also may thin respiratory secretions, says Kay A. Bauman, MD, MPH, of the department of family practice and community health at the John A. Burns School of Medicine at the University of Hawaii in Mililani.

Take acetaminophen. It's the best OTC remedy for reducing muscle aches, fever, head pain, and other cold symptoms. Unlike aspirin, it's unlikely to cause stomach upset. (It's also safer for children and teenagers, who may experience harmful reactions when they take aspirin or aspirin-like drugs.)

Reduce congestion with medications. Pharmacy shelves are packed with products that relieve nose and chest congestion. Antihistamines may dampen cough, sneezing, watery eyes and nasal discharge, while decongestants can open up a clogged nose. They all have side effects—many cause drowsiness and some can't be taken if you have high blood pressure—so ask your doctor to recommend something based on your symptoms.

alternative therapies

Try echinacea. Some research has shown that the herb echinacea may cut the duration of colds and also reduce the severity of symptoms; other studies have found that it works no better than a placebo. Some people swear by it. You can make echinacea tea with fresh or dried herb, but it's easier to take dried root tablets, available in health food stores. The recom-

Shake the On-the-Job Attitudes That Can Make You Sick

attitude on the job could affect your odds of getting a nasty cold or flu this winter, a current study suggests.

When researchers tracked more than 200 workers over a period of 3 months, they found that those who had control over how they did their work but either lacked confidence or tended to blame themselves when things went wrong on the job were more likely to catch the sniffles, flu, or other infections.

The reason behind this? For starters, people who lack confidence or tend to self-blame are more stressed on the job. "And the evidence is increasing that stress can lower your immunity, leaving you more susceptible to infections, particularly to upper respiratory infections," explains lead researcher John Schaubroeck, PhD, professor of management at Drexel University in Philadelphia. ∎

mended dose is two 500-mg tablets 3 times daily. If you prefer a tea, use ½ teaspoon of the dried root added to 2 cups of boiling water. Boil it down to 1 cup and drink 1 cup four times a day.

Try elderberry syrup or tincture. According to herbalists, elderberry (Sambucus nigra) can reduce the duration of colds by 30 to 40 percent—and it tastes a lot better than OTC remedies. Look for elderberry syrup and tinctures at your health food store. Take 1 teaspoon of syrup or 1 teaspoon of 1:5 tincture 3 times a day.

Get extra vitamin C. This is a controversial cold treatment, but there is some evidence that extra C can reduce the duration and severity of a cold. It seems to strengthen immune cells and also helps block the effects of histamine, the body chemical responsible for causing watery

eyes and runny noses. At the first sign of cold symptoms, take 2,000 mg of vitamin C daily. Divide it into several doses of 500 mg and take it throughout the day.

For Long-Term Prevention

home remedies

Wash your hands often. One reason that colds are so difficult to prevent is that the viruses spread widely every time you sneeze or blow your nose. Invariably, some of the viruses survive on the hands—and on doorknobs, light switches, and towels—and then find their way into the body. Washing your hands often—every few hours is best—is among the best ways to prevent colds from coming back. Make sure you wash them long enough. Sing two choruses of "Happy Birthday"—aloud or to yourself—while sudsing your hands with soap and warm water, suggests the Centers for Disease Control and Prevention (CDC). You can also use alcohol-based hand wipes and gel sanitizers when you're not near a sink.

Cover your mouth. But not with your hand! If you sneeze or cough, do it into a tissue that you throw away or slip into your sleeve. Most illnesses are passed one to the other by hand. Wash your hands afterward.

Get regular exercise. A study by researchers at Appalachian State University in North Carolina found that being physically active can cut your risk of getting a cold and reduce the severity of your symptoms if you do get one.

when to see a doctor

If your cold symptoms last more than 2 weeks, see your doctor right away. Persistent nasal congestion, sore throat, or coughing could mean you have sinusitis, a more serious bacterial infection that requires antibiotics or other medical treatments.

If your mucus is tinged with yellow or green. This often means that the initial cold infection, caused by a virus, has been replaced with a secondary bacterial infection. You may need treatment with antibiotics.

cold sores

t's seems like you can always count on one to pop out at the wrong time—when you're meeting someone new, making a presentation to a client, going out on the town in your best outfit. Colds sores (despite the name, they have nothing to do with the common cold) aren't serious, just painful and annoying. They usually clear up on their own in a week or two. If you're lucky, you'll never have more than one outbreak, but you can't count on that: The virus that causes cold sores lives in the body forever.

As many as 90 percent of adult Americans are infected with a virus called herpes simplex virus 1 (HSV-1), which is typically contracted during childhood. During the initial outbreak, the virus can cause a variety of symptoms, such as fever, blisters in and around the mouth, and enlarged lymph nodes. Once the infection is done, the virus retreats into the body's nerves, where it lies dormant. In most cases, it never causes another symptom. But for a minority of those infected, the infection periodically springs back to life, triggering painful sores that usually appear on the edge of the lip. A tingling, burning, or itching sensation on the skin usually precedes an outbreak.

You can't get rid of the virus once you have it, but there are ways to prevent outbreaks and to help the sores heal more quickly.

For Immediate Relief

home remedies

Apply an anesthetic. Cold sores can be intensely painful, especially when you're eating or drinking. One solution is to apply an OTC benzocaine cold sore gel, such as Colgate Orabase B Topical and Oral Anesthetic Gel, which contains a mild anesthetic, says Teresa Soriano, MD, associate clinical professor of dermatology at University of California at Los Angeles School of Medicine.

If the pain is unusually intense, you may want to ask your doctor to prescribe a stronger numbing agent. Dr. Soriano suggests a 2 percent viscous lidocaine solution, which can be swished around in the mouth and then spit out. This treatment is especially helpful in reducing pain when it's used before meals, she says.

Speed the healing time. An OTC cream that contains docosanol (such as Abreva) can reduce the duration of cold sore attacks by 1 to 2 days, says David H. Emmert, MD, a family physician in Millersville, Pennsylvania, who published a study about the treatment of cold sores. As soon as you notice tingling, burning, or other cold sore symptoms, apply the cream 5 times daily, and keep using it until the sore has healed, he advises.

Prescription antiviral pills such as pencyclovir (Denavir), acyclovir (Zovirax), or valacyclovir (Valtrex) are also effective in shortening the duration and severity of outbreaks. Ask your doctor about these medications, especially if you suffer from frequent outbreaks.

alternative therapies

Use lemon balm. German researchers have found that people who apply lemon balm cream to cold sores four times daily heal faster and have less discomfort. You can buy lemon balm creams and ointments in health food stores. To reduce pain and speed healing, apply the cream for up to 10 days.

Try zinc oxide cream. In one small study people who applied zinc oxide cream to their cold sores saw them heal slightly faster (5 days versus 6½ days) than those who used a nontherapeutic placebo cream.

For Long-Term Relief

home remedies

Coat the sore with petroleum jelly. It traps moisture and prevents the sore from drying or cracking. Coating cold sores with petroleum jelly also speeds the healing time, says Dr. Emmert.

Avoid cold sore triggers. Research has shown that exposure to wind, cold, or excessive sunlight may trigger attacks in some people. If you're prone to cold sore attacks, it's worth using a lip balm that will protect the lips from the environment, says Leslie Baumann, MD, director of the Baumann Cosmetic and Research Institute in Miami. Select a lip balm that has an SPF of 15 or greater and reapply it every hour.

Apply an antibacterial ointment. Triple antibiotic ointments such as Neosporin and Betadine don't kill viruses, but they can help ensure that you don't develop a secondary bacterial infection in the open sore, says Dr. Emmert. If you're using an antiviral cream at the same time, be sure to apply it before using the antibacterial ointment.

THREE THINGS I TELL EVERY FEMALE PATIENT

DAVID H. EMMERT, MD, *a family physician in Millersville, Pennsylvania, who has studied cold sores, offers this advice for women who get frequent outbreaks.*

1 THINGS WILL GET BETTER. The herpes virus tends to reemerge from nerve cells at times of physical or emotional stress, but for most people, the severity and frequency of the attacks diminish over time.

ALWAYS USE LIP BALM. The sun's ultraviolet rays are among the most common triggers of cold sores. If you spend a lot of time outside, always use a lip balm that contains sunscreen. Be sure not to share lip balm with others; the virus is contagious and could be spread this way.

2

3 WASH YOUR HANDS OFTEN. The virus particles in cold sores are highly contagious. If you touch the sores—and almost everyone does—the infection can be spread to other people or to other parts of your body. Touch the cold sore as little as possible, and wash your hands frequently until the sore has healed. ■

conjunctivitis

Few things clear out a schoolroom faster than pink eye, the common term for bacterial conjunctivitis. When irritation—dry air, pollution, pollen, viruses, bacteria—affects the conjunctiva, the membrane that lines the eyelids and the white portions of the eyes, you're in for a period of redness, pain, and itching.

It's not always easy to pin down the precise causes of conjunctivitis. If the redness and irritation last longer than a day, you may need to see an ophthalmologist, who will examine your eyes under a microscope. Other symptoms to watch out for are itching, excessive tearing, blurred vision, discharge, and pain.

"If you wake up in the morning and your eyes are crusted together, you probably have bacterial conjunctivitis," says Sandra Belmont, MD, clinical associate professor of ophthalmology at Langone Medical Center at New York University. "If your eyes are itchy, burning, and red, it may be allergic conjunctivitis. If you have swollen glands, or you've just gotten over an upper respiratory illness, you may have viral conjunctivitis."

Conjunctivitis usually clears up on its own, although bacterial infections need to be treated by a doctor. To relieve the discomfort right away, here's what doctors advise.

For Immediate Relief

home remedies

Use artificial tears. Available in pharmacies, artificial tears do the same job as natural tears:

They moisturize the eyes and relieve itching and irritation. You can use them 6 to 8 times a day until your eyes are feeling better.

For additional relief, keep artificial tears in the refrigerator. The coolness is very soothing, says Stephanie Marioneaux, MD, an opthalmologist in Chesapeake, Virginia.

When using the drops, don't let the tip of the bottle touch your eye, Dr. Belmont adds. If you have viral or bacterial conjunctivitis, the harmful organisms can get on the tip and reinfect you later.

Apply a cool compress. Moisten a washcloth, put it in the freezer until it's cold, then apply it to your eyes several times a day, suggest Dr. Marioneaux. Don't use the cloth to rub your eyes, however, which can make the problem worse.

Try boric acid. Boil 1 teaspoon of boric acid in one cup water and apply cooled solution with a sterile eyecup or washcloth.

Avoid over-the-counter drops that "get the red out." These products, referred to as redness relievers, whiten the eyes by constricting blood vessels. The drops aren't harmful, but they don't treat the underlying causes of conjunctivitis—and when you quit using the drops, your eyes may be redder than ever, says Dr. Marioneaux.

medical options

Ask your doctor about medications. There are a number of prescription eyedrops that can be used to treat conjunctivitis. If the infection is caused by bacteria, your doctor will write a prescription for antibiotic drops. If it's viral, you can use antiviral eyedrops such as Zovirax or Viroptic. For eye irritation caused by allergies, you may need drops that contain antihistamines or anti-inflammatories, says Dr. Marioneaux. Antihistamine eyedrops include OTC Vasocon-A (antazoline phosphate) or prescription Patanol (olopatadine), which can reduce any swelling or itching.

Consider allergy shots. If you get conjunctivitis as the result of allergy, you should get shots to reduce your sensitivity.

For Long-Term Relief

home remedies

Prevent recontamination. Anything that touches your eye when you have conjunctivitis, including contact lenses and makeup applicators, can potentially be contaminated with harmful organisms. Avoid using eye makeup until after the infection is healed. Your doctor may advise you to discard your old contact lenses as well.

Wash pillowcases, sheets, and towels. The viruses and bacteria that cause conjunctivitis can survive on almost any surface. To prevent yourself from getting reinfected—and to protect other members of the family—be sure to wash

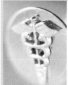

when to see a doctor

If eye irritation or redness persists for more than 24 hours, see your doctor right away. Conjunctivitis doesn't always require treatment, but sometimes it does—and acting quickly can prevent potential eye damage, says Sandra Belmont, MD, associate professor of ophthalmology at Cornell University in New York City.

If there's a discharge coming from one or both eyes, or if your vision is suddenly getting worse. Some forms of conjunctivitis, including those caused by bacteria, can cause permanent vision loss if they aren't treated promptly.

bedding, towels, or other linens that may have come into contact with your eyes.

Pillowcases—or anything else that may be exposed to fluids from the eyes—should be washed daily as long as the infection lasts, Dr. Belmont adds.

Wash your hands often. And scrub any surface that you've touched—doorknobs, computer keyboards, and even the steering wheel in your car—with a mild bleach solution, suggests Dr. Marioneaux.

constipation

"Anytime you're dissatisfied with your bowel movements—because you've strained too much, or the veins are popping out of your forehead—you're constipated," says Patricia Raymond, MD, gastroen-terologist and assistant professor at Eastern Virginia Medical School. But that doesn't mean you need to see a doctor. And not having bowel movements every day shouldn't send you reaching for a laxative.

"A generation ago, people were in the habit of giving children laxatives or enemas if they didn't go every day. But now we know that having a bowel movement anywhere from 3 times a week to 3 times a day is normal," says John W. Popp Jr., MD, clinical professor of medicine at the University of South Carolina School of Medicine in Columbia.

You only have constipation when you have stools that are infrequent, dry and hard, or difficult to pass, and if you have fewer than 3 bowel movements a week. There is, however, no "right" number of daily or weekly bowel movements. If you're constipated, the bowel movements may be painful. Some patients also complain of feeling sluggish, bloated, and uncomfortable.

Lack of fiber in the diet is one of the primary reasons for constipation, as is a fatty diet and a lack of exercise.

You may become constipated when you're pregnant, thanks to hormones and a growing uterus that compresses the intestines. Multiple sclerosis, lupus, Parkinson's disease, scleroderma, and stroke can all cause constipation. So can diabetes, an underactive or overactive thyroid, and spinal cord injuries. People with inflammatory bowel disease sometimes have bouts of constipation as well as diarrhea. Some medicines trigger constipation, too, including antidepressants, antihistamines for allergies, drugs for Parkinson's disease, pain medications (particularly narcotics), blood pressure drugs, diuretics (often called water pills), and antacids containing calcium or aluminum. Pain medica-

THREE THINGS I TELL EVERY FEMALE PATIENT

JOHN W. POPP JR., MD, *clinical professor of medicine at the University of South Carolina School of Medicine in Columbia, who has written about constipation for the American College of Gastroenterology, says that patients with bowel problems take their bowel movements very, very seriously.*

"I've had patients come in with photographs of their stool," Dr. Popp says with a chuckle. Yet going to the bathroom doesn't have to trigger anxiety. Here's some advice he gives his patients.

1

DON'T THINK OF HAVING A BOWEL MOVEMENT AS A COMPETITION. "The key is what's normal for you," Dr. Popp says.

2

ESTABLISH A BATHROOM ROUTINE. Set aside a regular time each day—after breakfast or when you've finished dinner—for a visit to the bathroom. Make sure you're not disturbed. "Every morning after breakfast, sit down, but don't become upset if you don't score the perfect 10 BM," Dr. Popp says.

3

ADD FIBER GRADUALLY. If you're currently eating 5 to 7 grams of fiber each day and set a goal of 25 grams, don't adjust your diet overnight. "It's a huge mistake to take too much too soon," Dr. Popp advises. "Always start with a very low dose. And make simple substitutions. Replacing a serving of white rice with brown rice will give you triple the amount of fiber." ■

tions, antispasmodic drugs, iron supplements, and anticonvulsants used for epilepsy can also slow your bowel movements.

Older adults are more likely to report problems with constipation than young people. That's because they're more likely to take constipating drugs, and they're less likely to exercise, eat adequate amounts of fiber, and drink enough fluids.

Constipation in older women may also be linked to pelvic muscles weakened as a result of pregnancy and childbirth.

For Immediate Relief

Answer nature's call. Yes, the kids are clamoring for breakfast–now. That doesn't mean it's prudent to ignore your urge to have a bowel movement. People who ignore the need to go to the bathroom may eventually stop feeling the urge–and that can lead to constipation. If you're already constipated, don't sit and strain. It's better to wait until you feel the urge to go, and then try.

Try a home remedy. Craig Rubin, MD, professor of internal medicine at the University of Texas Southwestern Medical Center in Dallas, suggests mixing ½ cup of unprocessed bran, available in most supermarkets, and ½ cup of applesauce with ⅓ cup of prune juice. Refrigerate the mixture, then take 2 to 3 tablespoons after dinner and drink a tall glass of water. If needed, increase your dosage to 3 to 4 tablespoons. The mixture will keep for about 2 weeks in the refrigerator.

Find flax. Two tablespoons of nutty-tasting flax each day may offer enough insoluble fiber to keep you regular. To make a flax-rich breakfast smoothie, combine 1 cup of orange juice, one banana, and 2 rounded tablespoons of ground flaxseed (317 calories, 11 grams of fat, 12 grams of fiber). Always refrigerate ground flaxseed.

Consider a little extra help. Metamucil and other over-the-counter fiber supplements may help ease symptoms. Miralax, a laxative that doctors prescribe, has been found to be effective. Other meds can help. Stool softeners (Colace and Surfak) moisten stool to make it easier to pass; saline laxatives such as Milk of Magnesia draw water into the colon to help stool move along; and lubricants such a mineral oil grease the stool.

Analyze your routine. Have you changed your diet, workouts, or work schedule? Any deviation from your routine can trigger a change in your bowel habits. Are you taking any medication that might be constipating? Ask yourself these questions to determine if you are truly constipated: Do I have a hard time passing stools? Am I having fewer bowel movements than I normally have each week? Do I have pain during bowel movements? Do I have other problems, such as bleeding? Always talk to your doctor about these symptoms. While occasional constipation is nothing to worry about, these can be symptoms of serious conditions.

Relax. Deep breathing can help you relax all over–including your digestive tract, says Lin

when to see a doctor

If you've had any change in your usual bowel habits, or if you notice blood in the stool, call your doctor right away. It's probably nothing serious, but these and other changes could be a sign of cancer or other grave illnesses.

"Blood in the stool, a change in bowel habits, a thinning of the stools—all are red flags to call your physician, especially if they occurred out of nowhere," says William J. Snape Jr., MD, medical director at the Center for Neurogastroenterology and Motility at California Pacific Medical Center.

Yet some patients procrastinate, fearing the truth—and the medical tests, says John W. Popp Jr., MD, clinical professor of medicine at the University of South Carolina School of Medicine in Columbia. "Patients will say, 'The doctor is putting a lighted tube where? No way.' The biggest fear is the fear of the unknown."

Several other symptoms should send you to a doctor, too. They include weight loss, severe abdominal pain, and a change in your bowel pattern—either the frequency or the consistency of your bowel movements.

Sometimes straining to have a bowel movement causes a small amount of the intestinal lining to protrude from the rectal opening in a condition known as a rectal prolapse. Mucus staining on the undergarments is a symptom.

Abdominal pain and bloating, combined with constipation, could signal an intestinal obstruction.

Chang, MD, co-director for the Center for Neurovisceral Sciences and Health at University of California at Los Angeles. For example, focus on how your stomach moves as you inhale for a count of 4 and exhale. Do this twice daily for 15 minutes.

Consider biofeedback for serious cases. Some patients suffer from abnormalities in the structure of the rectum and anus, conditions doctors call anorectal dysfunction or anismus. Women with anismus cannot relax the anal and rectal muscles used during bowel movements. Some people with these disorders may get relief by using biofeedback to retrain their muscles after they receive instructions on the procedure from their doctors.

For Long-Term Relief

home remedies

Drink when you're dry—and then some. Juices and other liquids such as water may help make bowel movements softer and easier to pass. Aim for eight 8-ounce glasses each day.

Fill up on fiber. "Fiber is very important, and a lot of people will say, 'But I eat bran cereal,' mistakenly thinking they're getting a whole day's worth," says Dr. Popp. Eat six servings of fruits and vegetables and three servings of whole grains every day, says James W. Anderson, MD, professor emeritus of medicine and clinical nutrition at the University of Kentucky and chair of the National Fiber Council. If you replace your cup of Rice Krispies (zero grams) with just ½ cup of Fiber One cereal, you start the day with

14 grams of fiber. Add a couple of apples after lunch and dinner (4 grams apiece), snack on an ounce of dried whole almonds in the late afternoon (3 grams), and down 1 cup of chopped, cooked broccoli at dinner (5 grams), and you'll easily exceed your daily goal. Don't forget to eat your vegetables. Brussels sprouts, carrots, potatoes, and sweet potatoes with their skins are especially helpful to people with constipation. Just don't stuff yourself with fiber while you're constipated, says Dr. Raymond. "Adding fiber is like adding straw to mud and making adobe bricks. Fiber is good when you are having bowel movements, albeit sluggish ones, but fiber and fiber supplements such as Metamucil are terrible when you're constipated."

Get physical. Doctors aren't sure why, but regular exercise might help your system stay regular. If you have heart disease, emphysema, or any chronic illness, ask your doctor before you start exercising or change your routine. Even if you are healthy, don't think you have to be a marathon runner. A 20- to 30-minute walk, every day, should be enough.

Use laxatives prudently. The key words are temporarily and occasionally. "If you're taking a constipating drug like an antihistamine or have an acute illness that causes constipation, it's perfectly acceptable to take a laxative," Dr. Popp says. When you finish the drug or recover from your illness, drop the laxative or risk becoming dependent. "The more you use laxatives, the more your bowel depends on them, and eventually the bowel may stop working," Dr. Popp says.

cough

Pollen. Dust. Hair spray. Dander from dogs and cats. Secondhand smoke. Every day you're breathing in these and other environmental particles as well as toxic or irritant gases or vapors. They're like sand in the sheets, itchy and bothersome, and your body tries to get rid of them with a good cough.

If you have allergies or a cold, of course, the problem comes from within. Coughing is your body's way of getting rid of mucus buildup that makes it hard for you to breathe. If you have gastroesophageal reflux disease—the backward flow of stomach acid into the esophagus—you may cough as your acid-bathed airways go into spasm. Some medications, including ACE inhibitors for high blood pressure, can also cause a chronic cough.

"Cough can be as trivial as a little water down the wrong pipe and as serious as pneumonia," says David L. Katz, MD, MPH, director of the Yale Griffin Prevention Research Center and author of *The Way to Eat*. "That's why it's so important to keep an eye on it."

There are two main types of coughs: "dry" coughs, which are usually caused by simple irritation, and mucus-filled, "productive" coughs, which are often a sign of colds or other upper respiratory infections or of inflammation occurring for noninfectious reasons. Some coughs are chronic and persistent, depending on the cause and treatment (or lack of it) received.

A persistent cough—one that lasts more than 3 weeks—and certain temporary coughs may be caused by a number of serious illnesses. A medical examination and laboratory tests may be necessary for diagnosis and specific therapy.

You can also practice a little diagnosing—at least, to tell you when it's time to call the doctor. "A dry cough might be totally benign," says Dr. Katz. "But if the cough is producing sputum with a color, it could be a sign of an infection. Add a fever and it's more serious still. Or layer on chest pain and blood and you need immediate emergency attention."

Coughs associated with a specific episode, such as a respiratory infection or a brief exposure to a toxic environmental substance, may also require medical treatment. They usually clear up on their own, but they can make women miserable in the meantime. Here are a few ways to soothe them fast.

For Immediate Relief

home remedies

Get plenty of fluids. Doctors usually advise drinking at least eight 8-ounce glasses of water, juices, or other nondehydrating fluids daily when you have a cough that produces secretions. The extra fluids thin mucus so it's easier to expel. If you're drinking fruit juices—it's a good idea to chose one that's rich in infection-fighting vitamin C, such as orange, grapefruit, or pineapple juice—reduce the amount of sugar by diluting the juice by half or stirring a small amount into a glass of water.

Suck on cough drops or lozenges. The juices will coat irritated cough receptors at the back of the throat, which can help suppress dry

---

THREE THINGS I TELL EVERY FEMALE PATIENT

WILLIAM J. HALL, MD, *Paul Fine Professor of Medicine and director of the Center for Healthy Aging at the University of Rochester School of Medicine in New York, advises women with pesky coughs to do the following.*

1 TRY TO AVOID DECONGESTANT NOSE SPRAYS. Even though they can reduce coughs caused by postnasal drip, they often increase symptoms as soon as you quit using them.

2 USE COUGH SUPPRESSANTS SPARINGLY. People who use these medications for long periods of time may experience high blood pressure, increased heart rate, or other side effects. Don't take them longer than 2 to 3 days without a medical examination.

3 DON'T INSIST ON ANTIBIOTICS. If you have a bacterial infection, your doctor will prescribe them, but most coughs are caused by viruses, which aren't affected by antibiotics. ■

coughs. (Make sure to brush your teeth afterward if you're sucking on sugared products.)

Try some honey. An old-time remedy for cough—honey in tea or warm water with lemon—may help. In one study, children with upper respiratory tract infections given 2 teaspoons of honey at bedtime reduced nighttime coughing and improved sleep—and worked as well as an OTC cough syrup.

Breathe some steam. Humidification may help if your house is very dry or if your sinuses are congested. It decreases the viscosity of mucus, which makes it easier to cough up. The easiest way to steam your airways is to enjoy a long shower or bath. At night, plug in a vaporizer or humidifier until you feel relief. The moist air will soothe your airways while you sleep. You can also boil a pot of water, remove it from the heat, and let it cool a little. Then put your head over the pot with a towel over your head and breathe deeply. You can always add a few drops of rosemary, eucalyptus, thyme, or peppermint essential oils. "This will help you get a steady flow of mucus over the whole mucus membrane, rather than having patches of mucus sticking around in certain areas," says Irwin Ziment, MD, professor emeritus of clinical medicine at the David Geffen School of Medicine at the University of California at Los Angeles and Olive View-UCLA Medical Center.

alternative therapies

Try an herbal soother. Some herbs contain mucilage, a slippery substance that coats irritated tissues in the throat. Two of the best are marshmallow root and slippery elm, which can be brewed into teas. Pour ½ cup of boiling water over 1 teaspoon of powdered herb. Sip throughout the day. You can also buy slippery elm lozenges at drugstores and health food stores.

Use a natural expectorant. Some herbs are nature's equivalent of over-the-counter expectorants. Herbal supplements and teas that may be helpful include horehound, thyme, and eucalyptus. Make thyme tea by steeping 2 teaspoons of the herb in 1 cup of water for 10 minutes. Drink this 3 times a day. If you want to try

when to see a doctor

 If your coughs are accompanied by blood in the mucus or by symptoms such as chest pain, wheezing, or shortness of breath, or if they persist or get worse, call your doctor right away. You could have a serious infection or other problem that won't clear up without proper diagnosis and medical treatment. Bacterial infections will require treatment with antibiotics. Just a few of the serious conditions that can cause long-term coughing are asthma, heart disease, and lung cancer.

If you're coughing a lot and also have persistent heartburn. A condition called esophageal reflux, in which stomach acid splashes into the esophagus, often causes chronic coughs.

If you've been coughing for more than 3 weeks. You may have a chronic cough caused by certain drugs you're taking, such as angiotensin-converting enzyme (ACE) inhibitors. Coughs may also be caused by nervousness or emotional and psychological problems.

eucalyptus leaf, 3 times a day take 6 drops of a 1:1 tincture or 30 drops of a 1:5 tincture.

Try ginger. Ginger tea can help to thin secretions when you have a thick, mucus-heavy cough. To make ginger tea, take an inch-long piece of fresh ginger root, cut it into very thin strips, and simmer covered in a cup of water for 7 to 8 minutes. Strain the mixture and add honey and lemon to taste.

Choose the right medicine. If you have a productive cough (it's annoying, but a good thing), you can speed it on its way by taking an OTC expectorant that contains guaifenesin (such as Robitussin). To suppress a dry cough, doctors usually recommend products that contain dextromethorphan (like Triaminic DM) or codeine.

dandruff

t isn't painful, but if you've ever flicked a sprinkle of white dead skin cells off your new black dress, you know that it's embarrassing. But dandruff isn't a sign that you're guilty of poor hygiene or a symptom of something more serious.

Dead skin cells are constantly flaking from the surface of the scalp, only to be replaced with new, identical cells. In people with dandruff, the cells proliferate at an abnormal rate, which is what produces the visible accumulation of white flakes.

About 20 percent of adults have dandruff. Doctors still aren't sure what causes the skin cells to go into overdrive. One factor appears to be a fungus called *Pityrosporum ovale*, which is thought to irritate the scalp and cause an increase in flaking, says Steven Mays, MD, associate clinical professor of dermatology at the University of Texas Medical School at Houston. Another irritant is a yeast-like fungus called malassezia that feeds on the oils in your hair follicles, irritating

your scalp and causing more skin cells to form.

There isn't a long-term cure for dandruff, but most people can control the flakes with a few simple strategies.

For Immediate Relief

Wash your hair daily. It's fine to use your regular shampoo at first. Frequent washing doesn't eliminate dandruff, but it will remove flakes before they have a chance to accumulate and become visible, says Dr. Mays.

One problem with frequent washing is that it may damage the hair shafts. This is especially true for African Americans, whose hair fractures easily. If you can't wash your hair daily, do it 3 or 4 times a week, Dr. Mays advises.

Wash with cool water. Hot water dries the scalp. This doesn't cause dandruff, but it does encourage dead skin cells to flake away and become visible.

Keep your blow-dryer at a distance. Hold it at least 10 inches from your hair, and use the low setting. The reduction in heat allows skin cells to stay moist, which makes them more likely to stay out of sight, on the surface of the scalp.

Switch to a medicated shampoo. If you can't control dandruff with a regular shampoo, use a dandruff shampoo. These products contain one of six active ingredients: ketoconazole, coal tar, sulfur, pyrithione zinc, or selenium sulfide, which help eliminate dandruff-causing fungi from the scalp; or salicylic acid, which breaks up clumps of skin cells and makes them easier to remove.

Dr. Mays recommends starting with a shampoo that contains ketoconazole (such as Nizoral). "It is available over the counter, and it's very effective."

Give shampoos time to work. It takes time for the active ingredients in medicated shampoos to soak into the surface of the scalp. When you take a bath or shower, lather your hair right away, then wait 1 to 3 minutes before rinsing out the shampoo.

Apply warm oil. Before you go to bed at night, massage 8 to 10 drops of olive oil or mineral oil on your scalp. "The scales are so thick sometimes that medicated shampoos can't get into the scalp," says Dr. Mays. "Applying oil will soften and remove scaly buildups."

After applying the oil, cover your hair with a shower cap, then wash out the oil in the morning with a regular or medicated shampoo.

when to see a doctor

If dandruff persists for several weeks even though you're using several medicated shampoos, see a dermatologist. "You'll probably need a prescription steroid solution to control scalp inflammation," says Steven Mays, MD, associate clinical professor of dermatology at the University of Texas Medical School at Houston. The dermatologist will also examine your scalp to ensure that there is not another cause for the excessive scaling.

If the flaking extends from the scalp to the eyebrows, the sides of the nose, or behind the ears. You may have a related skin condition called seborrheic dermatitis, which requires medical attention.

For Long-Term Relief

home remedies

Alternate shampoos. Skin cells on the scalp quickly become resistant to the active ingredients in medicated shampoos. "People should probably buy shampoos with three different active ingredients and alternate them daily," says Dr. Mays.

Test tar-based shampoos. They're very effective, but they often leave a brown stain in light-colored hair. Try other products first, Dr. Mays advises. If your hair is brown or black, a tar shampoo is probably a good choice to include in your hair-care routine.

Get a little sun. Ultraviolet rays in small doses are good for dandruff. No sunbathing, though. Just spend a little time in the sun with your head uncovered. Use sunscreen on your skin.

Deal with the stress in your life. Dandruff tends to flare up during stressful times, says Dr. Mays. You may be able to keep it from getting worse by relaxing a little more—going for long walks, leaving work at the office on weekends, and generally allowing yourself to unwind a little more.

depression

We all feel sad or discouraged from time to time, and usually we know why. It might be a troubled relationship, problems at work, or simply the winter blahs. As time passes, we work through the problems, and our moods begin to brighten.

Depression is an entirely different matter. "It's more than just a down mood," says depression drug researcher Jack G. Modell, MD, former professor of psychiatry at the University of Alabama in Birmingham and now a vice president at GlaxoSmithKline. "With depression, your feelings are controlling you, and you feel as though you just can't get past them."

Biological, hormonal, life cycle, and sociological factors may predispose women to depression. Women are twice as likely as men to suffer from depression and are particularly vulnerable after giving birth, when hormones and the responsibility of caring for a newborn can be overwhelming. Many women also suffer from depression before and during their periods, and later, in perimenopause, or when they have to juggle double caregiving duties—for children and aging parents—while in the workforce.

Signs of depression include loss of pleasure in daily activities, diminished appetite, difficulty concentrating, changes in your usual sleep patterns, and feelings of sadness, guilt, or worthlessness.

"If you start having three, four, or five symptoms every day for most of the day, and the feelings persist for more than 2 weeks, it's time for concern," says Kelly Conforti, PhD, a clinical psychologist in Albuquerque, New Mexico.

Depression can also contribute to other conditions, including heart disease, stroke, and diabetes, and may lead to suicide.

The treatments for depression—everything from medications and "talk therapy" to changes in lifestyle—can be surprisingly effective: Up to 80 percent of those who seek treatment will notice rapid improvement, usually within a few weeks.

For Immediate Relief

Put pleasure on your schedule. Every day, jot down a few enjoyable activities—going for a walk, enjoying a long bath, or simply perusing a magazine that you haven't had time to read—that you're going to do. Give them the same priority that you would a serious business appointment.

"We have too many 'shoulds' in our lives and not enough things that are enjoyable. That can lead to depression," says Dr. Conforti.

Walk off the pain. Study after study confirms that regular exercise can reduce depression in men and women across all age categories. In one study done at Duke University, people with major depression who exercised aerobically were just as like as people on antidepressants to have their moods lift. But 6 months later, those who kept up their exercise were more likely to be fully or partially recovered than those who took drugs.

Meditate. A 2010 Canadian study found that people who used mindfulness-based meditation—which teaches you to treat your thoughts nonjudgmentally and yourself with compassion—were just as likely as people on antidepressants to avoid a depression relapse after recovery.

Get enough calcium. Research suggests that women who experience premenstrual depression may feel better when they consume calcium. One study found that women who took 1,200 mg of elemental calcium daily in the form of calcium carbonate experienced more than a 50 percent reduction in their premenstrual syndrome symptoms.

The best sources of calcium are low-fat milk and cheese. Many juices and breakfast cereals are fortified with calcium, says Mary Lake Polan, MD, PhD, professor and chairperson of the department of gynecology and obstetrics at Stanford University School of Medicine.

Go to the light. During the fall and winter, some people suffer from a seasonal depression called seasonal affective disorder, or SAD, a biochemical brain imbalance caused by lack of sunlight in the winter. You can always winter in a sunny clime, but if that's not in the cards, exposure for 30 to 60 minutes a day to a very bright light from a special fluorescent lamp that mimics sunlight can help lift your mood.

THREE THINGS I TELL EVERY FEMALE PATIENT

JACK G. MODELL, MD, *a psychiatrist, depression drug researcher and vice president of GlaxoSmithKline, offers the following advice for coping with depression.*

1 **EXERCISE DAILY.** It boosts levels of chemicals in the brain that regulate mood. "If all you can do at first is 5 minutes, that's fine," he says. Research has shown that people who exercise regularly are less likely to stay depressed. They'll also recover more quickly when their moods head south.

2 **GET SOME SUN.** Exposure to sunlight triggers the release of melatonin in the brain. Melatonin regulates your sleep and wake cycles, and it can have a powerful effect on energy and mood.

3 **SHARE YOUR PROBLEMS WITH FAMILY AND FRIENDS.** Chances are, others have experienced the same feelings. Their understanding and emotional support will go a long way toward helping you feel better. ■

Try Saint-John's-wort. This herb appears to help maintain healthful levels of mood-regulating brain chemicals. Take 300 mg of Saint-John's-wort extract 3 times daily. It may interact with other medications, including some antidepressants. Don't combine it with other drugs without checking with your doctor first.

Consider electroacupuncture. One study found that acupuncture using needles that transmit a slight electric current were as good as some antidepressants at reducing depression symptoms.

Sniff some fragrances. A Korean study found that in 40 patients with arthritis who were also suffering from depression, using aromatherapy (the scents of lavender, marjoram, eucalyptus, rosemary, and peppermint blended with almond, apricot, and jojoba oil) reduced both pain and depression significantly. A similar study in which aromatherapy was combined with hand massage reduced depression in 28 patients with terminal cancer in a Korean hospice.

For Long-Term Relief

Stay in touch with your friends. It might be the best medicine for depression. A British study found that 65 percent of women with depression who met for 1 hour weekly with a volunteer "befriender" experienced a remission compared with 39 percent of those who didn't get the extra support. That's about the same success rate that's seen in conventional therapy or from taking drugs, says study author Tirril Harris, PhD, a researcher with the Socio-Medical Research Group in London.

Manage negative thoughts. You have a surprising amount of control over the ideas and beliefs that flit through your mind. People are more likely to suffer from depression when they embrace negative thoughts, such as "I've wasted my life" or "This is the worst thing that's ever happened."

Turn the thoughts around, Dr. Conforti advises. "When you tell yourself things like 'Things are getting better' or 'I've made

when to see a doctor

If you're feeling "blue" and are also experiencing physical problems, such as fatigue or unexplained changes in your weight, see your family doctor. Many symptoms of depression mimic those caused by underlying medical problems, says Kelly Conforti, PhD, a clinical psychologist in Albuquerque, New Mexico.

If your depressive feelings last longer than 2 weeks, or if you're thinking about suicide or death. These are symptoms of clinical depression, and you'll need professional help right away.

If you've had depression in the past, and you suspect that it's coming back. It is estimated that 50 to 60 percent of people who have had one episode of major depression will have another episode during their lives.

mistakes, but I think I can improve things,' you'll decrease your feelings of sadness or depression."

Stay in touch with your spirituality. "Studies have shown that people who are active in their churches or synagogues and feel a connection with God or some higher power have less depression," says Dr. Modell.

medical options

See a professional. Full-fledged depression is unlikely to disappear on its own. If your symptoms are mild, regular visits with a thera-pist are probably all you need. For more severe depression or low moods that linger (a condition called dysthymia), antidepressant medications may be added.

"The best treatment is often a combination of therapy and medications," says Dr. Modell. "Therapy will help you understand why you were having problems in the first place, and the medications will give you the energy and strength to make the most of the therapy."

For more information on depression. Visit the Web site of the National Institute of Mental Health at www.nimh.nih.gov.

diarrhea

Diarrhea. The runs. Montezuma's revenge. These are just a few of the terms used to describe the loose, watery stools that most people get, on average, about 4 times a year. Diarrhea is so common that it's second only to respiratory infections as the most commonly reported illness in the United States.

Doctors divide diarrhea into two categories. Acute diarrhea, which tends to clear up within a few days, is typically caused by minor intestinal infections, or by the hot peppers on your favorite, hold-nothing-back pizza. "Who hasn't gone to a summertime picnic and picked up something from the potato salad?" says Patricia Raymond, MD, gastroenterologist and assistant professor at Eastern Virginia Medical School. Chronic diarrhea, on the other hand, can last 3 weeks or more. It's also caused by infections or by more serious conditions, such as diabetes or inflammatory bowel disease.

Diarrhea rarely requires medical treatment, including the use of over-the-counter antidiarrhea medications. The drugs are effective, but they can trap bacteria or parasites in the intestine and slow your recovery.

Here are some better ways to reduce discomfort and speed diarrhea on its way.

For Immediate Relief

home remedies

Try yogurt. A cup of yogurt with live cultures, or probiotics, may bring you relief if your diarrhea stems from an infection. "It helps restore the balance of good and bad bacteria in your digestive tract," says Barbara Harland, PhD, professor in the department of nutritional sciences at Howard University College of Pharmacy, Nursing and Allied Health Sciences in Washington, DC.

Follow the BRAT diet. The letters stand for bananas, rice, applesauce, and toast. Each of these foods is very easy for your body to digest. Following the diet for a few days will give your intestines a chance to recover. "I like those microwaveable packets of Uncle Ben's rice," says Raymond. "You pop it in and in a few minutes you have a dish of rice flavored with chicken–and when everything is moving through you, it's awfully comforting to have something good stay in."

Drink a lot of fluids. Diarrhea removes a tremendous amount of water from the body. When you lose water, you also lose electrolytes, essential minerals that you need to be healthy. Plain water will replace fluids but it won't replace electrolytes.

"You need liquid with some substance to it, such as chicken broth," says Christine L. Frissora, MD, associate professor of medicine in the Division of Gastroenterology and Hepatology at the

Weill Cornell Medical College of Cornell University in New York City. Or you can drink rehydration solutions (available at drugstores), such as Pedialyte, which can also be used by adults.

For Long-Term Prevention

home remedies

Connect food with outbreaks. Do you find that you have diarrhea 30 minutes to 2 hours after you drink milk or eat dairy products? You may be lactose intolerant, meaning you lack an enzyme that helps you digest the sugar in dairy. You can take an over-the-counter tablet that contains the missing enzyme or buy dairy products developed for people like you.

Check out your sweeteners. If the product you're eating is sugar free, check to see if it's sweetened by sugar alcohols such as mannitol and sorbitol, which cause diarrhea in some people.

Take some of the heat out of your diet. Hot peppers add a lot of zest to pizzas, enchiladas, and other delicious foods, but they contain a fiery compound called capsaicin, which may trigger watery stools.

WHAT WORKS FOR ME

CHRISTINE L. FRISSORA, MD, *associate professor of medicine in the Division of Gastroenterology and Hepatology at the Weill Cornell Medical College of Cornell University in New York City, occasionally travels overseas. Here's how she protects herself.*

"I take Pepto-Bismol in tablet form to prevent diarrhea. I chew one tablet 2 times a day. It's so handy because you can just toss the package in your purse. People who take Pepto-Bismol sometimes get alarmed when their tongues or the stools temporarily turn black. It's the body's normal response to the medicine. It's nothing to worry about." ■

Wash your hands often. Your risk of getting intestinal infections will drop dramatically if you wash your hands often, especially before meals and after using the bathroom.

Travel wisely. It's not a coincidence that millions of Americans get diarrhea during the travel season. Water quality and food sanitation aren't always optimal in foreign countries, and your intestines may pay the price. Important travelers' guidelines include:

- Always use bottled water for drinking or brushing your teeth. Don't drink ice water unless you're sure the ice was made from sterilized water.

- Only eat fruits that you peel yourself, such as papayas, pineapple, or mangoes.

- Avoid raw vegetables or salad greens.

- Eat your meals in restaurants. Street vendors often sell delicious foods, but the risk of contamination is high.

diverticular disease

From the beginning of human history to the end of the 1800s, humans survived by eating whole grains, legumes, and other plant-based foods. They enjoyed meat, but it wasn't on the menu very often. And they certainly didn't eat the highly processed foods that we enjoy today.

Before thanking your lucky stars for progress, consider this: Diverticular disease, a condition in which portions of the intestinal wall weaken and bulge, used to be a rarity. Today, as many as half of older American adults (ages 60 to 80) have these intestinal pockets, and almost everyone over age 80 has diverticulosis. The disease is often silent; many people have it for decades without even knowing. But in some cases it results in cramps, diarrhea, bloating, or rectal bleeding. When the diverticula becomes inflamed or abscessed, it's called diverticulitis, meaning an inflammation of the diverticula, a serious condition that can cause perforation and internal bleeding.

What's the connection between the modern diet and diverticular disease? It all comes down to fiber. The kind found in plant foods absorbs water in the intestine. It makes stools larger as well as softer, which decreases the amount of pressure that's required to push them out of the body.

Americans today, however, only get about half of *Prevention*'s recommended 25 to 35 grams of fiber a day. A low-fiber diet produces stools that are smaller and harder than they should be, which means that the intestine has to exert more pressure to push them along. The increase in pressure may cause the intestinal wall to bulge, much like a weak spot on a tire. In addition, a low-fiber diet often results in constipation. The harder it is to move your bowels, the more you strain—and straining increases pressure in the intestine.

Once the bulges, or diverticula, form in the intestinal wall, you have them for good. However, there are a few ways to reduce the discomfort and also prevent them from forming.

For Immediate Relief

home remedies

Ease cramping with heat. One of the most common symptoms of diverticular disease is cramping, which often occurs after meals. A quick way to reduce the discomfort is to hold a hot-water bottle wrapped in a towel or a heating pad on your abdomen for 10 to 15 minutes. You can repeat the treatment as often as necessary to get relief.

Include more fiber in your diet. While the jury is still out on whether fiber can ease the painful effects of diverticular disease, the overall advantages of fiber make it worth while to give it a try.

when to see a doctor

If you're having severe abdominal cramps, or if the cramps are accompanied by fever, call your doctor immediately. People with diverticulosis sometimes develop an infection in one of the intestinal pockets, a potentially serious condition called diverticulitis. You'll probably need antibiotics to knock out the infection.

If you're having rectal bleeding. It's often caused by hemorrhoids, but it can also occur in those with diverticular disease. If the bleeding is severe, you could need surgery to correct the problem.

For Long-Term Prevention

home remedies

Eat more fruits and vegetables. Aim for eating five vegetables and four fruits a day. Along with legumes and whole grains, they're among the best sources of intestine-protecting fiber. In a study published in the *British Medical Journal*, researchers compared the stools of Africans, who primarily ate a very high fiber diet, with those of Europeans, who filled up mainly on a refined Western diet low in fiber. They found that the stools of the Africans were bigger and moved much more quickly through the intestine.

Buy whole grain breads and flour. Even if you don't eat a lot of fruits or vegetables, you can get substantial amounts of fiber just by eating whole grain breads. Try to incorporate three to six servings of whole grains into your diet every day. "Two-thirds of the fiber in flour is lost in modern milling," says Karen Heitzman, MD, an internist with a specialty in geriatrics in private practice in Manlius, NY. "Diverticular disease would be a disease none of us ever heard of if flour milling had not been invented."

Track fiber the easy way. Unless you walk around with a calculator in one hand and nutritional charts in the other, it's hard to tell when you're getting enough fiber to prevent diverticulosis. One way to make it easier is to follow these general rules.

▪ A serving of fruits or vegetables has at least 1 gram of fiber. If you have fruit at breakfast, lunch, and dinner, plus a couple of servings of vegetables at dinner and a high-fiber cereal–some of which provide more than 10 grams of fiber—in the morning, you'll almost automatically get all the fiber that you need.

- Consider a fiber boost. If you find that you're not getting a lot of fiber in your diet—a common problem for those who travel or who eat away from home a lot—you may want to take a fiber supplement. Found in the laxative aisle in pharmacies, fiber supplements such as psyllium (found in Metamucil and Hydrocil) and methylcellulose (found in Citrucel) are an excellent way to supplement the fiber in your diet. Find one that is pleasant tasting, and take it 1 to 3 times a day when you cannot get your usual food sources of fiber.

- Think about flax. Flaxseed contains fiber so it's a natural laxative.

Drink plenty of water. It's absorbed by the fiber in the stools, which makes them larger as well as softer. This can help prevent constipation and the straining that accompanies it. Doctors advise drinking eight full glasses of water every day.

Follow a regular routine. The urge to have a bowel movement, called the gastrocolonic reflex, is usually strongest in the morning after breakfast. If you sometimes suffer from constipation, it's worth listening to the body's "gotta go" signals. The longer you wait, the harder it may be to move your bowels later.

Slim down. Diverticular disease is associated with obesity.

medical options

Talk to your doctor if you overuse painkillers. Several studies have suggested that use of NSAIDs and acetaminophen on a regular basis is linked to a higher risk for bleeding and other severe symptoms of diverticular disease.

For more information on diverticular disease. Go online to visit the Web site of the National Institute of Diabetes and Digestive and Kidney Diseases at www.niddk.nih.gov.

dizziness and vertigo

Dancing in circles is fun. Ferris wheels and merry-go-rounds are fun. What isn't fun is feeling as though the world is whirling even when you're sitting still.

Dizziness that comes from out of the blue is surprisingly common, especially among older adults. Approximately 90 million Americans suffer from occasional dizziness, and about one in five adults ages 60 and older says that it interferes with their daily lives.

One common form of dizziness is called vertigo. Caused by inflammation or damage in the inner ear, vertigo can make you feel as though the world is spinning around you, says Gordon B. Hughes, MD, program officer for clinical trials for the National Institute on Deafness and Other Communication Disorders in Bethesda, MD.

Other forms of dizziness or light-headedness may be caused by poor circulation, side effects from medications, or a condition called orthostatic hypotension, in which blood pressure temporarily drops when you're changing position–while bending over to tie your shoes, for example, or getting out of bed in the morning. Meniere's disease, acoustic neuroma (a benign nerve tissue tumor), multiple sclerosis, and migraine headache can also cause vertigo. The most common form of the condition is benign paroxysmal positional vertigo (BPPV), which occurs when small calcium "stones" in your fluid-filled ear canal roll back and forth and throw off your body's system for letting your brain know how your body is positioned. You can also experience dizziness as the result of your emotions, a condition called psychogenic dizziness.

"Time alone cures most inner ear problems," Dr. Hughes adds. "But dizziness and vertigo can be disabling because they often occur without warning and can cause people to become reclusive or avoid their normal activities."

However, with a combination of medical care and home treatments, most people can reduce or even eliminate the discomfort.

For Immediate Relief
home remedies

Steady yourself. If you feel an attack of dizziness or vertigo coming on and you must walk, lightly rest your fingers on a table or another familiar piece of furniture. "The brain senses the touch and tells the legs what posture to maintain," says Dr. Hughes. Sit down or lie down, if possible.

Flex your legs. If you have orthostatic hypotension, the blood tends to pool in the legs and feet. Flexing your leg muscles before you stand up–by crossing and uncrossing your legs, for example–will help push blood back into circulation.

One study found that when men and women with orthostatic hypotension flexed their thigh and buttock muscles, their blood pressure upon standing rose by 30 percent, according to study coauthor Phillip Low, MD, professor of neurology and a researcher at the Mayo Clinic.

Hold your head still. Dizziness is often triggered by movement. Lying still for a few minutes will allow blood pressure to stabilize, and it also may reduce "confusion" in the inner ear.

THREE THINGS I TELL EVERY FEMALE PATIENT

GORDON B. HUGHES, MD, *program officer for clinical trials for the National Institute on Deafness and Other Communication Disorders in Bethesda, MD, offers this advice for people with dizziness or vertigo.*

1 **DON'T WALK IN DARKNESS.** "If you're having trouble with your inner ear or the balance in your legs, keeping a light on and using your vision will help keep you properly oriented."

2 **WEAR FLAT SHOES.** They allow your feet to maintain a firm platform on the ground, which sends posture information signals to the brain.

3 **AVOID RISKY ACTIVITIES.** Forget ladders: If you're having trouble with dizziness or vertigo, getting on a ladder or other unstable surface is an accident waiting to happen. ■

Be careful after hot baths or showers. "When you're in a hot bath, the blood vessels dilate in order to dissipate the heat," says Robert Peterka, PhD, an associate scientist at the Neurological Sciences Institute at Oregon Health and Science University in Portland. "If you get up too quickly, your brain may not get enough blood, which will make you temporarily feel light-headed."

Get out of bed slowly. This allows your blood pressure to adjust to the change in position, which can prevent dizziness in some cases, says Dr. Hughes. When you're ready to get up, swing your legs over the side of the bed and rise to a sitting position. Wait for a minute or two, then slowly stand up.

Use safety gear. To prevent falls around the house, make sure you have nightlights in every room and in the hallways and handrails on your stairs and tub. Make sure you put away area rugs that have edges you can trip over and tuck power cords or phone lines out of your way.

Drink up. Dehydration can make you feel lightheaded or dizzy, so make sure you stay hydrated throughout the day.

alternative therapies

Try ginger capsules. They can help prevent the nausea that sometimes accompanies dizziness or vertigo. "If you use herbal medicines, be sure to follow the directions on the label," Dr. Hughes says.

medical options

Review your regular medications with your doctor. Many prescription and even some over-the-counter drugs, such as medications for treating high blood pressure, may cause dizziness. Make a list of all the drugs you're taking and show it to your doctor. In some cases, switching drugs is all that's necessary to eliminate the symptoms, says Dr. Hughes.

Consider antidizziness drugs. A number of prescription and OTC drugs sedate the central nervous system and shorten the duration and severity of vertigo and dizziness attacks.

"You can take them around the clock if dizziness is frequent or severe," says Dr. Hughes. For quick relief, he recommends a prescription drug

when to see a doctor

 A yearly general checkup is always a good idea, says Gordon B. Hughes, MD, program officer for clinical trials for the National Institute on Deafness and Other Communication Disorders in Bethesda, MD.

If you're having chest pain, shortness of breath, loss of consciousness, or another new neurological symptom, call 911 or visit your emergency department at the hospital right away. These may be signs of potentially serious problems, such as a blocked coronary artery or a brain disorder.

If you've had a recent cold or flu. Dizziness is sometimes caused by inner ear viral infections, which commonly occur after these and other respiratory infections. If symptoms do not clear within several days, see your doctor for an examination and treatment.

called lorazepam (Ativan), which is placed under the tongue. It works much more quickly than oral drugs.

For inner ear problems, which can result in nausea, your doctor may prescribe medications such as meclizine (Antivert) and diazepam (Valium), or even Dramamine, which is available over the counter. Corticosteroid drugs may also improve your symptoms.

Ask your doctor about head position therapy. If you have benign paroxysmal positional vertigo, you may benefit from a technique called the canalith repositioning procedure, which should be done by a trained therapist. It involves moving the head into different positions until the calcium particles that come loose from the inner ear return to their proper locations. Many patients who undergo this procedure once will remain symptom free. For inner ear problems, your doctor may also discuss vestibular rehabilitation (balance retraining exercises), which you learn from either a physical therapist or occupational therapist and do yourself at home.

Long-Term Solutions

home remedies

Reduce your salt intake. Vertigo caused by Meniere's disease occurs when fluid accumulates in the inner ear. One way to reduce the fluid buildup is to follow a low-salt diet, getting no more than 2,000 mg of sodium daily. "People need to read food labels to keep track of how much salt they're getting," says Dr. Hughes.

Stay physically active. People with vertigo or dizziness often lose their physical confidence and become increasingly sedentary. This can reduce the ability of the brain to monitor and fine-tune your sense of balance. "The idea is to keep moving, either with physical therapy or by getting regular exercises," says Dr. Peterka.

mind-body techniques

Reduce the stress in your life. "Emotional stress aggravates inner ear disorders, although the mechanisms aren't known," says Dr. Hughes. Your symptoms may be a sign that you need to unwind—by taking long walks, meditating, or participating in counseling or a support group.

dry eyes

f you have dry eyes, you can blame your birth control pills, other medications, or even menopause. But ophthalmologists are seeing more and more patients who are in perfect health and aren't taking drugs that leave them dry-eyed.

"Dry eyes are almost an epidemic because of our energy-efficient environment," says Stepha-

nie Marioneaux, MD, an ophthalmologist in Chesapeake, Virginia. Modern homes, buildings, and cars are so airtight that people are exposed to filtered air that contains little or no moisture, she explains. The ultra-dry air pulls moisture from the skin, hair, and nasal passages—and, of course, from the eyes.

Dry air isn't the only reason that so many people are suffering from scratchy, irritated, desert-dry eyes. Staring at computer screens doesn't help. The American Optometric Association calls it computer vision syndrome. But concentrating intensely on a book, DVD, knitting, or driving at night can also strain your eye-focusing muscles because you forget to blink. When you don't blink enough, your cornea doesn't get enough lubrication, more tears evaporate, and your eyes dry out.

Other culprits: contact lenses, hair-dryers, and the never-ending exposure to air pollution and chemical vapors. Dry eyes are also a common complication of LASIK (laser-assisted in situ keratomileusis) surgery for correction of near-sightedness.

To moisturize your eyes and ease the irritation fast, here are a few things to try.

For Immediate Relief

home remedies

Use artificial tears. Available in pharmacies, artificial tears have a similar composition to your natural tears. You can use them 6 or 8 times a day to supplement your own tear production and to soothe and moisturize the surfaces of the eyes, says Dr. Marioneaux.

It's a good idea to avoid artificial tears made with preservatives because they can trigger allergic reactions in some people, she adds. Eyedrops that are preservative-free usually carry the label "PF."

Avoid eyedrops that remove the red. They're decongestants and can dry your eyes out even more.

Humidify the air. Indoor humidifiers can be inexpensive, and they fill the air with eye-protecting moisture.

Take a break from contact lenses. No matter what kind you wear, contact lenses dry the eyes and can make them sore and irritated. When your eyes are bothering you, switch to your regular glasses for a few days. Even a short break from contacts may be enough to eliminate the irritating dryness. Talk to your doctor about special contact lenses developed for dry eyes: They rest on the whites of your eyes and create a fluid-filled layer to keep your eyes from becoming parched.

when to see a doctor

If your eyes have been dry for more than 2 weeks, or if the dryness is causing considerable discomfort, make an appointment to see an ophthalmologist. There are a number of potentially serious conditions—such as Sjögren's syndrome, thyroid disease, or lupus—that can cause dry eyes, says Sandra Belmont, MD, associate professor of ophthalmology at Cornell University in New York City.

If you have eye dryness and you're also taking medications. Ask your doctor to review your medications to see if any of them might be responsible. A number of drugs—including antihistamines, birth control pills, decongestants, and medications for depression and high blood pressure—can cause eye dryness, as can hormone replacement therapy.

Don't rub. That will just irritate your eyes even further. If they're really uncomfortable, give them some rest and relaxation with a hot compress.

medical options

Save the tears. Normally, there are plenty of tears to coat the eyes and protect the delicate surfaces. After they've done their work, the tears leave the eye through a duct called the lacrimal punctum. If you're suffering from dry eyes, your doctor may recommend plugging the duct with silicone or collagen, which allows more of the tears to stay in the eyes, says Dr. Marioneaux.

Ask about serious eyedrops. If you have a severe case of dry eyes, talk to your doctor about autologous serum eyedrops. Made from your own blood serum, these drops contain ingredients such as vitamin A and growth factors that help heal the eye and increase lubrication.

For Long-Term Relief

home remedies

Remind yourself to blink. When you're engrossed in a movie or working on a computer, you probably keep your eyes open much longer than you normally would. The tears evaporate instead of lubricating the eye surface. Try to blink 12 to 15 times a minute, says Dr. Marioneaux. Blinking spreads tears over the surfaces of the eyes, which helps prevent dryness.

Don't blow it. Direct fans, hair-dryers, and car vents away from your eyes. Both heat and air conditioning dry the air, which can irritate your eyes. Tilt the vents so that the airflow is below, above, or to the sides of your eyes.

Wear sunglasses or goggles. Women who are active often suffer from dry eyes because the rushing wind wicks away moisture. An easy, long-term solution is to wear protective goggles when you ski, cycle, or run.

earaches and ear infections

Ear pain and infections are often considered to be childhood problems. In fact, ear infections are the most common reason children visit their doctor. Adults are less likely to get ear infections and the earaches that accompany them. But we're not immune.

Infections of the middle ear often follow on the heels of colds or allergies, which cause an increase in secretions that sometimes block the narrow passageway (the eustachian tube) that connects the back of the nose to the ear. The blockage prevents normal airflow, creating an environment that's ideal for infection.

Less common, but even more painful, is swimmer's ear, a condition that occurs when moisture in the external or outer ear canal causes breaks in the skin that allow harmful germs to move in. Despite the name, it isn't caused only by swimming. "It can occur when you get water in your ears when you shower, bathe, or wash your hair," says Gregory Bergman, MD, a family practice physician in Minster, Ohio.

In some cases, an earache is radiated pain from temperomandibular joint dysfunction, a pain originating in your jaw. An earache that doesn't quit may be related to cholesteatoma, an abnormal skin growth or infected cyst in the middle ear behind the eardrum, often the result of frequent ear infections.

Some ear infections, especially those involving the external ear canal, need to be treated promptly. Apart from the fact that ear infections can be extremely painful, they can potentially cause permanent hearing loss. Here are a few ways to get them under control.

For Immediate Relief

home remedies

Soothe the pain with heat. Applying heat to the ear improves circulation and quickly reduces the painful throbbing in the outer ear. The easiest approach is to rest your head on a heating pad or hot-water bottle wrapped in a towel, says Dr. Bergman.

Make the ears less hospitable with vinegar. There's no such thing as an "ear towel" for those prone to swimmer's ear, but the next best thing is to put in a few drops made from equal amounts of white vinegar and warm water. After putting in the drops, raise your head for 3 to 5 minutes and then tilt it so the excess runs out of your ears. The solution will change the acid level in the outer ear, inhibiting the growth of bacteria and fungi, says Dr. Bergman.

Reach for the hot sauce. "Food that is so spicy that it makes your nose run can ease earaches associated with congestion," says Evelyn Kluka, MD, associate professor of clinical otorhinolaryngology at the Louisiana State School of Medicine at New Orleans. "Try a good hot-and-sour soup or, better yet, an authentic New Orleans gumbo loaded with hot peppers."

Breathe away an ache. Qigong's deep-breathing techniques may offer help for earaches and other pain. They oxygenate the body, strengthen the immune system, and open blockages, says Effie Chow, RN, PhD, a certified acupuncturist and qigong master in San Francisco and director of the Global Integrative Medicine Network.

medical options

Take antibiotics. Most ear infections are caused by bacteria, and a course of antibiotics will usually stop the pain of a middle ear infection within 3 days. If you do need antibiotics, be sure to finish the prescription, adds Dr. Bergman. It's the only way to ensure that all the harmful germs are eliminated.

Pop a painkiller. To ease severe ear pain and reduce fever, take ibuprofen or acetaminophen according to package instructions, says Donna Jean Millay, MD, associate professor of otolaryngology at the University of Vermont in Burlington. If your symptoms are related to congestion, take a decongestant, according to package instructions.

For Long-Term Prevention

home remedies

Blow away moisture. If you sometimes get earaches because of swimmer's ear, an easy

when to see a doctor

If the pain is so bad that you're thinking about taking an analgesic, call your doctor. There's a good chance that an infection is developing in the outer or middle ear, and you'll probably need antibiotics, says Gregory Bergman, MD, a family practice physician in Minster, Ohio.

If you have ear pain and there's also blood or pus coming from the ear. Your eardrum may have ruptured, and you'll need immediate medical attention.

If you've been feeling dizzy and can't figure out why. Dizziness is a common symptom of ear infections, even in the absence of pain, says Dr. Bergman.

solution is to dry the inside of the ear with a hair-dryer, says Dr. Bergman. After swimming or showering, hold the hair-dryer 8 to 12 inches away from your ear. Set the heat on low, pull your ear back with one hand, and let the dryer run for a few minutes to thoroughly dry the ear.

Keep cotton swabs out of your ears. Women often use them for removing earwax, but they irritate the ear canal and increase the risk of earaches, says Dr. Bergman.

Blow gently. Aggressive nose blowing increases pressure in the middle ear, says Dr. Bergman, which can damage delicate tissues and make you more vulnerable to infections.

Prepare for takeoff. Every year, millions of travelers experience ear pain while flying, usually during takeoffs and, more likely, landings, when the changes in air pressure are greatest. To prevent the pain, equalize the pressure in the ears. One way to do this is to repeatedly say words with a "k" sound, like koala, says Dr. Bergman. Chewing gum or swallowing repeatedly will also help. Some experts also recommend you take a decongestant every 6 hours the day before you fly and continue 24 hours after you land to shrink membranes in the sinus and ear. You can also use a nasal spray once right before you board to open the eustachian tube.

Go Frenzel on your flight. The Frenzel maneuver can help move air through eustachian tubes that are clogged during flight, says Laura Orvidas, MD an otolaryngologist at the Mayo Clinic. Simply pinch your nose and push your tongue against the back part of the roof of your mouth.

eczema

The worst part about eczema isn't necessarily the painful sores or shedding skin flakes. It may not even be the itching, which people often describe as severe. The worst part about this persistent, inflammatory skin condition is that it often appears on the face, elbows, wrists, or other visible areas. Some people are so self-conscious during flare-ups that they're reluctant to leave the house.

Doctors aren't sure what causes eczema, although it's probably linked to defects in the immune system that makes skin hypersensitive, setting it up for long-term inflammation. It runs in families, and attacks can be triggered by changes in temperature, rising or falling humidity, or even the changes of seasons, says Thomas Helm, MD, clinical professor of dermatology and pathology at the University of Buffalo School of Medicine and Biomedical Sciences.

Eczema often appears in infancy and seems to be linked with asthma, which increases your risk. Although many children outgrow it by the time they're in their teens, about 30 to 50 percent carry it into adulthood. It's not uncommon for remissions to last for months or even years. Even though there isn't a cure for eczema, most people can control it with medications and simple home care.

For Immediate Relief

home remedies

Use steroid creams. The quickest way to reduce skin inflammation and itching is to apply an over-the-counter cream that contains hydrocortisone or other steroids, says Amy S. Paller, MD, Walter J. Hamlin professor and chair of dermatology and professor of pediatrics at Northwestern University Feinberg School of Medicine in Chicago. You can apply the creams up to 2 times daily to get relief.

Keep your hands busy. Doctors advise people with eczema not to scratch—but nearly everyone ignores the advice because the itching is so intense. Still, it's good advice because scratching irritates the skin and can make the itching worse. One solution is to keep your hands busy with enjoyable activities, such as knitting, quilting, or painting.

Use a cold compress. This will help reduce itching and keep you from scratching.

Take an antihistamine. OTC products can help you deal with itching. Many will help you sleep, but if daytime itching is a problem, choose one with an nondrowsy formula.

Use moisturizers daily. They keep the skin moist and pliable, which helps stop irritation and itching. The best time to apply a moisturizer is right after you bathe or shower because it will seal in water and give it a chance to be absorbed. Use products without alcohol, scents, dyes, fragrances, and other chemicals.

For Long-Term Relief

home remedies

Take quick baths and showers. The water should be warm, not hot. Extra-long baths in hot water may trigger flare-ups in some people.

when to see a doctor

If you have eczema and your usual treatments don't clear the rash, call your doctor for advice. It's common for medications and other treatments to lose their effectiveness over time, says Thomas Helm, MD, clinical professor of dermatology and pathology at the University of Buffalo School of Medicine and Biomedical Sciences.

If your skin develops moist patches or blisters. There's a good chance that you've developed an infection, probably as a result of scratching. You may need antibiotics or other medications to stop the infection and speed healing.

Pat yourself dry. After bathing, don't rub the skin vigorously with a towel. Air-drying is best, but if you can't take that much time, pat your skin with a towel for gentle drying.

Spend some time in the sun. Exposure to the ultraviolet light in sunshine sometimes prevents flare-ups. Your doctor may "prescribe" spending 10 to 15 minutes in the sun each day.

Of course, too much sun can be just as harmful as too little. Ask your doctor whether sunshine will be helpful for you and whether you'll need to use a sunscreen to prevent skin damage.

Breast-feed your baby. This may not help your skin problems but it might prevent them from being handed down to your children. Studies have found that children who are breast-fed are less likely to get eczema, especially if the nursing mother avoids cow's milk in the diet. You may also want to avoid eggs, fish, peanuts, and soy while breastfeeding.

medical options

Calm the immune system. When eczema doesn't respond to home treatments or OTC creams, your doctor may recommend a stronger steroid cream or ointment, or medications called immunomodulators. A study of more than 1,000 children and adults showed that an immunomodulating ointment called tacrolimus improved or completely eliminated eczema in more than 80 percent of the people who used it. "They have all of the benefits of topical or oral steroids, with few of the risks," Dr. Helm says. Protopic and Elidel are brand names of this ointment.

Ask about phototherapy. A fancy word for light exposure, phototherapy involves exposing the skin to precise amounts of ultraviolet light from specialized lamps. It's a very effective way to prevent flare-ups or to help skin rashes and inflammation heal more quickly.

fatigue

Actress Angelina Jolie says her secret to juggling six kids, a film career, and a bruising schedule of charity work is . . . insomnia. She has it so she can get more done. But the rest of us—even if we aren't "lucky" enough to be insomniacs—barely have enough energy to get through the day, and the problem is getting worse all the time.

Americans are spending more time working and less time sleeping or simply having fun. According to a survey conducted by the National Sleep Foundation, 60 percent of women don't get the 7 to 8 hours of sleep that they need to feel refreshed and energized.

"Most women need that much sleep in order to wake up feeling rested and to have energy throughout the day," says Lynn Mack-Shipman, MD, an endocrinologist and assistant professor of internal medicine at the University of Nebraska Medical Center in Omaha. "Sleep deprivation is a common cause of fatigue."

It's not the only one, however. Many women

of childbearing age are low in iron. That's the mineral essential for creating hemoglobin, the iron-based protein in blood that ferries the oxygen that the body needs for energy. Thyroid conditions can also lead to fatigue, says Dr. Mack-Shipman. So can depression, anxiety and stress, which is almost at epidemic proportions these days.

"The average woman today has many responsibilities, such as a full-time job, child rearing, housework, and taking care of aging parents," says Dr. Mack-Shipman. Both personal and professional responsibilities, along with the physical burden of trying to do too much, leaves many women feeling exhausted all the time.

If fatigue is bothering you, it's a good idea to check in with your doctor for an evaluation. That's because "every conceivable illness has fatigue as a symptom," says Michael Clark, MD, MPH, MBA, a psychiatrist and the director of the Chronic Pain Treatment Program at Johns Hopkins. In most cases, however, it's possible to recharge your batteries with a variety of at-home techniques.

For Immediate Relief
home remedies

Adjust your sleep schedule. Many women get into the habit of keeping late hours just to get things done or have time for themselves—but the alarm clock still goes off at the same time every morning. If you aren't getting enough sleep at night, unless you're Angelina Jolie, there's no way you're going to feel energetic during the day.

A Hidden Cause of Fatigue

the thyroid is a small gland at the base of the front of the neck. It uses iodine from the blood to produce and store thyroid hormone, which plays a major role in the body's metabolism. Women who produce too little thyroid hormone, a condition called hypothyroidism, will feel tired, weak, or depressed.

Doctors estimate that 17 percent of women will have thyroid problems by the time they reach 60. "The condition often comes on gradually, over months or years, so it's not always diagnosed right away," says Gay Canaris, MD, assistant professor of internal medicine at the University of Nebraska College of Medicine in Omaha. As a result, the symptoms often go unnoticed by either the patient or her doctor and are easily attributed to other medical problems, overwork, or stress, Dr. Canaris adds. Hypothyroidism is diagnosed by a blood test that measures thyroid gland function.

Women with a family history of thyroid disorders, or those with autoimmune conditions such as lupus, have a higher risk of developing hypothyroidism. Women who have recently given birth are also at risk, Dr. Canaris says.

Hypothyroidism is easy to treat with medications. Once your hormone levels are back to normal, most thyroid symptoms will improve. "You just have to take one small pill a day of synthetic thyroid hormone. "It's really very simple." ▪

The solution is simple: Try to go to bed a little earlier. You can't shift your body's internal clock all at once, so you have to work in increments. Go to bed about 15 minutes earlier than usual. Do this for a few weeks until it feels like the right time. Then move your bedtime back another 15 minutes. Keep doing this until you're getting a full 8 hours of sleep. Most women can make the transition easily, and you'll find that your energy levels will be higher throughout the day.

Get your body moving. Exercise doesn't produce energy directly; as a matter of fact, it consumes energy. But women who walk, jog, work in the yard, or are otherwise physically active generally notice that fatigue is much less of a problem.

"Physical activity stimulates the release of beta-endorphins, hormones that make you feel alive, refreshed, and energized," explains Dr. Mack-Shipman. Exercise is also beneficial because it tires the muscles, which in turn will make it easier to sleep at night.

A 2006 paper in the journal *Sports Medicine* compiled the results of 12 previous studies—involving 137,000 people—that were done during the previous half-century. It found that people who choose to be physically active are about 40 percent less likely to have low energy and fatigue compared to people who are sedentary. According to the authors, people who are physically active are also about half as likely to have depression.

THREE THINGS I TELL EVERY FEMALE PATIENT

LYNN MACK-SHIPMAN, MD, *an endocrinologist and assistant professor of internal medicine at the University of Nebraska Medical Center in Omaha, sees a lot of women whose main symptom is fatigue. Here's what she advises.*

1

DO EVERYTHING YOU CAN TO RELAX. "Stress can zap anyone of their energy," says Dr. Mack-Shipman. "Practice relaxation techniques. I've actually written a prescription for one of my patients to enroll in a yoga class."

Some women cut back on their work hours. Others practice relaxation techniques such as meditation or visualization. Exercise is a great stress-reducing technique because it stimulates the releases of calming chemicals in the brain.

2

ON COMPLEX CARBOHYDRATES. Whole grains, legumes, and other plant foods are rich in complex carbohydrates, which are broken down slowly during digestion. This allows glucose (blood sugar) to be produced at a steady pace, which helps maintain energy.

3

AVOID SIMPLE CARBOHYDRATES. There's nothing wrong with having a sweet snack on occasion, but the sugars in snacks and sodas, known as simple carbohydrates, cause blood sugar levels to spike. The body responds by releasing large amounts of insulin, which can make you feel tired. ■

Vary your routine. Women who are new to exercise often complain that doing the same things every day is too boring to stay motivated. That's why many people who start exercise plans drop out within a few weeks or months. The solution is to identify a dozen or more physical activities that you enjoy—it could be swimming, working in the garden, bicycling, or even walking through the mall—and to swap them around so that you never get bored.

"Try running one day and lifting weights the next. Or do something entirely different, like tai chi or ballroom dancing," Dr. Mack-Shipman suggests.

alternative therapies

Energize with essential oils. "Smelling certain scents can invigorate your body and mind and help you feel more energetic," says Alan Hirsch, MD, neurologic director of the Smell and Taste Treatment and Research Foundation in Chicago. The scents of peppermint and jasmine essential oils are especially energizing, he says.

In fact, a researcher at Wheeling College in West Virginia found that basketball players who used peppermint inhalers had more energy, motivation, speed, and confidence.

The easiest way to use scent therapy is to put a few drops of essential oil on a handkerchief then take a few minutes to enjoy the aroma. Another option is to use an aromatherapy diffuser, available from mail order catalogs and some health food stores. It will fill the air with the special scents. You can also buy a peppermint inhaler at many sporting goods stores.

For Long-Term Prevention

home remedies

Get enough iron. Millions of American women don't get enough iron in the diet. This is especially common during the childbearing years because women lose a little blood each month during menstruation. Even when a woman doesn't have full-fledged iron-deficiency anemia, low levels of this mineral can result in fatigue.

"Some women don't consume enough iron-rich foods, such as red meats, because they are concerned about gaining weight," says Dr. Mack-Shipman. Without sufficient amounts of iron, the red blood cells can't carry as much oxygen, which results in fatigue.

The best sources of iron are lean red meats, poultry, eggs, and fish, says Dr. Mack-Shipman. Other options include fortified breakfast cereals, potatoes, and beans. The Daily Value for iron is 18 mg, she says.

Drink plenty of water. "Dehydration, even in its earliest stages, can make you feel tired and weak," says Dr. Mack-Shipman. Try to drink eight full glasses of water daily, she advises.

Lose weight sensibly. Women who are trying to lose weight often depend upon restrictive diets such as those high in protein and low in carbohydrates, and others that are very low in calories. These diets aren't very effective for weight loss, and they're even worse for maintaining healthful energy levels, says Cindy Polich, RD, a medical nutritionist at the University of Nebraska Medical Center in Omaha.

"Following one of these 'starvation' diets can lead to fatigue and weakness," she says. "When you don't get enough carbohydrates, you deplete your short-term energy supplies."

Whether or not you're trying to lose weight, you want to choose a variety of foods from the food guide pyramid, focusing on carbohydrates such as whole grains, legumes, and fruits and vegetables. "The body converts carbohydrates into glucose, which is used for energy," Polich explains.

Avoid caffeine. "I'm a believer in getting people off caffeine," says Mary Ann Bauman, MD, medical director for women's health and community relations for Integris Family Care Central in Oklahoma City. Caffeine stimulates you, making you feel happy, energetic, and alert. For someone with fatigue, those may be appealing rewards. But when its effect wears off, you may feel sluggish and groggy again. Drink it too close to bed, and it can keep you awake–but if you don't drink it, you might have withdrawal symptoms overnight that keep you from sleeping, Dr. Bauman says. It's best just to avoid it.

If you drink a lot of caffeine, don't stop all at once. Gradually reduce the amount you drink each day to minimize the unpleasant symptoms of withdrawal–such as headaches, fatigue, and mental fogginess. Slowly replace the caffeinated sodas, coffee, and tea you drink with alternatives like water, low-fat milk, and decaffeinated green tea.

Maintain a healthful weight. Women who are above a healthy weight are more likely to experience fatigue. Extra weight can also increase your risk for a sleep disorder called apnea, in which breathing is reduced at night.

Your body responds by waking up momentarily in order to take a deep breath. You might not be aware of the disturbance in your sleep, but your energy levels are sure to suffer the next day.

when to see a doctor

If you feel as though you sleep well at night, but you're still exhausted during the day, make an appointment to see your doctor. You could have a sleep problem that's preventing you from getting all the rest you need, says Lynn Mack-Shipman, MD, an endocrinologist and assistant professor of internal medicine at the University of Nebraska Medical Center in Omaha.

Insomnia is probably the most common sleep disorder, but it's not the only one. Your doctor might advise you to have a sleep test, which will measure brain waves, respiration, and other factors that can affect the quality of your sleep, she explains.

If you've been fatigued for months, and nothing you try seems to help. You should ask your doctor about getting tested for iron-deficiency anemia. If you are anemic, getting adequate amounts of iron will reverse the symptoms within weeks or even days.

If the fatigue is accompanied by weight gain, intolerance to cold, and constipation. These are classic symptoms of an underactive thyroid, says Dr. Mack-Shipman.

If you have increased thirst and you're also urinating frequently. You could have diabetes, which is often accompanied by severe fatigue.

fever

When you're feeling hot and bothered because you're sick, try to remember that fever is your friend. The rise in temperature that occurs when you're ill may enhance the body's defense mechanisms against viruses and bacteria. When it does, you recover more quickly.

If your fever isn't too high, you may want to put up with it for a while, says Philip Mackowiak, MD professor of medicine at the University of Maryland School of Medicine and chief of medical service at the Baltimore Veterans Affairs Medical Center. Major studies have shown that when you have a viral infection, such as a cold or possibly the flu, taking over-the-counter remedies to lower your fever can help make the illness last longer.

Fevers can be caused by dozens of conditions, from ear or urinary tract infections to simple colds and flu, as well as certain inflammatory, immunologic, or malignant disorders, and some medications. As long as fever is your main symptom, and your temperature doesn't spike above 102°F, it's fine to treat it at home. Here are a few helpful strategies.

For Immediate Relief

home remedies

Decide whether to stop it or not. If your fever doesn't seem to be related to a serious problem that needs treatment—for example, you don't have symptoms of a urinary tract infection and the fever isn't dangerously high—it's up to you whether to bring it down, Dr. Mackowiak says. You'll feel more comfortable if you lower the fever, but your illness may linger a day or two longer.

Some doctors recommend letting a fever do its job, while others point out that doctors are in the business of making people feel better, thus they recommend lowering the fever. "If I have a cold or influenza, I try not to take aspirin or Tylenol, but almost invariably I do, because of how much better they make me feel," Dr. Mackowiak says.

Drink enough water. Your body loses a lot of water when you have a fever, which can dehydrate the brain and other tissues and leave you feeling weak and tired. Try to drink a sufficient amount of water so that you will need to urinate once every 1 to 2 hours—that's about eight glasses of water a day—until the fever is gone. Caffeine-free, nonalcoholic beverages and 100 percent fruit juices diluted by half with water are also helpful.

Take an over-the-counter painkiller. In addition to their pain-relieving properties, aspirin, ibuprofen, and acetaminophen are very effective at lowering fever, says William J. Hall, MD, professor of medicine and director for the Center for Healthy Aging at the University of Rochester School of Medicine in New York.

Be careful which drugs you choose since they

all have side effects, some of which, accompanying fever, are serious. For example, acetaminophen is less likely to cause stomach upset than aspirin or ibuprofen. And doctors warn that children with the flu or other respiratory infections should never be given aspirin because it can increase the risk for Reye's syndrome, a potentially serious neurological disorder. If you have a chronic disease or are taking other medications, consult with your doctor before using any OTC drug.

Stay warm. Although keeping warm when your body is already too hot may seem like a strange choice, you should do just that for run-of-the-mill fevers, Dr. Mackowiak recommends. If you get in a cool shower or turn on the air conditioner, your body will try to keep your temperature up, and you'll start shivering, which is uncomfortable.

You don't want to make yourself hot—just keep comfortably warm. Sip some hot soup, drink hot tea, and cover yourself with a blanket if necessary.

Forget about that number you've heard. "The idea that 98.6 degrees is normal should be discarded," Dr. Mackowiak says. That's not a magic number that you need to reach in order to feel well. Instead, most peoples' "normal" temperature actually ranges from about 96 to a little less than 100. Usually your temperature is lower in the morning and higher in the afternoon. Your body follows this cycle when you're sick, too. So if you have a fever that's a few degrees higher in the afternoon, it doesn't necessarily mean you're getting sicker; you're just following your usual routine.

Take one by mouth. When taking your temperature, use a thermometer that you put in your mouth, Dr. Mackowiak says. It gives a more accurate measurement than the kind you place into your ear.

Get your Zzzs. Your body needs more sleep when you have a fever. All that extra heat it's producing uses extra energy. So if you have a fever, cut back on your activities and allow yourself plenty of bed rest.

when to see a doctor

If your temperature climbs to 102°F or higher. It's common for children to develop high fevers, but adults rarely do unless they have something more serious than a simple cold or flu.

If you have underlying medical problems, such as heart or lung disease. Any fever, even a low-grade one, should be taken seriously, especially in older people, because fever increases the body's oxygen demands, which can put a strain on the heart and other already damaged organs.

If the fever is accompanied by teeth-chattering chills that last more than 10 minutes at a time. This is a sign that bacteria may have entered the bloodstream, which can result in a serious infection. Call your doctor immediately.

fibromyalgia

People with fibromyalgia hurt all over. When they say they're tired, they mean bone weary and exhausted–too tired to go out, socialize, even stay up. Most have a sleep disorder that keeps them from getting deep, restorative sleep, the kind that leaves them refreshed in the morning. They can have a variety of other symptoms too, from headaches and migraines, to rashes, dry eyes, anxiety, dizziness, and even poor coordination.

This syndrome affects as many as 10 million Americans, and is most common in women of childbearing age, but children, the elderly, and men can also be affected.

How can you tell if your symptoms are caused by fibromyalgia? The telltale sign is "tender points"–extremely sensitive areas that generally appear in the neck, spine, shoulders, and hips, says Lenore Buckley, MD, a rheumatologist and professor of internal medicine and pediatrics at Virginia Commonwealth University School of Medicine in Richmond. Depression is another common symptom. Research has shown that between 18 and 36 percent of people with fibromyalgia suffer from depression at any given time.

Scientists still aren't sure what causes fibromyalgia. A number of studies have found some striking abnormalities in patients, including increased levels of a pain chemical called substance P in the spinal cord, low levels of blood flow to the thalamus region of the brain (relay stations for nerve impulses carrying messages to the brain), and low levels of the brain chemical serotonin and amino acid tryptophan, which help regulate mood and sleep.

Fibromyalgia is a challenge to diagnose because many of the symptoms are similar to those caused by other disorders. If you have tender points and widespread pain that has lasted more than 3 months, and tests show that you don't have lupus, arthritis, or Lyme disease, you could have fibromyalgia.

So far, there isn't a cure for fibromyalgia. That doesn't mean you have to live with it forever. The severity of the symptoms tends to come and go, and it's not uncommon for fibromyalgia to spontaneously disappear. In the meantime, here are a few ways to reduce the pain and discomfort.

For Immediate Relief

home remedies

Get a massage. "I have found in my patients with fibromyalgia that a massage stops the pain," says Denise Borrelli, PhD, a nationally certified massage therapist and clinical director of A Healing Touch Holistic Healing Center in Medford, Massachusetts.

Massage is relaxing, which makes it much easier for people with fibromyalgia to get the sleep they need. "Some of my patients have been able to cut back on their sleep medications after they started getting massages regularly," says Dr. Borrelli.

Tender Spots Signal
Fibromyalgia

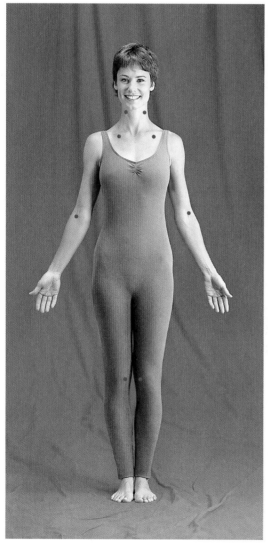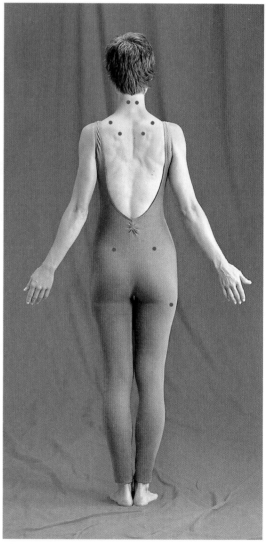

According to the American College of Rheumatology, people with fibromyalgia have widespread pain, along with tenderness in at least 11 of 18 "tender point" locations, shown here.

There are a bewildering variety of massage techniques to choose from. "I recommend Swedish massage because the long, gentle strokes are very soothing," Dr. Borrelli says. "I advise against deep muscle tissue massage because it can irritate nerve endings and cause more pain," she adds.

Depending on where you live, massage can cost anywhere from $30 to $100 per hour. To find a massage therapist in your area, contact the American Massage Therapy Association at (877) 905-0577. Or go to the association's Web site at www.amtamassage.org.

Enjoy pool therapy. Warm-water pool therapy is a great way to relax the muscles and reduce the pain, says Dr. Buckley.

Exercise as much as you can. Walking, biking, water exercise, and other forms of aerobic exercise have been shown to reduce muscle pain and tenderness. Regular exercise also stimulates the production of endorphins, chemical messengers in the brain that promote feelings of relaxation and well-being.

If you have fibromyalgia, it probably won't be easy to start an exercise program because your muscles will be sore and achy. But it's worth pushing through the initial discomfort. As your muscles get stronger, you'll find you have more energy and endurance, and the intensity and frequency of the pain will gradually diminish.

If you haven't been physically active, you'll want to start out with stretching exercises before launching into full-fledged workouts. "Walking is more of an intermediate exercise for women to work up to," says Dr. Buckley. "Take a brisk 5-minute walk, then gradually increase the time and intensity until you're walking briskly for 40 minutes three times a week."

Avoid caffeine. Coffee, tea, and other caffeine-containing beverages are America's favorite pick-me-ups, but people often forget just how stimulating they can be. If you have fibromyalgia, consuming caffeine close to bedtime can make it difficult to get the deep, restorative sleep that you need.

Your doctor may advise you to limit your consumption of caffeine-containing beverages to one or two servings daily—and to avoid them altogether in the afternoon and evening.

For Long-Term Relief

home remedies

Take a yoga class. Even though regular exercise is among the best ways to ease the discomfort of fibromyalgia, people are often too tired or sore to get started. One way to get the muscles primed for action is to practice yoga. "If yoga is the exercise you choose, start with a beginning class," says Dr. Buckley. A small study done at Oregon Health and Science University in Portland found that most of the women who practiced yoga for 2 hours a day once a week for 8 weeks felt less pain, fatigue, and depression.

Learn tai chi. A study published in the August 19, 2010, issue the *New England Journal of Medicine* found that people with fibromyalgia who practiced tai chi—a practice combining meditation with flowing poses—twice a week for 12 weeks felt dramatically better. Their pain lessened, and they had less fatigue, depression, anxiety and improved function than people who did stretching exercises and attended a health education class. In fact, 35 percent of the tai chi participants were able to stop taking their medications as a result.

Sign up for aquacise. "Warm-water exercises are very beneficial for fibromyalgia patients because they relax the muscles and decrease pain," says Dr. Buckley. "The water supports the muscles, so you're not working against gravity."

Some people head straight to a local pool, but it's better to sign up for an aquacise program tailored for those with fibromyalgia. "It's important to make sure that you're doing the moves correctly so you don't hurt yourself," says Dr. Buckley. Your doctor can refer you to a physical therapy program that includes water exercises. Many health clubs and YMCAs and YWCAs also offer aquacise classes in cooperation with the Arthritis Foundation.

Try to think positively. It's hard to be upbeat and positive when you're hurting, but it's worth making the effort. Studies have shown that people who dwell on their pain and unhappiness experience a lot more stress, which in turn increases pain.

In one large study, researchers at the University of Missouri in Columbia compared drug and nondrug treatments for fibromyalgia. They found that people who exercised or practiced cognitive-behavioral therapy—in which they learned to substitute positive thoughts for negative ones—experienced less pain and fatigue.

THREE THINGS I TELL EVERY FEMALE PATIENT

LENORE BUCKLEY, MD, *a rheumatologist and professor of internal medicine and pediatrics at Virginia Commonwealth University School of Medicine in Richmond, offers this special advice for women with fibromyalgia.*

1 **FOCUS ON SLEEP.** "It's hard for doctors to help people with fibromyalgia until we take care of the sleep problem," Dr. Buckley says. "Many people don't get the 7 or 8 hours of deep, uninterrupted sleep that they need, which leaves them feeling tired and unable to concentrate."

DO EVERYTHING POSSIBLE TO RELAX. The more stress you have in your life, the more anxiety and pain you'll experience. "Stress reduction helps people feel better overall, and it also helps them sleep better at night," says Dr. Buckley. Everyone relaxes in different ways, and you'll have to experiment to find what works best for you. "I advise people to do whatever appeals to them, whether it's walking, water exercise, deep breathing, meditation, or yoga." **2**

EXERCISE IS CRITICAL. "It's very difficult for fibromyalgia patients who are not part of an exercise program to get better," says Dr. Buckley. "Regular, gentle exercise such as walking or warm-water exercises can help loosen up stiff muscles and get the blood flowing again—all of which will help ease pain." ■ **3**

They also performed daily tasks more easily than those who only took drugs.

A good place to start is to make an appointment with a psychological therapist. In the meantime, do everything you can to relax. Set aside time each day to meditate, listen to music, or simply unwind.

Take some SAM-e. According to the National Center for Complementary and Alternative Medicine, this pain-relieving supplement often recommended for people with arthritis shows some promise in easing fibromyalgia symptoms as well.

medical options

Consider antidepressants. Even if you aren't suffering from depression, tricyclic antidepressant medications such as amitriptyline (such as Elavil or Endep) and selective serotonin reuptake inhibitors (SSRI) such as fluoxetine (Prozac), paroxetine (Paxil) and sertraline (Zoloft) increase the amount of sleep, and the mood-regulating hormone serotonin can reduce muscle pain and make it easier to sleep, which will significantly boost energy and help you to stay active. Today's antidepressants are safe and effective, but they may cause side effects, such as a dry mouth or grogginess.

Ask your doctor about drug combinations. In a study at Newton-Wellesley Hospital in Newton, Massachusetts, people with fibromyalgia were treated with Elavil, Prozac, or a combination of the two drugs. Those who took both drugs experienced twice the improvement of those taking the drugs separately. In fact, 12 of

when to see a doctor

If you've had widespread pain for 3 months or more, see your doctor right away. It's one of the classic signs of fibromyalgia, says Lenore Buckley, MD, a rheumatologist and professor of internal medicine and pediatrics at Virginia Commonwealth University School of Medicine in Richmond.

If you feel pain at specific "tender points." People with fibromyalgia typically have tender areas on the shoulders, elbows, hips, or buttocks.

If you're always fatigued and you can't figure out why. Fibromyalgia isn't the only condition that can result in low energy or lethargy. If you're exhausted all the time and there doesn't seem to be a good reason for it, see your doctor.

the 19 participants in the study reported improvements of at least 25 percent.

Researchers suspect that the combination of Elavil and Prozac may change pain perception in people with fibromyalgia. The medications also affect blood flow to pain-receptive regions of the brain, and they enhance the body's production of feel-good chemicals such as serotonin.

There are also mixed reuptake inhibitors, which raise levels of serotonin and norepinephrine, that are being studied as fibromyalgia treatments. They include venlafaxine (Effexor) and nefazadone (Serzone).

Take a sleep aid. "The main goal in the pharmaceutical treatment of fibromyalgia is to help people get some sleep," says Dr. Buckley. "The pain often keeps people up at night, and even when they do fall asleep, the pain often wakes them up." Your doctor may recommend other drugs to treat symptoms of restless legs syndrome (such as benzodiazepine drugs including Valium) and irritable bowel syndrome, which sometime occur with fibromyalgia.

Ask about the newest drugs. The drug pregabalin (Lyrica) reduces pain and aids sleep; milnacipran HCL (Savella) and duloxetine HCL (Cymbalta) are FDA-approved for people who don't respond to other drugs.

For more information on fibromyalgia. See the Web site of the National Institute of Arthritis and Musculoskeletal and Skin Diseases at www. nih.gov/niams. Other helpful Web sites include the Fibromyalgia Network at www.fmnetnews. com and the Arthritis Foundation at www. arthritis.org.

flu

Swine flu. Bird flu. H1N1. Flu has been garnering headlines over the last decade as air travel makes it possible to pick up a flu germ in Taiwan and infect New York City. It's not just a cold on steroids. Short for "influenza," the flu is a highly contagious illness that's responsible for more than 20,000 deaths in the United States every year. It's so dangerous that the Centers for Disease Control and Prevention urges everyone over the age of 6 months to get a flu shot every year before flu season (November through May, peaking in February).

It's a different shot every year. The problem with the flu virus is that it's constantly changing, or mutating, in order to outfox the body's immune system, so you can't build up an immunity to it. The virus changes so rapidly that vaccine manufacturers have to design new formulas every year to combat the newest strains.

A mild case of the flu bears some resemblance to a serious cold, causing coughs, achy muscles, and a sore throat. More often, the flu feels like no cold you've ever had. In fact, you may feel like you have been hit with a giant pile driver.

Utter exhaustion is usually the first symptom. After that, you may have intense head and muscle aches, a high fever, chest congestion, and a severe cough. While most people recover in a few days or a couple of weeks, some people, particularly those with chronic health problems, the very young and very old, and pregnant women, can develop life-threatening complications from the flu.

There isn't a miracle cure for flu. Medications can help, but mainly you need to take it easy until the infection passes. In addition, it's important to boost your body's defenses and take a few steps to ease the worst of the discomfort.

For Immediate Relief
home remedies

Eat immune-boosting foods. When you're sick, more than ever it's important to choose foods that shore up the immune system, such as green leafy vegetables (which are rich in vitamins A and C), citrus fruits, tomatoes, strawberries, carrots, and pumpkin. Even small amounts of produce can make a big difference: One study found that eating about one medium carrot or two small carrots significantly boosted immune cell activity.

Remember that old rule: An apple a day just might keep the doctor away! When invading viruses go chomping and chewing their way through your healthy cells, they leave behind a trail of free radicals, tiny land mines that can blow up your immune system's defenses. Quercetin, a natural plant chemical found in apples as well as in onions, berries, and tomatoes, is one of the top technicians on the bomb-defusing squad.

"Quercetin disarms free radicals, disrupting the tricks those pathogens use to sabotage us," says David L. Katz, MD, director of the Yale-Griffin Prevention Research Center. Try to get nine servings of quercetin-containing fruits and vegetables every day.

Make an antiviral soup. To stimulate your body's defenses, chop up fresh vegetables, add plenty of onions and garlic, and cook them in 8 ounces of steaming chicken broth per serving. Both onions and garlic contain compounds that have antiviral properties.

Don't forget yogurt with live active cultures. In a Swedish study, those who drank a daily supplement of "good" bacteria found in Stonyfield Farm yogurt had a third fewer sick days than those given a placebo.

Cut back on fat and sugar. Until the virus is gone, try to eat as little fat as possible—no more than 25 percent of daily calories—because it reduces the ability of the immune system to work efficiently. It's also important to avoid sweet foods because sugar undermines phagocytosis, the process by which viruses are destroyed by white blood cells.

Drink hot tea. It's an old folk remedy for the flu, and there's good evidence that it works. Drinking several cups of steaming tea daily will thin mucus and help relieve congestion. Studies at Harvard Medical School also found the people who drank five cups a day of black tea had 10 times more virus-fighting interferon in their blood than those who drank a hot drink that served as a placebo. This tea also contains theophylline, a natural bronchodilator that will help keep your airways open. Add some honey to coat the throat to soothe irritation.

Breathe moist air. Take a long, hot shower or plug in a humidifier. Moisture in the air soothes irritated tissues in the throat and airways.

alternative therapies

Enjoy herbal teas. A number of herbal teas contain compounds that soothe sore throats and break up congestion in the airways. Some of the best include slippery elm bark and marshmallow root, which relieve sore throats; and thyme and eucalyptus leaf, which help loosen congestion. Teas made from boneset or yarrow are especially good because they have immune-boosting properties.

To make a tea, pour 1 cup of boiling water

when to see a doctor

If you suspect you have the flu, call your doctor right away. Antivirals work best when you take them a day or two after symptoms appear.

If your symptoms seem unusually severe. High fever, difficulty breathing, and other common flu symptoms can also be caused by other conditions, including pneumonia and heart disease. In addition, some strains of flu can make people so ill that they require hospitalization, so call your doctor right away if you're suffering from any severe symptoms.

If you start feeling better, then take a turn for the worse. The original flu infection could have set the stage for a secondary bacterial infection, which means you'll need to take antibiotics as soon as possible. Call your doctor immediately if you suspect an infection.

over crushed, dried herbs as indicated for each: slippery elm bark (powdered only) or marshmallow root, steep 2 teaspoons for 10 minutes; thyme, eucalyptus leaf, or yarrow, steep 1 teaspoon for 10 minutes; or boneset, steep ½ teaspoon for 30 minutes. Strain the leaves and drink the tea while it's hot. You can drink several cups of herbal tea a day—but drink only 3 cups daily of thyme or eucalyptus leaf.

Get some ginseng in you. This ancient herb boosts levels of infection-fighting white blood cells and immune system proteins called interleukins. It may also boost the effectiveness of the flu shot. In one study, the number of colds and flu were two-thirds lower for people who took Asian ginseng (Panax ginseng) for 12 weeks and got a flu shot after 4 weeks than those who took a placebo.

medical options

Ask about antivirals. The CDC recommends two antiviral drugs, Tamiflu, (in liquid or pill form) and Relenza (inhaled powder), which can shorten duration of flu symptoms by one or two days, help relieve symptoms and, most important, prevent complications.

food allergy

n the last decade or so we've gotten used to the vanishing peanut. No more peanuts on the plane or peanut butter sandwiches in the cafeteria. Why? Because they can cause food allergies that can kill. Some people who are allergic to peanuts can have a life-threatening reaction to even the scent molecules that waft from a newly opened bag.

Fortunately, most food allergies aren't this serious. People who eat the wrong foods may break out in hives or welts. Or offending foods—milk, eggs, fish, shellfish, nuts, soy, and wheat are the most common—may cause nausea, diarrhea, or other digestive problems. Once they clear the system, the symptoms rapidly disappear.

But whether your allergies are minor or severe, there's only one long-term solution: Avoid the foods that make you sick. This isn't always easy because people with food allergies are rarely allergic to just one food. They usually react to whole groups of foods, such as shellfish or certain grains. Identifying the culprit and avoiding it can take some work. As little as $1/5{,}000$ teaspoon of an allergy-causing food can trigger a reaction. Women who are allergic to peanuts, for example, could have problems if a cook uses the same spatula when baking different types of cookies, one of which contained peanuts. If you're allergic to a certain food or foods, you have to avoid them entirely—in some cases, for the rest of your life.

Food allergies occur when the immune system mistakes an entirely innocent protein for a harmful intruder. It overreacts and launches a full array of immune cells to counteract the "attack," which is what causes the symptoms, says Clifton T. Furukawa, MD, medical advisor to the Food Allergy and Anaphylaxis Network and an allergist at Northwest Asthma and Allergy Center in Washington.

Although most food allergies cause only minor symptoms, people with extreme sensitivities may experience a life-threatening reaction called anaphylaxis, which can literally shut down the airways and cause blood pressure to plummet.

Food allergies often begin in childhood, although adults can develop them. Children sometimes outgrow food allergies, but if you developed the problem as a grown woman, it's unlikely to go away, says Dr. Furukawa.

Researchers are investigating ways to reverse the body's sensitivity to potential allergens in foods, but for now there isn't a cure for food allergies. All you can do is make sure to avoid the wrong foods, and know what to do should an emergency strike.

WHAT WORKS FOR ME

ANNE MUNOZ-FURLONG *is chief executive officer of the Virginia-based Food Allergy and Anaphylaxis Network and the parent of a daughter who once suffered from severe food allergies. She quickly learned to be especially vigilant when they enjoyed meals away from home.*

We never went to restaurants during their busiest times. We usually ate at 5:00 p.m., not 7:00 p.m., because that's when restaurant staffs are fresh and we could get their attention.

When I ordered, I would carefully explain to the waiter what would happen if we were accidentally served the wrong food. Once they understood the consequences, they were much more willing to work with us.

Sometimes the waiter would accidentally bring the wrong dish. I would order a new serving, but I would keep the old serving on the table. Otherwise, the chef might merely remove the offending item—for example, the cheese on a hamburger. He would think he'd done the right thing, but the food would still be contaminated with the offending protein. ∎

For Immediate Relief

Act quickly. If you have a minor food allergy and you accidentally eat what you shouldn't, most reactions can be treated with an antihistamine, and you can simply wait for the symptoms to pass. But for those with severe allergies, waiting can cost them their lives. You have to be prepared to take immediate action–by giving yourself an antianaphylaxis injection and getting to an emergency room immediately.

Always carry a self-injector. Women with severe food allergies are advised to keep a self-injector handy. Products such as the EpiPen or Twinject contain a medication called epinephrine. It helps reverse anaphylaxis by stimulating the heart, opening the airways, and reducing swelling of the throat.

If you have a history of food allergies but haven't had a serious reaction for years, it's easy to get complacent and leave the injector at home–either because you forgot it at the last minute or because you figured you wouldn't need it. Don't take that chance. When researchers looked at 32 people who died from food allergy reactions, they found that only three of them were carrying their injectors.

"I tell patients they should always carry three doses of epinephrine," says Sandra M. Gawchik, DO, clinical associate professor of pediatrics at Thomas Jefferson University Medical College in Philadelphia and co-director of the division of allergy and clinical immunology at Crozer-Chester Medical Center in Upland, Pennsylvania. "They have one extra in case they drop one, another to buy them time until they get medical help, and a third in case they need another dose."

Use the medicine at the first sign of symptoms. Even if you're not completely sure whether you're having an allergic reaction, give yourself the injection anyway. "I advise patients to inject the epinephrine first and ask questions later," says Dr. Furukawa. The sooner you get the injection, the better your chances of making a full recovery.

The advantage of the EpiPen is that it's fully automatic: Just remove the safety cap, push the spring-loaded tip against the outer thigh to release the medicine, and hold it in place for 10 seconds. Then get to an emergency room right away.

Practice. It takes time to learn to use self-injectors properly, so it's important to practice ahead of time. "You need about 30 pounds of pressure to trigger the EpiPen, so if you just tap it lightly, it won't work," says Ira Finegold, MD, chief of the division of allergy and immunology at St. Luke's-Roosevelt Hospital Center in New York City. "That's why it's important to practice using it."

If you experience an allergic reaction and need to give yourself a shot, it's fine to raise your skirt slightly and put the shot into your thigh through panty hose, Dr. Finegold adds. If at all possible, avoid injecting yourself through thick fabric because you could get an infection when the needle goes through dirty clothing.

Avoid alcohol when eating out. Alcoholic beverages can increase the body's absorption of allergy-causing proteins, says Marianne Frieri, MD, PhD, attending chief of allergy and immunology in the department of medicine at Nassau University Medical Center in East Meadow, New York, and professor of medicine and pathology at the State University of New York at Stony Brook.

At home, where it's easier to control your exposure to potential allergens, it's fine to enjoy a beer or a glass of wine. But when you're eating away from home, avoiding alcohol will give you an extra measure of protection.

Never take chances. Many people with food allergies don't take their condition seriously. They may assume that "just a tiny taste" won't hurt. Or they may depend on medication to get them out of a tight spot. This is a dangerous

mindset, says Dr. Frieri. "Food allergies can be life threatening. People need to take their symptoms seriously."

For Long-Term Prevention

home remedies

Keep a food diary. It can be tricky to know what food or foods you're allergic to. The only way to find out which foods are friends and which are foes is to keep a comprehensive food diary. Every day, jot down everything you eat. Be specific: Don't write "salad" when you really ate lettuce, onions, tomatoes, and grated cheese.

Stay on Guard for Hidden Allergens

harmful ingredients lurk in some unexpected places. Food is the main offender, of course, but food allergens can also be found in cosmetics, shampoos, and other items you'd never think of eating.

It's possible, for example, for a woman who is allergic to nuts to develop a severe reaction if she uses a shampoo made with almond oil, says Hugh A. Sampson, MD, dean for Translational Biomedical Research, chief of the Division of Allergy and Immunology in the department of pediatrics, and director of the Elliot and Roslyn Jaffe Food Allergy Institute at Mount Sinai School of Medicine in New York City.

"One of my patients was allergic to nuts, and he developed wheezing and hives when the shampoo, which contained nut oils, got near the lips and eyes," he says.

Shaving creams, moisturizers, and lipsticks are often made with oils made from peanuts, almonds, or soybeans, adds Clifford W. Bassett, MD, assistant clinical professor of medicine at the State University of New York Health Science Center in Brooklyn, New York, and an attending physician and faculty member of New York University School of Medicine.

Even chewing gum is a potential problem for some people because it may contain cow's milk proteins, Dr. Bassett says.

Reading the labels may not always help because nonfood items rarely list all the ingredients, and those that are listed may be in scientific terms that are difficult to interpret. Although nothing is completely foolproof, in some cases it may be helpful to call the manufacturer—use the Internet to find the number—to inquire about ingredients before using any product that can potentially get into the nose, mouth, or eyes. ■

At the same time, note any physical symptoms that occur. If you keep the diary for several months, you'll start to narrow down the possible suspects.

Talk to your doctor about an elimination diet. This involves giving up, one at a time, the foods that you suspect are causing symptoms. If you felt that you had a reaction after eating shrimp, for example, you would give up shrimp for a few weeks. If you don't have additional symptoms, you may have discovered the culprit.

Of course, you might be allergic to more than one food, so you might have to repeat the process several times. Once you have a good idea what's causing the problems, the solution is obvious: You'll have to give up the foods completely.

Because there are so many ingredients in packaged foods, and because people with food allergies may react to similar proteins that are found in different foods, you'll need to work with your doctor to ensure that you're eliminating the proper foods. and to make sure that you're getting adequate nutrition while the elimination diet is under way.

Read food labels carefully. Packaged foods can contain dozens of ingredients, and sometimes you'll find ingredients where you least expect them. Surprising numbers of packaged foods contain soybeans, for example. Milk proteins are commonly used in packaged foods, even some that you wouldn't suspect of containing dairy, such as the artificial butter flavorings in popcorn or syrup, caramel candies, nougat, and even lunch meat.

The terms on food labels can be confusing,

so you'll need to work with your doctor to identify possible offenders. For example, many products contain "casein" or "caseinates." These include milk protein, and foods that contain them can cause allergic reactions. Suspect wheat if you see the words "cereal extract" or triticale, among others. You may even encounter shellfish in glucosamine supplements.

Check labels frequently. Food manufacturers often change the ingredients in their recipes. A food that was safe in the past might contain allergy-causing ingredients in the future. The only way to be safe is to read the labels every time you shop.

Keep foods and utensils separate. Some people with food allergies are so sensitive that the merest brush with an offending food can trigger anaphylaxis, says Dr. Gawchik. If you are at risk, you have to be careful that you don't inadvertently breathe, taste, or touch the foods you're allergic to.

If you're allergic to peanuts, for example, make sure that family members don't use "your" cutting board when making peanut butter sandwiches. If you're allergic to shrimp, eating foods that were fried in the same oil could be just as harmful as eating the shrimp itself, says Dr. Finegold.

Clean up correctly. Wash all surfaces with soap and water. Studies have found that conventional cleaning methods effectively wash away food allergen proteins. Bar and liquid soap can remove them from your hands, but one study found that alcohol-based hand sanitizers don't. Use commercial cleaning preparations rather than dishwashing liquid to clean tabletops if you or a family member has a peanut allergy.

Call restaurants ahead of time. Eating away from home can be risky for people with food allergies. Asian restaurants, for example, typically use the same woks to cook all the dishes. Even if the chef assures you that your dish doesn't contain a certain ingredient, traces of it might remain on the utensils. Doctors refer to this as cross-contamination.

Rather than trusting a waiter to communicate your concerns to the chef, it's worth calling the restaurant ahead of time to express your concerns and to find out if they're willing to accommodate you, says Anne Munoz-Furlong, chief executive officer of the Food Allergy and Anaphylaxis Network, based in Virginia.

Even if you call ahead, be sure to explain the issues to the waiter. If you're allergic to shellfish, for example, let the waiter know that the steak you've ordered can't be cooked in the same pan or section of the grill that's used to prepare shellfish, explains Dr. Gawchik.

Order simple foods. When you're eating out, it's a good idea to order foods that undergo minimal preparation. A baked potato, for example, is unlikely to be cross-contaminated with other foods, whereas french fries are prepared in oil that may be used to fry other foods.

Wear a medical alert bracelet or necklace. Anaphylaxis and other food allergy symptoms can come on very quickly—too quickly, in some cases, for people to care for themselves. Teach your friends and family about your self-injector so that they can help during a time of crisis. It's also helpful to carry a personalized card that lists your name, your doctor's name and phone number, and a list of foods that you're allergic to.

For more information about food allergies. Visit the Web site of the Food Allergy and Anaphylaxis Network at www.foodallergy.org.

gallstone attacks

The gallbladder is a small pouch that's connected to the liver at one end and the small intestine at the other. It's like a squeeze bottle; every time you eat, the gallbladder contracts and pushes out bile, a digestive fluid that breaks down fats, into the small intestine.

Bile consists of cholesterol, minerals, and other substances. Trouble begins when some of these substances form hard little deposits, or stones. The stones themselves don't cause problems unless they lodge in the tiny openings, or ducts, that lead to the small intestine. When that happens, the bile flow is interrupted and tension builds up, causing fierce abdominal pain.

Gallstones, which are 3 times more likely to affect women between the ages of 20 and 60, are potentially serious because the blockages can cause an infection in the gallbladder. The gallbladder could even burst open, causing even more problems, some life threatening. Most gallstones are silent, however. About 60 percent of those who have them never get sick.

But if you've had one gallstone attack, you know once is enough. Here are a few ways to reduce the discomfort and prevent future problems.

For Immediate Relief

Avoid dietary triggers. One way to prevent gallstone attacks is to avoid foods that are high in fat. Fat in the diet signals the gallbladder to contract more than usual, which can trigger attacks in some cases. "The things that usually give people the most trouble are fried foods," says Thomas R. Gadacz, MD, professor emeritus in the department of surgery at the Medical College of Georgia in Augusta.

when to see a doctor

If you have unexplained abdominal pain or nausea, especially after meals, call your doctor right away. There's a good chance that you have gallstones, says Thomas R. Gadacz, MD, professor emeritus at the Medical College of Georgia in Augusta.

If you have a history of gallstones and the attacks have become more frequent or severe. Gallstones are often silent, but frequent or severe attacks mean that you're probably going to need medical treatment, says Dr. Gadacz.

Talk to your doctor about surgery. If you're having frequent attacks of gallstone pain, your doctor may recommend that you have your gallbladder removed, usually in a minimally invasive procedure called laparascopic cholecystectomy, after which you're often able to leave the hospital the same day or the next morning. More than 500,000 Americans have gallbladder surgery every year, for good reason: We can function just fine without it.

Consider nonsurgical options. If the gallstones are small and consist mainly of cholesterol, your doctor may be able to eliminate them with medication. Prescription drugs such as chenodeoxycholic acids (CDCA) and ursodiol (Actigall) dissolve the stones, but they can take as long as 2 years to work and more stones may form.

Another nonsurgical approach is extracorporeal shock wave lithotripsy (ESWL), a procedure in which shock waves are transmitted through the abdomen to crush the stones. Once the stones are small enough, they will pass through the bile ducts without causing blockages.

For Long-Term Prevention

Maintain a healthy weight. Research has shown that middle-aged women who are overweight or obese may be twice as likely to develop gallstones as those who are leaner. Maintaining a healthful weight is among the best ways to prevent gallstones from forming, says Dr. Gadacz.

Lose weight slowly. Dropping a few pounds can prevent gallstone attacks, but losing weight too quickly can make the problem worse. Crash diets typically call for restricting fat intake to fewer than 10 grams daily. With so little fat in the diet, the activity of the gallbladder slows too much, which can make stonelike deposits more likely to form, says Dr. Gadacz. So-called yo-yo dieting, in which women repeatedly lose weight and gain it back, increases the risk for gallstones even more. (For a complete guide to healthy weight loss, see Chapter 6.)

Get regular exercise. A study of more than 3,000 women found that those who walked briskly for 20 minutes 5 to 7 days a week were 20 percent less likely to get gallstones than those who were sedentary. (To start an exercise program, see Chapter 5.)

gas

Passing gas elicits giggles from 9-year-olds, but for millions of American adults, it's no laughing matter.

Every day, our bodies produce 1 to 4 pints of intestinal gas—and people pass it, on average, about 14 to 23 times a day. All perfectly normal.

There are three main sources of intestinal gas, says Henry C. Lin, MD, director of the gastrointestinal motility program and professor of medicine at the University of New Mexico in Albuquerque. The first is the air we swallow when we eat, drink, chew gum, or talk, which makes up the average belch. The second is stubborn carbohydrates, including beans, that are difficult for the body to digest. The third is bacteria that move from their normal abode in the colon into the small intestine.

What you probably didn't realize is that gas is made up of primarily odorless vapors. The unpleasant odor comes from bacteria in the large intestine that release small amounts of sulfur.

It isn't possible to eliminate gas completely, but there are ways to reduce the volume. Here's what experts advise.

For Immediate Relief

home remedies

Identify gas-producing carbohydrates. The worst offenders include beans, cabbage, brussels sprouts, broccoli, and asparagus. They contain a sugar called raffinose, a major trigger of gas. You don't want to give up these foods completely because they are very good for your health, but it may be worth eating them a little less often if you find they're causing you problems. And no, they don't bother everyone.

Avoid sugar-free products. Products containing sorbitol, mannitol, and other sugar alcohols cause gas and gastric upset in some people.

Switch to rice. Most starch-containing foods—such as wheat, corn, and potatoes—produce gas during digestion. Rice, however, doesn't have this effect.

Drink from a glass. All carbonated beverages, including beer and sodas, contain gas—and gas that goes into the body will eventually come out. One solution is to pour carbonated drinks into a glass, which allows some of the gas to escape.

Eat small quantities. Don't overload your stomach at one meal, which can cause gas and bloating.

Avoid restrictive clothing. A tight waistband, belt, or pair of Spanx can also contribute to gas.

Walk after eating. It does have to be a brisk walk—even a leisurely stroll will help relieve the bloat and help release the gas into the great outdoors.

For Long-Term Relief
medical options

Talk to your doctor. If gas is making you uncomfortable and nothing you do seems to help, ask your doctor if you should be tested for bacterial overgrowths, Dr. Lin advises. It's possible that eliminating the troublesome bacteria will eliminate much of the gas as well.

You should also see your doctor if you're belching a lot or if you have heartburn or stomach pain. Along with gas, these are common symptoms of gastritis (inflammation of the stomach), ulcers, and a condition called gastroesophageal reflux disease, says Dr. Lin.

gastroesophageal reflux disease

Nearly everyone suffers from heartburn sometimes, that uncomfortable feeling in your chest and throat that may feel like pain or burning. As long as it doesn't happen often, it's more of an annoyance than a serious medical problem.

But if you have it twice a week or more, you may have gastroesophageal reflux disease (GERD), which occurs when a ring of muscle at the base of the esophagus (the tube that carries food to the stomach) weakens or opens at the wrong times. This allows harsh stomach acids to splash upward into the esophagus, causing the characteristic burning.

There's no reason to suffer from the discomfort of GERD, says Joshua Ofman, MD, former assistant professor of medicine in the division of gastroenterology at Cedars-Sinai Medical Center in Los Angeles and now vice president of Amgen, a biotech company. It's usually easy to control with simple measures, including avoidance of certain foods, and medication if needed.

For Immediate Relief
home remedies

Take over-the-counter relief. Antacids containing magnesium or aluminum compounds provide quick relief from heartburn. Other helpful medications include famotidine (Pepcid-AC) and cimetidine (Tagamet), which reduce stomach acid. Medications called H2 blockers (Zantac) actually block the amount of acid your stomach makes. They don't work as quickly as antacids but they work longer. A proton pump inhibitor such as Prilosec is best for people who have heartburn often as it substantially reduces stomach acid and works for a longer period than other OTC medications.

For Long-Term Relief
home remedies

Take small servings. They put less pressure on the stomach than large amounts all at once, says Dr. Ofman. It's also helpful to loosen your belt or clothing: Tight clothes increase pressure on the stomach and can force the acid upward, he explains.

Raise the head of your bed. It's harder for stomach acid to flow upward when your torso is slightly elevated. Elevate the head of your bed 6 to 8 inches with blocks.

Maintain a healthful weight. It's one of the best ways to prevent GERD, says Dr. Ofman. "For most women, even a loss of 10 to 15 pounds can relieve the symptoms."

Cut back on chocolate. And on coffee, alcohol, and fatty foods. They weaken the esophageal muscle, causing painful symptoms for hours later. And don't necessarily reach for an after-dinner mint; it too can cause acid reflux.

Skip the acid foods. Citrus and tomato products are already acidic so can cause even more pain.

Don't have midnight snacks. In fact, don't eat or drink 2 to 3 hours before bedtime since lying down with a full stomach can put more pressure on your esophageal sphincter.

Stop smoking. Nicotine can also relax the esophageal sphincter and smoking promotes the production of stomach acid.

gout

Once known as the "disease of kings," gout is rare in women, though your risk for this particularly painful form of arthritis increases after menopause.

Gout occurs when there are high levels of uric acid in the blood. Uric acid is a waste product formed by the breakdown of proteins, especially proteins called purines. When uric acid reaches high concentrations, it may begin to form sharp little crystals, which literally stab into joints, often in the big toe, causing intense inflammation.

People who eat a lot of purine-rich foods, such as shellfish and organ meats, have a high risk of getting gout. Some people have a genetic tendency to produce abnormally high amounts of uric acid, or their bodies are unable to eliminate it efficiently. Other risk factors for gout include a history of kidney disease, high blood pressure, heavy drinking, and the use of blood pressure medications. It can be triggered by drinking large amounts of alcohol or eating too much rich food.

"Gout is often inherited," says Elizabeth Tindall, MD, clinical professor of medicine at Oregon Health Sciences University in Portland. If someone in your family had it, you're at a higher risk of getting it, too, she adds.

Gout is known as a male disease, and for good reason: Men are at a significantly higher risk of getting it than are women, who generally produce lower amounts of uric acid than men do.

But that doesn't mean you're safe. "Women can be slowly building up high amounts of uric acid in their bodies for 20 years. They'll have no symptoms—until they wake up in the middle of the night with severe pain in their large toe," says Dr. Tindall. "The pain can make a grown woman cry."

During an acute attack, the joint will be red, hot, and painful, Dr. Tindall adds. "Some of my patients say they couldn't walk and they couldn't even stand to have the bed sheet touching their foot."

Although gout usually affects the big toe, it can also strike the elbow, ankles, or other joints in the body. The pain only lasts a day or two, but it can feel like forever. Here are some tips for stopping gout fast and making sure that it doesn't come back.

For Immediate Relief

home remedies

Take ibuprofen. When gout first strikes, take ibuprofen or another over-the-counter pain reliever right away, advises Dr. Tindall. The drugs curtail the body's production of prostaglandins, chemicals that cause pain and inflammation. But stay away from aspirin. It can block the excretion of uric acid from the kidneys, thereby worsening a gout attack.

Pamper your foot. "Lie on the bed and make sure the foot doesn't have any weight on it. Remove your shoes and socks as well as the sheet or blanket," says Dr. Tindall. "All those things can cause pain just by touching the area."

Apply ice—or heat. Different things work for different people, says Dr. Tindall. Cold is often helpful because it reduces swelling. Wrap some ice cubes in a washcloth and hold it on your toe for 10 to 15 minutes. If you don't like the sensation of cold, it's fine to apply a heating pad or hot-water bottle wrapped in a towel.

medical options

Ask your doctor about colchicine. Available by prescription, it will stop the pain of gout within an hour or two. However, it works best if you take it within 12 hours after an attack begins. If you wait much longer, it won't be as effective.

Consider corticosteroids. Given orally or by injection, corticosteroids are powerful drugs that are considered the gold standard for stopping inflammation. Because of the risk of side effects, however, they're usually used only when other treatments don't work.

Talk about other drugs. Drugs called xanthine oxidase inhibitors (Zyloprim, Aloprim) block uric acid production. Your doctor may recommend them, but after your current gout attack has passed. If taken during an acute attack, they can trigger another one. Taking colchicine before starting the drug can reduce that risk. Probenicid (Probalan) boosts your kidneys' ability to remove uric acid. The first new gout drug in 40 years, febuxostat (Uloric), was FDA approved in 2009; it also lowers uric acid in the blood.

For Long-Term Prevention

home remedies

Stop drinking alcohol. "Alcohol is the number-one dietary-related cause of gout because it interferes with the ability of the kidneys to excrete uric acid," says Dr. Tindall. Some women

when to see a doctor

If the joint in one of your big toes is red, swollen, and warm to the touch, call your doctor. There's a good chance you're suffering a gout attack, says Elizabeth Tindall, MD, clinical professor of medicine at Oregon Health Sciences University in Portland.

If symptoms similar to those caused by gout are affecting joints besides the big toe. It could be gout, or it could be a different form of arthritis or even an infection, says Dr. Tindall.

If the attacks are happening frequently. Take prescription drugs that will help prevent attacks of gout. It's important, however, to use the drugs exactly as they're prescribed. "People will take the drugs in the beginning, but as the pain goes away, they'll tend to forget," says Dr. Tindall. "If you're taking prescription drugs for gout, you must take them every day in order to prevent future attacks."

can get away with drinking small amounts of alcohol, but others may have to give it up altogether.

Get purines out of your diet. Foods that are high in purines include anchovies, shellfish, gravies made with organ meats, and red meats.

Women do need some red meat in the diet in order to get enough iron, Dr. Tindall adds. "I recommend keeping the serving to about the size of a deck of playing cards. It's fine to have that much twice a week."

Drink a lot of water. Eight to 16 cups daily is ideal. Water increases the amount of uric acid excreted by the kidneys, Dr. Tindall explains. It's especially important to drink water when you're exercising or working hard. "You don't want to get dehydrated, because that can trigger a gout attack."

Exercise regularly. It will keep your weight down, which reduces the amount of uric acid that the body produces. Dr. Tindall advises her patients to get aerobic exercise—jogging, swimming, riding a bike, or aerobic dancing, for example—most days of the week.

In addition to regular exercise, women with a history of gout should think about controlling their weight by following a plant-based diet, one that includes only a small amount of meat, and is rich in fruits, vegetables, whole grains, and legumes. "If you limit red meat, you'll automatically consume less fat and fewer calories, along with cutting down on the purines."

Have some coffee. Studies have linked coffee drinking with lower levels of uric acid in the body. Decaf also seems to work.

Sip cherry juice. One recent small study of 24 patients with gout found that those who had a tablespoon of cherry juice concentrate twice a day for at least 4 months had a more than 50 percent reduction in attacks. The researchers said they didn't see a drop in levels of uric acid, so the effect may be the result of cherries' ability to reduce inflammation.

For more information about gout. Visit the Web sites of the Arthritis Foundation at www. arthritis.org and the National Institute of Arthritis and Musculoskeletal and Skin Diseases at www.nih.gov/niams.

gum problems

Your mouth is a hotbed of bacteria. Hundreds of species of bacteria make their home in the human mouth. Some are harmless; others cause gum disease and tooth decay. Gum disease affects about 75 percent of adults over age 35 to some degree. In recent years, it's been linked to increased risk of heart disease, diabetes, and Alzheimer's disease. The common denominator: inflammation.

Every time you eat, bacteria in the mouth feed on food particles and form a sticky gel called plaque, which adheres to the teeth and wedges beneath the gum line. The bacteria in plaque release toxins that irritate and break down gum tissues, causing gum disease. This condition (also called periodontal disease) is an infection of the tissues surrounding and supporting teeth and a major cause of tooth loss in adults.

The mildest form of gum disease is gingivitis, which causes bleeding and swelling around the gums. This is a signal that your immune system is kicking in, trying to fight the infection with inflammation. "If you catch it early, gingivitis is a fully reversible condition," says Jonathan Korostoff, DMD, PhD, associate professor of periodontics at the University of Pennsylvania School of Dental Medicine in Philadelphia. But if gum disease advances to periodontitis, the gums and bone that support the teeth can become seriously damaged and the localized inflammation can become systemic, predisposing you to more serious disease.

Here's what you need to do.

For Immediate Relief

home remedies

Brush at least twice daily. Brushing your teeth removes plaque and takes away the nourishment that bacteria need to thrive. It's especially important to brush before bedtime because the cleansing flow of saliva is reduced at night. Use a fluoride toothpaste or one contain triclosan/copolymer (such as Colgate Total), which studies have found are better at killing the bacteria that cause cavities and gum disease.

Use soft-bristled brushes. They're less likely to damage the gums than hard brushes. "Brush with more of a gentle circular motion rather than an aggressive up-and-down motion," says Dr. Korostoff. "Studies have shown that to brush effectively, it takes 4 to 5 minutes to do your entire mouth," he adds.

Switch on an electric brush. This kind requires less strength and coordination than manual brushes, so people tend to brush their teeth longer, says Dr. Korostoff. Studies have found that rotating brushes reduced plaque by 17 percent or more over manual toothbrushes.

Rinse in a pinch. Between regular brushings, rinse your mouth with an OTC antimicrobial mouthwash. "I'm not sure they have a dramatic effect on plaque buildup, but the physical action of rinsing does remove particles and plaque," says Dr. Korostoff.

Floss daily. It's the only way to remove plaque and bacteria that hide between the teeth. Don't use a lot of force; it can damage the gums. "You want to do it in a nice, controlled fashion," says Dr. Korostoff. Guide the floss along both sides of each tooth. "You want to go up and down about 6 times on each tooth surface," he adds.

Use an oral irrigator. People don't always have enough manual dexterity (or patience) to floss correctly. Oral irrigation devices such as Waterpik or Hydro Floss direct a strong jet of water between the teeth and around the gums, which removes food particles as well as plaque and bacteria, says Dr. Korostoff.

medical options

Have your teeth professionally cleaned. Your dentist (or a dental hygienist) will remove plaque and tartar from the teeth and beneath the gums. If this doesn't eliminate the infection, you may need antibiotics. They're usually taken

One More Reason to Keep Flossing

a s we've noted, left unchecked, gum disease is more than a mouth problem. It can boost the risk of other health conditions, including heart disease, stroke, diabetes, respiratory infections, and even premature birth.

"Women with gum disease are 3 to 8 times more likely to go into premature labor than those with healthy gums," according to Marjorie Jeffcoat, DMD, professor of periodontics at the University of Pennsylvania School of Dental Medicine, who has studied the link between gum disease and preterm birth. "The more severe the disease is, the greater your odds are of premature labor."

Meanwhile, experts are discovering that some health woes can make gum disease worse. "Diabetes inhibits immune response, leaving you more vulnerable to infection," explains Jack Caton, DDS, a professor of periodontology at the University of Rochester in New York and former president of the American Academy of Periodontology.

And as osteoporosis thins your bones, it can leave your jawbone more vulnerable to erosion from gum disease, explains Dr. Jeffcoat.

So what is the best gum protection plan? Brush twice a day, floss once a day, and have a dental checkup and cleaning twice a year, Dr. Jeffcoat says. ■

when to see a doctor

If your gums are swollen, red, or bleeding, you need to see your dentist right away. These are early signs of gum disease, says Jonathan Korostoff, DMD, PhD, associate professor of periodontics at the University of Pennsylvania School of Dental Medicine in Philadelphia.

If your gums are inflamed and you also have diabetes. Diabetes increases the risk of gum disease. Research also suggests that people with oral infections may have difficulty controlling their glucose (blood sugar) levels.

orally, although your dentist may insert an antibiotic gel directly into parts of the gums.

"People rarely need medications for gum problems," Dr. Korostoff adds. "I usually clean the teeth, and that's enough."

Ask about periodontal pockets. If you have gum disease, these pockets form where tooth meets gum. Ask your dentist how your gums are doing. The earlier that gum disease is diagnosed and treated, the better.

Long-Term Solutions

home remedies

Quit smoking. The American Academy of Periodontology has found that smokers are almost 3 times as likely to suffer gum damage as nonsmokers. Giving up cigarettes is the best solution, but if you're not ready to quit, at least cut back. Research suggests that people who smoke fewer than ten cigarettes daily have half the risk of developing serious gum disease of those who smoke more than thirty cigarettes daily.

hay fever

For 30 percent of all Americans, hay fever is an annual rite of spring. Your eyes well up, your nose springs a leak, and your ears and throat start itching.

"There's a reason they call it hay fever, even though it doesn't cause a fever and it isn't triggered by hay," says Harold S. Nelson, MD, an immunologist and professor of medicine at the National Jewish Medical and Research Center in Denver. "The term was coined in the 19th century because people with hay fever have

fatigue and difficulty thinking, as if they had a feverish illness."

People with hay fever are usually sensitive to pollen, and pollen is everywhere. Ragweed plants, for example, can release up to 1 million pollen granules a day.

Other common causes of hay fever are grasses, which release their eye-watering payload in summer; a variety of weeds, which cause problems in summer and early fall; and trees, which come into bloom in the spring.

Hay fever may also be caused by dust mites, molds, and pet dander, adds Sandra M. Gawchik, DO, codirector of the division of allergy and clinical immunology at Crozer-Chester Medical Center and clinical associate professor of pediatrics at Thomas Jefferson University Medical College in Philadelphia.

It's impossible to avoid all of the allergens that nature throws at you, but reducing the amount that you breathe will help keep your symptoms at manageable levels. In addition, there are a variety of medications that can dramatically reduce the discomfort.

For Immediate Relief
home remedies

Take an antihistamine. Available over the counter, antihistamines that contain chlorpheniramine (Chlor-Trimeton) or diphenhydramine (Benadryl) are very effective at relieving allergy symptoms. The problem with these drugs is that they often cause side effects, including drowsiness or dry mouth. Try nonsedating antihistamines, such as loratadine (Claritin), fexofenadine (Allegra), cetirizine (Zyrtec), and azelastine (Astelin Nasal Spray). They are as effective, more long-lasting, and much less likely to cause side effects.

Time your antihistamines. If your allergies keep you up at night, your doctor may advise you to take one of the sleep-inducing antihistamines at night, when drowsiness isn't a problem. Then, in the morning, you can take one of the nonsedating drugs. However, the drowsiness from the bedtime dose may continue into the next day, so this strategy may not work for everyone, says Dr. Nelson.

Unclog with a decongestant. They won't control your allergies, but they will shrink the swollen membranes in your nose that make it hard to breathe. Don't use decongestant sprays for more than 5 days or you risk rebound congestion, a worsening of your symptoms.

Wash your hair before going to bed. Pollen particles that cling to your hair will coat the pillows at night, giving you an extra 8 hours to breathe them in. Washing your hair at night will remove the pollen before it has a chance to get into your airways.

Close the windows and use the air conditioner. It will trap pollen before it has a chance to get inside. It's also a good idea to use the clothes dryer instead of hanging your laundry outside. Fabrics are natural traps for pollen, especially when they're damp.

Substitute washable throw rugs for wall-to-wall carpets. Carpets trap a tremendous amount of pollen, which can leave you sneezing and rubbing your eyes long after the allergy season is gone. Washing carpets will remove pollen as well as pet dander and other potential allergens.

Use the hot cycle. Cool water will remove pollen, but it won't kill allergy-causing dust mites, which accumulate on rugs, shower curtains, sheets, and bedspreads. Water hotter than 130°F will kill the mites, along with their eggs.

Stay inside in the morning. "Pollen counts are highest between the hours of 6:00 a.m. and 10:00 a.m.," says Dr. Gawchik.

Keep the grass cut short. Mowing the lawn every few days, especially in the spring, will prevent the grass from sprouting pollen-producing flowers.

Keep your work clothes outside. When it's time to come back inside, change into clean clothes, and leave your pollen-laden jeans on the porch. Washing your "outside" clothes after every wearing will help keep their pollen loads low.

Wear a microfiber mask when working outside. Available at hardware stores, the masks slip over the nose and mouth and are held in place with a rubber band. They'll prevent large amounts of mold or pollen from getting into your airways.

alternative therapies

Take stinging nettle. A natural antihistamine, stinging nettle has been used around the world to combat allergies. In one study, 57 percent of people with allergies who took it experienced relief from stuffy nose, sneezing, and sniffles. Start off by taking 20 drops of a 1:1 tincture or 1 teaspoon of a 1:5 tincture once a day for the first few days. Then begin taking this dose 3 times a day. Stinging nettle is available in health food stores and some pharmacies.

Add onions to recipes. And eat plenty of apples. They're among the richest sources of quercetin, a natural plant nutrient that appears to inhibit allergic reactions. In one recent study, it even quashed peanut-induced anaphylactic reactions in lab rats. You can also buy quercetin supplements in health food stores. The recommended dose is 600 mg, taken 2 or 3 times daily.

when to see a doctor

If your hay fever symptoms are accompanied by a fever or a bad headache, call your doctor. Persistent nasal congestion sometimes results in sinusitis, a bacterial infection in the sinuses that may require antibiotics, says Sandra M. Gawchik, DO, codirector of the division of allergy and clinical immunology at Crozer-Chester Medical Center and clinical associate professor of pediatrics at Thomas Jefferson University Medical College in Philadelphia.

If the nasal discharge is greenish or yellowish instead of clear. This can be a sign of a bacterial infection, which may require medical care.

For Long-Term Relief

home remedies

Track pollen counts. When pollen counts are high—usually between 20 and 100 grains per cubic meter—you may want to stay indoors. You can get the latest information on pollen and spore counts in your area on the Web site of the National Allergy Bureau at www.aaaai.org/nab.

Use a nose spray. One of the most effective over-the-counter sprays contains cromolyn sodium (Nasalcrom). If you start taking it a few weeks before allergy season begins and continue using it 4 times daily during the spring and summer, you'll have a dramatic reduction in sneezing and other allergic nasal symptoms.

If nothing seems to help, keep a food diary. The allergy-causing particles in pollen may be similar to proteins found in common foods. If your symptoms include itching in the mouth or swollen lips, it's possible that allergens in carrots, celery, cantaloupe, or other foods are partly responsible. Unfortunately, there isn't a cure for this condition, called "oral allergy syndrome," but avoiding the wrong foods will eliminate the problems, says Dr. Gawchik.

Ask your doctor about steroid nasal sprays. Available by prescription, nasal sprays that contain steroids will lessen nasal itching and reduce nasal swelling that increases congestion. Some people will see an improvement in as little as 12 hours, but others may need 3 to 10 days of use before they see relief of these allergy symptoms, adds Dr. Gawchik. The drugs are usually used in combination with antihistamines.

headaches

Every year, 90 percent of men and 95 percent of women have at least one headache. For some it's just a mild twinge, for others it's skull-pounding agony. Most people—78 percent—have tension headaches, which doesn't meant they're caused by stress, but they could be. What they usually have in common is muscle tightness—tension—at the back of the neck or scalp, but they may also involve chemical and nerve imbalances in the brain.

If you have a tension headache, your whole head can be involved—including the small muscles around the eyes and behind the ears. The pain is usually mild or moderate, and it can be triggered by emotional factors, such as stress, anxiety, fear, or anger.

About 13 percent of population suffers—and that's an accurate description—from migraines. These powerhouse headaches can actually be disabling. They cause moderate to severe throbbing or pulsing pain, usually on one side of the head. The pain of migraines, which can last as long as 3 days, is often accompanied by nausea and sensitivity to light or sound. About 20 percent of migraines are preceded (or accompanied) by visual disturbances that include wavy lines, dots, flashing lights, or blind spots. Some people experience changes in their usual sense of touch, taste, or smell prior to the attacks.

Doctors still aren't sure what causes migraines. The prevailing theory is that a migraine starts when, for some reason, the arteries leading to the main part of the brain close. That decreases blood flow, which may be responsible for the aura or visual hallucinations that some people experience. When those arteries relax, they become overly relaxed, which causes the headache. Serotonin and dopamine, two of the brain's chemical messengers, also appear to be involved. Genes may also play a role: If one parent had migraines, there's a 50 percent chance you will too. That rises to 75 percent if both parents had them.

Women are 3 times more likely than men to get migraines, possibly because changing hormone levels affect the brain. In fact, 60 percent of women report that attacks coincide with their menstrual cycles.

"Some women get migraines from the falling estrogen levels associated with their menstrual cycles," says Stephen D. Silberstein, MD, director of the Jefferson Headache Center and professor of neurology at Thomas Jefferson University Hospital in Philadelphia.

Another hormonal factor that contributes to migraines is pregnancy. "Some women find that they get more migraines during the first trimes-ter, when their levels of estrogen and progesterone change," Dr. Silberstein explains. "The migraines usually go away during the second and third trimesters, when hormones level off. Then, after women give birth, they often return within the first week because of falling estrogen levels."

Hormonal fluctuations are just one migraine trigger. Doctors have identified dozens of things that can set them off, including stress, bright lights, food preservatives (such as nitrites and nitrates), even changes in the weather.

There are several kinds of medications for migraines—ones to relieve pain and others that reduce the severity or frequency of the headaches. In general, they tend to be tougher to tame than tension headaches, but nearly all

THREE THINGS I TELL EVERY FEMALE PATIENT

STEPHEN D. SILBERSTEIN, MD, *director of the Jefferson Headache Center at Thomas Jefferson University Hospital in Philadelphia, offers the following advice for women coping with headaches.*

DON'T WAIT TO GET HELP. Women often assume that headaches are "normal"—and they suffer for years or decades without getting help. "Most women with tension or migraine headaches can get successful treatment that will keep them under control," Dr. Silberstein says. Before your doctor's appointment, keep a journal noting the dates, severity, and duration of the headaches, any possible triggers, and the headache's impact on your life, such as missed workdays, suggests Dr. Silberstein.

THEY'RE NOT "ALL IN YOUR HEAD." In the past, doctors sometimes dismissed headaches as a sign of emotional problems. Nothing could be further from the truth. "Headaches are a biological disorder of the brain, and we can usually control them," says Dr. Silberstein.

TAKE TIME FOR YOURSELF. "Write a prescription for yourself to relax," Dr. Silberstein advises. "Schedule time to do anything you want, whether it's listening to relaxing music, meditating, or reading a book. Everyone needs this special time to relax, and it may prevent headaches." ∎

headaches, regardless of the type, can be managed with a combination of medications and self-care strategies.

For Immediate Relief

home remedies

Use over-the-counter painkillers. They're very effective at stopping tension headaches, says Dr. Silberstein. Aspirin, ibuprofen, naproxen, and acetaminophen are all equally effective.

There are a number of FDA-approved OTC products for treating migraines, he adds. A product called Excedrin Migraine, for example, contains aspirin, acetaminophen, and caffeine. Other migraine medications contain ibuprofen. All these products work for a nondisabling migraine, so you can take them if your pain is not so severe that you are unable to function. Everyone responds differently, so you may have to try several medications to find the one that works best.

Take a hot shower. "It may relieve tension headaches because the warm water loosens and relaxes muscles in the back of the neck and head," says Dr. Silberstein.

Ice it down. Cold compresses are helpful for all types of headaches because they numb the area and also constrict blood vessels, which can reduce the painful pounding. Apply an ice pack or a plastic bag filled with ice cubes and wrapped in a towel to the painful area for about 10 to 15 minutes. Or wrap a bag of frozen peas in a towel and place it on your forehead, Dr. Silberstein suggests.

Have a cup of coffee. There's a reason OTC migraine medications contain caffeine: Studies show it can short-circuit a headache and enhance the painkilling effects of acetaminophen or aspirin. Stick to one cup: Too much caffeine can give you a withdrawal headache when you stop drinking it. (That's true even if you don't have migraines.)

alternative therapies

Try feverfew. It's been used for thousands of years to treat headaches, and there's some evidence that it's effective. A common herb, feverfew contains compounds called sesquiterpene lactones, which reduce spasms in blood vessels in the brain. The research isn't conclusive, but feverfew appears to be more effective at preventing migraines than at stopping them once they begin. The recommended doses vary, depending on the form. If you're using fresh feverfew, take one leaf once daily; for freeze-dried feverfew tablets or capsules, take 300 mg daily; for fresh plant tinctures, take 40 drops daily; and for standardized extracts in tablet form, take a daily dose that provides the equivalent of 0.25 to 0.50 mg of parthenolide.

One more point about feverfew: Many herbs are dried with traditional methods, but this destroys the active compounds in feverfew. It's best to use tinctures made from fresh leaf, or tablets or capsules that contain freeze-dried herb.

Take some butterbur. There have been several studies finding that this little-known herb can reduce the frequency and duration of migraines. Ask your doctor about a safe product to use; butterbur contains dangerous alkaloids that can harm your liver so you want to make sure you use an extract that lowers the alkaloid levels.

For Long-Term Prevention

home remedies

Drink more fluids if you're active. Some people get migraines mainly when they exercise, possibly because they allow themselves to get dehydrated, says Dr. Silberstein. "To prevent dehydration, be sure to drink eight 8-ounce glasses of water each day," he advises. "If you're working out and perspiring, you're losing water, and it needs to be replaced."

Take riboflavin. Researchers have found that brain cells in some people with migraines produce insufficient amounts of energy. One way to boost energy production and prevent headaches might be to flood the cells with vitamin B_2, also known as riboflavin.

In a study in Belgium, 55 migraine sufferers were given either 400 mg of riboflavin or a placebo. At the end of the 3-month study, 56 percent of the riboflavin group reported a decrease in the frequency of their migraine attacks. In the placebo group, only 19 percent had a similar benefit.

The amount of riboflavin used in the study was much higher than the amount that most people get—235 times the Daily Value of 1.7 mg, to be exact. "It's difficult to get that much riboflavin from foods, and the study wasn't recommending that all migraine sufferers take the study amount in supplement form," Dr. Silberstein says. "But women with migraines might consider asking their doctors for advice on whether to try a supplement and the dosage that's right for them," he adds.

A recent study found that riboflavin when taken with a beta-blocker drug, usually prescribed to help prevent migraines, significantly reduced the frequency, intensity, and duration of migraines and decreased patients' need for medicine.

Keep a food journal. Many people believe that when they quit eating the "wrong" foods, their migraines disappear, and there is some

when to see a doctor

If you're experiencing headaches more than usual, or if the pain seems to be getting worse, see your doctor right away. Headaches can be caused by a variety of potentially serious neurological problems, including tumors, says Stephen D. Silberstein, MD, director of the Jefferson Headache Center at Thomas Jefferson University Hospital in Philadelphia.

If the pain mainly occurs on one side of the head. You're probably suffering from migraines, which are a lot more serious (and painful) than garden-variety tension headaches.

If the headaches that you experience are accompanied by nausea or vomiting or if you're experiencing auras or visual disturbances that may include waving lines, flashing lights, or blind spots in your vision that precede or accompany (or both) the headache. You may be experiencing the classic form of migraines, and you'll probably need medications to get them under control.

evidence for that. In one study, 60 patients who went on an elimination diet—banning certain suspected foods—stopped having headaches after 5 days. The number of headaches they experienced fell from 402 to 6 per month, and 85 percent of the study participants became headache free. The foods that appeared to be the likely culprits were wheat, orange, egg, tea and coffee, chocolate, milk, beef, corn, cane sugar, yeast, mushrooms and peas.

For some migraine sufferers, the desire to eat particular foods can be a warning sign of an impending migraine attack, adds Dr. Silberstein.

The next time you get a migraine, take a few minutes to jot down everything you ate in the past 48 hours, Dr. Silberstein suggests. If you keep the journal consistently, you may discover that the headaches are consistently preceded by a craving for certain foods.

Some of the foods that are commonly associated with migraines include:

- Ripened cheeses such as cheddar, Stilton, Brie, and Camembert

- Fermented, marinated, or pickled foods

- Chocolate

- Sour cream

- Nuts or peanut butter

- Sourdough breads or crackers

- Broad beans, lima beans, fava beans, or snow peas

- Foods with monosodium glutamate (MSG), such as soy sauce, seasoned salt, or meat tenderizer

- Papayas, figs, raisins, or avocados

- Citrus fruits

- Processed meats, such as bologna and pepperoni

- Alcoholic beverages

Keep a regular sleep schedule. Women who keep irregular hours—by staying up late on weekends, for example, then sleeping until noon the next day—are more likely to suffer from headaches than those who keep regular hours. "Make sure that the bedroom is dark, peaceful, and quiet," Dr. Silberstein adds. "When your body is resting, your brain is resting."

Exercise regularly. Your body has its own painkillers and they're released when you exercise. Studies have found that exercise helps reduce stress and boost mood, so it can help ease tension as well as migraine headaches. Don't skip meals. About 50 percent of people will get a migraine when they fast.

mind-body techniques

Take up yoga or meditation. Stress probably doesn't cause headaches, but it does act as a trigger in those who are susceptible to migraines or tension headaches. Some of the best ways to relax and reduce stress include yoga, deep breathing, and meditation, says Dr. Silberstein. The U.S. Headache Consortium's treatment guidelines for migraines includes relaxation training, thermal biofeedback combined with relaxation training, EMG biofeedback, and cognitive behavioral therapy, a form of psychological counseling.

Try progressive relaxation. This relaxation technique calls for tensing and then relaxing every muscle in your body, starting with your toes and working upward to your skull. It can take 20 minutes or more to complete a session, but it's worth it. People who practice progressive relaxation say it helps them feel rested and relaxed—and less likely to suffer from headaches.

medical options

Ask about prescription relief. Medications for migraines are divided into two main groups: those that prevent migraines and those that can quickly reduce the pain of attacks.

Doctors have found that medications—such as divalproex sodium (Depakote) and topiramate (Topamax)—used to control some types of seizures can also prevent migraines. Propranolol (Inderal) a beta-blocker used to treat high blood pressure, tremor, and abnormal heartbeats, is also a preventative, as are some other antihypertension medications, antihistamines, antidepressants. and many others. To stop migraines that are already under way, doctors usually prescribe a class of drugs known as triptans, which include sumatriptan (Imitrex), rizatriptan (Maxalt), naratriptan (Amerge), and zolmitriptan (Zomig). The medications work by attaching to a receptor for serotonin, a neurotransmitter in the brain. Some, like Treximet, combine sumatriptan with naproxen sodium, an NSAID. Your doctor may also prescribe antinausea medications, ergot drugs (for recalcitrant pain), other combination drugs such as Bupap and Phrenilin Forte, which mix the sedative butalbital with aspirin or acetaminophen, or others that include caffeine or codeine, as well as opiates.

For the fastest relief possible, doctors often advise people with migraines to use sumatriptan in an injectable form, Dr. Silberstein adds.

Talk about Botox. It's not just for wrinkles. Studies have found that people who get Botox injections have fewer headaches. It's an expensive option, but it's mainly used in those who, for whatever reason, can't take or don't get relief from other medications.

Consider biofeedback. It's a technique that teaches people to control muscle tension, lower blood pressure, and even divert blood away

WHAT WORKS FOR ME

STEPHEN D. SILBERSTEIN, MD, *director of the Jefferson Headache Center at Thomas Jefferson University Hospital in Philadelphia, says, "When I get a bad headache, I take an over-the-counter analgesic or migraine-specific medication.*

"If I'm at work, I take a break by closing the door to my office, shutting off the lights, and unwinding," he adds. "I go into a mild trance, a very calm, relaxing state." ∎

from the head at the first signs of headaches. Biofeedback is simple to learn, but it requires the use of sophisticated equipment that allows patients to monitor changes in their physical signs. Ask your doctor if a referral to a biofeedback specialist would be helpful.

For more information about headaches. Visit the Web site for the National Headache Foundation at www.headaches.org. The telephone number is (888) NHF-5552. Or go to the Web site for the American Council for Headache Education at www.achenet.org.

hemorrhoids

They're the proverbial pain in the butt, but you don't hear much about them. And it's not that a lot of women don't have them About 75 percent of people have hemorrhoids at some time in their lives, but who wants to talk about them? Hemorrhoids occur when veins in the rectum become stretched, swollen, and inflamed. Basically, they're like the varicose veins you see on people's legs, except they are in a much more sensitive area.

Most hemorrhoids occur inside the anus, where there aren't many nerve endings. These internal hemorrhoids aren't painful, but if they protrude outside the anus they can become sensitive and sometimes cause bleeding. Hemorrhoids that start on the outside of the anus, on the other hand, can swell or form a hard lump caused by a blood clot. This type of hemorrhoid, called a thrombosed external hemorrhoid, causes acute pain.

Constipation is the main cause of hemorrhoids. When you strain to have a bowel movement, the increase in internal pressure damages the walls of the veins. If you're pregnant, you're especially vulnerable because the growing uterus also causes an increase in vein-damaging pressure. Many women never experience hemorrhoids until they have a baby.

Hemorrhoids usually go away in a few days to a week, but they can make your life miserable in the meantime. Here are some quick ways to reduce the discomfort and prevent hemorrhoids from coming back.

For Immediate Relief

home remedies

Use baby wipes for a few days. Toilet paper can feel like sandpaper when you have hemorrhoids. "The best thing people can use is alcohol-free baby wipes," says Bruce A. Orkin, MD, chief of colon and rectal surgery and professor of surgery at Tufts University School of Medicine in Medford, Massachusetts.

Take baths instead of showers. Soaking the area in warm water for 10 minutes 2 or 3 times a day will shrink swollen tissues and reduce the discomfort.

Soften the stools. When you have hemorrhoids, having a hard bowel movement can be agony. To soften stools in a hurry, use an over-the-counter stool softener or a fiber supplement that contains psyllium (like Metamucil) or methylcellulose (like Citrucel), following the directions on the label. Stool softeners may be taken twice a day. Fiber supplements with psyllium (Metamucil and Fibercon), should be taken one or two times per day with plenty of fluids, adds Dr. Orkin.

For Long-Term Prevention

home remedies

Increase the fiber in your diet. Found in fruits, vegetables, whole grains, and other plant foods, fiber helps prevent hemorrhoids—and reduces discomfort if you already have them. Gradually increase your fiber intake to avoid bloating.

"Fiber acts like a sponge and soaks up water," Dr. Orkin says. The water makes stools softer, which reduces straining during bowel movements.

According to *Prevention*, everyone should eat 25 to 35 grams of fiber daily. "I tell patients to choose cereals with 5 to 7 grams of fiber per serving," Dr. Orkin says. Add to that a few servings of fresh fruits, raw or lightly steamed vegetables, and fiber-rich foods such as whole grains and legumes, and you'll automatically get all the fiber that you need.

Drink a lot of water. It's absorbed by stools in the intestine, which makes them softer. Plan on drinking eight full glasses of water daily. If

when to see a doctor

If you're having rectal bleeding, even if it's just a few drops on the toilet paper, see your doctor right away. Most bleeding is caused by hemorrhoids, but it can also be caused by colon cancer, says Heidi Nelson, MD, professor of surgery and a member of the division of colorectal surgery at the Mayo Clinic.

If the discomfort is accompanied by changes in bowel habits or unusually thin stools. These are other common symptoms of colon cancer.

If a hemorrhoid is causing excruciating (not just annoying) pain. The hemorrhoid could have a blood clot inside that may need to be removed by your doctor.

you drink coffee, tea, or a caffeinated soft drink, only count that as two-thirds of a serving toward your fluid intake for the day, recommends *Prevention* magazine. These drinks can pull water out of your stool.

Use the bathroom right after breakfast. That's when the body's urge to go is strongest. If you wait until later in the day, you'll probably have to strain more, which increases the risk of hemorrhoids.

Don't dawdle. The more time you spend on the toilet, the more likely you are to suffer from hemorrhoids. "You shouldn't need to sit there for more than a few minutes to have a bowel movement," says Dr. Orkin.

Get a move on. Exercise can help move things along and prevent constipation.

hepatitis

epatitis, an inflammatory disease of the liver, has been called a silent illness because many people don't even know they have it until it's discovered during a routine blood test—sometimes years after they were first infected. If symptoms are present, they are likely to be mild and intermittent. They may include fever, dark urine, light-colored stools, loss of appetite, nausea, vomiting, abdominal pain, and jaundice (yellowing of the skin and whites of the eyes).

Even when it doesn't cause symptoms, hepatitis can result in serious and sometimes permanent damage. It is usually caused by a virus, and the severity of the disease depends on the type of virus that's involved.

The main types of hepatitis are labeled A, B, and C. Hepatitis A, the mildest form of the disease, is often caused by exposure to something that's been contaminated with the stool of someone who's infected. Typically, it is spread by household members or food handlers who fail to wash their hands after using the bathroom. Hepatitis B is often spread by sexual contact or the transfer of contaminated blood—by an accidental needle stick, for example. Hepatitis C, the most serious form of the disease, is spread mainly by tainted blood; it's common among drug addicts who share hypodermic needles.

Hepatitis A almost always clears up on its own, says Samuel Meyers, MD, a gastroenterologist and clinical professor of medicine at Mount Sinai School of Medicine in New York City. Types B and C, however, may become chronic and may require a combination of medications and lifestyle adjustments to keep the infection and symptoms under control and to prevent liver failure or cancer.

For Immediate Relief

home remedies

Drink plenty of water. Vomiting is a common symptom of hepatitis in the early stages, says Dr. Meyers. Drinking a lot of fluids—doctors usually recommend drinking at least 64 ounces daily—will help prevent dehydration.

Rest, and keep resting. "The classic symptom of hepatitis is fatigue and weakness," says Dr. Meyers. "You don't have to stay in bed, but it's important to rest or take naps whenever you feel tired."

Avoid ibuprofen or other painkillers. They're processed by the liver, so taking them can slow your recovery time or lead to further damage.

"If you're feverish, you can put a cold compress on your head," says Dr. Meyers. "The less medication you use, the better off you'll be."

Don't drink alcohol. When you have hepatitis, the effects of alcohol on the liver are magnified: A single beer or glass of wine is the equivalent of having four or five drinks when you're healthy, Dr. Meyers explains. Even small amounts of alcohol are likely to increase damage to the liver.

alternative therapies

Take milk thistle. It contains a chemical compound called silymarin, which is thought to

when to see a doctor

If you have flulike symptoms, such as fatigue, fever, loss of appetite, and nausea, that linger more than 2 weeks, see your doctor. Hepatitis is often confused with the flu in the early stages, says Samuel Meyers, MD, a gastroenterologist and clinical professor of medicine at Mount Sinai School of Medicine in New York City.

If you have dark urine or pale stools. These are classic signs of hepatitis. They indicate that the liver isn't working properly and may be inflamed.

If you develop symptoms about 2 weeks after having unprotected sex. Hepatitis B is commonly spread by sexual contact.

reduce damage to liver cells and help the cells regenerate. In fact, in a 2011 study of 1,049 patients in the Hepatits C Antiviral Long-Term Treatment against Cirrhosis (HALT-C) study, those who took silymarin (34 percent) and had advanced hepatitis C-related liver disease saw a reduced progression in their disease.

Look for supplements that contain 150 mg of milk thistle extract that's been standardized to contain 70 percent silymarin. Take one capsule 3 times daily for as long as the infection lasts. It can be used for both acute and chronic hepatitis.

Boost immunity with maitake. A type of mushroom, maitake stimulates the body's defensive white blood cells and may reduce symptoms of hepatitis, according to Douglas Schar, PhD, an herbalist and author. A study done at Pennsylvania State University found that mushrooms do have anti-inflammatory properties. He recommends taking 4 to 6 grams of tableted powdered maitake daily as long as you're having symptoms.

medical options

Take immune globulin immediately. If you suspect you've been exposed to hepatitis B—because your spouse is infected, for example—a prescription medication called immune globulin may eliminate the virus and prevent infection.

"You have to take it very early," Dr. Meyers adds. "If symptoms have already appeared, immune globulin won't help."

Treat chronic hepatitis with drug therapy. About 6 percent of those infected with hepatitis B and nearly everyone who gets hepatitis C are unable to eliminate the virus from their bodies, says Dr. Meyers. Your doctor may recommend taking interferon, which may eradicate the virus in some cases. Interferon, a synthetic version of a substance that is naturally produced by the body's cells, stimulates immunity, but may cause depression, hypothyroidism, loss of appetite, and flulike symptoms. It's often combined with antiviral drugs to reduce the amount of virus in your system. This dual therapy can result in elimination of the virus in 50 percent of the people who take it.

Prevent it. There are vaccines to prevent hepatitis A and B. The hepatitis B vaccine is now routinely given to all babies in their first year, but it's advisable for anyone who is at high risk, including health care providers, travelers who will be in areas where it's widespread, and people who have multiple sex partners or use IV drugs to get both A and B vaccines.

Long-Term Solution

Exercise if you can. Walking, biking, and other forms of exercise can help restore some of the energy that hepatitis takes away. But don't overdo it, Dr. Meyers advises. "If you get tired, rest. You have to use common sense."

For more information about hepatitis. Visit the Web site of the American Liver Foundation at www.liverfoundation.org.

hives

Stress. Food. Heat. Cold. Whatever the cause, hives can leave your skin with a mass of inflamed, itchy bumps.

One out of five people will get hives at least once. If you've had them before, chances are you'll have them again, especially if you have a family history of hives or suffer from hay fever, food allergies, eczema, or asthma, says Gillian Shepherd, MD, an allergist/immunologist and clinical associate professor of medicine at Weill Cornell Medical College of Cornell University in New York City.

Hives usually come and go within a few hours; they're intensely itchy, but relatively brief. In rare cases, though, they become chronic, lasting for months and even years.

"Hives can be caused by everything under the sun—and even the sun itself," notes dermatologist Wilma F. Bergfeld, MD, section head in the department of dermatology at the Cleveland Clinic Foundation in Cleveland. "Your body is visibly reacting to something."

The most common triggers are things you ingest: foods such as nuts, chocolate, shellfish, berries, and tomatoes; and medications like antibiotics, pain relievers, and sedatives. A trigger prompts mast cells in the skin to release chemicals, called histamines, that cause swelling and itching, notes Mary Ruth Buchness, MD, chairperson of the dermatology section of the New York Academy of Medicine and a dermatologist in private practice in New York City.

"Some people also get them from stress or chronic infections, like hepatitis B," adds Dr. Buchness. "Others react to something physical, like heat, exercise, air conditioning, and even pressure from a tight belt or the elastic on their underwear."

If you have hives, the first order of business is to relieve the itching and inflammation, then take steps to avoiding what gets under your skin. Here's what doctors recommend.

For Immediate Relief

Cool the itch. To reduce swelling, constrict blood vessels, and slow the release of histamines, place a few ice cubes inside a wet towel or paper towel and apply to the affected area. Let it melt there for 1 or 2 minutes, then take it off. Reapply within minutes or as needed until the itching subsides, says Dr. Bergfeld. Cold baths and showers lasting 15 to 30 minutes will also provide relief from itching.

Choose your anti-itch lotion carefully. Try over-the counter anti-itch treatments available at your local drugstore, says Dr. Buchness.

when to see a doctor

 If hives last longer than 24 hours, cover approximately 10 percent of your skin (one whole arm, a thigh, or your entire stomach, for example) or don't blanch (turn white) when you press them. Contact your doctor, advises allergist-immunologist Gillian Shepherd, MD, clinical associate professor of medicine at Weill Cornell Medical College of Cornell University in New York City.

If hives worsen rapidly or if you have difficulty breathing, feel light-headed, or grow nauseated, you may be suffering from anaphylactic shock, an extreme drop in blood pressure and other problems, which is a sign of a severe, body-wide allergic reaction. Go to the nearest emergency room. You may need a shot of epinephrine (a drug similar to the natural adrenaline in your body) to open your breathing passages and keep your blood pressure from dropping dangerously low. If your response to an allergen is this serious, you will want to carry an EpiPen, an OTC product containing epinephrine, with you at all times.

Avoid creams containing antihistamines or those ending in "caine," such as benzocaine, which may cause an allergic reaction when applied to the skin.

Bathe in oatmeal. For additional relief, Dr. Buchness recommends natural colloidal oatmeal powder, available OTC in various brands, added to a lukewarm bath.

Take an antihistamine. If needed, try 25 mg of diphenhydramine (Benadryl) every 4 hours, advises Dr. Buchness. If this makes you too drowsy, take a nonsedating alternative, such as fexofenadine (Allegra), cetirizine (Zyrtec), astemizole (Hismanal), or loratadine (Claritin), Dr. Bergfeld suggests. If they aren't working well enough for you, ask your doctor about combining them with other drugs, including antacid pills, anti-inflammatory antibiotics, nifedipine (a blood pressure medicine), Accolate (an asthma drug), and colchicine (a gout drug), all of which are nonstandard therapies that work for some, according to the American Osteopathic College of Dermatology.

alternative therapies

Try herbal antihistamines. If drugstore antihistamines bother you, consider antihistamine alternatives, such as stinging nettle. This remedy may surprise you since rubbing against stinging nettle plants in the wild irritates the skin and causes hivelike welts. When taken orally, however, it contains substances that heal hives. Studies have found that it reduces the amount of histamine the body produces in response to contact with an allergen. Take one or two capsules of freeze-dried nettle leaf extract every 2 to 4 hours until symptoms disappear.

Quercetin, a bioflavonoid from citrus fruits and buckwheat, is another effective antihistamine. Take 400 mg of quercetin tablets twice daily until symptoms disappear, suggests Andrew Weil, MD, director of the program in integrative medicine and clinical professor of medicine at the University of Arizona College of Medicine in Tucson and author of *8 Weeks to Optimum Health*.

mind-body techniques

Calm yourself. Not only does stress sometimes cause hives, particularly chronic cases, but it can aggravate an outbreak you already have, notes Dr. Buchness. She recommends stress-busting activities, such as biofeedback, acupuncture, meditation, or anything that calms you.

(For additional steps you can take to handle stress, read Chapter 7.)

Long-Term Solutions

home remedies

Avoid known triggers. "Hives usually show up within a couple of hours after contact with a stimulus," says Dr. Buchness. So once you discover the cause, it makes sense to avoid it in the future.

Play detective. For chronic hives, keeping a food diary may help scout out the source. But if you're not having luck, your doctor may order some tests. "With chronic cases, we seldom find the cause," Dr. Buchness admits. "But most hives eventually go away as mysteriously as they came."

For more information on hives. Visit the American College of Allergy, Asthma and Immunology) at www.acaai.org.

THREE THINGS I TELL EVERY FEMALE PATIENT

WILMA F. BERGFELD, MD, *a dermatologist and the section head in the department of dermatology at the Cleveland Clinic Foundation in Cleveland, offers this special advice.*

1 **LIQUID ANTIHISTAMINES BRING FASTER RELIEF.** They're absorbed into the blood in only 15 to 20 minutes, compared with 30 to 45 minutes for pills, but they also contain more sugar. If you're obese or have diabetes, you'll need to remember to factor in the additional sugar to your diet.

2 **HIVES AND HEAT DON'T MIX.** Avoid hot showers or intense workouts. Heat increases blood flow to the skin, encouraging the release of more histamines.

3 **CONSIDER ALL CAUSES.** Not only can you have multiple allergies at once, but the source of your hives may change over time. ■

inflammatory bowel disease

Unpredictability is one of the biggest challenges of inflammatory bowel disease. You can go for months, even years, without symptoms, then one day you're heading to the bathroom 6 or 7 times a day or more with abdominal cramps and diarrhea, which leads to weight loss and other painful (and frightening) symptoms.

There are two main types of inflammatory bowel disease, or IBD: Crohn's disease, which can damage any part of the digestive tract, and ulcerative colitis, which affects only the top layer of the large intestine, explains Theodore M. Bayless, MD, professor of medicine and director emeritus of the Meyerhoff Inflammatory Bowel Disease Center at Johns Hopkins Hospital in Baltimore and author of 13 books for physicians and patients.

Despite these differences, the conditions have many things in common. During flare-ups, patches of the intestine become raw and irritated. The inflammation is usually limited to the intestinal surface, but sometimes the damage extends all the way through the intestinal wall.

No one's sure what causes IBD, but it appears to be an immune disorder—a condition that occurs when the immune system mistakenly attacks the body's tissues. In this case, it may lead to an imbalance in the normal bacteria found in the digestive system. More women than men have the disease.

There's no cure for IBD, but most people can manage it successfully with medications, lifestyle changes, surgery, or a combination of these treatments.

For Immediate Relief

home remedies

Keep track of what you eat. For some people, eating fatty foods can result in cramping or diarrhea; for others, spicy foods or caffeine is a problem. Still others have a tough time with the high fiber content of nuts and raw fruits and vegetables. When the disease is active, use a food diary to figure out which foods make your symptoms worse. Many physicians recommend avoiding dairy products. However, these are excellent sources of calcium, so don't eliminate them from your diet if you can tolerate them.

Eat smaller meals. It's usually easier for the intestines to handle small, frequent meals than single large servings.

Ease discomfort with a hot-water bottle. Place it on your abdomen when you're experiencing cramps to reduce some of your pain, suggests Sunanda V. Kane, MD, associate professor of medicine at the Mayo Clinic College of Medicine.

Take extra calcium. Evidence suggests that it reduces the severity and frequency of abdominal cramps, says Dr. Kane. She advises taking 1,200 to 1,500 mg of calcium daily, based on the amounts used in studies.

Drink chamomile or peppermint tea. The herbs contain compounds that reduce spasms in the intestine, which can help ease gas and painful cramps. To make a tea, pour 1 cup of boiling water over 1 to 2 teaspoons of dried herb, cover, and let steep for 10 to 15 minutes. Keep in mind that peppermint taken close to bedtime may cause heartburn by relaxing the esophagus.

For Long-Term Relief

Avoid aspirin or ibuprofen. They're a very common cause of IBD relapses because they weaken the mucosa, the protective coating that lines the intestine.

If you smoke, try to quit. "For people with Crohn's disease, smoking increases relapses," Dr. Bayless says.

Exercise—and relax. Emotional stress doesn't cause IBD, but it can make the symptoms worse. An excellent way to reduce stress is to get regular exercise. As a bonus, exercise helps prevent weight gain in those taking steroids to control their symptoms, says Dr. Kane. (For step-by-step details on starting an exercise program, see Chapter 5.)

Take some deep breaths. Learn meditation, yoga, or tai chi, or just do simple muscle relaxation exercises to keep your tension in check.

Drink plenty of water. If you're doing regular exercise, you need to avoid dehydration, so make sure you drink both before and after you exercise.

Say no to the big three. Caffeine, alcohol, and tobacco may increase or worsen symptoms.

Have some probiotics. The active live cultures in yogurt provide your gut with some of these good bacteria, but they're also available as supplements. One small study found that taking *Saccharomyces boulardii* (250 mg 3 times a day to 500 mg 4 times a day) reduced the incidence of diarrhea in people with Crohn's, though other

---

THREE THINGS I TELL EVERY FEMALE PATIENT

WILLIAM TREMAINE, MD, *professor of medicine at the Mayo Clinic College of Medicine, has some special advice for patients with inflammatory bowel disease.*

1 TALK TO YOUR FAMILY AND FRIENDS. People with intestinal disorders are often too embarrassed to discuss their conditions with others, but the support you get from family will help you cope with this difficult condition.

2 JOIN A SUPPORT GROUP. It's a great place to get emotional support as well as practical tips for controlling IBD. The Crohn's and Colitis Foundation of America Web site (www.ccfa.org) will steer you to a support group in your area.

3 DO YOUR HOMEWORK. The more you learn about the disease, the better you'll be able to manage it, says Dr. Tremaine. ∎

studies have had mixed results. Still, it's a promising line of investigation. In a 2010 study, scientists found that butyric acid–an anti-inflammatory chemical secreted by certain gut bacteria–may help restore normal levels of digestive system bacteria and reduce symptoms. Many IBD patients have reduced levels of the butyric acid-producing bacteria.

medical options

Control IBD with medications. Not so long ago, the main treatment for IBD was corticosteroids–drugs that are rife with side effects. There are many more options today, including drugs that modify the immune system and get the inflammation under control, says Stephan R. Targan, MD, director of the Inflammatory Bowel Disease Center at Cedars-Sinai Medical Center in Los Angeles.

Talk to your doctor about supplements. People with IBD often have decreased appetite and malabsorption issues so they may be lacking in some vitamins and minerals, such as vitamin D, B_{12}, K, folic acid, calcium, and zinc. Your physician may recommend you take a daily multivitamin.

For more information about IBD. Visit the Web site of the Crohn's and Colitis Foundation of America at www.ccfa.org. Or look up "digestive diseases" at the Web site of the National Institute of Diabetes and Digestive and Kidney Diseases at www.niddk.nih.gov.

irritable bowel syndrome

f you ever want to know where the restroom is, ask a woman with irritable bowel syndrome (IBS). She scouted it out the minute she walked into the room. She had to, because the symptoms of IBS–usually abdominal pain, cramping, and diarrhea–can come on with very little warning.

Before leaving the house, women with IBS invariably ask themselves, "Is my bowel going to act up today?" says Nancy Norton of Milwaukee, founder of the International Foundation for Functional Gastrointestinal Disorders.

IBS is unpredictable. Some women will have sudden attacks of diarrhea, sometimes several times a day. For others, diarrhea may alternate with constipation, painful gas buildups, or other digestive upsets.

There's still a lot of mystery surrounding IBS. Normally, the muscular walls of the intestine contract and relax in a predictable and rhythmic way. Research has shown that in people with IBS, the contractions are stronger and last longer–although it's not yet clear if this is the underlying cause of the condition, says Marie Borum, MD, professor of medicine in the Division of Gastroenterology at George Washington University in Washington, DC. Other speculation: People with IBS have colons that are hypersensitive to certain foods or stress; there may also be immune system involvement.

Since doctors haven't discovered what causes IBS, there still isn't a cure. However, there are a number of medications that can control the symptoms. In addition, there are a number of home-care strategies that will go a long way toward reducing the discomfort.

For Immediate Relief

home remedies

Be prepared. Many people with IBS have a condition called exaggerated gastrocolic reflex—the very act of eating sends a premature signal to your colon to stimulate contractions while you're eating or, more likely, just after you finish a meal. Sometimes it's related to a particular food. Some people report it after eating at restaurants—not the best place when a sudden urge to go happens. For short-term control of diarrhea, take over-the-counter diarrhea remedies such as loperamide (Imodium), says Eugene Bozymski, MD, professor of medicine at the University of North Carolina at Chapel Hill. It may also help to do an elimination diet—drop out the foods your gut tells you are problems and see if you have fewer episodes. If so, avoid those foods.

Cut back on coffee and tea. Caffeine may irritate the digestive tract, so it's a good idea to avoid anything containing caffeine.

Take fatty foods off the menu. They're difficult for the body to digest, which can result in more gas and indigestion.

Choose soluble fiber supplements over bran. Some IBS sufferers find that bran and other foods rich in insoluble fiber worsen their condition. If you're one of them, switch to a soluble fiber supplement, such as psyllium.

Apply heat. Electric heating pads, a nice soak in a warm tub, or a hot-water bottle can all help relieve abdominal discomfort. Heat wraps designed for menstrual cramps (such as ThermaCare HeatWraps) may also help, and you can wear them under your clothes.

Reduce gas. Bloating or distention resulting from intestinal gas is one of the most common symptoms of IBS and can also lead to cramping and abdominal pain. Over-the-counter products that contain simethicone may help relieve intestinal gas. Or you may want to try an OTC product called Beano. Taken with gassy foods, such as broccoli or beans, its enzyme action helps you digest the sugars in these foods that give you trouble and actually prevents gas from forming.

Eat less dairy. Millions of Americans have a condition called lactose intolerance: They don't produce enough of the enzyme (lactase) that's needed to digest a sugar (lactose) found in dairy foods. If you're lactose intolerant and also have IBS, even small amounts of milk, cheese, or other dairy foods may cause symptoms.

when to see a doctor

If diarrhea or other common symptoms of IBS are accompanied by weight loss, see a doctor right away. You could have a more serious digestive condition, called Crohn's disease, says Marie Borum, MD, professor of medicine in the division of gastroenterology at George Washington University in Washington, DC.

If you notice rectal bleeding or if you've had recent changes in your symptoms. Some of the same signs of IBS can also be caused by colon cancer. You'll want to get a checkup right away.

If you're lactose intolerant, you might be able to enjoy small servings of dairy foods, especially if you have them with other foods. You can try adding lactase enzyme (Lactaid) to dairy products or buying dairy products that already come with it. Or you may have to avoid dairy products altogether. You may have to experiment a bit to find out which approach works for you.

Consider probiotics. The "good" bacteria in products such as active culture yogurt and supplements—particularly *Lactobacillus acidophilus* and *Bifidobacterium*—have helped relieve the symptoms of IBS in some, though not all studies.

Turn to flax. If your IBS manifests as constipation, 6 to 24 grams of flaxseed a day may help. In one study, 55 people who used flaxseed reduced constipation, bloating, and stomach discomfort.

alternative therapies

Relax the intestine with herbs. Chamomile and valerian relax intestinal contractions. Valerian may be especially helpful because it also reduces stress, a common trigger of IBS. Pour 1 cup of boiling water over 1 to 2 teaspoons of dried chamomile flowers. Cover and let steep for 10 to 15 minutes. For valerian, take two 500-mg root tablets 30 minutes before bed.

You can buy herbal teas and supplements at pharmacies and health food stores.

Try peppermint. Another herb that relaxes the intestinal muscles, it appears to be very helpful for those with IBS, says Mark Stengler, NMD, a naturopathic physician at the Stengler Center for Integrative Medicine in La Jolla, California.

In one study, of the 52 people with IBS who took one peppermint capsule before meals for 1 month, most reported having less abdominal pain, bloating, and diarrhea. If you decide to try peppermint capsules, look for products that are enteric-coated: They dissolve in the intestine instead of in the stomach, thereby reducing stomach upset. Look for capsules with 0.2 to 0.4 milliliter of oil.

Try cognitive therapy. Studies have shown that using a type of "talk therapy" can help you feel better by changing the way you view your problems. Cognitive therapy involves keeping a diary of your symptoms and your feelings about them. A therapist can help you reframe your feelings so you gain control over your IBS symptoms.

Take a yoga class. A few small studies have found that people who practice yoga have fewer IBS symptoms.

Get hypnotized. If you're hypnotizable, there's good scientific evidence that hypnotherapy can help reduce your IBS symptoms. In one study of 81 people with IBS, those who received five weekly sessions with a hypnotherapist and also used a self-hypnosis tape had significantly fewer symptoms than those who didn't get the mind-body treatment. To find a trained hypnotherapist, contact the American Association of Professional Hypnotherapists at (503) 533-7106 or go to their Web site, aaph.org.

For Long-Term Relief

home remedies

Include more fiber in your diet. It's among the best strategies for controlling IBS, says Dr.

Borum. *Prevention* recommends getting 25 to 35 grams of fiber daily. If you start the day with a high-fiber cereal, snack on fruit throughout the day, and include several servings of vegetables with meals, you'll almost automatically get all the fiber you need.

There are several types of fiber, and they aren't quite interchangeable. If your main symptom is diarrhea, try to increase your intake of soluble fiber, found in fruits, oatmeal, rice, barley, and psyllium, says Elaine Magee, MPH, RD, author of *Tell Me What to Eat If I Have Irritable Bowel Syndrome*. If constipation is the problem, you'll do better focusing on the insoluble fiber found in legumes, whole wheat, and vegetables.

Keep a regular meal schedule. Having breakfast, lunch, and dinner at the same time every day will help regulate digestion and prevent sneak attacks of IBS.

Eat cooked vegetables. They're easier to digest than raw vegetables, says Dr. Stengler.

Eat smaller meals. Overdoing it at the table has been linked to a worsening of IBS symptoms.

medical options

Talk to your doctor about antidepressants. Patients with more severe symptoms may benefit from antidepressants. They have been shown to relieve some of the symptoms of IBS, especially when people are also suffering from pain and depression.

Your doctor may recommend one of the tricyclic antidepressants, such as imipramine (Tofranil) or amitriptyline (Elavil). Apart from reducing stress and depression, these drugs may decrease stool frequency, which is helpful for some people with IBS.

Other medications that may be helpful to some people include fluoxetine (Prozac) or paroxetine (Paxil). These drugs tend to be used when people with IBS are suffering from constipation as well as depression.

THREE THINGS I TELL EVERY FEMALE PATIENT

MARK STENGLER, ND, *a naturopathic physician at the Stengler Center for Integrative Medicine in La Jolla, California, suffered from IBS for years. Here are his strategies for getting the symptoms under control.*

1 EXERCISE REGULARLY. There's no scientific evidence that it controls IBS, but many patients report that it helps. "Choose an exercise that you really like, such as taking walks with a friend," Dr. Stengler advises.

TAKE CONTROL OF STRESS. "When you're under stress, the sympathetic nervous system gets stimulated and the normal contractions of the intestines are altered," he explains. Some of the best ways to reduce stress include yoga, prayer, and meditation. "You'll have to experiment to find what works best for you," he says.

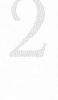

TRY PASSIONFLOWER. An herb, it reduces digestive discomfort, Dr. Stengler explains. If you're using a 1:1 tincture, take 20 drops three times daily. If you're using capsules, take two 500-mg tablets three times daily. ∎

Ask about other treatment options. In a study of 800 people with IBS, those who took a medication called tegaserod (Zelnorm) daily for 12 weeks had 20 percent less abdominal pain and 25 percent less constipation. For severe diarrhea symptoms that don't respond to other treatments, your doctor may prescribe alosetron hydrochloride (Lotronex), which has serious side effects, including reduced blood flow to the colon. A large 2011 study found that a 2-week course of the antibiotic rifaximin (Xifaxan) stopped the symptoms of IBS and that relief last for 10 weeks after stopping the drug. The study, which looked at 600 IBS patients whose main symptom was diarrhea, found that more than 40 percent experience symptom relief after the first 4 weeks compared to around 30 percent of those on placebo. The researchers believe the drug eliminates the bacteria in the bowel that may cause diarrhea.

kidney infections

Even women who get frequent urinary tract infections are surprised—and dismayed—by how sick they feel when the infection moves upward from the bladder to the kidneys.

The kidneys are the body's main filters. They remove waste products from the blood and ship them to the bladder for disposal. An infection in the kidneys, called pyelonephritis, can result in excruciating pain. There's also a risk that the infection will spread to other parts of the body.

"Women get kidney infections more than men because they tend to ignore bladder infections, instead of getting them treated right away," says urologist Larrian Gillespie, MD, former medical director of the Pelvic Pain Treatment Center in Beverly Hills and author of *You Don't Have to Live with Cystitis.*

Kidney infections tend to occur when bacteria that have multiplied in the bladder travel upstream through the ureters, the tubes that connect the kidneys to the bladder. It's common, in fact, for women to have infections in the kidneys and bladder at the same time. You know you have a traveling infection when you feel pain in your back, side, and groin, you have a fever, you feel nauseous or vomit, and you have pain when you urinate.

Kidney infections don't get better with self-care treatments. Once you have one, you'll need antibiotics not only to kill the infection but to prevent it from spreading, a rare complication but one that can lead to sepsis and kidney failure. While you're waiting for the drugs to work, there are a number of ways to reduce the discomfort. You can also take steps to prevent future infections.

For Immediate Relief

home remedies

Drink as much as you can hold. Water helps flush the infection from the kidneys, and it also dilutes the concentration of bacteria in the bladder, which can prevent kidney infections from getting started, says Dr. Gillespie. For long-term protection, *Prevention* recommends drinking at least eight 8-ounce glasses of water daily.

Use pain relievers as needed. While you're waiting for antibiotics to work, taking aspirin or ibuprofen will help reduce fever and muscle aches, says Dr. Gillespie. Just follow the directions on the label.

Apply heat. Women with kidney infections often feel better when they apply a hot-water bottle to the abdomen or below the ribs, says Dr. Gillespie.

medical options

Get a prescription. Kidney infections always require antibiotics and cannot be treated with herbs, says Dr. Gillespie. Some women get so sick that they're given the drugs intravenously, but oral medications are usually effective. The antibiotics—such as trimethoprim with sulfamethoxazole, ciprofloxacin, amoxicillin, Augmentin, doxycycline or fluoroquinolones—are usually taken for anywhere from 3 to 14 days, depending on the severity of the infection.

Reduce bladder irritation. Women with kidney infections often experience intense urges to urinate, even after they've just used the bathroom. An over-the-counter medication called phenazopyridine (such as Pyridium) reduces the "gotta go" symptoms and the burning pain, says Dr. Gillespie.

For Long-Term Relief

home remedies

Inhibit bacteria with baking soda. If you have a bladder infection and want to ensure that it doesn't spread to the kidneys, mix ¼ teaspoon baking soda in a glass of water and drink it once a day. It makes the urine more alkaline, which helps prevent bacteria from thriving, says Dr. Gillespie.

Keep bacteria away from the urethra. Women often get kidney or bladder infections when germs from the anal area get inside the urethra, the tube that carries urine from the body. When you use the bathroom, always wipe from front to back, which pushes bacteria out of harm's way, says Mary Jane Minkin, MD, clinical professor of obstetrics and gynecology at Yale University School of Medicine.

when to see a doctor

If you have pain in the flank (below the ribs toward the back), fever, or nausea and vomiting, see a doctor right away. These are classic symptoms of kidney infections, says urologist Larrian Gillespie, MD, former medical director of the Pelvic Pain Treatment Center in Beverly Hills and author of *You Don't Have to Live with Cystitis.*

If the urine is cloudy or tinged with blood or if it has an unpleasant smell. You probably have an infection somewhere in the urinary tract—either in the bladder or the kidneys.

Wash before sex. Washing the genital area—with soap and water, or simply warm water—removes bacteria that might otherwise slip into the urethra, says Dr. Minkin. Urinating after sex is also helpful because it flushes away bacteria that were lucky enough to get inside.

Use sanitary pads. Tampons may make you more susceptible to infection. Make sure you change the pads every time you use the bathroom.

Avoid anything perfumed. Stay away from douches, sprays, powders, and bubble baths since they can create irritation and increase infection risk.

Drink cranberry juice daily. Research has shown that cranberry juice contains chemical compounds that make it more difficult for bacteria to stick to cells in the urinary tract. Women who get a lot of infections will often drink one or two glasses of cranberry juice daily as a preventive measure. Dried cranberries, which contain the same infection-fighting chemicals, are also a good choice.

kidney stones

Kidney stones are so painful, more than a half a million people every year drag themselves to an emergency room to have one treated. "I've known people who were involved in car accidents because they were so distracted by the severe pain of their kidney stones," says Howard Heller, MD, an endocrinologist in Dallas, Texas. Conversely, some people may experience little or no pain, but this is fairly rare.

Are you at risk? Check the color of your urine: The darker it is, the more concentrated it is—and the greater your risk for developing kidney stones.

Here's how they happen: When minerals and other substances in urine become too concentrated, they may form hard little crystals on the kidney walls. You won't have a problem as long as the rough little stones stay in place. But sometimes a stone breaks free and squeezes through one of the ureters, the tubes that connect the kidneys to the bladder, or the urethra, which carries urine from the bladder out of the body.

Kidney stones can often cause extreme pain, usually on either side of the lower back, when they're lodged or passing. They can also be accompanied by blood in the urine, nausea or vomiting, fever or chills, or urine that smells bad or looks cloudy. Large kidney stones can cause bleeding, infection, and severe kidney damage. Sometimes they get stuck in the ureters or other parts of your urinary tract and have to be removed in the hospital. And having one stone doesn't guarantee it won't happen again. Quite the opposite: People who have had one kidney stone once have a 50 to 70 percent chance of a repeat performance.

You're also at higher risk if you have high blood pressure, diabetes, are obese, have osteoporosis, or have a family history of stones. Scientists aren't sure why, but the incidence of kidney stones is on the rise. In the late 1970s, less than 4 percent of the population had kidney stones; now it's climbed to more than 5 percent and some of them are children.

For Immediate Relief

home remedies

Dilute the urine. You can help kidney stones pass more quickly—and prevent them from coming back—by drinking nine to ten 8-ounce glasses of water daily. To accomplish this, Dr. Heller recommends drinking two glasses with meals, one between meals, one at bedtime, and, for people who frequently get stones, one more during the night. "Increasing fluid intake can significantly reduce the risk of stones," says Dr. Heller. "It's the cheapest medicine we have."

Enjoy lemonade. It counts toward your water total, and it also contains citrate, a chemical that inhibits the formation of kidney stones. Medical researchers recently found that drinking lemonade every day is an effective way for people prone to kidney stones to slow the development of new stones. To try your own lemonade therapy, mix 1 cup of concentrated lemon juice with 7 cups of water and sweeten with a noncaloric sweetener. Then pucker up and drink as much as you can.

Take something for pain. Kidney stones can be excruciatingly painful until they pass—which can take anywhere from a few minutes to hours or even days. To reduce the pain, take acetaminophen, or, if that doesn't work, try ibuprofen or another over-the-counter analgesic, Dr. Heller advises. Just follow the dosage directions on the label. For severe pain, your doctor may prescribe stronger medications.

medical options

Crush the stones. When a kidney stone is too large to pass by itself, your doctor may crush the stone with a procedure called extracorporeal shock wave lithotripsy (ESWL). Sound waves pass through the abdomen and are absorbed by the stone, which often crumbles. The smaller fragments then pass out of the body in the urine.

Go in after them. If your stone is stuck in mid- or lower-ureter, your doctor can reach it with a small fiber optic instrument called a ureteroscope inserted through your urethra and bladder. He or she then shatters the stone with a

when to see a doctor

If you have pain that began around the flank (the area under the ribs toward the back) and then moved toward the groin, call your doctor. You're probably passing a kidney stone, says Howard Heller, MD, an endocrinologist in Dallas. This pain can be severe and may be accompanied by fever, nausea, burning with urination, blood in the urine, or the inability to urinate.

If you've had kidney stones along with a rapid heartbeat, insomnia, or increasing irritability. You could be producing too much thyroid hormone, which increases calcium levels in the urine.

If you get frequent urinary tract infections. They're a common cause of a class of kidney stones called struvite stones.

laser or shock wave, or removes the stone whole with a small cage-like device.

See a surgeon. Stones that don't respond to sound waves may need to be surgically removed. With a recently developed procedure called percutaneous nephrolithotomy, a surgeon can remove stones with a tiny tube that's inserted through the back into the kidney.

Long-Term Solutions

home remedies

As always, drinking plenty of water is an important factor in the prevention of kidney stones. For some people, the following changes in diet may also be helpful—but be sure to consult your doctor first to make sure that these changes are right for you.

Reduce the oxalates. If you have calcium oxalate stones—the most common kind of kidney stone—you may want to reduce your intake of meats (especially organ meats), spinach, rhubarb, beets, chocolate, and many other foods that contain oxalates.

"Brewed tea is also high in oxalates," says Dr. Heller. "The darker the tea, the more oxalates it contains." You may want to consider switching to green tea. Some studies suggest it may help the body rid itself of oxalate and reduce the risk of these common kidney stones.

Talk to your doctor about calcium. It was once thought that calcium contributed to kidney stones, but studies are suggesting otherwise. The more calcium in your diet, the less your risk because calcium binds with the oxalate before it

reaches your kidneys and helps get rid of it. But with one caveat: Calcium supplements are still linked to kidney stone risk, so get your daily dose of calcium in food.

Enjoy beer on occasion. According to the research of Pirjo Pietinen, DSc, professor at the National Public Health Institute in Helsinki, Finland, beer increases the amount of water in urine, which reduces the concentration of stone-forming calcium. In his 3-year study, Dr. Pietinen found that the risk of kidney stones dropped 40 percent with each beer drunk daily. However, excessive alcohol consumption can lead to health problems, so limit your drinks. Men can have one or two 12-ounce glasses, and women should stick to one glass a day.

Give up antacids. Both calcium- and aluminum-based antacids increase the concentration of stone-forming calcium in the urine. People with a history of kidney stones should switch to H2 blockers (such as Tagamet), medications that control stomach acid without increasing the risk of stones, says Dr. Heller.

Eat less meat. The protein in beef, chicken, and pork breaks down in the body to form uric acid, a common cause of kidney stones. For patients with high uric acid or with high urine calcium, eat no more than 3 ounces of meat at each meal.

Eat more citrus fruits. Like lemonade, citrus fruits and juices such as oranges, grapefruit, and orange juice contain stone-inhibiting citrate.

Cut back on sodium. Salt in the diet increases the amount of stone-forming calcium in the urine. People who get kidney stones from high urine calcium should reduce their salt intake to fewer than 2,500 mg daily. To do this, Dr. Heller recommends using fresh or frozen foods instead of canned or processed ones, eating at home rather than in restaurants, and avoiding the temptation to add salt to your food.

medical options

Prevent stones with medications. People at high risk for kidney stones often take medications to prevent them. If you tend to form calcium stones, your doctor may prescribe a thiazide diuretic (water pill).

For uric acid stones, you may need a medication called allopurinol (Zyloprim), which prevents stones from forming by lowering uric acid production. Potassium citrate (Urocit-K) has also been shown to prevent stones in patients with high uric acid, and, by raising pH levels, it may actually help to dissolve small stones.

For more information about kidney stones. Go online to visit the Web site of the National Institute of Diabetes and Digestive and Kidney Diseases at www.niddk.nih.gov.

laryngitis

The human voice produces sounds when air from the lungs causes folds in the larynx, or voice box, to vibrate. When tissues in the larynx swell, usually from inflammation, allergy, or an infection, they don't vibrate the way they should. This causes the most melodious voice to get raspy or even disappear for a few days.

If you develop laryngitis and you also have a sore throat or stuffy nose, you probably have a minor viral infection and will get your voice back in a week or two, says Gregory Grillone, MD, an associate professor and vice chairman of the department of otolaryngology-head and neck surgery at Boston University Medical Center.

Anything that irritates the vocal cords—smoking, a chatty night with girlfriends, or cheering your kid's soccer team—can cause temporary inflammation and voice loss, Dr. Grillone adds. Long-term laryngitis, on the other hand, is more likely to be caused by underlying problems, such as heartburn (in which acids from the stomach irritate tissues in the throat) or polyps (growths on the vocal folds).

Persistent laryngitis should always be evaluated by a doctor. In most cases, however, you can soothe the larynx and regain your voice with some simple home remedies

For Immediate Relief

home remedies

Rest your voice. It's the best way to help the vocal cords recover. Talk as little as possible, and don't whisper—it irritates the larynx even more than talking.

Drink warm liquids. Water is fine, or you can brew cups of decaffeinated tea. Warm liquids soothe irritated tissues in the throat and may help the irritation heal more quickly, says Dr. Grillone. Add a little honey, a traditional remedy for an irritated throat.

Suck on a lozenge. Or a hard candy or cough drop. The idea is to keep your throat moist.

Take long showers. Or plug in a humidifier. Breathing humid air will soothe and moisturize the injured tissues, says Dr. Grillone.

Avoid alcohol and caffeine for a few days. They remove water from the body and will make the larynx even drier.

Take care of heartburn. You'll feel—and talk—a lot better if you get your stomach acid under control. There are many strategies for reducing heartburn. They include:

■ Elevate the head of your bed a few inches. That will make it harder for acids in the stomach to travel upstream.

■ Take antacids or acid-reducing drugs.

■ Avoid fatty foods, and those containing caffeine, including chocolate. They weaken the circular muscle that prevents acid in the stomach from getting into the esophagus.

alternative therapies

Drink cinnamon tea. It reduces inflammation as well as pain. To make a tea, pour a cup of boiling water over 1 teaspoon of powdered cinnamon. Let it steep, covered, for 20 minutes, and drink it down.

You may want to add honey to the tea, which will soothe the throat, and a squeeze of lemon, which stimulates saliva production and will help keep the tissues lubricated.

Try goldenseal. Taking goldenseal in a tincture form can focus its antibiotic and anti-inflammatory properties directly on the throat. But be wary. "It's pretty bad-tasting," says Jill Stansbury, ND, a naturopathic physician in private practice at Battle Ground Naturopathic Family Practice in Battle Ground, Washington. "You'd be unlikely to have a small child do this, but somebody else can put the tincture in a sip of water and just gargle and swallow that. It's not so bad. It's just bitter." Take a dropperful every one to two hours for an acute infection, or a dropperful 2 to 3 times a day as a preventive measure.

THREE THINGS I TELL EVERY FEMALE PATIENT

GREG GRILLONE, MD, *is associate professor and vice chairman of the department of otolaryngology-head and neck surgery at Boston University Medical Center. He advises women with laryngitis to do the following:*

1 **DRINK AS MUCH WATER AS YOU CAN HOLD.** It hydrates the vocal cords, speeds healing, and reduces the raspy irritation.

2 **FOLLOW THE "ARM'S-LENGTH" RULE.** To preserve (or restore) your voice, don't talk to anyone who's more than an arm's length away.

3 **AVOID OVER-THE-COUNTER COLD REMEDIES.** The same active ingredients that ease congestion will remove moisture from the vocal cords. ■

Combine with echinacea. Whether used as a tincture or in a tablet, echinacea's immune-stimulating effects make a nice complement to goldenseal as part of your laryngitis treatment plan. For the tincture, follow the dosage instructions listed above for goldenseal. For the dried root tablets, take two 500-mg tablets 3 times daily.

Get your voice back with ginger. Brewing up ginger in a mug of hot tea is excellent for a hoarse voice. Its anti-inflammatory properties soothe the throat, and its diaphoretic properties help you sweat out an infection. To make a mean cup of ginger tea, cut roughly 1 inch of fresh ginger root into very thin slices. Then simmer in 8 ounces of water for 7 or 8 minutes covered. Strain it and drink as needed.

Long-Term Solutions

home remedies

If you smoke, try to quit. Cigarette smoke is irritating and a common cause of hoarseness.

Can the caffeine. The caffeine found in coffee, teas, and colas can dry your throat out and prolong laryngitis.

when to see a doctor

When laryngitis lasts longer than 2 weeks, make an appointment to see your doctor. Persistent hoarseness may be a symptom of vocal cord damage or even cancer, says Gregory Grillone, MD, associate professor and vice chairman of the department of otolaryngology-head and neck surgery at Boston University Medical Center.

If the hoarseness is accompanied by trouble swallowing, or if there's a lump in the throat. These are also warning signs of cancer.

Wear a protective mask. Pollen, mold, high office humidity, and even simple yard dust can irritate the larynx and lead to hoarseness or full-fledged laryngitis.

A paper surgical mask will filter out the coarsest particles. But a protective respirator, available in hardware stores, is a better choice when you're doing things like refinishing furniture, laying carpet, adding a pressed-wood door to a shed, or working with power tools or paints or other chemicals like varnishes and adhesives.

lupus

Lupus has been called the "disease with a thousand faces" because it causes an incredible variety of symptoms, ranging from fatigue, achiness, and swollen joints to persistent fever, anemia, sensitivity to sunlight, and skin rashes. In severe cases it can damage the heart, lungs, kidneys, and other vital organs.

Lupus is an autoimmune condition, which means that the immune system "mistakenly" attacks healthy tissues throughout the body, resulting in inflammation. It's difficult to estimate how many Americans suffer from lupus because its symptoms vary widely, even in the same individual over time, and its onset is often hard to determine. Studies have shown, however, that lupus is much more common among women, affecting them about 8 to 10 times as often as men. It usually strikes during the childbearing years, but older women, too, can get it. It's also more common in African Americans and Asians.

"Researchers aren't sure why more women than men are diagnosed with lupus, but one possibility is that it's a result of environmental exposure to toxins," says Michael Lockshin, MD, director of the Barbara Volcker Center for Women and Rheumatic Disease at the Hospital for Special Surgery in New York City. Many scientists think that some people are born with the genetic predisposition to lupus and it's turned on by some kind of environmental exposure, including ultraviolet radiation from the sun or sun-sensitizing drugs such as penicillin. It's also possible that lupus is triggered by bacteria or viruses. Physical and emotional stress may play a role. Because so many more women than men get the disease, researchers are also exploring a hormonal connection, specifically the role of estrogen. There appears to be no dietary cause, though a popular Internet rumor fingers the artificial sweetener, aspartame. There is no scientific evidence to support that.

There's no way to prevent lupus, nor is there a single test to diagnose it. If your doctor suspects that you have lupus, you may be given a blood test called an immunofluorescent antinuclear antibody (ANA) test. A positive result doesn't necessarily mean that you have lupus;

other diseases and some drugs can cause false positives. In fact, only a minority of patients with positive ANA have lupus, but the test is almost always positive in lupus. Another test is the erythrocyte sedimentation rate. This is a blood test that examines how fast the red blood cells settle to the bottom of the test tube and is a marker of inflammation. If they settle faster than normal, it could indicate a systemic disease, including lupus. Your doctor may also order a blood count test because people with lupus can have low numbers of white blood cells. Low platelets or red blood cells and low hemoglobin are also common signs of lupus.

Because lupus causes so many possible symptoms, and because the disease is so unpredictable—it's common for women to experience extended periods of remission, followed by sudden flare-ups of symptoms—there isn't a one-size-fits-all treatment plan. Here are some of the strategies your doctor may recommend.

For Immediate Relief

home remedies

Take aspirin or ibuprofen as needed. Many women with lupus will experience joint pain or swelling, which can significantly reduce their ability to get around. Aspirin and ibuprofen can help because they reduce inflammation as well as pain, says Dr. Lockshin.

Always use sunscreen. Two-thirds of people with lupus are photosensitive. Even small amounts of sun exposure can trigger a flare-up of symptoms. "Use a sunscreen with an SPF of at least 30," he adds. Choose one that blocks both UVA and UVB rays and apply it liberally to your neck, temples, and ears, areas often affected by lupus-related skin problems. Be sure to reapply it often, especially if you're swimming or perspiring, which will wash the sunscreen off the skin.

Avoid the sun's peak hours. "Stay out of the sun between 10:00 a.m. and 4:00 p.m.," Dr. Lockshin advises. That's when the sun's rays are strongest. "If you're doing outdoor activities, such as walking or gardening, do them first thing in the morning or later in the evening." Indoor fluorescent lighting can also emit UV rays, but a simple light shield, available from a number of manufacturers and retailers online, can help protect you.

Exercise as much as you're able. As many as 80 percent of people with lupus have fatigue, and that can discourage them from exercise.

when to see a doctor

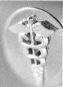 **If you have unexplained fatigue, muscle or joint pain, low-grade fever, hair loss, or a facial rash, such as spots about 1 to 2 inches in diameter on the cheeks or eyebrows, call your doctor right away.** These are the classic symptoms of lupus, and you should get tested for it right away, says Michael Lockshin, MD, director of the Barbara Volcker Center for Women and Rheumatic Disease at the Hospital for Special Surgery in New York City. A butterfly-shaped rash across the nose or cheeks, while an important sign doctors use to diagnose lupus, is relatively uncommon, at least at the onset of the disease.

Even if you'd rather take a nap, exercise anyway. Regular exercise can help reduce muscle stiffness, relieve stress, increase your range of motion, and keep your heart and bones healthy. Some of the best exercises are bicycling, swimming, and walking. You'll probably want to avoid pounding exercises such as running, which can put additional stress on joints that are already tender. But before you start an exercise program, ask your doctor to recommend a type and level of activity that's right for you.

medical options

Get the immune system under control. When lupus is active, the immune system can destroy tissues throughout the body. Sooner or later, your doctor will probably give you prescription medications to suppress immunity and reduce inflammation and pain. Some of the medications commonly used for lupus include corticosteroids, azathioprine (Imuran), and cyclophosphamide (Cytoxan).

The drugs can be very effective, but they're also rife with side effects. If your doctor prescribes corticosteroids, you will be given tapering doses, in which the amounts of medication are slowly reduced over time, which gives the body a chance to adjust to the change. The other medications don't require tapering.

Long-Term Solutions

home remedies

Eat as well as you can. There aren't specific dietary guidelines for people with lupus, but eating a well-balanced diet is essential to keeping the immune system healthy. Doctors usually advise women to restrict their consumption of red meat and other fatty foods and to eat a variety of whole grains, legumes, and fruits and vegetables. This is a good plan for anyone, even if you don't have lupus, notes Dr. Lockshin.

Get plenty of rest. "Physical exhaustion tends to trigger flare-ups," says Dr. Lockshin. "Getting a good night's sleep, and doing that on a regular basis, is one of the things women can do to help manage the disease. It's believed that sleep is also the time the body repairs cellular damage, so it may be helpful for the immune system."

Beware of colds or the flu. Even though lupus puts the immune system into overdrive, women with this condition are actually more susceptible to infections of all kinds, including colds and the flu, from the treatments and the disease itself. And when they do get sick, it may take them longer to recover.

It's impossible to avoid cold and flu viruses totally, of course (though it's a good idea to avoid the people who have them), and certain treatments for lupus may weaken the effectiveness of the immune system, reducing your ability to fight any infection. If you do get infected, be sure to see your doctor. Even minor infections can be much more serious when you're also dealing with lupus. Consider getting an annual flu shot, now recommended for everyone over 6 months. Studies have found that people with lupus develop antibodies to the flu after being vaccinated, though their antibody levels tend to be lower than in those who are

healthy. Just avoid the inhaled flu prevention treatment (FluMist) because it contains a weakened by still live virus.

Do everything you can to reduce stress. Women with lupus have been known to have flare-ups when they're going through difficult times. "Everyone experiences stress, but people with lupus should try to avoid it," Dr. Lockshin says. "Professional counseling to help the woman and her family deal with this chronic illness may be helpful." Friends and family can also provide emotional and social support. Many organized groups for lupus also exist. To locate a support group in your area, check with your doctor or local hospitals.

Some women with lupus ask Dr. Lockshin whether they should practice stress reduction techniques, such as deep breathing, biofeedback, meditation, or yoga. Since these can sometimes be helpful, he usually advises anyone who wants to try them to go ahead.

Get out of the "lupus fog." Almost everyone who has lupus knows what this is—the difficulty you may have remembering things you need to do, names, dates, all those things that people write off to "senior moments." You may get some help from a cognitive therapist or another kind of psychologist who can help you build the skills for dealing with "the fog," such as writing to-do lists, jotting down names and information you need to remember, learning memory techniques, and staying organized.

For more information about lupus. Visit the Web site of the Lupus Foundation of America at www.lupus.org.

lyme disease

Ever since Lyme disease was first identified in the United States in 1975, millions of Americans have been nervous about being in the great outdoors, where they might encounter tiny, sesame-seed-sized deer ticks or western black-legged ticks, which transmit this sometimes painful bacterial infection.

It's reasonable to be concerned about Lyme disease, especially if you live in a high-risk region, such as the northeastern, upper midwestern, and Pacific coast states. The incidence of Lyme disease has been rising steadily, with nearly 30,000 new cases identified in 2009, the last year for which there are statistics. But there's no reason to limit your activities because of it.

"There's a lot of unwarranted anxiety in this country about Lyme disease," says Robert T. Schoen, MD, a leading Lyme disease researcher and clinical professor of medicine at Yale University School of Medicine in Connecticut, where the first cases were diagnosed. The number of ticks infected with the bacterium *Borrelia burgdorferi* varies by region. The greatest incidences of Lyme disease occur in states along the east coast from Virginia to Maine. Even if you do get bitten, it takes more than 24 hours for the tick to transmit the bacteria into a human. You can greatly reduce your chances of getting the disease simply by removing the tick as soon as you see it.

Unfortunately, removing ticks isn't always easy—they're not much larger than a sesame seed, so even when you're looking for one, you won't always spot it. The only way many people know they've been exposed to the Lyme bacterium is when they develop symptoms, such as fatigue, fever, joint pain, and a skin rash that looks like a bull's-eye.

For Immediate Relief
medical options

Take antibiotics. For all the worries about Lyme disease, it's usually easy to treat. If you are diagnosed with Lyme disease, your doctor will give you a course of antibiotics consisting of amoxicillin or doxycycline. In most cases, that will knock out the infection for good. People who are treated early in the infection usually recover rapidly. However, if your infection is discovered in the later stages, you may be at risk for chronic Lyme disease, which has more serious complications, so you may need a second course of antibiotics.

For Long-Term Prevention
home remedies

Dress properly. If you live in an area that's known to harbor deer ticks, wear a long-sleeved shirt and pants when you go outside. Tuck the pants into your socks or boots. You may want to wear light-colored clothing, which makes it easier to spot any ticks that climb on board.

Avoid high-risk areas. There's no reason to stay inside during the spring and summer months, when tick season is at its height, but it's a good idea to steer clear of areas where ticks are likely to thrive, especially high-grass areas thick with leaf litter or low-lying vegetation. If you must be in those areas, stay to the center of the paths.

Use repellent. Before going outside, spray insect repellent on your clothing and any exposed skin. Adults should use an insect repellent that contains 20 to 30 percent DEET. Don't use any DEET-containing products on children under age 2. If you want to use DEET on a child over 2, never use a product that contains more than 10 percent, and always consult a pediatrician first. Another repellent, permethrin, kills ticks on contact. Just one application to pants, socks. and shoes typically lasts through several washings. It's not meant to be sprayed on skin.

when to see a doctor

If you develop a persistent fever or joint pain during the warm months, or if you have an unexplained rash, see your doctor right away. Even if you never saw a tick, you could be infected with the Lyme bacterium, says Robert T. Schoen, MD, clinical professor of medicine at Yale University School of Medicine.

Keep up with yard maintenance. Even if you live in the suburbs, deer ticks probably aren't far away. To keep them from getting too cozy, keep your grass cut short and clear leaves or brush from around the house and yard. If you live in a heavily wooded area, thinning the trees to let more sunlight through will also cut down on ticks by reducing the amount of habitat available for the deer and mice that carry the pests.

Remove ticks promptly. Before you go into the house, check your clothing for ticks and remove them. Wash all clothing in hot water and dry with high heat to kill any remaining hangers-on. Ticks that haven't started feeding can be flicked off the skin with a washcloth or towel. Once they're embedded in the skin, however, they really hang on—and your risk for developing Lyme disease begins to rise.

To remove a tick, grip it close to the skin with a pair of fine-tipped tweezers. Pull with steady pressure, and the tick will pop right out. Try not to squeeze the body, which could cause the bacteria that are in the tick to be injected into the skin. After removing the tick, disinfect your skin and wash your hands with soap and water.

medical options

For more information about Lyme disease. Visit the Web site of the Centers for Disease Control and Prevention at www.cdc.gov. Click on the banner "A–Z Index" and scroll down to "Lyme Disease."

macular degeneration

As the Baby Boomers age, more and more attention is being focused on this once little-known condition that is the leading cause of blindness in people over 60. If you're over 50, chances are your eye doctor is already looking for signs of macular degeneration, which occurs when the macula, the central area of a thin membrane at the back of the eyes called the retina, breaks down. The retina contains light-sensitive cells that send visual signals to the brain. The macula processes sharp straight-ahead vision. The first symptom of this breakdown is blurry or distorted vision. Eventually, the damage causes blind spots in your central vision.

By 2050, nearly 22 million Americans are expected to have some form of macular degeneration, nearly double the number that have it today. There's a strong genetic component to the condition but lifestyle factors, such as diet, weight, and smoking, all play a role.

There are two main forms of macular degeneration. The "dry" form, known as age-related macular degeneration (AMD), is thought to be caused by free radicals in the body that are formed whenever you're exposed to sunlight, cigarette smoke, and air pollution; they're also a natural by-product of your body's metabolic processes. The less common, "wet" form of the disease occurs when there's leakage from abnormal blood vessels in the eyes. The risk for both forms increases with age.

"You can repair some of the damage by improving circulation to the eyes and getting the appropriate nutrients," says Robert Abel Jr., MD, an ophthalmologist on staff at Christiana Health Care System in Delaware and author of *The Eye Care Revolution.*

Just as important, there are steps you can take that will protect your eyes from both forms of this free radical free-for-all.

For Immediate Relief

home remedies

Fill up on spinach. Along with other leafy greens, such as kale and Swiss chard, it's rich in a plant pigment called lutein, which prevents eye-damaging blue light in sunshine from harming the eyes. It also "neutralizes" free radicals, says Dr. Abel.

One study found that people who ate ½ cup of cooked spinach 4 to 7 times a week for a year had significant improvements in night vision. "One man told me that he was thrilled to be able to read a clock after years of struggling with blank spots in his vision," says study leader Stuart Richer, OD, PhD, a vision researcher with the Veterans Administration in Chicago.

Other studies have found that people who eat vegetables high in lutein and zeaxanthin (they travel together in the same leafy green foods) have lower risk of AMD. The highest accumulation of both those chemicals is in the retina.

Add a little fat to your greens. Your body can't absorb much lutein unless you consume it with a little fat. Adding a teaspoon of olive oil to lutein-rich vegetables will boost blood levels of the nutrient by as much as 88 percent.

Give your vision a boost. Women with mild forms of macular degeneration will see clearly most of the time, but they may need a little help when they're reading or watching TV. "Aids for low vision in the later stages of the disease, such as magnifiers, telescopic lenses, and closed-circuit reading devices, can make a real difference," says Dr. Abel.

For reading, an inexpensive pair of reading glasses may be all you need. "If you wear glasses, make sure your prescription is up-to-date," Dr. Abel adds.

Be careful when driving at night. Some people with macular degeneration have perfectly good vision during the day but lose some of their ability to see after dark, says Dr. Abel.

alternative therapies

Have a daily cup of bilberry tea. It's rich in chemical compounds called anthocyanosides, which strengthen blood vessels in the eye and inhibit the effects of free radicals. "Bilberry is especially good for improving night vision," says Dr. Abel. "You'll notice the difference very quickly."

Use ginkgo supplements. Available in health food stores, ginkgo improves circulation in the eyes. Better circulation means that you'll get additional nutrients into the damaged areas, says Dr. Abel. He recommends taking 15 drops of ginkgo extract, dropped into a sip of water, once or twice daily for a month.

For Long-Term Relief

home remedies

Take special eye supplements. The Age-Related Eye Disease Study (AREDS), sponsored

---

THREE THINGS I TELL EVERY FEMALE PATIENT

ROBERT ABEL JR., MD, *an ophthalmologist on staff at Christiana Health Care System in Delaware and author of* The Eye Care Revolution *offers the following advice for keeping the eyes healthy.*

1 DRINK EIGHT GLASSES OF WATER DAILY. "The eye is basically a bag of water with two lenses," Dr. Abel says. "Most of us don't drink enough water to replenish the fluids and get an improved circulation of nutrients."

2 EAT LIVE-CULTURE YOGURT. Or take probiotic supplements. Levels of stomach acid decline with aging, which reduces the absorption of important nutrients. Yogurt and digestion-friendly supplements will help the eyes stay nourished.

3 TAKE OMEGA-3 SUPPLEMENTS. They help repair damaged tissues in the eyes. Fish contains some omega-3s, but supplements—especially those containing a high concentration of an omega-3 called DHA—give a more concentrated dose. Take 400 to 500 mg daily, Dr. Abel advises. ∎

by the National Eye Institute, found that people who take high levels of antioxidants and zinc can reduce their risk of macular degeneration by about 25 percent. If you're at high risk for developing advanced AMD, talk to your doctor about the benefits and risks of taking 500 mg of vitamin C, 400 IU of vitamin E, 15 mg of beta-carotene, 80 mg of zinc oxide, and two mg of copper as cupric oxide, the latter of which was added to the formula to counteract the anemia-causing effects of high zinc intake.

Wear sunglasses. Wraparound shades are your best choice because they provide the most protection from ultraviolet (UV) light in sunshine. "Everyone should wear sunglasses when they go outside," says Dr. Abel.

Get extra vitamin C. It accumulates in the watery portions of the body, including in the eyes. It's extremely effective at blocking the effects of free radicals, says Dr. Abel. He recommends supplementing your diet with 1,000 mg of vitamin C daily.

Eat a variety of fruits and vegetables. They contain a variety of antioxidant compounds, including lycopene and zeaxanthin, which have been shown to mop up free radicals in the eyes.

Put fish on the menu. A study of 2,900 people found that those who ate fish once or more a month had half the risk of developing macular degeneration than those who ate fish less often.

Limit your consumption of fat. Studies have shown that people who get a lot of fat in the diet, especially the saturated fat that's found in meats and full-fat dairy foods, have a much higher risk of macular degeneration. "Saturated fat contributes to blocked arteries, which reduces circulation in the eyes," Dr. Abel explains.

To protect your eyes as well as your heart and arteries, doctors advise limiting fat consumption to 25 percent (or less) of total calories.

Control high blood pressure and obesity. Both conditions increase your risk of macular degeneration. If your BMI, a measure of body fat, is greater than 30, your risk goes up 2½ times.

Have a little wine. Or red grapes. Or blueberries. They contain a phytochemical called resveratrol that might help block the growth of abnormal blood vessels in the eye that occurs in

when to see a doctor

If your vision is a little blurry, or if you see a small blind spot in the middle of your field of vision, or notice that straight lines appear to be distorted, see an ophthalmologist. These are classic symptoms of macular degeneration, says John D. Hunkeler, MD, clinical professor of ophthalmology at the University of Kansas School of Medicine in Kansas City.

If the change in vision occurred suddenly. You could have a leakage of blood in the brain that's affecting the optic nerve.

If your vision is blurry and you also have diabetes. You could have a potentially serious condition called diabetic retinopathy that, without prompt treatment, can lead to blindness.

macular degeneration, say researchers at the Washington University School of Medicine in St. Louis.

Talk to an ophthalmologist. There have been many advances in the treatment of macular degeneration, including drugs that stimulate the growth of new blood vessels in eye, and small, implantable "telescopes" that magnify central images for the retina which reduces the size of the blind spot. An ophthalmologist can talk to you about all your options.

For more information on macular degeneration. Visit the Web site of the National Eye Institute at www.nei.nih.gov.

memory problems

Don't be too hard on yourself the next time you lose the car keys or forget the name of someone you just met. Many people begin experiencing memory lapses as they turn 50, and in adults 70 years and older, declines in memory are nearly universal. Blanking out occasionally is exasperating, but no big deal.

Occasional forgetfulness isn't a sign of Alzheimer's disease. It doesn't mean you're destined to spend the rest of your life wondering why you put the mail in the freezer. What it probably means is that cells in your brain aren't getting all the nourishment or stimulation that they need to withstand the normal wear and tear of aging.

"Some people, whether because of their behavior or their genetic makeup, are able to avoid or slow the usual declines in memory function," says Stanley Birge, MD, director of the Older Adult Health Center at Washington University School of Medicine in St. Louis.

Stress can cause momentary lapses. Health problems such as high blood pressure and high cholesterol may also contribute, so it's important to talk to your doctor if you find you're forgetting things more than you used to.

But in most cases occasional forgetfulness doesn't mean you're losing your mental faculties. There's a good chance you can significantly improve your memory—and reduce the risk of further declines—with a variety of mental tactics and simple lifestyle changes.

For Immediate Relief

Exercise your mind. "People who remain active socially and are engaged in demanding cognitive activities may be able to reduce the usual aging of the brain," says Dr. Birge. Crossword and Sudoku puzzles and games of Scrabble will keep the brain challenged. Volunteer work is helpful. So are hobbies, or simply reading magazines and newspapers. The Internet can also keep your brain in gear. UCLA researchers even found that people who did Internet searches had three times more brain activity than ordinary Web surfers, largely because Googling uses brain circuitry not activated by just reading.

"You don't want to do just one thing," Dr. Birge adds. "You want to keep the brain operating at a multitude of activities."

Review important information. The brain has more trouble taking in new information as you get older. You can overcome this by mentally reviewing information that you want to retain.

The next time you meet someone new, for example, repeat the name in your mind several times. If you tend to lose the car keys, keep them in the same place and mentally visualize where they are.

"The better the preparation, the stronger the memory," says James McGaugh, PhD, research professor of neurobiology and behavior at the School of Biological Sciences at the University of California Irvine.

Reinforce your memory with a cup of coffee or tea. Laboratory studies suggest that the caffeine in coffee, tea, and sodas may enhance long-term memory when it's consumed shortly after learning new things.

Drink more water. People who don't drink enough can get dehydrated, which affects blood flow to the brain, leading to fatigue and making it harder to remember things. Try to drink at least eight 8-ounce glasses of water daily.

Check your meds. If you're having troubling memory lapses, put all your medications and

THREE THINGS I TELL EVERY FEMALE PATIENT

STANLEY BIRGE, MD, *director of the Older Adult Health Center at Washington University School of Medicine in St. Louis, gives this important advice.*

BE SURE TO EXERCISE REGULARLY. Walking, biking, and other forms of exercise increase blood flow to the brain. In addition, exercise stimulates different parts of the brain. When people engage in physical activity, their risk of cognitive impairment is dramatically reduced.

TALK TO YOUR DOCTOR ABOUT HORMONE REPLACEMENT THERAPY. The hormone estrogen protects memory in several ways. It

reduces free radical damage, increases blood flow, and stimulates growth factors that are involved in the repair of damaged neurons. Supplemental estrogen may help after menopause, when a woman's natural supply of the hormone declines.

TAKE CONTROL OF STRESS. Sustained high levels of cortisol and other stress hormones may block the ability to remember important information, such as names or telephone numbers. People who reduce their levels of cortisol—with exercise, meditation, or other pleasurable activities—are less likely to experience degenerative damage in the brain. ∎

supplements into a brown bag and take them to your doctor for review. Some drugs, such as statins, antidepressants, Parkinson's medications, even ordinary painkillers, can affect memory and cognition. If you're older, drugs tend to linger in your system longer, which increases the risk of problem interactions, especially if you take many drugs.

Don't sweat your memory problems. Stressing out about a lapse here and there will actually make your memory problems worse, found a study done at North Carolina State University. When a group of healthy older people were told that aging caused forgetfulness, they scored poorly on memory tests. Another similar group who were told that memory didn't decline much with age scored 15 percent higher.

when to see a doctor

If your memory is progressively getting worse, see your doctor immediately. Memory declines may be caused by potentially serious—and treatable—conditions, such as depression, thyroid disorders, or nutritional deficiencies, says Stanley Birge, MD, director of the Older Adult Health Center at Washington University School of Medicine in St. Louis.

If your memory gets worse and you're taking a new medication. Many prescription drugs, including those used to control high blood pressure, may cause impairments in memory. Changing to a new drug will often resolve the problem.

Drink sage tea. Folk healers have traditionally recommended sage for improving memory, and new research suggests it could work. Sage contains two chemical compounds—1,8-cineole and alpha-pinene—that block an enzyme that may be linked to Alzheimer's disease. One 2010 British study found that sage improved both cognitive performance and mood in a group of healthy subjects.

The problem with sage is that is also contains a compound called thujone, which may be toxic in large doses. It's fine to enjoy sage tea on occasion, but you don't want to drink it every day.

Boost cell communication with huperzine A. A supplement based on a Chinese herbal remedy, huperzine A (HupA) is thought to protect the brain's supply of acetylcholine, a chemical messenger that may break down over time. Studies of people with Alzheimer's disease have shown that 60 percent of those who took HupA had significant improvements in mental function, says Alan Kozikowski, PhD, former director for the drug discovery program at the Institute for Cognitive and Computational Sciences at Georgetown University Medical Center in Washington, DC, and now a professor in the department of medicinal chemistry and pharmacognosy at the University of Illinois at Chicago.

Improve your memory with PS. Short for phosphatidylserine, PS is a component of brain cells that regulates chemical messengers, or neurotransmitters. One study showed that people who took PS found it easier to recall the names of people they'd recently been introduced to.

Long-Term Solutions

Eat brightly colored fruits and vegetables. They contain chemical compounds called flavonoids, antioxidant compounds that blunt the effects of free radicals, unstable oxygen molecules in the body that may damage blood vessels in the brain and increase the risk of memory decline. In one study, animals that were given flavonoid-rich blueberries or spinach daily were able to reverse memory impairments.

"If you want to slow down the free radical aging process, blueberries are the leader of the pack," adds Ronald Prior, PhD, head of the USDA Phytochemical Laboratory at Tufts University in Boston. "With $\frac{1}{2}$ cup of blueberries, you can just about double the amount of antioxidants that most Americans get in one day." Lab studies involving rats have found that blueberries can increase cell growth in the hippocampus region of the brain and seem to help rats better navigate a maze. Think finding where you parked your car in the mall lot.

Have an apple. Or two. "Apples have just the right dose of antioxidants to raise levels of acetylcholine, a neurotransmitter that's essential to memory and tends to decline with age," says Tom Shea, PhD, director of the University of Massachusetts Lowell Center for Cellular Neurobiology and Neurodegeneration Research. An apple's antioxidants protect brain cells from damage by the free radicals created by normal metabolism.

Exercise at least 3 days a week. Regular aerobic exercise not only builds muscles, it increases the volume of brain tissue, says researchers from the University of Illinois's Beckman Institute. That can boost the speed and sharpness of your thought processes. As little as 50 minutes of brisk walking 3 days a week can help. And take a walk in the park: Another study found that people who walked through a tree-lined environment performed 20 percent better on memory and attention tests than those who walked on a city street.

Enjoy citrus fruits. They're among the best sources of vitamin C, an antioxidant nutrient that promotes healthy blood flow by preventing cholesterol and other fatty substances from accumulating in blood vessels in the brain. Vitamin C also makes vitamin E work more effectively and improves its ability to block cell-damaging free radicals, says Dr. Birge.

Add some folate. In new research, older people with lower levels of the B vitamin folate in their blood found it harder to hold on to new information that was coming at them quickly.

"Folate is one of the most valuable nutrients you can take for healthy memory function throughout life," says Jay Lombard, MD, director of the Brain Behavior Center in Nyack, New York. Dr. Lombard thinks that folate helps memory by "recycling" chemicals that brain cells need to communicate and by fighting artery plaque, which can reduce blood flow to the brain.

Get your B_{12} checked. Memory loss is one of the symptoms of B_{12} deficiency, a problem easily remedied with a supplement or a daily serving of fortified cereal containing 100 percent of the daily requirement for this vitamin. Although you can have a deficiency at any age, as you get older, the small intestine loses some of its ability to absorb vitamin B_{12}. Lean meats, eggs, and low-fat dairy foods provide abundant amounts of B_{12}. Vegetarians, however, may need to take a supplement or eat fortified foods. The Daily Value for vitamin B_{12} is 6 micrograms.

Keep alcohol consumption moderate. Stick to no more than one drink a day. A Wellesley College study found that the more alcohol you drink, the smaller your total brain volume becomes. This link was stronger in women than men because smaller people tend to be more susceptible to alcohol's effects.

Pick the right pain reliever. If you take over-the-counter nonsteroidal anti-inflammatory medications such as ibuprofen for the treatment of arthritis, it may delay the effects of memory loss. Although these drugs are readily available OTC, they should not be taken without medical supervision. Older people are particularly sensitive to the drugs' effects on the stomach, which can result in bleeding ulcers.

Battle depression. It can make people feel tired, unfocused, and mentally slow. In fact, depression in the elderly is often mistaken for Alzheimer's disease.

"Antidepressant medications do more than relieve the symptoms of depression," says Dr. Birge. They seem to affect the region of the brain (the hippocampus) that plays a key role in memory. "They also may stimulate the generation of nerve cells," he adds. By aiding in the repair of nerve cells, antidepressants may help restore memory and other mental functions that have degraded over time.

Meditate. Experienced meditators have bigger brains. One study at Massachusetts General Hospital in Boston found that meditators experience growth in the cortex, the part of the brain that controls memory, language, and sensory processing. In another study, meditators performed better than their nonmeditating counterparts on a series of mental acuity tests.

For more information on memory loss. Visit the Web site of the American Geriatrics Society at www.americangeriatrics.org. Or go to the Alzheimer's Association at www.alz.org.

multiple sclerosis

The symptoms seem mild at first. A little fatigue or weakness. An increase in frequency of urination. A "funny" feeling in the arms and legs that doesn't go away.

"For some, multiple sclerosis remains a relatively mild disease," explains Thomas Leist, MD, director of the Comprehensive Multiple Sclerosis Center at Thomas Jefferson University Hospital in Philadelphia. Even when the disease takes a more serious course, symptoms tend to flare briefly, then improve or go into remission for long periods of time.

Multiple sclerosis (MS) is thought to occur when the immune system's defensive cells attack the sheath, or myelin, that insulates nerve fibers. The damage results in inflammation and scarring (sclerosis), which blocks nerve signal transmission.

The disease usually strikes people between the ages of 20 and 40, and more than three-fourths of those newly diagnosed are women, who experience a higher rate of autoimmune diseases than men. It may be linked to viral infections, and people with affected relatives may be more susceptible than those without a family history. There may also be environmental factors involved.

There's no cure for MS, but with a combination of medications and home-care strategies, most people can manage the symptoms.

For Immediate Relief

home remedies

Allow time for rest. Bone-weary fatigue is the hallmark of MS. "People have to figure out what their stamina levels are and make the necessary adjustments," says Dr. Leist. Get help with your physical household chores. Make arrangements to adjust your work schedule. "I advise people to have 40 minutes or an hour of quiet time at lunch in order to recharge their batteries," he adds.

Keep temperatures on the cool side. MS reduces the body's ability to tolerate heat. You'll probably find yourself setting the thermostat at a lower setting than you used to. If you get too hot when you do your usual exercise, switch to swimming or aquatherapy, Dr. Leist advises. The water will help lower your body temperature.

Eat whole grains and other fiber-rich foods. Fiber helps to prevent constipation, a common symptom in those with MS.

Enjoy regular massages. Massage may help fight the muscle spasms that are often a symptom in MS, says Dr. Leist.

alternative therapies

Take vitamin C supplements. Women with MS have a high risk of urinary tract infections because the bladder doesn't always empty completely. Dr. Leist recommends taking 1,000 mg of vitamin C daily, unless there is a history of kidney stones. "It acidifies the urine and helps prevent infections," he says.

Try cranberry caplets. Available in health food stores, they contain substances that help reduce frequent urination, a bothersome symptom

when to see a doctor

If you have muscle weakness, persistent numbness, pins and needles, or persistent fatigue, see a doctor. These are among the earliest symptoms of multiple sclerosis, says Thomas Leist, MD, director of the Comprehensive Multiple Sclerosis Center at Thomas Jefferson University Hospital in Philadelphia.

If new or old symptoms occur after a period of remission. It's important to make sure that you don't have an infection. If you're having a relapse, you may need intravenous injections of anti-inflammatory drugs. The drugs are usually given for 3 to 5 days, says Dr. Leist. If this happens often, your doctor may want to review your immune-regulating regimen.

in those with MS. Dr. Leist recommends following the directions on the label. "You can't drink enough cranberry juice to get the same effects," he adds.

mind-body techniques

Join a support group. Or make an appointment to see a counselor. Research suggests that people with MS suffer from depression more than the general population. Remaining active and keeping a positive outlook on life will give you the energy you need to cope with the illness.

medical options

Take symptom-targeted medications. During flare-ups, your doctor may give you injections of corticosteroids, medications that reduce inflammation and help decrease the severity and duration of symptoms. There are also prescription drugs that can quell muscle spasms, urinary problems, depression, sexual problems, and fatigue.

Ask about bladder and bowel symptom relief. MS can cause bladder symptoms such as urine leakage, a strong and frequent need to urinate, difficulty initiating urination, as well as bowel problems such as constipation and stool leakage. Along with medication, your doctor can teach you exercises to strengthen your pelvic floor muscles as well as train you in techniques to help you maintain bowel control, including biofeedback.

Make sure you sleep well. If your sleep quality is good and the fatigue persists, medication can help. A study of 72 people with MS found that 85 percent had less fatigue when they took a prescription medication called modafinil (Provigil).

Long-Term Solutions

home remedies

Exercise often. It boosts energy, may help relieve urinary and bowel symptoms, and also increases bone density. People with MS are often sedentary, which weakens bones and raises the risk of fractures, says Dr. Leist. Low-impact aerobic exercises, such as walking or swimming, are good choices, he adds. Make sure you stretch; it will help prevent muscle stiffness.

Get the good fats. Some studies have found that a diet high in omega-3 (fish, flax, walnuts) and omega-6 fatty acids (sunflower or safflower seed oil) may be beneficial—especially if your diet is low in saturated fat, the kind found in meat and full-fat dairy.

medical options

Control relapses with immune-regulating drugs. "Interferon beta-1a (Avonex), interferon beta-1b (Betaseron), and glatiramer (Copaxone) reduce the number of attacks by about a third and impact the course of the disease," says Dr. Leist. Other drugs in this category are mitroxantrine (Novantrone), natalizumab (Tysabri), and fingolimod (Gilenya).

For more information on multiple sclerosis. Visit the Web site of the National Multiple Sclerosis Society at www.nationalmss.org, or go to the Web site of the Multiple Sclerosis Foundation at www.msfacts.org.

nausea and vomiting

L iterally hundreds of illnesses and conditions—from food poisoning and stomach "flu" to pregnancy—can result in nausea or vomiting. Most of the time, these miserable sensations are simply your body's way of saying "no thanks."

If you ate tainted food at a greasy spoon–type diner, for example, your stomach would do everything possible to expel the offending substances. Even morning sickness in pregnancy is thought by researchers to be one of the body's defense mechanisms against contaminants in the diet.

You may feel nauseated and vomit in response to medications administered during labor, surgery, or chemotherapy, although significant strides have been made in prescription medications that counteract these sometimes violent reactions. Motion sickness, migraines, kidney stones, and a number of other illnesses can make you vomit—as can seeing someone else vomit.

In the vast majority of cases, nausea and vomiting will get better on their own. Usually the most serious consequence is dehydration, which is easily remedied, "It's horrible, but you just have to ride it out," says Alan L. Melnick, MD, associate professor for the department of family medicine and department of public health and preventive medicine at Oregon Health Sciences University in Portland.

Depending on the cause of the queasies, here's what doctors advise.

For Immediate Relief

home remedies

Sip slowly. If you've been vomiting, you're probably losing important electrolytes, the minerals in the blood that regulate muscle contraction, suggests Miriam Erick, a registered dietitian at Brigham and Women's Hospital in Boston and author of *No More Morning Sickness*.

You need to replace the liquids and minerals that were lost—but slugging down water or juice will make the nausea worse. It's better to sip small amounts of liquids—juice or broths—until your stomach is better. "Lemonade seems to work for some women," she says. "It could be the small amounts of potassium or its calorie content."

Clear the air. Nausea can be worsened by strong odors. This is especially true during pregnancy, when many women become hypersensitive to smells. When your stomach is tossing and turning, open a few windows and keep the fresh air flowing. You may even want block the bottom of the bedroom door with a rolled towel or blanket to prevent odors from coming in, says Erick. Even if your favorite meal is in the oven, try to avoid all food smells while you're still nauseated.

Eat lightly. When your stomach is upset, eating large portions will trigger muscular contractions that will make the nausea worse. It's a good idea to eat just a few mouthfuls at a time until you're feeling better. If you're vomiting, wait 6 to 12 hours after you stop before eating, then try a little clear soup, salted crackers, dry

when to see a doctor

If nausea or vomiting persists for more than 48 hours, or if you're having other symptoms such as abdominal pain or blood in the vomit, see your doctor right away. You could have a more serious problem that requires medical attention, says Scott A. Fields, MD, vice chairman of family medicine at Oregon Health Sciences University in Portland.

toast or bread, or sherbet. Or follow the BRAT diet: bananas, rice, applesauce and tea. Keeping a little food in your stomach will help absorb acids and reduce nausea-causing spasms, says Erick.

Indulge your food desires. Ask yourself whether any food or type of food seems remotely appealing during bouts of queasiness. Erick divides potential foods into categories such as salty, crunchy, sour, spicy, and cold, and lets women find choices they can stomach. Even snack foods are fine for 1 to 2 days, says Erick.

Wear a wristband. Available from mail order catalogs and outdoor supply stores, acupressure wristbands put pressure on the inside of the wrist, which may prevent or stop nausea. In a Norwegian study of 97 women suffering from morning sickness, those who wore the bands recovered more quickly than those who didn't use them. In a study from England, doctors found that acupressure help significantly reduce nausea caused by chemotherapy. In the test, acupressure was applied using Sea-Band wristbands worn for 5 days following the chemotherapy administration.

Take a stomach soother. Products that contain phosphorated carbohydrate solution (such

as Emetrol) will reduce stomach contractions and make the nausea more bearable.

Ask for a massage. In a recent Swedish study, researchers evaluated if massage therapy could reduce nausea among 39 women who were undergoing chemotherapy for breast cancer. All the women had reported nausea and anxiety. They were randomly assigned to get five 20-minute effleurage (soft massage) sessions or five 20-minute sessions of unstructured conversation with a hospital staff member. Massage significantly reduced symptoms of nausea.

Take OTC motion sickness drugs. Cruising? Driving? Take along OTC dimenhydrinate (Dramamine) or diphenhydramine (Benadryl), which can counteract motion sickness.

alternative therapies

Give ginger a try. A traditional remedy for motion sickness, ginger may also relieve nausea caused by morning sickness. The easiest way to use ginger is in supplement form: The recommended dose is two 500-mg tablets 3 times daily. Or you can drink ginger tea, made by steeping 1 cup of boiling water over a teaspoon of freshly grated ginger for 10 minutes.

Eat peppermint candy. Or drink peppermint tea. It contains a chemical compound called menthol, which eases digestion and calms the stomach.

To make peppermint tea, crush 1 teaspoon of fresh peppermint leaves, cover with a cup of boiling water, and let it steep 10 minutes. You can drink the tea as often as necessary to get relief.

Learn to relax. Morning sickness and chemotherapy-associated nausea and vomiting may be calmed when you are calmed. Meditation, visual imagery, hypnosis, massage, and progressive relaxation techniques (systematically tensing and relaxing muscle groups) are options that may make you feel better emotionally and physically.

For Long-Term Prevention

medical options

Ask your doctor about vitamin B$_6$. If you experience severe nausea during pregnancy, your doctor may recommend taking vitamin B$_6$ supplements. There's some evidence that it's helpful, and dosages up to 50 mg daily have been shown to be safe during pregnancy.

Talk to you doctor about medications. If you've suffered from motion sickness in the past, you may want to ask your doctor for a prescription drug to help alleviate the symptom, says Scott A. Fields, MD, vice chairman of family medicine at Oregon Health Sciences University in Portland. There are several to choose from that you can take before embarking on cruises or long drives, including a patch of scopolamine.

overactive bladder

The bladder's job is simple. It stores urine, a mixture of water and wastes excreted by the kidneys, then squeezes it out of the body when it's full.

The bladder's signaling mechanisms are equally simple. When it starts filling up, pressure on its muscular walls triggers nerve signals, which tell you that it's time to use the bathroom. Most people's bladders hold about 15 to 18 ounces, and the "empty" signal can occur at around 6 ounces.

In women with overactive bladders, also known as urge incontinence, there's often a problem with the nerves or with the bladder muscle itself. Rather than wait until it's full, the bladder sends out "gotta go" signals when even a tiny amount of urine trickles in. This creates an overwhelming need to urinate, even if you've just used the bathroom.

Many things can cause a hair-trigger bladder, including urinary tract infections and injuries (which may occur during vaginal childbirth) that affect the muscles or nerves, says Abraham N. Morse, MD, instructor at Harvard Medical School in Cambridge and a urogynecologist in private practice in Brookline, Massachusetts.

Doctors estimate that fewer than 50 percent of women with bladder control problems get help from their doctors. This is unfortunate because nearly everyone can achieve good bladder control with a few simple strategies.

For Immediate Relief

home remedies

Cut back on caffeine. A study of 259 women with overactive bladders found that those who consumed the most caffeine had the highest risk of experiencing bladder instability, or urge incontinence.

"Caffeine is a major bladder irritant," explains Dr. Morse. "When people switch to decaf, they usually get a lot better."

Carbonated drinks may also irritate the bladder so go easy on them too.

Quit smoking. The nicotine in cigarettes affects more than the lungs. "The nerve receptors in the bladder that stimulate contractions are called nicotinic receptors," says Dr. Morse. "You can imagine what smoking does to them."

Avoid spicy foods. Eating high-octane salsa or other spicy foods can stimulate bladder contractions and cause uncomfortable sensations of urgency, says Gary Lemack, MD, professor of urology at the University of Texas Southwestern Medical Center in Dallas.

Pass up cranberry juice. "A lot of women drink cranberry juice because they've heard that it prevents urinary tract infections," says Dr. Morse. "The problem with cranberry juice is that it can irritate the bladder and make it more sensitive." Acidic fruit juices and fruits can also cause bladder irritation.

Drink loads of plain water. It can help reduce leakage and prevent urine odors. Don't drink large quantities of fluid at meals but try to distribute your fluids at regular intervals during the day to make it easier to manage your bladder.

Squeeze the urge away. The next time you feel as though you have to urinate immediately, tighten the same muscles that you'd use to stop urine in midflow, says Dr. Morse. If you do this several times in succession, the feelings of urgency will often go away.

Don't drink at bedtime. It's not uncommon for people with overactive bladders to wake up on damp sheets in the morning. "I advise people to stop drinking water or other beverages after 8:00 p.m.," says Dr. Lemack.

THREE THINGS I TELL EVERY FEMALE PATIENT

ABRAHAM N. MORSE, MD, *professor of urogynecology at Harvard Medical School in Cambridge, Massachusetts, gives the following advice for coping with an overactive bladder.*

1 **SEE A "BLADDER TRAINER."** Ask your doctor to refer you to a physiotherapist who specializes in pelvic floor exercises. You'll also receive instruction in bladder drill training to help your bladder hold urine longer.

2 **DON'T LOOK FOR AGGRESSIVE TREATMENTS.** Women with overactive bladders rarely require surgery. They often have success with simpler approaches, such as Kegel exercises and bladder training.

3 **PUT YOUR MIND AT EASE.** Poor bladder control is embarrassing and uncomfortable, but it doesn't have to be permanent. Nearly all women who work with their doctors will gain full or partial control, usually within weeks. ■

Try acupuncture. There's some evidence that stimulating an acupuncture point above the ankle can override intense urges to urinate. The treatment makes sense in theory because there's a nerve above the ankle that has branches leading to the bladder, Dr. Morse explains. In one study of 85 women, those who received acupuncture had significant increases in bladder capacity, reduced incidences of urgency and frequency, and reported that their quality of life had improved compared to a similar group of women who received a sham treatment as a placebo.

Quiet your mind. The next time you experience a sudden urge to urinate, "breathe deeply, calm yourself down, and have confidence that you're not going to make a mess," says Dr. Morse. If you can calm yourself for about 30 to 60 seconds, there's a good chance that the urge will go away, he explains.

For Long-Term Relief

Put your bladder on the clock. "The best treatment for urge incontinence is what we call bladder drill training," says Dr. Morse. Urge incontinence occurs when you are unable to hold back urinating when the urge to void is present. The rules are simple: Rather than rush to the bathroom when your bladder tells you to, you go only at certain times.

"You would start out by going to the bathroom every 20 minutes, whether you need to go or not," says Dr. Morse. "In between, you have to try to hold it, even if it means leaking a little. Most people can make it for 20 minutes, and it gets you thinking more about the time than about your discomfort."

Once women can comfortably hold their urine for 20 minutes, they begin increasing the time. "People feel that if they don't go to the bathroom immediately, they're going to leak later. Breaking this behavior cycle is very important and very effective," says Dr. Morse.

when to see a doctor

If the need to urinate interferes with your daily activities or your sleep, see a doctor.

If you're having large accidents rather than small leaks, see your doctor right away. Losing large amounts of urine may be a sign of nerve damage or other neurological problems, says Gary Lemack, MD, professor of urology at the University of Texas Southwestern Medical Center in Dallas.

If you see blood in the urine. You might have a urinary tract infection that is irritating the bladder. Tumors in the urinary tract can also cause bleeding along with urgency.

If you feel as though your bladder never completely empties. This means that the nerves or muscles that control the bladder probably aren't working the way they should. You're also more likely to develop urinary tract infections.

Most women can get to the point where they're urinating, by the clock, about every 3 hours. "When you get to that point, you're done," says Dr. Morse.

Do Kegel exercises. They're a powerful strategy for calming an overactive bladder because they strengthen the pelvic floor muscles, the same muscles that give you urinary control, says Dr. Lemack.

Kegels are done by squeezing the muscles that you use to stop and start the flow of urine. Clench and relax the muscles about 10 times, and repeat this exercise several times daily. "Women who do these exercises daily almost always gain a significant amount of control," says Dr. Lemack.

Use biofeedback. Biofeedback can make sure you're doing the Kegel exercises properly. In some cases, therapists will actually place a sensor in the vagina to measure muscle contractions. When you view the results on a monitor, you can perfect your form so you get the most out of the workout.

mind-body techniques

Reduce the tension in your life. "We're not sure why, but in younger women especially, those who have very stressful lives often suffer from urgency," says Dr. Lemack.

Take a hint from your bladder: Unwind. Give yourself an hour each day to do something that's just for you, like taking a long walk, watching some television, or going to a movie or museum. "Doing whatever it takes to reduce stress is probably the best solution for many women," Dr. Lemack adds.

medical options

Calm the bladder with medication. Anticholinergic drugs (oxybutynin, tolterodine and tropsium) relax the bladder muscle and also reduce irritation.

Give the bladder a jolt. Research has shown that it may be possible to stop irregular bladder contractions by hitting them with precise amounts of electricity for 20 to 30 minutes. This technique is known as functional electrical stimulation. A probe is inserted into the vagina, where it releases an electrical current that stimulates nerves that lead to the bladder. "It can dramatically reduce the way the bladder responds to signals," says Dr. Morse.

Ask your doctor about InterStim therapy. You've heard of pacemakers for the heart, but now there are similar devices for controlling urinary urges. A surgically implanted InterStim system sends electrical signals to the nerves that regulate bladder function.

"The electrical pulses act as a distraction to a trigger-happy bladder," explains Rodney Anderson, MD, professor emeritus of urology at Stanford University.

The patient is given a remote control to turn stimulation up or down as needed. In studies, Dr. Anderson and others found that it completely eliminated incontinence in almost half of the patients studied.

For more information on urge incontinence and an overactive bladder. Point your browser to the Web site of the Simon Foundation for Continence at www.simonfoundation.org.

overactive thyroid

You can think of hormones produced by the thyroid gland as the fuel that keeps you going. When the thyroid gland produces the proper amount of hormones, your vital functions hum along at the proper speed. If the gland is overactive, on the other hand, it's like stepping on the accelerator. Your heart rate goes up, you may be nervous or excitable, and your body will gobble calories in order to fuel your high-speed metabolism. You may welcome the weight loss, but this is not a condition you can ignore because it can lead to serious complications.

The most common cause of an overactive thyroid gland, called hyperthyroidism, is Graves' disease, an immune system disorder that disrupts the gland's ability to regulate its hormone output. Hyperthyroidism can also be triggered by a viral infection called viral thyroiditis.

"Viral thyroiditis clears up on its own, although we may give medications to temporarily reduce the heart rate and reduce the pain of the inflammatory process," says Shahla Nader-Eftekhari, MD, professor in the department of obstetrics, gynecology and reproductive sciences at the University of Texas Medical School at Houston. However, most people with hyperthyroidism will need medical treatment to get their hormones under control.

For Immediate Relief

home remedies

Have your doctor review your medications. Some prescription medications, including a heart drug called amiodarone (Cordarone), contain large amounts of iodine. This can stimulate the thyroid gland to produce excessive amounts of hormone, says Dr. Nader-Eftekhari.

Get plenty of calcium. People with high levels of thyroid hormone in the blood may lose bone calcium at an accelerated rate. Your doctor may advise you to eat plenty of leafy greens, fortified juices or cereals, low-fat dairy products, and other calcium-rich foods. The loss of calcium doesn't occur quickly, however. It's mainly an issue for people whose hyperthyroidism has gone untreated for a long time, Dr. Nader explains.

alternative therapies

Take an herbal combination. In Europe, a common treatment for early-stage thyroid problems is to drink an herbal tea that combines bugleweed with lemon balm. Used in combination with medical treatment, the tea can help control the amount of hormone produced by thyroid cells.

To make a tea, combine 2 teaspoons of lemon balm with 1 teaspoon of bugleweed in a cup of hot water. Let the herbs steep for 10 minutes, and drink the tea several times a day.

medical options

"Burn out" the gland. When hyperthyroidism is caused by Graves' disease, your doctor will probably recommend treatment with radioactive iodine. Taken orally, the iodine is absorbed by the gland, where it releases radiation that destroys hormone-producing cells. "Usually a single dose will correct the overactivity," says Dr. Nader-Eftekhari.

The one problem with radioactive iodine is that it typically destroys so much of the gland that levels of thyroid hormone drop too low. Most people who undergo the treatment will take thyroid-replacing hormones for the rest of their lives.

Consider surgery. Some people aren't able (or willing) to take radioactive iodine. Surgery to remove the gland is an effective alternative, says Dr. Nader-Eftekhari. Again, however, you

when to see a doctor

If your appetite has increased but you're losing weight, see your doctor right away. This is one of the first signs of an overactive thyroid gland, says Shahla Nader-Eftekhari, MD, professor in the department of obstetrics, gynecology and reproductive medicine at the University of Texas Medical School in Houston.

If your eyes are protruding, or if you feel as though there's sand in your eyes. These may be symptoms of Graves' disease.

If you're experiencing depression or mood swings and you've never had these problems before. It's not uncommon for people to be diagnosed with depression when they actually have an unrecognized thyroid problem, and it is worthwhile to check out the thyroid.

will have to take thyroid medication for the rest of your life.

Stop the symptoms. Because high levels of thyroid hormones can put excessive strain on the heart and circulatory system, your doctor may give you medications—usually beta-blockers such as Inderal or Lopressor—to slow the heart rate and take the strain off the arteries until other treatments take effect.

For Long-Term Relief

home remedies

If you smoke, give it up. People with Graves' disease who smoke appear to have a higher risk of developing blindness or other eye problems related to this condition, says Dr. Nader-Eftekhari.

medical options

Take antithyroid drugs as directed. They gradually reduce symptoms by curtailing the thyroid gland's output of hormones. "We advise pregnant women to use medications and absolutely avoid exposure to radioactive iodine," says Dr. Nader-Eftekhari.

The drugs propylthiouracil (which is suitable for pregnancy) and methimazole (Tapazole) are generally taken for a year and then discontinued. In some cases, this eliminates the problem for good. In about 50 percent of cases, however, Dr. Nader-Eftekhari says, people will have relapses that will require additional treatment.

parkinson's disease

Though actor Michael J. Fox has become the public face of Parkinson's disease and Parkinson's research's staunchest ally, this motor system disorder marked by tremors and poor balance is more likely to strike people over the age of 50. And "strike" is too aggressive a word. Parkinson's disease doesn't strike as much as sneak. The symptoms are so mild at first that many people don't bother calling their doctors. They may be a little shaky, or tired more often. Their handwriting may change, or they may be irritable or depressed for no apparent reason. If they have trouble getting out of a chair, they just assume that they're getting a little creaky with the passing years.

Even though Parkinson's disease often progresses at a snail's pace, there's no stopping it. Over time, nerve cells in a part of the brain called the substantia nigra become impaired or die. They're unable to produce a chemical called dopamine, which allows the brain to direct the body's complex movements. The result can be muscle stiffness or tremors that gradually get more and more severe.

No one's sure what causes the neurons to die off. Some people may have a genetic tendency to develop Parkinson's disease. For example, one study published in 2010 identified a gene variant in a significant number of people with Parkinson's that controls the activity of an enzyme that helps convert dietary vitamin B_6 into its active form. The body needs that raw material to create dopamine. It's one of 13 genes linked to the disease. But there are likely also environmental triggers. What these triggers might be, however, remains largely a mystery, says Richard B. Dewey Jr., MD, professor of neurology and director of the Clinical Center for Movement Disorders at the University of Texas Southwestern Medical Center in Dallas. Studies have identified potential risk factors, including exposure to pesticides, herbicides, living in rural areas, and drinking well water, but what role they play is still unknown.

There isn't a cure for Parkinson's disease, but there are a number of strategies for relieving symptoms and supplying the brain with the dopamine that it needs.

For Immediate Relief
home remedies

Exercise as much as you can. One study found that people with early- to mid-stage Parkinson's disease who exercised twice a week had strength increases of 41 percent and improvements in coordination of 42 percent, according to lead researcher Iris Reuter, MD, of the department of clinical neurosciences at King's College Hospital in London. One reason it helps: As dopamine-producing cells are lost, your brain compensates for their loss, basically reshaping itself, as it does in childhood, by experience. So if you're exercising regularly, your brain is able to restore lost connections and even form new ones that, according to the Parkinson's Disease Foundation, "may actually outweigh the effects of neurodegeneration."

Stay active, both socially and physically. "There's a tendency for people with Parkinson's to get very sedentary," says Dr. Dewey. "They need to stay active because it will help them maintain their normal lifestyles as long as possible."

Eat a high-fiber diet. It helps prevent constipation, a common symptom in those with Parkinson's disease.

Get regular massages. Massage reduces muscle pain and stiffness, and it also helps people relax. "Anything that people with Parkinson's can do to relax is helpful because stress can aggravate the symptoms," Dr. Dewey explains.

Talk to your doctor about supplements. Several substances have shown promise for PD relief, though there's no conclusive evidence they work. Coenzyme Q10 helps fuel the mitochondria—considered the "powerhouse" of the cell—and recent studies have found that high doses (up to 1,200 mg) slowed progression of the disease in a small group of patients. Likewise, creatine, best known for its ability to create phosphocreatine, a brain and muscle energy source, and glutathione, an antioxidant, are now under study, as are the use of fermented papaya and blueberries to delay nerve cell death.

when to see a doctor

 If you have persistent, involuntary trembling or quivering that seems to be getting worse, see a neurologist right away. This is known as a tremor, the classic symptom of early-stage Parkinson's disease, says Richard B. Dewey Jr., MD, professor of neurology and director of the Clinical Center for Movement Disorders at the University of Texas Southwestern Medical Center in Dallas.

If you're having symptoms on one side of the body, Both Parkinson's disease and stroke tend to occur "unilaterally." If you're having symptoms on both sides of the body, you may have a different type of neurological problem.

If you're taking medications and notice an increase in symptoms. People with Parkinson's may need to have their dosages of medication adjusted as often as every 3 months.

medical options

Start drug treatment immediately. If you've recently been diagnosed with Parkinson's disease, your doctor will probably give you a prescription for dopamine agonists, medications that simulate the effects of dopamine in the brain, and/or a medication called levodopa (or L-dopa), the oldest drug in the Parkinson's armament and still the most prescribed. The brand name is Sinemet.

People who take a dopamine agonist will often have a complete remission of symptoms for 1 to 3 years. As the drugs become less effective, your doctor will probably supplement your treatment with L-dopa.

"Most people will eventually wind up taking a combination of the two drugs," Dr. Dewey says.

Another drug that may help is anticholinergic medications that increase the activity of acetylcholine, another brain messenger that, like dopamine, controls movement. If you have mild PD, this may be the drug your doctor tries first.

MAO-B inhibitors (Eldepryl) block an enzyme that breaks down L-dopa. It's often prescribed by itself to delay the need for L-dopa and in late-stage PD to boost L-dopa's effects.

If you're taking L-dopa, your doctor may also prescribe entacapone (Comtan), a drug that also prevents the breakdown of L-dopa, allowing more of the drug to reach the brain, raising dopamine levels and prolonging symptom relief.

Talk to your doctor about surgery. People with severe tremors, or who develop a resistance or adverse reactions to PD medications, may be candidates for what's called deep brain stimulation surgery, in which a pacemaker-like device is implanted under the collarbone to send electric impulses to the parts of the brain involved in motor function. It's not a cure and provides only temporary relief (about 5 years), but the results can be dramatic.

For Long-Term Relief

home remedies

Eat protein late. Dietary protein blocks some of the effects of levodopa therapy. Your doctor may recommend that you follow a protein "redistribution" diet, in which most of the protein in your diet is consumed at night, when a temporary loss of mobility won't be as bothersome.

For more information on Parkinson's disease. Visit the Web site of the National Parkinson Foundation at www.parkinson.org.

phlebitis

The Greek language is unusually precise. Take the word "phlebitis": It's derived from the Greek word for vein (phleb), and the suffix for inflammation (itis). It's hard to get clearer than that.

Phlebitis usually occurs when a blood clot inside a vein causes painful inflammation, says John Blebea, MD, codirector of the Heart and Vascular Institute, University Hospitals Case Medical Center and professor of surgery at Case Western Reserve University School of Medicine in Cleveland. When the inflammation occurs in veins deep beneath the skin, it's called deep venous thrombosis (DVT); this condition is extremely serious since a blood clot can form and block the vein. NBC newsman David Bloom died of DVT in 2003 while embedded with troops in Iraq. It's a condition associated with long airplane flights, car or train rides, or any activity in which you have limited movement that can impair circulation to the legs. More often, the problem occurs in veins that are closer to the skin. Known as superficial phlebitis, it may cause pain, redness, or localized swelling. The area may be warm to the touch and feel painful when you're walking.

Women with varicose veins have a higher

risk of developing superficial phlebitis because the blood in their legs flows more slowly and irregularly, making it more likely to form clots, says Dr. Blebea. Women are more likely than men to get phlebitis because they tend to be more likely to have varicose veins.

Anything that interferes with circulation can potentially cause phlebitis. Hormone replacement therapy or the use of birth control pills can be risk factors, as can smoking, especially in combination with birth control pills, or a sedentary lifestyle. "Pregnancy also puts a woman at risk for phlebitis or deep venous thrombosis," Dr. Blebea

adds. The levels of estrogen and progesterone then are higher than normal, which increases the risk of clotting. In addition, as the uterus gets larger and heavier, it puts pressure on veins in the abdomen, which decreases blood flow to the legs.

Superficial phlebitis is more of an annoyance than a serious health problem, but the pain in the legs can be very uncomfortable and in some cases take weeks to clear up. It also increases the risk that clots will occur in deeper veins in the future. To reduce inflammation and get blood moving again, here's what doctors advise.

when to see a doctor

If you have an area on a leg that is red, swollen, or painful, see your doctor right away. Even if you don't have varicose veins, these symptoms could mean that you have phlebitis or deep venous thrombosis, says John Blebea, MD, co-director of the Heart and Vascular Institute, University Hospitals Case Medical Center and professor of surgery at Case Western Reserve University School of Medicine in Cleveland.

"You cannot distinguish between superficial phlebitis and a clot in the deep-vein system, which is potentially life threatening, without the appropriate treatment."

If you do have a blood clot in a deep vein, your doctor will most likely give you a prescription for blood-thinning medications, which will keep the clot from getting bigger while your body works to dissolve it. Surgery or clot dissolution is usually required only when leg swelling is severe.

For Immediate Relief

home remedies

Cool the area. When the veins first start to act up, applying an ice pack or a cool compress will temporarily reduce inflammation and relieve the pain, says Dr. Blebea. He recommends using compresses made with an aluminum acetate solution (Domeboro), which is available at pharmacies. "Such compresses to the affected area are often useful for the first several days," he says.

Take ibuprofen. "It will reduce the inflammation, which will improve the pain," says Dr. Blebea. For the first week that your legs are hurting, take 400 mg of ibuprofen 3 times daily, or every 4 to 6 hours, he advises.

Put your feet up. In order to reduce the swelling and lessen your discomfort, elevate your legs when you're not walking. This can be done by simply putting a pillow under them while you relax on the couch or in bed, or using a step stool when sitting on a chair. A recliner-type chair is ideal for phlebitis patients, says Dr. Blebea.

Walk, run, dance, or swim. In fact, any type of exercise that flexes the calf muscles can help prevent the progression of phlebitis. When muscles in the legs contract, they put pressure on the veins that can literally push blood uphill, says Dr. Blebea. He warns, however, to hold off on most activity for about a week, or until the pain has diminished.

For Long-Term Relief

home remedies

Wear compression stockings. The best ones are available by prescription. They apply precise amounts of pressure to the legs, which can reduce swelling and pain. "If you're on your feet a lot, compression stockings can sometimes improve blood flow and help to prevent recurrent phlebitis," Dr. Blebea adds. "If you already have it, you should be wearing them every day once the worst of the pain is over and you are able to put them on comfortably." Just avoid regular knee-high stockings, garters, tight socks, and pantyhose.

Wear flats instead of heels. The problem with high heels is that they restrict the movements of muscles in the legs. When you wear flats or shoes with low heels, every step you take pushes blood upward to the heart.

Don't cross your legs. This can also cut circulation to your lower extremities.

Take a mile-high walk. If you're on a long flight, make sure you get up and move about the cabin every 15 to 30 minutes to keep your circulation moving. Take many breaks during any other kind of long trip. When you can't take a walk, do some simple exercises such as rotating you ankles, lifting your knees, heels, and toes, and curling your toes.

Drink lots of water. Combine dehydration with immobility (sound like a flight?) and blood can start collecting in your legs. Make sure you have plenty to drink, which will also remind you to get up now and again.

For more information about phlebitis. Point your browser to the Web site of the American Venous Forum at www.venous-info.com.

phobias and panic attacks

Fear can save your life. When you see a suspicious stranger on the street or when a large, angry dog is coming your way, fear makes your heart beat faster and prepares your mind and muscles for action.

But irrational fear can wreak havoc on your life. Millions of women (and men) suffer from panic attacks—overwhelming sensations of anxiety that come without warning and for no good reason. Others are terrified by things that shouldn't be all that scary, like riding in elevators or browsing in a shopping mall. In some cases, fears can be debilitating. People with agoraphobia are often afraid to leave the house in case they have a panic attack.

Doctors aren't sure what causes panic attacks and phobias, though they're both part of a larger group of emotional illnesses called anxiety disorders.

They're probably linked to disruptions in a part of the brain called the hippocampus. "These are people who may be more sensitive than they should be to perceptions of potential danger," says Jack G. Modell, MD, vice president of clinical psychiatry at GlaxoSmithKline in North Carolina.

If one or both of your parents suffered from phobias, you're more likely to have them, too. Women may experience phobias more than men and generally tend to feel more vulnerable. About 40 million Americans have some kind of anxiety disorder, making anxiety the most common psychiatric disorder in the United States.

Don't allow your fears to take control of your life. With a combination of therapy, medications, and a variety of coping strategies, almost everyone can get them under control.

For Immediate Relief

home remedies

Hold your breath for 10 seconds. "It allows carbon dioxide to build up in the body, which reduces hyperventilation and other symptoms of anxiety for some people," says Kelly Conforti, PhD, a clinical psychologist in Albuquerque, New Mexico.

Take some deep breaths. When you're anxious, your breath tends to be quick and shallow, and that tells your brain that you're in panic mode, which makes things worse. When you find yourself feeling anxious, take a deep breath through your nose to the count of 4, then exhale to the count of 4. Pay attention to your stomach. It should rise a little as you breath in, then sink as you breathe out. Do this until you feel a sense of calm.

Get up and leave. People tend to experience panic attacks at certain times or in certain situations, such as when they're in a crowded place. "Just leaving the situation and going somewhere else can reduce levels of panic," says Dr. Modell.

In the long run, it's better to get the problem under control than to "run" when you start feeling anxious, Dr. Modell adds. "But to get relief from a particular attack, getting away is a reasonable thing to do."

THREE THINGS I TELL EVERY FEMALE PATIENT

KELLY CONFORTI, PhD, *a clinical psychologist in Albuquerque, New Mexico, gives the following advice for stopping panic attacks.*

1 **BREATHE SLOWLY AND DEEPLY.** "A lot of panic symptoms are triggered by hyperventilation," Dr. Conforti says. When you force yourself to breathe no more than 8 to 12 times a minute, you'll reduce the amount of oxygen in your body, which will help stop you from hyperventilating.

2 **BREATHE INTO A PAPER BAG.** It increases blood levels of carbon dioxide, thereby reducing feelings of anxiety and panic.

3 **DRINK LESS COFFEE.** For some people, as little as 200 mg of caffeine—about the amount in two cups of coffee—can stimulate the feelings of panic attacks. ∎

Take a 10-minute walk. Many people get immediate relief from a brief spell of activity, and it can last for hours. You can certainly exercise longer, but for anxiety relief, frequency is the key.

mind-body techniques

Play a mind game. Nearly everyone gets anxious when they feel that people around them are judgmental or dominant. "Try imagining that the person is a turkey, or even the back end of a horse," Dr. Modell advises. "You'll be less nervous when you take the situation less seriously and see the person in a different light."

Sample many alternatives. Meditation, particularly mindfulness meditation, which encourages you to avoid judging and labeling your thoughts, and yoga, prayer, biofeedback, and arts therapies (art, dance, music) may help ease your fears.

medical options

Sedate your fears. If you occasionally need to get your fears under control—because you're about to take a plane trip, for example—ask your doctor if a sedative would help, Dr. Modell suggests. Prescription sedatives won't eliminate fears, but they will temporarily reduce feelings of anxiety and help you cope with the moment. Sedatives that are commonly used for phobias and panic attacks include lorazepam (Ativan), diazepam (Valium), clonazepam (Klonopin), and alprazolam (Xanax). These medications may cause drowsiness and driving impairment, so use with care, cautions Dr. Modell.

Block panicky feelings. Many people avoid sedatives because they dislike feeling less alert than usual. An alternative is to take a prescrip-

tion drug called a beta-blocker. "Beta-blockers don't do much from the neck up, but they block the body's response to fear," says Dr. Modell. They may cause dizziness, he adds.

For Long-Term Relief

home remedies

Get into therapy. There are many kinds of psychological therapy that have been shown to be effective for anxiety issues, including cognitive-behavioral therapy, which focuses on identifying and altering thinking patterns.

when to see a doctor

If your heart is racing, you're perspiring, and you're having trouble breathing, seek urgent care immediately. The symptoms of panic attacks and heart attacks are very similar, says Jack G. Modell, MD, vice president of clinical psychiatry at GlaxoSmithKline in North Carolina.

If you've just started having panic attacks, and you've never had them before. A number of medical problems, including hypoglycemia (low blood sugar), can trigger symptoms that feel like panic. The side effects from medications, including decongestants, can also simulate the sensations of panic attacks.

If you're having panic attacks more than a few times a month or if you've avoiding normal activities because you're afraid of attacks. You'll want to see a mental health professional, who will help you find ways to prevent anxiety from interfering with your life.

Get to know what scares you. People are most frightened by things that seem unfamiliar and alien. Dr. Modell advises women to learn everything they can about the things that frighten them most.

If you're afraid of flying, read up on how airplanes work and what pilots do to control them. If you're afraid of spiders or snakes, learn about their natural habits. "When you understand that snakes aren't going to run up and chase you, you'll realize that the fears may be excessive and unreasonable," Dr. Modell says.

Exercise regularly. Do whatever it takes—an iPod crammed with your favorite tunes, a walking buddy, a fun exercise routine like salsa-inspired Zumba classes—to build physical activity into every day.

medical options

Confront your fears. One of the best ways to overcome phobias is with a technique called exposure and response prevention. You'll work with a therapist or psychologist, who will expose you, in a slow and controlled way, to the things that scare you most.

Suppose you're afraid of spiders. Your therapist might begin by talking about spiders. Then she'll show you pictures of spiders. Finally, she might ask you to be in the same room with a spider.

"You gradually increase the intensity of the exposure while teaching coping skills," Dr. Conforti explains. About 80 percent of those who practice this technique will experience partial or even total relief from their fears.

Consider SSRI antidepressants. Even if you don't suffer from depression, this type of medication (selective serotonin reuptake inhibitor) can help reduce the frequency and intensity of panic attacks and phobias. The drugs are usually taken for about 6 months, at which point your doctor may wean you from the medication. In some cases, the panic attacks will stop for good, although many people will continue to take small doses of the medication to prevent recurrences.

For more information on phobias and panic attacks. Visit the Web site of the National Institute of Mental Health at www.nimh.nih.gov.

pneumonia

A generation ago, people were terrified of pneumonia, and for good reason. It was the leading cause of death in the United States until the mid-1930s, and even today, it's the eighth leading cause of death (along with flu) among adult women, although numbers are dropping because of vaccines to prevent it.

Pneumonia isn't one disease, but refers to a number of infections and inflammatory conditions that affect the lungs. Many cases of pneumonia are caused by bacteria, but they also can be caused by pollutants, viruses, fungi, or tiny organisms called mycoplasmas. The flu virus is the most common cause of pneumonia in adults, likely occurring because the lungs are already inflamed and weakened. Bacterial pneumonia can also follow a bout of the flu. The most common cause of bacterial pneumonia in adults is *streptococcus pneumoniae*, for which a vaccine is available.

Pneumonia can cause shaking chills, a high fever, chest pain, difficulty breathing, and discolored mucus. It's essential to see a doctor because pneumonia can potentially cause permanent lung damage and can be fatal.

The only way to definitively diagnose pneumonia is to have a chest x-ray, along with laboratory tests to determine what type of pneumonia you have. You'll probably need medications to knock out the infection. In the meantime, here are a few ways to reduce the discomfort right away.

For Immediate Relief

home remedies

Eat chicken soup. It's not just an old wives' tale. Chicken soup really does help ease respiratory infections, including pneumonia. It helps thin airway secretions so you can breathe more easily. It's wise to get plenty of fluids of any kind to help loosen and bring up phlegm.

Inhale steam. It moisturizes dry tissues in the airways and helps loosen mucus in the chest. The easiest way to steam your airways is to take a long, hot shower or bath. Or you can fill a pot with water and bring it to a boil. Carefully, remove the pot from the stove and place it on a protected table or counter. Drape a towel over your head to create a type of sauna and breathe in the steam. Be sure to keep your face a safe distance from the scalding hot water so you don't get burned.

To make the steam even more effective, add a few drops of eucalyptus oil to the pot. Eucalyptus has been used for centuries as a natural expectorant. Look for it at a health food store or pharmacy.

Take it easy. When you have pneumonia, your lungs can't absorb as much oxygen as they should. It's a good idea to avoid strenuous activity until you're completely better.

Watch out for relapses. It's not uncommon for pneumonia to get better for a while, then suddenly get worse. If you find that you're getting short of breath after you've been recovering, or if you have a recurrent fever, see your doctor right away.

alternative therapies

Breathe easier with thyme. Herbalists recommend this flavorful kitchen herb for treating coughs caused by pneumonia and other respiratory infections. It thins mucus in the airways and makes coughs more "productive."

To make a tea with thyme, steep 2 teaspoons of dried herb in a cup of hot water for 10 minutes. You can drink the tea several times a day.

medical options

Call your doctor. When pneumonia is caused by bacteria, you're going to need antibiotics. They work very quickly and will usually start easing symptoms within a few days. You'll have to take them longer than that—usually for 10 days—to ensure that all the bacteria are destroyed. You may also need oxygen if you're having trouble breathing.

For Long-Term Relief

home remedies

Eat a lot of fruits and vegetables. Some of the best are spinach and kale, which are rich in vitamins A and C, and tomatoes, broccoli, and strawberries, which provide even more vitamin C. These and other nutrients in these foods strengthen the immune system, which may help you heal more quickly.

While you're shopping for vegetables, be sure to stock up on carrots. Researchers at the USDA Human Nutrition Research Center on Aging at Tufts University found that eating as little as $1\frac{1}{2}$ to 2 carrots daily significantly increased immune cell activity.

Avoid cigarette smoke and alcohol. Both of them tend to suppress the ability of the immune system to cope with the infection.

medical options

Get shot. Both the flu shot and the pneumonia shot can help protect you from two of the leading causes of pneumonia—the flu virus and the strep germ.

raynaud's phenomenon

t hardly takes courage to pull a tray of ice cubes from the freezer or pluck a newspaper from a snow-covered lawn—unless you have Raynaud's phenomenon, a mysterious condition in which changes in temperature cause the fingers or toes to turn cold and tingly—even look blue—sometimes for hours at a time.

It's natural for blood vessels to constrict temporarily when you're exposed to cool temperatures. In those with Raynaud's, however, the vessels overreact and stay shut longer than they should. The prolonged lack of circulation causes the skin to turn white from a lack of blood, then blue as the tissues run out of oxygen, and then pink when circulation eventually resumes. Stress can also cause Raynaud's. There are two forms of Raynaud's: the primary form, which means that there isn't an underlying disease that's causing the symptoms, and the secondary form, in which the symptoms are caused by other problems, such as scleroderma, a connective tissue disorder, lupus, or even carpal tunnel syndrome.

Most people with primary Raynaud's don't mind it all that much, says Filemon Tan, MD, PhD, professor of internal medicine at the University of Texas Medical School at Houston.

"It can be bothersome, but it's rarely serious," says Dr. Tan. "It doesn't take people long to learn how to prevent the attacks."

For Immediate Relief

home remedies

Stick your hands under warm running water. It will stop an attack almost instantly. "By the time you get your hands under the tap, the attack may have just about run its course anyway," Dr. Tan adds. If you're not near a sink, stick your hands under your armpits, massage your hands or feet, wiggle your finders or toes, or make wide circles with your arms to stimulate circulation.

Use a cup holder. Holding a cold can of soda or even a glass of ice water can trigger attacks in some people with Raynaud's. You may want to spend a few dollars for a plastic or foam cup holder, which will keep your fingers from getting chilled.

Buy a pair of lined mittens. They trap body heat better than gloves. Pull them on whenever you're going outside in cold weather—or, if necessary, when you're taking something out of the refrigerator or freezer, says Dr. Tan.

Bundle up. It's not enough just to protect your hands and feet. For people with Raynaud's, the blood vessels may shut down when any part of the body is exposed to cold, says Dr. Tan. Dressing in layers is the best way to stay warm during the cold months. Wear a T-shirt under a shirt under a sweater under a jacket.

alternative therapies

Warm your feet with hot pepper. It doesn't work for everyone, but you may want to try an old folk remedy for Raynaud's: Mix a little red pepper with talc and cornstarch and sprinkle it in your socks, or use a cream that contains the hot chemical in peppers, called capsaicin, which may help to stimulate blood flow and keep your feet warm. If your mouth or eyes come in contact with the pepper, burning and irritation may result. People sensitive to capsaicin may develop a rash, Dr. Tan cautions.

Consider niacin supplements. Vitamin B_3 causes your blood vessels to dilate, which increases circulation to your skin. The most common side effect is flushing of the face and body. Talk to your doctor first.

Give ginkgo a go. One small study found that people who took 160 mg a day of this herb had less pain. Ginkgo can interact with other herbs and drugs and cause bleeding, especially if you're taking a blood thinner. Talk to your doctor before you try this.

when to see a doctor

If emotional stress triggers Raynaud's attacks even when your hands or feet are warm, or there's swelling, joint redness, muscle weakness, tight or puffy skin over the hands, or unusual skin rashes. You may have secondary Raynaud's, a potentially more serious form of the disease, says Filemon Tan, MD, PhD, professor of internal medicine at the University of Texas- Medical School at Houston. These symptoms may indicate an underlying tissue disease, Dr. Tan says.

If the attacks happen more than once a day or if the symptoms persist for more than a few minutes. The persistent lack of blood flow could lead to serious tissue damage, including gangrene.

If the fingertips have turned black, ulcerations have developed on the tips, or you've lost all feeling. You may have suffered tissue damage, and need to see a doctor immediately.

Try biofeedback. With training, you can learn to control your own temperature, which could decrease the number and severity of your Raynaud's attacks.

medical options

Get prescription relief. If you have frequent Raynaud's attacks or if the attacks are unusually painful, your doctor may prescribe a medication that will help keep the blood vessels open. These might include oral medications, such as calcium channel blockers, alpha-blockers, or vasodilators, such as nitroglycerin cream (topical) or losartin, a blood pressure drug, or even Viagra, an erectile dysfunction medication.

"People who live in warm climates, such as here in Houston, may only have to take the medication in winter," Dr. Tan adds.

For Long-Term Relief

home remedies

If you smoke, try to quit. The nicotine in cigarettes causes blood vessels in the hands and feet to constrict, which may increase the frequency of attacks, says Dr. Tan.

Avoid caffeine. When you consume caffeine, your blood vessels constrict, which can worsen symptoms.

mind-body techniques

Reduce the stress in your life. Exposure to cold may be more likely to trigger an attack if you're already tense and anxious. In rare cases, stress alone is enough to trigger an attack, says Dr. Tan.

There are dozens of effective ways for reducing stress, such as yoga, meditation, and feel-good activities such as going to the movies or gardening.

repetitive strain syndrome

f you've ever slept with your arm in an uncomfortable position and awakened to feel tingling as blood returns to the hand, you've experienced one of the classic symptoms of repetitive strain syndrome.

Repetitive strain syndrome is an umbrella term for a group of conditions that includes carpal tunnel syndrome and tennis elbow. Carpal tunnel syndrome is the most serious form of repetitive strain, and it's very common in women.

The carpal tunnel is a narrow passage in the wrist, with the wrist bones on one end and the carpal ligament on the other. Within the tunnel are the flexor tendons and the median nerve. Problems begin when the outer layer of the flexor tendons, the synovium, swells and thickens.

"As it thickens, it takes up space in the carpal tunnel and starts to block the blood supply to the median nerve," explains Mary Lynn Newport, MD, orthopedic surgeon at the University of Connecticut Health Center in Farmington. Without adequate blood flow, nerve damage begins.

The first symptoms of carpal tunnel syndrome include tingling, numbness, burning, or pain in the hands. The symptoms tend to be worse in the morning. In some cases, the hands get so weak that some people can't hold a cup of coffee.

Many things can cause carpal tunnel syndrome. Women who repeat the same motions over and over again—typing, for example, or working on cash registers or assembly lines—have a high risk of developing carpal tunnel syndrome. In fact, women are 3 times more likely than men to get it, in part because the carpal tunnel is smaller in women than men and in part because of hormonal fluctuations that lead to fluid retention. "When tissues in the hands retain fluid, the synovium swells, which pinches the median nerve," Dr. Newport explains.

Carpal tunnel syndrome can often be reversed as long as it's treated before permanent nerve damage occurs. Here are some of your options.

For Immediate Relief

home remedies

Ice it right away. As soon as you start having wrist pain, put a cold pack or ice cubes wrapped in a towel on the back of the wrist. Applying cold for 10 to 15 minutes at a time, several times a day, will constrict blood vessels and reduce inflammation in the wrist, says M. Patricia Howson, MD, an orthopedic surgeon at Kaiser Permanente Medical Center in Redwood City, California.

Take over-the-counter pain relievers. Aspirin, ibuprofen, and other analgesics reduce the body's production of prostaglandins, chemicals that increase pain and inflammation.

Use wrist splints. Available in drugstores, splints keep the wrists flat and straight, which reduces strain and helps the injury heal more quickly. "Wear the splint as often as possible," says Dr. Howson. "It's especially important to wear it at night because many people sleep with their hands curled up."

Massage your arm and hand. It can also help to do regular stretching.

when to see a doctor

If you have persistent numbness or tingling in the hands, or if pain doesn't go away, contact your doctor right away. There's a good chance you have carpal tunnel syndrome, and quick treatment will help ensure that it doesn't get worse, says Mary Lynn Newport, MD, an orthopedic surgeon at the University of Connecticut Health Center in Farmington.

If the pain gets progressively worse or if it interferes with your normal activities. Your doctor may recommend injecting steroids into the injured area to reduce inflammation. Steroid injections sometimes cure the problem, but more often they're used to provide short-term relief (up to 3 months, in some cases).

If steroids or other medications don't bring relief. You may need surgery to cut and release the band of ligaments at the bottom of the carpal tunnel. This provides more space for the nerve and tendons to move freely, without compression of the nerve.

Long-Term Solutions

Stretch your hands. Stretching increases blood flow and flushes out accumulated fluids. "Use one hand to stretch and pull the fingers back on your other hand," Dr. Newport suggests.

Avoid prolonged wrist motions. "If you're sitting in front of a computer all day, get up every hour and make a few phone calls or do some filing," says Dr. Newport. "The key is to use different muscles in your hands and fingers."

Make your workstation wrist-friendly. If you spend a lot of time at a desk or workstation, take a few minutes to arrange things in a strain-reducing manner. For example:

- Adjust the computer monitor so that it's at eye level. If it's too low or too high, you'll hold your body in unnatural positions that can increase strain on the wrists, says Dr. Newport.

- Relax your shoulders, keep your feet comfortably flat on the floor, and sit in a chair that helps to hold your back straight.

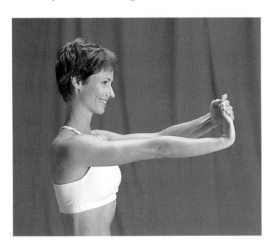

- Hold your wrists straight when you type; your elbows should be bent at a 90-degree angle.

Cut back on dietary salt. The average American consumes more than 3,000 mg of salt daily, a lot more than the upper limit of 2,400 mg that doctors recommend. High intakes of dietary salt can lead to fluid retention, which increases pressure on the median nerve responsible for carpal tunnel pain, says Dr. Howson.

Some of the saltiest foods include cheeses, chips, fast food, and packaged and convenience foods. It's worth reading food labels and stocking up on low-sodium foods whenever possible, says Dr. Howson.

Keep your wrists in neutral. When you're doing things that seem to be causing pain, take a look at your hands. There's a good chance that they're tensed, with the wrists bent, says Dr. Howson. "Try to keep the wrists straight whenever possible," she advises. "You want to avoid keeping them in a bent, flexed, or twisted position for long periods of time."

Use your entire hand for gripping. When you hold items with just your thumb and fingers, you're working muscles that share the same nerve supply as the carpal tunnel, which further fatigues the area. "Use your whole hand, including the palm and fingers, when gripping an object," says Dr. Howson.

Get your body moving. "We don't exactly know why, but studies have shown that regular aerobic exercise may prevent carpal tunnel syndrome, in addition to slowing its progress," says Dr. Newport.

Take vitamin B$_6$. "We don't have scientific studies to prove it, but vitamin B$_6$ does seem to help some people," says Dr. Newport. If you're having wrist pain, try taking 50 mg of vitamin B$_6$ twice daily for 6 weeks to see if it helps, she advises.

For more information about repetitive strain syndrome. Visit the Web site of the American Academy of Orthopedic Surgeons at www.aaos.org.

respiratory allergy

I f women with respiratory allergies spent their lives in a bubble—if their kids never brought home stray pets and dust disappeared with a dirty look—then sneezes and watery eyes would be as rare as winning the lottery.

But we live in the real world. Indoors and out, allergy-causing substances are everywhere. Dogs and cats are covered with dander. There are dust mites, molds, and pollen-filled winds, any one of which can put your respiratory system on red alert. Unfortunately, most times your immune system is responding to a false alarm, mounting a defense against an enemy that's pretty benign, like your kitty's skin.

"Most people believe that outdoor allergens cause the biggest problems, but indoor allergens actually have the greatest impact because people spend most of their time inside," says William Berger, MD, clinical professor at the College of Medicine, Division of Allergy and Immunology at the University of California Irvine, and author of *Allergies and Asthma for Dummies*. In fact, indoor air can sometimes cause greater symptoms than the air outside, he adds.

Some women suffer from respiratory allergies only during hay fever season, but for many others, the misery persists all year. Doctors call this perennial allergic rhinitis, and it's easy to diagnose because women with allergies often have "allergic shiners"—dark circles under the eyes that are caused by increased blood flow near the sinuses.

You can't cure respiratory allergies, but there are many ways to ease the symptoms, or even stop them entirely.

For Immediate Relief

Take advantage of antihistamines. They block the effects of histamine, the body chemical that causes sneezing, wheezing, and other respiratory symptoms. Over-the-counter products that contain antihistamines—such as diphenhydramine (like Benadryl) and chlorpheniramine (like Chlor-Trimeton or Dristan Cold Multi-Symptom Formula)—can be very effective, although they may cause drowsiness or a dry mouth in many people who use them.

To get the benefits of antihistamines with few

or no side effects, your doctor may advise you to use a prescription nonsedating product, such as loratadine (Claritin) or fexofenadine (Allegra).

Use decongestants as necessary. Decongestant sprays relieve nasal congestion by shrinking blood vessels in the nose and reducing swelling. These medications are very effective for short-term relief–but don't use more than the recommended dosage, and certainly not on a regular basis, and never for more than 3 to 5 days in a row. People who overuse nasal decongestants often experience a rebound effect, in which the stuffiness comes back with a vengeance as soon the medications are discontinued. In some states you'll need to ask your pharmacist for decongestants because they're not out on shelves, as some of the ingredients can be used in the manufacture of illicit drugs. They can cause nervousness, sleeping problems, heart palpitations, and high blood pressure.

Get dust mites out of your life. These tiny creatures live in house dust, and they thrive in sheets, pillowcases, mattresses, drapes, and carpets. In fact, many people with allergies also test positive for sensitivity to dust mites. To get rid of mites:

- Dust thoroughly at least once a week. Wipe every surface with a damp cloth, including the tops of door and window frames. Be especially vigilant about cleaning the bedroom because you spend more time there than in any other room.

- Cover heating and air conditioning vents with filters, available at home supply stores. Look for HEPA filters, which will trap mites and other allergy-causing particles.

- Vacuum the house once a week, preferably with a vacuum cleaner equipped with a HEPA filter. Hardwood, tile, and linoleum floors are easier to keep dust free than is carpeting.

- Wear a dust mask whenever you're cleaning or raising dust in the house.

- Wash your bedding weekly in hot water. Dust mites can't survive high temperatures. As long as the hot water in your house is 130°F or hotter, it will kill mites as well as their eggs. A Korean study found that laundering cotton sheets at 140°F killed 100 percent of dust mites, but a warm 104°F setting only wiped out 6½ percent.

Keep pollen out. To keep allergy-causing pollens out of the house, you may want to keep the windows closed in the spring and summer, and use the air conditioner instead. If you've been outside, jump in the shower. You can carry pollen inside on your hair, skin, and clothes which will continue to trigger symptoms, says allergist Stanley Fineman, MD, of the Atlanta Allergy and Asthma Clinic.

Move the plants outside. Studies have found that more than 75 percent of people with allergies are allergic to at least one common houseplant. The most common culprits are ficus, ivy, yucca, palm orchid, and fern.

Stay inside during peak hours. During the allergy season, airborne pollen counts are highest in the early morning and in the evening. You may want to schedule your days so that you're inside during those times.

Use a nasal wash. Mix ½ teaspoon of uniodized salt in an 8-ounce glass of warm water, add a pinch of baking soda, and, using a squirt bottle, eyedropper, or neti pot (a small teapot-like container), pour or squeeze about 4 ounces of the solution in one nostril. It will come out of the opposite nostril or the mouth. Then blow your nose slightly. Repeat with other nostril. This method can help clear nose secretions, remove allergens and irritants, bacteria and viruses, and may help make medication more effective.

medical options

Talk to your doctor about nasal sprays. If you can't seem to control your allergies with home care, you may want to consider using a steroid nasal spray such as Flonase, Nasonex, or Rhinocort. Within the first 24 hours, steroid nasal sprays reduce inflammation and irritation in the lining of the nose, which can reduce nasal congestion and sniffles and make it easier to breathe.

Another nasal spray commonly used is cromolyn sodium (Nasalcrom). Nasalcrom is available without a prescription and is used to prevent or treat the symptoms of seasonal and chronic allergic rhinitis. Your doctor may decide to prescribe a nasal antihistamine spray called azelastine (Astelin), which is used to treat the symptoms of allergic rhinitis.

Consider immunotherapy. If your allergies are severe and you can't seem to get relief, your doctor may recommend a procedure called immunotherapy, or allergic desensitization. You'll work with an allergist, who will give you a series of injections that contain tiny amounts of the allergens that bother you. Over time, your body will become less and less sensitive. Immunotherapy therapy won't necessarily eliminate allergies, but it can make your symptoms much more tolerable. Allergy shots work best for pollen, eye, bee

"False" Allergies

I f your nose starts running every spring or if your symptoms tend to get worse during the semiannual housecleaning, you can be pretty sure you have respiratory allergies. But what if your symptoms flare up even when you haven't been around pets, pollen, or dust?

You could have a condition called nonallergic vasomotor rhinitis, which basically means that your nose is overly sensitive, even in the absence of allergies.

"Just as some women blush more easily than others, some get stuffy or congested when they're exposed to things such as spicy foods or cold air," says William Berger, MD, clinical professor at the College of Medicine, division of allergy and immunology at the University of California Irvine, and author of *Allergies and Asthma for Dummies*.

Many things can trigger nonallergic vasomotor rhinitis. Possible culprits include changes in temperature or weather, tobacco smoke, paint fumes, even the smell of newspapers.

Oral antihistamines and other oral allergy medications may not help if you have nonallergic vasomotor rhinitis, says Dr. Berger. Your doctor will probably advise you to use a nasal antihistamine spray that has been approved by the FDA for the treatment of this condition. ∎

sting, and some drug allergies. It usually takes 6 months or more of shots before you notice relief.

For Long-Term Relief

home remedies

Keep a distance from dogs and cats. Millions of Americans are allergic to proteins found in the saliva, urine, and skin cells of dogs and cats. All pets produce these proteins. There's no

when to see a doctor

If you can't control sneezing, a runny nose, or other allergy symptoms with home care, make an appointment to see an allergist. You may need skin tests to determine what, exactly, you're allergic to, says William Berger, MD, clinical professor at the College of Medicine, division of allergy and immunology at the University of California Irvine, and author of *Allergies and Asthma for Dummies*. Once you've identified the problem, it will be easier to find ways to avoid it, he explains.

If your symptoms include persistent headaches, fever, or fatigue. What appear to be allergy symptoms may be caused by an underlying ear or sinus infection.

If you've had allergies for years, and they seem to be getting worse. Long-term allergies can increase the risk for nasal polyps, growths in the nasal passages that can interfere with breathing. Your doctor will examine the inside of your nose to make sure that the breathing passages are clear.

such thing as a hypoallergenic pet—although cats with dark coats do appear to cause more symptoms than those with white- or light-colored coats.

If your dog or cat sleeps in the bedroom with you, chances are you're inhaling tremendous amounts of allergens every night, says Frank Virant, MD, an allergist and clinical professor of pediatrics at the University of Washington School of Medicine in Seattle. At the very least, you should put your pet's bed in another part of the house.

You'll do even better if your dog or cat spends more time outside, adds Linda B. Ford, MD, an allergist in Papillion, Nebraska, and a past president of the American Lung Association.

If possible, wash your pets every 1 to 2 weeks. A plain-water wash may reduce the number of allergic-causing particles from the coats of dogs and cats, says Clifford W. Bassett, MD, medical director of Allergy and Asthma Care of New York.

Wash up after pet owners. Even if they leave their pets at home, visitors can bring animal hair and dander with them on their clothes and shoes and that can make you cough and sneeze. Vacuum your furniture after guests leave.

Keep your furnishings simple. Overstuffed chairs and couches are wonderful to sit on, but over time they trap and hang on to large amounts of dust mites, animal dander, and other allergy-causing particles. The same is true of heavy drapes, feather pillows, and textile wall hangings. In fact, animal dander sticks to your clothing, your hair, and the walls of your house.

You'll do better if you furnish your home with

products made from wood, leather, plastic, or vinyl, says Laurie Blevins Fowler, MD, an allergist in Columbia, Missouri. Be aware that some people with chemical sensitivities may have reactions to plastic or vinyl products as well.

Make cotton the fabric of your life. Rub a couple of synthetic fabrics together and they create an electrical charge that attracts pollen, says Gailen D. Marshall, MD, director of clinical immunology and the division of allergy at the University of Mississippi.

Control stress. A 2008 study at Ohio State University College of Medicine found that allergic people had more symptoms after they took an anxiety-provoking test than when doing something that didn't make them tense. The reason: Stress hormones may stimulate the body to produce IgE, a protein in the blood that causes allergic reactions.

Avoid smoke—and smokers. Allergy sufferers are particularly sensitive to cigarette smoke, says the National Institute of Environmental Health Sciences. In one study, more than 80 percent of students who came from homes where family members lit up had nasal allergy symptoms.

Plant wisely. Some plants are just more pollen-y than others. Flowering trees and azaleas produce a waxy pollen that's actually too heavy to surf the breeze, making them a better choice than maples and beeches.

For more information about respiratory allergies. Visit the Web site of the American Academy of Allergy, Asthma and Immunology at www.aaaai.org.

restless legs syndrome

Some people call it "jimmy legs," the creeping, crawling, burning sensation that can jerk you awake from a sound sleep and make you want to move your legs. Instead of snoozing, you can spend a good part of the night stretching, pacing, or marching in place just to make it go away.

Doctors aren't sure what causes restless legs syndrome. They suspect that it's a neurological condition linked to an imbalance of chemicals in the brain or spinal cord, or possibly to problems with peripheral nerves in the legs or feet, says Nancy Foldvary-Schaefer, DO, a neurologist and director of the Sleep Disorders Center at the Cleveland Clinic Foundation in Cleveland. A recent study from the Mayo Clinic identified a particular mutated gene linked to RLS, indicating that in at least some people, there's a strong genetic component to the condition that affects as many as 11 percent of people worldwide.

Restless legs syndrome is more common in women, and it tends to worsen over time. At one time, medical experts believed RLS didn't cause serious problems, but a study done at Harvard Medical School in Boston involving 3,433 people found that having the condition makes you twice as likely to have a stroke or heart disease. The possible link: The 200 to 300 periodic leg movements many RLS sufferers have each night increase blood pressure and heart rate. Sleep deprivation may also play a part.

To give your legs the "rest" they need, here's what doctors advise.

For Immediate Relief

home remedies

Massage your legs. It's probably the quickest way to relieve the sensations, especially if you use vigorous pressure to knead and rub the muscles. "Stimulation of the legs seems to be effective in some people," says Dr. Foldvary-Schaefer.

Take a warm bath. Not only does it help your muscles relax, it helps you relax, and stress can make RLS symptoms worse.

Stretch your muscles. Any kind of leg movement will help reduce the uncomfortable sensa-

tions, says Dr. Foldvary-Schaefer. One helpful exercise is to stand briefly with your back against a wall and your knees bent, as though sitting in a chair. This stretches and tires the muscles, which will often temporarily relieve the feelings.

"It's very helpful for people just to stretch their ankles by extending their feet while they're lying in bed," Dr. Foldvary-Schaefer adds. "It's also helpful for some people to get out of bed and move. The movement somehow inhibits the uncomfortable sensations."

Avoid caffeine and alcohol. It's not clear why, but people who quit drinking alcoholic or caffeinated beverages sometimes have a significant reduction in restless legs symptoms.

Drink tonic water before bed. This fizzy drink contains quinine, which can stop muscle contractions.

mind-body techniques

Keep your mind busy. The next time your legs get restless, try giving your full attention to mental activities, such as doing crossword puzzles, Sudoku, or playing a video game. It may reduce or eliminate the discomfort.

For Long-Term Relief

home remedies

Get more iron in your diet. Studies have shown that people with low blood levels of iron may be more likely to develop restless legs syndrome—and the lower their iron levels, the worse the symptoms get.

"There are people whose symptoms go away after they start taking iron supplements," says Dr. Foldvary-Schaefer.

when to see a doctor

If you're extremely tired during the day even though you felt as though you slept well the night before, or if you have insomnia, call your doctor. People with restless legs syndrome often experience jerky leg movements while they sleep, which can prevent them from entering the deeper sleep stages, says Nancy Foldvary-Schaefer, DO, a neurologist and director of the Sleep Disorders Center at the Cleveland Clinic Foundation in Cleveland.

If your leg discomfort is accompanied by persistent fatigue, or if you're also having heavy menstrual bleeding. You could be suffering from iron deficiency anemia, which may cause or contribute to the discomfort.

People with low levels of iron may be advised to take 45 mg of iron daily until their blood levels of this important mineral return to normal. After that, you'll want to make sure to get the Daily Value of 18 mg of iron, by taking a multivitamin and also by eating lean meats, fortified cereals, or other iron-rich foods.

Take a B-complex supplement. People who don't get enough folate, vitamin B$_{12}$, or other B vitamins may experience nerve problems (neuropathies), which have been linked to restless legs syndrome, says Dr. Foldvary-Schaefer. Follow the directions on the label.

medical options

Ask your doctor about medications. As recently as 10 years ago, sedatives were the main drugs used to treat restless legs syndrome. The medications helped, but people who took them often felt tired and hung over in the morning. Today there are many more choices available, says Dr. Foldvary-Schaefer.

Your doctor may prescribe a medication called ropinirole (Requip). This drug is very effective at controlling symptoms in some people. Your doctor may also prescribe levadopa (Sinemet), gabapentin, and pregabalin. Used to treat Parkinson's disease, they also can relieve restless legs syndrome by increasing brain levels of a chemical called dopamine. Low doses of narcotics can sometimes relieve RLS symptoms, but they can't be used indefinitely.

For more information on restless legs syndrome. Visit the Web site of the Restless Legs Syndrome Foundation at www.rls.org.

rheumatoid arthritis

Rheumatoid arthritis can strike at any age, even in childhood, and women are its usual targets. They're two to three times more likely than men to get this autoimmune disease, and their numbers are growing. Scientists at the Mayo Clinic have been tracking RA trends and were surprised to find that the incidence of the disease in their study population had jumped more than 50 percent between 1995 and 2004. The rates among men were unchanged.

The researchers don't know why, but speculated in published reports that there was an environmental cause: possibly smoking, potentially use of low-estrogen oral contraceptives, even deficiencies in vitamin D which are more common in women.

Rheumatoid arthritis has been called a whole-body illness. In addition to causing joint pain, it may result in fatigue, fever, weight loss, anemia, and joint deformity that leads to disability. In later stages, inflamed cells produce an enzyme that literally eats away bone and cartilage. The trigger that turns the body's immune system against its own tissue by causing widespread inflammation can also affect tissues and organs as well as the joints.

It's not clear what causes rheumatoid arthritis. There are genetic factors. One gene that occurs in only 20 percent of the general population has been identified in more than two-thirds of Caucasians with RA. It may be triggered by infection. People with RA also have high levels of an antibody called rheumatoid factor, which, in smaller quantities, regulates normal antibodies. Hormones may play a role. Women develop RA often after pregnancy and women with RA can go into remission while they're pregnant.

Symptoms may be limited to pain and stiffness, although in many cases the joints will also be swollen and warm to the touch, says Michael Lockshin, MD, director of the Barbara Volcker Center for Women and Rheumatic Disease at the Hospital for Special Surgery in New York City. Rheumatoid arthritis can worsen very

when to see a doctor

 If you're experiencing pain or swelling in three or more joints and the symptoms persist for more than a week, see a rheumatologist. There's a good chance you have rheumatoid arthritis, and quick treatment is essential to slow the progression of the disease, says Michael Lockshin, MD, director of the Barbara Volcker Center for Women and Rheumatic Disease at the Hospital for Special Surgery in New York City.

If joint pain is accompanied by fever, fatigue, or other whole-body symptoms. You may need prescription medications to help reduce the body's overactive immune response.

quickly. In some cases, in fact, it can permanently damage joints in as little as one year. Quick treatment is important, both to halt the progression of the disease and to ease the painful symptoms.

For Immediate Relief

home remedies

Use over-the-counter painkillers. A class of medications called nonsteroidal anti-inflammatory drugs (NSAIDs), which includes aspirin and ibuprofen, is considered the first-line treatment for arthritis-related pain and stiffness, says Dr. Lockshin.

Warm the joints. Applying heat to the sore joints can be very soothing, especially in the morning, when joints are stiffest and range-of-motion restricted. The easiest way to heat the joints is to lounge in a hot bath or shower. Or, using warm water (not above 90°F), you can moisten a towel or fill up a hot-water bottle and hold it to the affected area. When the towel or hot-water bottle cools, wet or fill it up again and repeat the treatment.

Ease pain with wax. If you're having trouble with joints in the hands or feet, you may want to try a paraffin bath, in which the joints are coated with a warm, waxy coating. The wax delivers long-lasting heat to relieve stiffness and pain. Mail order catalogs and some pharmacies sell Crock-Pot–like devices that heat paraffin to the appropriate temperature.

Exercise as much as you can. Regular exercise improves circulation to the joints, increases strength, and raises levels of brain chemicals that reduce pain. It's among the best treatments for rheumatoid arthritis, says Dr. Lockshin.

"You don't want to do aggressive exercise right away," he adds. "In the beginning, a woman could do gentle range-of-motion exercises, such as stretching. If she has neck pain, she could slowly roll her head around in a circle 10 times twice a day. If she has wrist pain, she could simply open and close her hands slowly 10 times twice a day. As she becomes more limber, she could move to more aerobic exercises." Try doing some stretching in the morning before you get out of bed to help you feel more limber.

Consider modest weight lifting. When combined with range-of-motion and aerobic exercises, weight lifting can reduce pain and possibly help prevent long-term damage. However, be sure to talk to your doctor before lifting weights. He may advise you to work with a physical therapist, who will design a workout to strengthen the areas where you need the most help.

alternative therapies

Take ginger. A recent study found that a ginger extract can dampen the effects of inflammation-causing chemicals in the body, including two targeted by arthritis medications. Take up to 2 grams in three divided doses, or up to four cups of ginger tea daily.

Give ashwagandha a try. A traditional Indian herb, it contains chemical compounds that reduce inflammation. The recommended dose is 3 to 6 grams of dried ashwagandha root daily in a decoction (boiled down), or 6 to 12 milliliters of liquid extract per day.

Or try guggul. A resin extracted from an Indian desert-dwelling tree, guggul supplements

---

THREE THINGS I TELL EVERY FEMALE PATIENT

MICHAEL LOCKSHIN, MD, *director of the Barbara Volcker Center for Women and Rheumatic Disease at the Hospital for Special Surgery in New York City, offers this advice for women with rheumatoid arthritis.*

1

BE PERSISTENT. Because rheumatoid arthritis can cause so many different symptoms, it may take months before it's identified with certainty. "If you're in pain and your regular doctor isn't helping, see a rheumatologist, who will examine you for rheumatoid arthritis," says Dr. Lockshin.

2

REPORT ALL CHANGES IN SYMPTOMS. It's normal for women with rheumatoid arthritis to have periods of relatively little pain, followed by flare-ups. It's important to report all changes to your doctor, such as having persistent fever when in the past you've only had joint pain. Changes in symptoms may mean that you need different medications or treatments to get the problems under control.

3

BE PREPARED FOR UPS AND DOWNS. "There will be good times and bad times," says Dr. Lockshin. "We can usually minimize the bad times by using the proper medications." ∎

have been shown to have powerful antiarthritic and anti-inflammatory effects. The recommended dose is 500 mg of standardized guggul extract (standardized to guggul lipids), taken internally twice daily.

Use capsaicin. The ingredient that makes hot chile peppers so fiery can, when applied topically, temporarily reduce the amounts of substance P, which contributes to pain and inflammation in people with arthritis. It's available in OTC creams.

Turn to turmeric. This ingredient found in ballpark mustards is also an anti-inflammatory. Take 400 mg three times a day.

Drink three to four cups of green tea every day. It's rich in polyphenols, chemical compounds that appear to prevent inflammatory cells from getting into joints to do damage. Green tea also is rich in the antioxidant vitamins C and E, nutrients that neutralize joint-damaging molecules in the body called free radicals.

The polyphenols in green tea may help prevent the condition from getting started. In a study at Case Western Reserve University in Cleveland, laboratory mice were given the amount of polyphenols found in three to four cups of green tea. Fewer than half of the animals developed rheumatoid arthritis, compared with 92 percent of those given plain water.

medical options

See a rheumatologist at the first sign of symptoms. A UCLA study concluded that seeing a specialist is the gold standard strategy for treating rheumatoid arthritis. Among patients whose care did not include a rheumatologist, only 50 percent received the level of care recommended by the American College of Rheumatology, such as annual doctor visits, blood tests, and drug monitoring.

Use the heavy hitters. Many people with rheumatoid arthritis can control their symptoms for years or even decades with OTC analgesics. As the disease progresses, however, prescription medications are often essential—either to calm the immune system or to relieve painful and joint-damaging inflammation in a variety of ways, says Dr. Lockshin. There are three classes of drugs used to treat RA, including nonsteroidal anti-inflammatory medications, corticosteroids, and disease modifying antirheumatic drugs (DMARDS). Some your doctor will likely mention include prednisone, methotrexate (Rheumatrex), hydroxychloroquine (Plaquenil), sulfasalazine (Azulfidine), leflunomide (Arava), etanercept (Enbrel), inflicimab (Remicade), adalimumab (Humira), abatacept (Orencia), rituximab (Rituxin), cyclosporine (Sandimmune, Neoral), and injectable gold salts (Myochrysine, Solganal). Since joint-damaging effects occur early in the disease process, you may wind up on a DMARD along with analgesics and anti-inflammatory drugs shortly after your diagnosis.

For Long-Term Relief

home remedies

Eat more fish. Or talk to your doctor about taking fish oil supplements. Studies have shown that the omega-3 fatty acids in fish oil can help relieve joint swelling and morning stiffness. Your doctor may advise you to take 8 to 10 capsules of fish oil daily—about the amount that you'd get in a 6-ounce serving of salmon or other fatty fish. Fish oils don't work overnight, however. Research has shown that they have to be used daily for about 12 weeks to get results.

Go Mediterranean. In a 2007 study, women with RA who went on a Mediterranean-style diet—consuming more fruits, vegetables, beans, and monounsaturated fat like that found in olive oil—had less pain and morning stiffness and felt in better overall health than a matched group that didn't follow the diet.

Cut out most animal products. Studies have found that people who have RA who become lacto-ovo vegetarians—they don't eat meat but do consume eggs and dairy—or vegans (who don't eat any animal products at all) experience fewer symptoms.

Stretch out with yoga. It's among the best ways to improve your range of motion by restoring flexibility and improving circulation to the joints. Improved circulation is important because it brings more oxygen and nutrients to the damaged joints.

Yoga has other benefits as well. It relaxes muscles and stimulates the release of endorphins, painkilling chemicals produced by the body. Mentally, yoga has a calming, relaxing effect.

Most health clubs offer yoga classes, from beginning to advanced. If you're just starting out, check with your doctor before signing up for yoga. You'll be advised to start out slowly in order to build strength and flexibility. Eventually, you'll want to work up to 40 to 60 minutes of yoga daily. That may sound like a lot, but rheumatoid arthritis is a serious condition, and the time you spend doing yoga will be time well spent.

For more information about rheumatoid arthritis. Visit the American College of Rheumatology Web site at www.rheumatology.org, or go to the Web site of the Arthritis Foundation at www.arthritis.org.

sciatica

Back pain is part of the human condition. Sciatica, a painful, often unrelenting irritation of the lumbar nerves in the lower back, is its curse.

"The most common symptoms of sciatica are numbness, tingling, and weakness or pain in the leg or foot," says Stephen Hochschuler, MD, clinical instructor at the University of Texas Health Science Center in Dallas, cofounder and chairman of the Texas Back Institute in Plano, and author of *Treat Your Back without Surgery*.

Sciatica is associated with pressure or inflammation of nerves—which in turn is often associated with a bulging or herniated disk, spinal stenosis, or piriformis syndrome, a pain condition involving the piriformis muscle in the buttocks.

Surgery is sometimes required to relieve pressure on the nerves, but often you can ease the painful inflammation with a combination of medications and simple home remedies.

For Immediate Relief

home remedies

Ice the injury. As soon as sciatica pain begins, apply ice wrapped in a towel to the lower back for 15 minutes several times a day. Continue applying ice for 48 hours. It numbs the area and constricts blood vessels, reducing swelling and inflammation, says Dr. Hochschuler.

Follow cold with heat. "After 48 hours, apply heat to the area," Dr. Hochschuler advises. It increases circulation and removes pain-causing toxins from the tissues. Put a heating pad or hot-water bottle wrapped in a towel on your lower back for 15 minutes at a time, and repeat the treatment throughout the day, he advises. Be careful not to burn the skin.

Drink 8 to 10 glasses of water daily. It's another way to help remove the inflammatory (and painful) toxins from the body, says Dr. Hochschuler.

Exercise in water. Swimming or simply wading in a heated pool is probably the best exercise for sciatica. "The warmth of the water prevents the muscles from going into spasm and putting more pressure on the nerves," says Dr. Hochschuler. Stop if pain increases, however.

Take one to two regular-strength aspirins or ibuprofen 4 times daily. The drugs relieve inflammation as well as pain, says Dr. Hochschuler.

Sleep like a baby. Lie in a curled-up fetal position with a pillow between your legs, or, if you sleep on your back, place a pillow or rolled up towel under your knees to take the pressure off.

medical options

Take oral steroids, if prescribed. Available by prescription, steroids are considered the gold standard for reducing inflammation. They have side effects, however, so they're used only when home treatments aren't effective.

WHAT WORKS FOR ME

STEPHEN HOCHSCHULER, MD, *is a clinical instructor at the University of Texas Health Science Center in Dallas, cofounder and chairman of the Texas Back Institute in Plano, and author of* Treat Your Back without Surgery. *He's suffered from sciatica for 16 years. Here's how he keeps it under control.*

"I take ibuprofen whenever I feel the leg pain. I avoid any lifting during that time, and I try to avoid any stresses or strains on my back.

"When I do have to lift something, I always bend at the knees, no matter what the object is. I also wear a back support because I have to stand and operate for up to 7 hours at a time. I also keep my weight down, drink lots of water, and exercise. I vary my exercise routine by riding a bike, hiking, and skiing." ■

Ask your doctor about injection therapy. When sciatica doesn't get better on its own, your doctor may recommend injections that combine an anesthetic with a powerful anti-inflammatory drug. Injected around the injured nerve, the medications reduce pain and swelling and may eliminate the need for surgery.

Long-Term Solutions

home remedies

Get physical therapy. It's among the best ways to prevent future episodes of sciatica because it strengthens the back and makes it less prone to injuries.

Rest before you lift. "If you've been on a long car ride, don't get out of the car right away and unload your luggage," says Dr. Hochschuler. "You don't want to add stress by lifting heavy objects. Get out of the car, stretch, and relax a bit. Then unload your luggage."

Lift with your legs. "Many women bend at the waist to lift heavy objects, which stresses the lower back," says Dr. Hochschuler. "Get close to the object and bend your knees. Don't stoop over." Lift using your legs and knees, not your back.

when to see a doctor

If the numbness, tingling, or leg pain lasts more than 2 weeks, see your doctor. Long-term sciatica may not get better without medical treatment, says Stephen Hochschuler, MD, clinical instructor at the University of Texas Health Science Center in Dallas, cofounder and chairman of the Texas Back Institute in Plano, and author of *Treat Your Back without Surgery.*

If the pain is accompanied by a loss of bladder or bowel control. This means the nerve injury is potentially serious, and you may require surgery to prevent it from getting worse. It is an emergency and needs treatment immediately.

shingles

Chicken pox is a common disease of childhood. Once the itchy red spots disappear, most of us just assume that the infection is gone for good and rarely give it a second thought.

But the herpes zoster virus that causes this childhood disease doesn't go away. It lies dormant in certain nerves of the body and can return many years later, rise to the surface, and cause a painful, blistering rash known as shingles.

During its first stage, shingles causes a deep, burning pain somewhere in the skin. You may also have a fever or headache. As the infection progresses, you develop red skin lesions, which quickly blister. The rash and blisters most commonly appear on the trunk of your body, but they may also occur around one eye, on the face or scalp, inside the mouth, or down an arm or leg. The blisters develop over several days and last 7 to 10 days before crusting. They may be very painful. You may also experience intense pain even if there isn't any rash.

"One of my patients told me that the pain was so bad that she wanted to jump off the roof," says John W. Edelglass, MD, associate clinical professor of dermatology at Yale University School of Medicine.

The one good thing about shingles is that this second bout of the chicken pox virus will probably be your last. However, women whose immune systems are weaker than they should be—because of underlying medical problems, for example—can get shingles again. And the big problem with shingles is that the pain often persists long after the sores have healed. This nerve pain, called postherpetic neuralgia, can drag on for months or even years.

Once you're infected with the virus, there's no way to get rid of it since it lives in the nerves forever. You can, however, reduce the pain of outbreaks with simple home care. There are also a number of medications that can dramatically reduce the pain and shorten the duration of the illness, says Dr. Edelglass.

For Immediate Relief

home remedies

Relieve pain with a cool wet compress. The quickest way to soothe rashes or sores caused by shingles is to apply a compress made with Burow's solution (like Domeboro). The solution reduces pain and also dries the sores,

THREE THINGS I TELL EVERY FEMALE PATIENT

JOHN W. EDELGLASS, MD, *associate clinical professor of dermatology at Yale University School of Medicine, gives women this advice for reducing the discomfort of shingles.*

1 **GET PLENTY OF REST.** Shingles can take quite a toll on the body. You will need plenty of rest in order to recover. Take it easy and let others pamper you for a while.

KEEP YOUR DISTANCE—SOMETIMES. Shingles itself is not contagious, so you can't give or catch it. However, shingles is caused by the chicken pox virus, which means that a child or adult who has not had chicken pox in the past could poten-

2 tially be infected by someone with shingles. When you have the rash or blisters, avoid close contact with anyone who has never had chicken pox, Dr. Edelglass advises. Once the blisters have crusted over, the danger has passed.

3 **SEE A DERMATOLOGIST.** Internists and family practice physicians may not be as familiar with shingles as dermatologists are, which means they could miss the diagnosis and delay treatment, says Dr. Edelglass. You're better off seeing a dermatologist as soon as symptoms begin, when you feel a persistent one-sided burning or pain in the skin, and especially if blisters begin to appear. ■

which helps them heal more quickly, says Dr. Edelglass. Prepare the compress by first mixing Domeboro powder or tablets with water according to the package directions. Dr. Edelglass recommends using a clean cloth, such as a piece of old linen, saturating it in the solution, and gently squeezing out the excess. Apply the compress to the affected area repeatedly over 10 minutes, resaturating the cloth if necessary. If the solution stings the skin, dilute it with more water. Repeat the compresses 2 to 4 times a day, as needed for comfort.

Cool the skin. "In addition to the Burow's solution, you may apply a lotion called Sarna," says Dr. Edelglass. "It contains menthol, which can cool and soothe the skin."

Enjoy an oatmeal soak. If you don't want to bother with compresses or lotions, you can ease rashes and sores by taking a lukewarm (not hot) bath. Sprinkle a cup or two of colloidal oatmeal (like Aveeno) into the water, Dr. Edelglass advises. Soak for 10 to 15 minutes, two to four times a day, until you feel better. "You can also use oatmeal bar soap," he adds. "Oatmeal is very soothing to the skin."

Take a painkiller. Aspirin, ibuprofen, naproxen, and other over-the-counter analgesics reduce skin inflammation as well as pain, says Dr. Edelglass.

medical options

Take antiviral medication. The severity and duration of shingles attacks can be significantly reduced if you take prescription antiviral drugs within 1 to 2 days after the blisters erupt. Drugs such as valacyclovir (Valtrex) and famciclovir (Famvir) help prevent the virus from reproducing, which can reduce or even eliminate postherpetic neuralgia, says Dr. Edelglass.

Get the vaccine. A herpes zoster vaccine, which reduces complications from shingles, is recommended for everyone over 60. The condition is more likely to strike this age group.

For Long-Term Relief

home remedies

Apply hot pepper cream. If you still feel pain after the blisters have healed completely, your doctor may recommend an OTC topical analgesic cream containing capsaicin (like Zostrix and Capzasin). Capsaicin is a chemical compound made from hot pepper extract. "You will feel a temporary burning or tingling sensation, which may last for 3 to 4 days," Dr. Edelglass explains. "Capsaicin essentially swamps the nerve endings, thereby gradually reducing the deeper nerve pain caused by the virus."

Apply a thin coating of the cream to the affected area, gently rubbing it into the skin, three to four times a day as needed. Wash your hands when you're finished to avoid getting the cream into your eyes or other sensitive areas. Do not use on sensitive skin, such as the face or groin, or on open sores. If you experience too much irritation or if the burning sensation lasts longer than 3 to 4 days, stop using it and consult your doctor.

For more information about shingles and postherpetic neuralgia. Visit the Web site of the National Institute of Neurological Disorders and Stroke at www.ninds.nih.gov.

sore muscles

Muscles are tough, flexible bands of tissue. They can stretch and contract to a remarkable degree, but they aren't impervious to damage. When you've done something too vigorously and feel sore the next day—like digging up your flower bed in the spring—it's because the muscles have developed tiny tears.

"The muscle becomes inflamed, and the inflamed tissue releases histamines and prostaglandins, chemicals that irritate nerves and cause soreness, says Priscilla Clarkson, PhD, professor of exercise science and associate dean of the School of Public Health and Health Sciences at the University of Massachusetts in Amherst.

As you would expect, soreness usually occurs when you've worked your muscles harder than they're accustomed to—either because you're doing a new activity, such as playing tennis for the first time in 20 years, or because you did too much too fast, such as sprinting when you usually jog.

Muscle soreness isn't likely to be serious, and it usually fades within a few days. But it can have long-term consequences: Among women who begin a new exercise program, soreness is among the reasons for giving it up. So if you're hoping to achieve long-term fitness goals, or simply want to move without grimacing, it's worth taking quick action to relieve soreness and protect the muscles from additional damage.

For Immediate Relief
home remedies

Take aspirin or ibuprofen. Don't assume that these medications are lightweights just because you can buy them over the counter. They're among the best remedies for stopping muscle pain as well as swelling.

Ice the area. "As soon as you feel the soreness, immediately place an ice pack—or even a bag of frozen vegetables—on the area for about

---

WHAT WORKS FOR ME

WILLIAM O. ROBERTS, MD, *a professor in the department of family medicine at the University of Minnesota Medical School, editor-in-chief of the* journal Current Sports Medicine Reports, *and medical director of the Twin Cities Marathon, is serious about getting regular exercise—and sometimes he overdoes it. Here's his secret for relieving soreness fast.*

"When I cross-country ski out West, I give my muscles a strenuous workout, and sometimes I get a little sore. I soak in the hot tub at the spa or at the hotel I'm staying at. I also take 400 IU of vitamin E and 250 mg of vitamin C. The research is scant on this, but I suspect that taking antioxidant nutrients reduces damage to the muscles when you're doing unaccustomed exercise." ∎

20 minutes," says William O. Roberts, MD, a professor in the department of family medicine at the University of Minnesota Medical School, editor-in-chief of the journal *Current Sports Medicine Reports,* and medical director of the Twin Cities Marathon. You can protect your skin by putting a damp cloth between it and the ice pack or bag of frozen vegetables. "Ice reduces swelling and soreness, slows bleeding from muscle tears, and reduces bruising."

If you don't have an ice pack, it's fine to apply ice cubes wrapped in a damp washcloth or towel. Repeat the treatment once an hour until the pain is better, Dr. Roberts advises.

Give muscles some time off. If you keep doing whatever made your muscles sore in the first place, tears will get larger and you'll hurt even more later on. "Rest your sore muscles for 24 to 48 hours after they start to ache," says Dr. Roberts.

Speed healing with heat. Within a day or two after the soreness begins, it's a good idea to apply a heating pad or a hot-water bottle wrapped in a washcloth or towel to the area for about 20 minutes at a time. Heat increases circulation, which helps flush toxins from the area. It also speeds the body's natural repair process.

"I'm a big fan of sitting in a hot bath or a hot tub," says Dr. Roberts.

You can also use a therapeutic heat wrap that contains small pads of iron that create heat as it starts to oxidize (which it does once it hits the air). It maintains heat at a constant, low temperature over an 8- to 12-hour period and can be worn under clothing. Pain relief lasts for around 24 hours.

Use a counterirritant. A topical capsaicin product, one that produces a cold feeling, or those that make you feel hot, can help give you temporary relief from muscle pain. Examples include Capsaicin, Icy Hot, or Ben-Gay.

Look for distractions. Studies have shown that when people concentrate on pain, the muscles contract even more, increasing soreness. So don't dwell on the discomfort. Get your mind off the pain—by listening to music, watching TV, or simply curling up with a good book.

Get a massage. "It breaks up scar tissue and helps remove waste products, such as lactic acid,

when to see a doctor

If you have muscle soreness that doesn't get better in a few days or if there's an unusual amount of swelling or pain, call your doctor. You could have torn a ligament or even fractured a bone, says Priscilla Clarkson, PhD, professor of exercise science and associate dean of the School of Public Health and Health Sciences at the University of Massachusetts in Amherst.

If your urine is brown, see your doctor immediately. A severely damaged muscle resulting from overexertion can cause excessive proteins to leak out into the blood and tax your kidneys, sometimes causing them to shut down.

If the muscle pain is accompanied by a fever, a rash, or whole-body aches and pains. It's not uncommon for muscle pain to be a sign of Lyme disease, a bacterial infection that requires treatment with antibiotics.

from the site," says Dr. Roberts. This is important because lactic acid increases pain and slows the time it takes for injured muscles to heal.

To find a qualified massage therapist near you, go to the American Massage Therapy Association Web site at www.amtamassage.org.

For Long-Term Prevention

home remedies

Get regular exercise. The muscles are more likely to stay loose and limber when you exercise regularly, which can prevent painful tissue tears, says Dr. Roberts.

"Try to work out for at least 30 minutes 5 days a week," he advises. For overall muscle fitness, aerobic exercises—such as walking, biking, and swimming—are hard to beat. "Activities that involve jumping or pounding, such as jumping rope, can be uncomfortable and may lead to injury," he adds.

Give the muscles time to adjust. "Start a training program gradually," says Dr. Clarkson. "Listen to your body. If you feel pain or discomfort, stop. Don't overexert yourself."

Warm up and cool down. Even if you're in good shape, plunging right into physical activity without giving the muscles time to warm up may increase the risk of soreness.

Start by doing your usual activity at a lower intensity than usual, says Michele Stanten, fitness director at *Prevention* magazine. For example, if you normally jog at a 10-minute-mile pace, slow it down at first. This gets your body ready for exercise by stretching the muscles and increasing blood flow. After about 5 minutes, you can pick up the pace to your regular intensity.

THREE THINGS I TELL EVERY FEMALE PATIENT

WILLIAM O. ROBERTS, MD, *a professor in the department of family medicine at the University of Minnesota Medical School, editor-in-chief of the journal* Current Sports Medicine Reports, *and medical director of the Twin Cities Marathon, treats a lot of women with muscle pain. He always gives his patients this special advice.*

EAT SMART. "If you eat a healthful diet, you will have an adequate energy supply for the muscles to work properly," he advises. For optimal muscle health, he advises minimizing the intake of meat and saturated fat and eating more fish, legumes, whole grains, and fruits and vegetables.

ALWAYS STAY ACTIVE. "You decrease your chances of damaging the muscles if you exercise regularly," says Dr. Roberts.

PACE YOURSELF. A lot of women get hurt when they've been less active than usual then overdo it. During the winter, for example, it's common for women to be somewhat sedentary. Then, on the first warm day, they charge outside and tear up the yard or go for a long run. The muscles aren't used to the exertion, which can result in painful tears. Always start slowly to give your muscles time to adjust, Dr. Roberts advises. ■

Whole-Body Stretch

This is one of the best all-around stretches for relieving tight muscles.

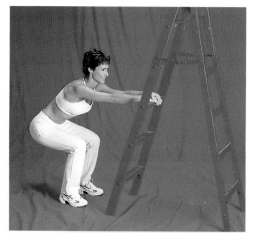

Hold on to a doorknob, a pole, or something else sturdy. Your feet should be shoulder-width apart, with the toes pointing forward. Slowly sit back into a squat, keeping your knees over your ankles. Lower yourself as far as you comfortably can, but don't bend your knees beyond 90 degrees (left).

Slowly drop your chin toward your chest and round your back (below). Hold the position, take 6 to 8 slow breaths, then slowly return to the starting position.

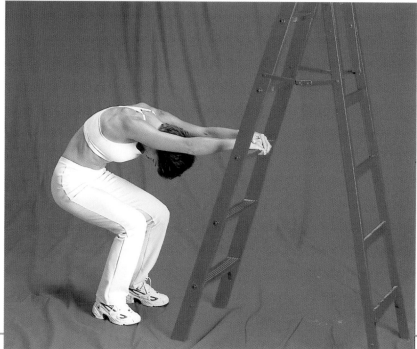

When you're ready to call it quits, don't just stop. If you do, lactic acid and other waste products of metabolism will remain in the muscles. Instead, gradually decrease the intensity of the exercise for about 5 minutes—for example, by dropping down to a slower jog, then to a brisk walk, and finally to a plain walk.

For more information about muscle soreness. Visit the Web site of the American College of Sports Medicine at www.acsm.org.

sore throat

Everything from viruses to air pollution to cheering too loud and too long for your favorite football team can give you a store throat. Most of the time, though, you can blame a virus or bacteria, including cytomegalovirus and *streptococcus*. Many clear up on their own; some need a dose of antibiotics. Here's how to reduce the discomfort.

For Immediate Relief

home remedies

Gargle with salt water. It's an old folk remedy, but it's still one of the best ways to soothe a sore throat. Mix ¼ teaspoon of salt in ½ cup of warm water, and gargle several times a day.

Suck on hard candy. It increases the flow of saliva and helps moisturize irritated tissues in the throat. Medicated lozenges are even better because they contain a mild anesthetic that temporarily numbs the throat.

Add honey to your tea. It soothes tissues in the throat and helps prevent further irritation, and there's good evidence that it's also antimicrobial—effective against bacteria and viruses. The tea itself is beneficial because it helps moisturize dry, irritated tissues.

Drink a lot of water. One reason sore throats hurt so much is that the inflamed tissues have lost their usual moisture, making them dry and irritated. The best way to remoisturize tissues is from the inside: Drink at least eight full glasses of water daily, and more if you can.

Freeze it up. This is one time that sucking on a sugary popsicle is good for you. Or try ice water—it has fewer calories.

Eat plenty of citrus fruits. They might sting a bit going down, but they're rich in vitamin C, which has been shown to shorten the severity and duration of colds. Vitamin C also strengthens the body's ability to resist pain-causing viruses.

Breathe steam. It fills the throat and airways with moisture and provides almost instant relief. The easiest way to inhale steam is to take a long, hot shower. Or you can plug in a vaporizer. To make the steam even more effective, add a few drops of eucalyptus oil to the diffuser. It breaks up congestion, which makes it easier to breathe when you have a cold or the flu. Look for eucalyptus oil at health food stores and pharmacies.

Take acetaminophen. It quickly reduces pain and swelling when you have a sore throat, says William J. Hall, MD, Paul H. Fine Professorship in Medicine at the Department of

when to see a doctor

If your throat is so sore that swallowing is extremely painful or if your voice is wheezy or you're having trouble breathing, call your doctor immediately. Sore throats are sometimes caused by a condition called epiglottitis, a dangerous throat infection that can shut down the airway and make it impossible to breathe.

If your throat is sore and you also have a high fever. You could have strep throat, a bacterial infection that requires treatment with antibiotics.

If you've recovered from a sore throat but then relapse with achy joints, fever, or a sharp pain that may mimic cardiac trouble. It's possible that you had strep throat, and it's now causing a secondary condition called rheumatic fever. Rheumatic fever can damage the heart, so it's essential that you see a doctor right away.

Medicine, University of Rochester School of Medicine, New York. Aspirin and ibuprofen are also helpful, but they're more likely to cause stomach upset or other side effects, says Dr. Hall.

Use an anesthetic spray. There are many over-the-counter products that contain small amounts of local anesthetics. Sprays such as Chloraseptic are short-lasting, but they reduce pain almost instantly, says Dr. Hall.

alternative therapies

Coat your throat with slippery elm. It's been used for hundreds of years to ease sore throat pain. Taken in tea or lozenge form, slippery elm coats tissues with a smooth, slick barrier that reduces irritation. To make the tea, pour $\frac{1}{2}$ cup of boiling water over 1 teaspoon of powdered slippery elm bark. Sip tea throughout the day to soothe the irritated throat. Purchase lozenges at the health food store, and follow the label instructions. Make certain the primary ingredient is slippery elm; some products are slippery elm in name only.

sprains

The joints in your body are held together with tough, fibrous cords of tissue called ligaments. Ligaments, which support the joints and keep them stable, have a certain amount of give. But when they're stretched too hard or suddenly, they get inflamed and irritated—sprained, in other words.

"Ligament sprains are always related to some form of injury," says Kim Fagan, MD, a sports medicine physician in Birmingham, Alabama. "The most common ligament injuries involve the ankle, and they're generally the result of twisting types of injuries, such as when you jump and land on the side of the foot."

Sprains are rarely serious, but they're painful and slow to heal. You may find yourself limping and grimacing for a week or more. To reduce the discomfort and help sprains heal more quickly, here's what experts advise.

For Immediate Relief

home remedies

Take a rest. Whether you sprained an ankle while playing tennis or jammed your wrist while working in the yard, the most important thing is to stop what you're doing immediately. If you keep putting pressure on the joint, you'll increase the pain and inflammation, and lengthen the time it takes to heal.

Apply ice. "The key to treating a sprain is to get ice on it immediately. Ice reduces the swelling, which will reduce pain," says Dr. Fagan.

If you don't have a cold pack, fill a plastic bag with ice cubes or take an unopened bag of frozen peas, wrap it in a thin towel, and hold it on the area for 20 minutes at a time. Repeat the

when to see a doctor

If you've sprained a joint and the pain is severe, or if the pain doesn't get better in a few days, make an appointment to see your doctor. You may have torn a ligament or even broken a bone, and surgery might be needed to repair the damage, says Kim Fagan, MD, a sports medicine physician in Birmingham, Alabama.

If you notice little or no improvement in the swelling or the ability to move or use the joint after a couple of days or if you're unable to bear weight on the affected joint, consult your doctor. These are red flags that mean the sprain might not get better without medical treatment, says Dr. Fagan.

treatment four times a day until the pain is gone, says Dr. Fagan.

Wrap it tightly. Use an Ace bandage or elastic wraps to bind the area over the sprain, says Dr. Fagan. This technique, called compression, helps reduce swelling and pain. Don't make the bandage so tight that you cut off circulation, Dr. Fagan adds. It should be just tight enough that you can barely lift the edge to look underneath.

Elevate the joint. If you've sprained your wrist, try to keep your hand elevated above chest level to reduce swelling. For your ankle, put a pillow underneath the calf.

Continue following the rest, ice, compression, and elevation therapy for 24 to 48 hours or for as long as there is swelling, advises Dr. Fagan.

Take aspirin or ibuprofen. Apart from reducing pain, they also decrease the inflammation associated with the injury, which may help the sprain heal more quickly, says Dr. Fagan.

For Long-Term Prevention

home remedies

Strengthen the joints. When muscles in the ankle and other joints are strong, there's less stress on the ligaments, which reduces the risk of sprains. Because ankle sprains are so common, it's worth focusing on this area to build up your strength.

"Simple heel raises are a good form of ankle strengthening," says Dr. Fagan. Stand with your toes on the edge of a stair or a curb, your heels suspended over the edge. Rise on your toes, pause at the top, then lower your heels. Try to repeat the exercise 10 to 15 times, once or twice a day. "As you get stronger, you can do one leg at a time," says Dr. Fagan.

Watch where you're going. Sprains often occur when people accidentally step off a curb or into a hole in the yard. "Walk on familiar territory so you can avoid the pitfalls," says Dr. Fagan. "Also, try to walk where it's well lit so you can see where you're going."

Stretch first. Before you exercise, it's a good idea to warm up slowly—by going up and down on your toes, for example, or bending your wrist backward and forward.

Abandon the high heels. And make sure the shoes you wear fit properly and offer your ankles support so you can avoid sprains in the first place.

temporomandibular disorder

Of all the joints in the body, the jaw probably has the heaviest workload. Every time you eat, drink, talk, or yawn, this joint moves smoothly up and down.

At least, that's what's supposed to happen. "If there is uneven stress because the muscles and joint are out of alignment, the muscles can shorten, tighten, and go into spasm, causing temporomandibular joint disorder," says Richard H. Price, DMD, spokesperson for the American Dental Association and former clinical instructor at Boston University Dental School. Apart from jaw pain, temporomandibular joint disorder (TMD) can result in clicking or popping sounds, pain that extends to the neck or shoulders, and sometimes headaches or hearing problems. It's not clear why, but studies suggest women are $1\frac{1}{2}$ to 2 times as likely as men to suffer from TMD.

Many things can cause the disorder. A severe injury to the jaw or joint and arthritis resulting from an injury are two clear causes. Habits such as resting your chin against your hand or another object may lead to TMD. That's why violin players may be prone to the disorder, notes Dr. Price. Some experts suggest that stress can cause or aggravate TMD since people who clench or grind their teeth can develop long-lasting jaw pain. It can also be caused by a misalignment between the upper and lower teeth. Sometimes the problem is as simple as a cap or filling that isn't fitted properly: Your bite will be uneven, which puts uneven (and painful) pressure on the jaw joint, Dr. Price explains. Researchers now say TMD may be the result of a combination of behavioral, psychological, and physical factors.

TMD can be a chronic problem that requires dental treatment. But usually it's a temporary condition related to stress, says Dr. Price. When the stressful times are past, and you quit clenching your jaw or grinding your teeth, the pain will often disappear as well.

To relieve the discomfort right away, and to reduce the chances that it will become a long-term problem, here's what you can do.

For Immediate Relief

home remedies

Take some pain relief. When TMD comes on suddenly, the best approach is to take ibuprofen or naproxen. Both of these medications reduce inflammation as well as pain, says Dr. Price.

Chill the area. When you first start having jaw pain, hold a cold pack or a plastic bag filled with ice cubes on the area to relieve pain and inflammation. "You can also use a bag of frozen vegetables," says Dr. Price. The advantage of this approach is that the bag will mold itself around the contour of your jaw, putting the cold right where you need it, he explains. Whatever method you choose, just make sure to keep the bag wrapped in a thin towel to protect your delicate skin. Hold it on the area for 20 minutes. Continue the ice treatments three or four times a day for 2 to 3 days, or until the pain is relieved.

Apply heat for chronic TMD. "Ice works for people with acute pain, but moist heat works better for those with chronic pain," says Dr. Price. "Stand in a comfortably hot shower and let the water run over your jaw. You can also put a hot-water bottle or a heating pad on the jaw until you feel relief." Applying heat to the area will increase circulation and relax painful muscle spasms and is sometimes a part of the therapy to manage a chronic condition, he says.

when to see a doctor

If you're having jaw pain and it's getting worse despite home treatments, or if the symptoms come back over time, make an appointment to see your dentist. Since most TMD problems are temporary, the goal of therapy is to let the body heal itself through stress management and self-care practices. Your dentist may recommend anti-inflammatory drugs to help you deal with pain. But sometimes the joint itself is damaged, and surgery may be the only way to relieve the pain, says Richard H. Price, DMD, spokesperson for the American Dental Association and former clinical instructor at Boston University Dental School.

For Long-Term Prevention

home remedies

Limit jaw movements. Opening the mouth too wide strains the joint and surrounding muscles, which can trigger TMD. It will also make the pain worse if you already have the disorder.

"If you feel a yawn coming on, try not to open your mouth so wide," says Dr. Price. Cut up sandwiches and other types of food into smaller pieces. If you have the disorder, choose foods that are easy to chew, such as fish or whole wheat bread instead of a steak or a bagel.

Quit chewing gum. Every time you chew gum, your jaw moves up and down far more than usual, and the extra movements can aggravate TMD symptoms. If you don't already have the condition, the added motions may be a contributing factor resulting in TMD, says Dr. Price.

Use a bite guard when you sleep or anytime you're under stress. Available from dentists, bite guards are made from heavy-duty acrylic, and they're customized to fit your mouth exactly. They more equally distribute force when you grind or clench your teeth, which reduces stress on the jaw joint, Dr. Price explains.

"Some people only need to wear them at night during stressful times, when they're having pain in the jaw," Dr. Price says. "Others may need to wear them every night." The guards can also be worn during the day. "If you always feel anxious and frustrated when you're stopped in traffic, wearing a guard will help 'untrain' the joint that's moving incorrectly as you clench or grind your teeth," he adds.

Check your drugs. Some antidepressants can cause teeth-clenching and nighttime grinding. Talk to your doctor about switching you to a different medication.

See an acupuncturist. In one recent study, 85 percent of TMD patients who got acupuncture treatments experienced a 75 percent reduction in their symptoms.

mind-body techniques

Control the stress in your life. When you're tense, you may grind your teeth while you sleep or clench your jaw more than usual. Most people aren't even aware they're doing it, but over time it can lead to joint pain, says Dr. Price.

There's no easy way to unwind when life's pressures are getting to you. Dr. Price often refers people with the disorder for biofeedback training. "Specialists will teach you techniques that concentrate on relaxing and becoming more aware of what's happening in your body so that you can change an unconscious habit into a conscious action," he explains. "If you usually clench your teeth while waiting in the seemingly endless line at the toll booth, biofeedback will teach you to put yourself at ease and stop the movement." Other techniques that may be helpful include deep breathing, yoga, meditation, and listening to relaxation tapes. Regular exercise is an excellent way to dispel stress. So is taking time by yourself to just sit and think pleasant thoughts.

thinning hair

n some ways, women are luckier than men. Nearly all women will lose some of their hair over time, but they rarely develop bare spots. Even when their hair gets thinner, they can often disguise the changes by styling their hair differently or using shampoos and conditioners that bulk the hair and make it look thicker. Another plus is that when a woman's hair thins, the front hairline isn't lost, as with the telltale receding hairline that many balding men experience.

Despite these benefits, however, thinning hair can be a devastating experience for many women. "Even though they lose their hair differently, thinning hair may be more of a trauma for women because it is less socially acceptable," says Diana Bihova, MD, a dermatologist in New York City. A number of different factors can contribute to hair loss in women, but fortunately there are options that can help slow, stop, or reverse thinning hair, or at least minimize its appearance.

It's normal for a woman to lose anywhere from 100 to 150 hairs daily. The hairs are usu-ally replaced by new ones, which grow at the rate of about $\frac{1}{2}$ inch a month. As women get older and their estrogen levels fall, the rate of hair loss may slightly exceed the pace of replace-ment. Known as androgenic alopecia, this type of hair loss is caused by a combination of genetic factors and high levels of androgens—hormones that affect hair follicles—in the blood, says Dr. Bihova.

Trauma from accidents, divorce, and other stressful events—as well as physical problems, such as anemia, liver, or hypothyroid disease—may cause hair to get thinner. Solving hair loss problems involves addressing the underlying medical problem, as well as caring for your hair to minimize the visual impact of your condition.

when to see a doctor

If your hair is thinning and you're premenopausal, see a dermatolo-gist. Younger women who experi-ence hair loss may have medical problems, such as hypothyroid disease or dermatological problems, says Diana Bihova, MD, a dermatologist in New York City.

If you're taking a new medication and you're losing hair. A number of prescription and over-the-counter drugs—including diuretics, thyroid medication, and ibuprofen—may trigger hair loss in some people.

If the hair loss occurs suddenly and you've developed bare patches. You could have a con-dition called alopecia areata, which is thought to be linked to family history as well as stress. This condition is often temporary, and your hair may start to grow back within a few months.

If your hair loss is a serious concern to you. According to Dr. Bihova, the stress some women experience due to thinning hair problems can create a vicious cycle that only contributes to increased hair loss.

For Immediate Relief

home remedies

Change your hair color. The chemicals in hair colors slightly roughen the surface of each hair. This gives hair more body, makes it look fuller, and helps disguise thin spots, says Linda Tam, owner of Linda Tam Salon in New York City.

Women who have fine hair to begin with will want to choose lighter hair colors, Tam adds. Light browns or blondes will blend with the color of the scalp and make the hair appear thicker.

Add highlights. "I often advise women to highlight their hair because it creates a sense of depth and makes the hair appear fuller," says Anelka Szaruga, owner of Anelka Szaruga Beauty Shop in Philadelphia.

Or low-lights. Adding streaks of a color that are a shade or two darker than your natural hair color creates the illusion that your hair is thicker than it really is.

Wash your hair less often. Every time you shampoo your hair, the cleansing agents remove oils and cause the hair to lie flatter. "If you wash your hair a little less often, maybe two or three times a week, it will have a little more body and fullness," Tam says. This is most effective if you have normal or dry hair. If it tends to be oily, wash your hair daily, as usual, and add styling gel before blow-drying to give extra body.

Use protein-based conditioners. Check the label for ingredients called hydrolyzed animal proteins. Known as thickeners, the proteins coat the hair shafts and give the hair more thickness and heft.

"Women whose hair is thinning should use a lightweight conditioner," says Szaruga. "The lighter products don't bring the hair down next to the scalp as much as heavier conditioners."

Finish with a cold rinse. After washing and conditioning your hair, adjust the temperature so that cool water soaks your hair for a few minutes. A cold rinse seals in some of the conditioner, which will give your hair additional body and shine.

Put hair mousse to use. Mousse is a lightweight styling gel that adds a thin, oily coating to the hair shafts and makes them appear fuller, Tam says.

Wear your hair shorter. "One of the best things women can do is wear a shorter cut and style it with a body wave," Tam says. "When the hair is 2 or 3 inches long, it's a little more curly and is less likely to lie against the scalp and reveal the thin spots."

Go for a natural look. "I recommend that women wear their hair a little more messy and tousled, rather than always having it smoothly combed," Szaruga says. "They should definitely wear their hair above the shoulders, either for a layered look or in a shorter blunt cut. That will make it look fuller than before."

Use a blow-dryer. It roughens up the hair shafts and also causes the hair to rise higher off the scalp. To avoid damaging the hair shafts, set the dryer on low and hold it 6 to 10 inches away from your hair, Szaruga says.

Long-Term Solutions

home remedies

Eat a balanced diet. Women who go on crash diets, or those with eating disorders or other conditions that affect the body's intake of nutrients, may experience hair loss, says Dr. Bihova. Protein and iron are especially important for the hair to grow normally.

The best sources of protein include lean meats, low-fat dairy foods, legumes, and whole grains. For iron, enjoy lean meats and fish, and fortified cereal products.

medical options

Use minoxidil. Available over the counter, minoxidil (such as Rogaine and generic brands) is an effective treatment for androgenic alopecia.

"About a third of the people who use it will

grow new hair, and another third will maintain the hair they have," says Dr. Bihova.

Available as a liquid, minoxidil is rubbed into the scalp twice daily. It's not an instant cure, Dr. Bihova adds. In fact, she recommends seeing a dermatologist for a correct diagnosis of your hair-thinning problem because while minoxidil works for many people, it won't help at all if you don't have androgenic alopecia. Some women who use minoxidil may start to see results in about 3 months, but for others it may take as long as a year, says Dr. Bihova.

When using minoxidil, be careful to keep it off your face, Dr. Bihova warns. "It may cause facial hair growth if you get it on your skin."

mind-body techniques

Unload some of the stress in your life. In order to conserve energy during stressful times, your body may slow the rate of hair growth. If you're burning the candle at both ends or dealing with stressful life events, you may want to spend some time unwinding with meditation, regular exercise, and other relaxing activities.

tinnitus

T innitus means "to ring," but that doesn't begin to describe the buzzing, clicking, roaring, or other sounds that people with this condition hear inside their heads.

Experts aren't sure what causes tinnitus, a condition in which the brain perceives sounds when no real sounds exist. Recent studies suggest that it may be the result of the brain overcompensating for frequencies lost to ear damage—from loud noises, circulatory problems, and some medications. In some cases it can be caused by something as minor as earwax and as serious as a tumor. Certain conditions, such as Meniere's disease, which also causes hearing loss and vertigo, are marked by tinnitus. If your ear ringing pulses in rhythm with your heartbeat, you may have a condition caused by high blood pressure, atherosclerosis, or another vascular condition in which blood flow through your veins and arteries is impeded.

"It's also part of the aging process," says Gordon B. Hughes, MD, program officer for clinical trials for the National Institute for Deafness and Other Communication Disorders. "For the vast majority of people, it's mild, occasional, and not especially bothersome."

Tinnitus can sometimes be eliminated by treating underlying medical problems. More often, people have to find ways to cope with the persistent noise. Here are various strategies to try.

For Immediate Relief

home remedies

Cut back on coffee or tea. The caffeine in these and other beverages constricts blood vessels and temporarily raises blood pressure, which can make the sounds of tinnitus louder, says Dr. Hughes. Alcohol and smoking may have a similar effect.

Mask the sounds. A hearing aid–like device called a masker creates sounds that are matched in pitch to the sounds of tinnitus. "At least half the people who use a masker find that it's more acceptable to listen to an external sound than the spontaneous internal noise," says Dr. Hughes.

Listen to nature. A study in the *Journal of the American Academy of Audiology* found that masking sounds with white noise or music reduced ringing in the ears better than no noise at all. But when they tested some specific programs, the ones that masked tinnitus the best were water and nature sounds.

Use a hearing aid. About 90 percent of those with severe tinnitus also suffer from hearing loss. Wearing a hearing aid makes the tinnitus less noticeable by boosting the real sounds around you.

Clean out the wax. Excessive earwax can impair hearing and make the sounds of tinnitus louder. One solution is to use over-the-counter eardrops that contain carbamide peroxide. "Used as directed on the label, they're a reasonable approach," says Dr. Hughes.

Get more sleep. Researchers at Washington University in St. Louis gave a group of people with tinnitus a melatonin supplement (3 grams) every day for a month to help them sleep, then tracked them for a month without the supplement. By the end of the study, tinnitus symptoms had dropped by 30 percent (and sleep went up!).

medical options

See an audiologist. Since hearing loss plays a role in some cases of tinnitus, an audiologist should check your hearing.

Make a dental appointment. If your ringing is accompanied by popping and clicking, your tinnitus may be related to a temperomandibular joint disorder. Treating that condition may relieve your tinnitus.

Long-Term Solutions

home remedies

Protect your ears. Because tinnitus may be triggered by loud noises, any additional assaults on your ears could worsen it. Try to avoid noisy activities, such as mowing the lawn or attending loud concerts. It's also helpful to wear earplugs. Music stores sell earplugs that are designed for musicians: They let in music and voices, but at a lower volume.

when to see a doctor

If you're taking medications and start experiencing tinnitus, talk to your doctor or pharmacist. A variety of OTC and prescription drugs, including aspirin and some antibiotics, may cause ringing or other noises, says Gordon B. Hughes, MD, program officer for clinical trials for the National Institute for Deafness and Other Communication Disorders.

If you've just started hearing ringing or other sounds. You may have an underlying medical problem that's causing tinnitus. Causes can include inner ear conditions and, in rare cases, tumors. Scientists have found a link between tinnitus, Lyme disease, and hyperacusis, a heightened sensitivity to normal sounds.

Reduce the sodium in your diet. Tinnitus is sometimes caused by a condition called Meniere's disease, which occurs when excessive amounts of fluid accumulate in the ear. People with this condition should restrict their daily sodium intake to 2,000 mg by limiting the use of table salt and buying low-sodium soups, condiments, and other packed foods, says Dr. Hughes. "There's no question that physical and emotional stress aggravates tinnitus," he says. "If there's an obvious source of stress in your life, get counseling or find some other way to deal with it."

medical options

Ask your doctor about tinnitus retraining therapy. A combination of therapy and low-level noise helps patients get so used to the ringing in their ears that they no longer hear it. It works for as many as 80 percent of patients treated at the Tinnitus and Hyperacusis Center at Emory University in Atlanta, headed by Pawel J. Jastreboff, PhD, who developed the treatment. Since about 75 percent of people with tinnitus eventually treat their condition like any other sound that can be tuned out, Dr. Jastreboff designed his program to help patients basically ignore the sounds in their ears. Therapy helps train patients to regard the sounds as neutral and nonsignificant so they cease paying attention to them.

Consider antidepressants. Drugs that are used to treat depression may relieve tinnitus in some people. The medications don't work for everyone, however. They're effective only in those who are also suffering from depression, Dr. Hughes explains.

For more information on tinnitus. Go online and visit the Web site of the American Tinnitus Association at www.ata.org.

tooth discoloration

When you hear people describe teeth as pearly whites, you have to wonder if their eyesight isn't quite what it should be.

It would be nice if teeth stayed white and unblemished, but that's not the way nature made them. As the years go by, the teeth naturally take on a yellowish or grayish hue, says Lawrence Wolinsky, DMD, PhD, professor of oral biology and oral medicine and associate dean for academic programs and personnel at the University of California at Los Angeles.

Part of the problem is the foods we eat. The outer layer of the teeth, the enamel, is more porous than it appears. When you eat highly pigmented foods or beverages, such as tomato sauce, red wine, and coffee, some of the color is absorbed by the enamel. "They'll slowly but surely cause the teeth to stain," says Dr. Wolinsky. Enamel can also be discolored by exposure to fluoride-rich water during the early years of tooth development.

Staining occurs in deeper portions of the tooth as well. These types of stains, which are commonly caused by childhood exposure to tetracycline antibiotics, are not easily removed and usually require the attention of a dentist.

Dentists have developed a variety of techniques to bring back the original white, though they usually require care to maintain. There are also things you can do at home to make your smile brighter than ever. Choose what works best for you.

For Immediate Relief

Use whitening toothpastes. They may contain peroxides, which act as bleaching agents. "These pastes are good for minor surface stains," Dr. Wolinsky says.

Brush away the stains. Toothpastes that contain silica act as abrasives and help remove dingy stains, Dr. Wolinsky says. Baking soda mixed with a little water has a similar effect. "You don't want to use these products too often because they can wear away portions of the teeth," Dr. Wolinsky adds.

Use a bleaching gel. You can buy home bleaching kits at pharmacies. The kits include a bleaching agent, usually carbamide peroxide, and a mouthpiece. You fill the mouthpiece with gel and wear it for an hour or two a day, or overnight for quicker results. For the first couple of weeks after treatment, you should avoid foods and beverages that can stain your teeth. You can also use strips that have the bleaching agent hydrogen peroxide to boost lightening, or an at-home laser treatment that uses a built-in light to activate peroxide foam strips that sit on your teeth for 20 minutes each treatment over the course of 5 days.

Home bleaching will brighten the teeth somewhat, but it may require a long time, usually several weeks, before you'll notice the results, Dr. Wolinsky says. Also, the mouthpieces rarely fit well. Some people experience gum irritation or other side effects from the chemicals.

Get a power bleaching. Some dentists perform in-office bleaching, in which the teeth are coated with a highly concentrated bleaching gel. The gel is activated when it's exposed to special lights. It can lighten your teeth by as much as eight shades in five sessions, though a study done at Tufts University found that you experience an average shade rebound of about two shades in a week.

when to see a doctor

If your teeth get sensitive when you use a bleaching gel, call your dentist. Some bleaches contain chemicals that remove water from the teeth, which irritates the nerves, says Lawrence Wolinsky, DMD, PhD, professor of oral biology and oral medicine and associate dean for academic programs and personnel at the University of California at Los Angeles.

If there's a burning sensation in the gums that doesn't go away. The mouthpiece probably doesn't fit properly and is allowing the chemicals to irritate the gums.

If there's a generalized redness that extends to the cheeks or tongue. You may be having an allergic reaction to a chemical in the bleach.

Use a home treatment provided by your dentist. Unlike OTC bleaching kits, those provided by dentists use stronger chemicals, and the mouthpiece is customized for a precise fit. "You usually apply them for an hour a day for 7 days," says Dr. Wolinsky. There are also special pretreatments that reduce or eliminate sensitivity afterward.

Cover the stains. If your teeth are damaged or badly stained, your dentist may recommend covering them with veneers, ultrathin porcelain or plastic shells that are permanently attached to the teeth. The one drawback to veneers is cost: You can expect to pay as much as $1,000 per tooth.

Long-Term Solutions

home remedies

Always brush after meals. "It takes a long time for staining to occur," says Dr. Wolinsky.

"If you're constantly removing film from the teeth by brushing, it will reduce the possibility of staining."

Rinse your mouth. When you don't have time to brush, a quick rinse will help prevent staining chemicals in coffee, wine, and other foods and beverages from penetrating the enamel.

Finish meals with a carrot. Along with apples, celery stalks, and other raw fruits and vegetables, carrots contain fiber, which gently brushes the teeth with every crunch, says Dr. Wolinsky.

Avoid staining foods. Instead of drinking red wine, switch to white. Drink green or herbal teas instead of black tea or coffee. "Avoiding or having smaller amounts of staining foods can make a difference," says Dr. Wolinsky.

For more information on tooth discoloration and other dental issues. See the Web site of the American Dental Association at www.ada.org.

ulcers

For a long time, ulcers were thought to be caused by stress. Hard-driving executives were almost proud to have them because ulcers supposedly meant that they were working long hours and putting the company's success above all else.

Then, about 20 years ago, researchers discovered that the vast majority of ulcers are caused by infection with the bacterium *Helicobacter pylori*. Using its spiral shape as a microscopic bore, the bacterium burrows through the protective mucus that coats the stomach and part of the small intestine, allowing powerful stomach acids to damage the delicate layers underneath.

The result is an ulcer—a sore that's usually no larger than a pencil eraser but can cause a great deal of pain.

Most ulcers are caused by infections, but they can also be caused by the long-term use of aspirin, ibuprofen, and similar drugs. Known as nonsteroidal anti-inflammatory drugs, or NSAIDs, the medications inhibit the body's production of chemicals needed to protect the stomach lining.

Most people with ulcers require treatment with antibiotics or other medications, says David Peura, MD, professor emeritus of medicine at the University of Virginia in Charlottesville. Whether or not you take drugs, however, there are a number of strategies for easing the pain of ulcers and helping them heal more quickly.

For Immediate Relief

home remedies

Avoid acidic or spicy foods. While an ulcer is healing, the acids in oranges, grapefruit, and other foods can cause a temporary burning sensation, just as they can with any wound, says Dr. Peura. Fiery chili can make things worse. So can alcohol and caffeine. Once your ulcer is healed, however, you should be able to eat anything you want, Dr. Peura says.

Suppress the acid. Over-the-counter medications called H2 blockers, such as cimetidine (Tagamet) and ranitidine (Zantac), cause the stomach to produce less acid, which can reduce the pain of ulcers and help them heal more quickly once the underlying infection is treated.

Try to relax. Even though emotional stress doesn't cause ulcers, it does increase the stomach's output of acids, which can make the pain of ulcers worse, says George Sachs, MB, professor of physiology and medicine director of the Membrane Biology Lab at UCLA.

You can't eliminate life's stresses, but you can find ways to cope with them a little better—by exercising regularly, practicing yoga or meditation, or simply giving yourself a little more time to relax. (For step-by-step action plans for starting an exercise plan and relieving stress, see Chapters 5 and 7.)

medical options

Eliminate the infection. If tests show that your ulcer is caused by *H. pylori* bacteria, your doctor may recommend treatment with antibiotics. Once the organisms are gone, the ulcer will heal within a few weeks, and there's a good chance that it will never come back.

In addition to antibiotics, your doctor may prescribe H2 blockers or another type of medication called proton pump inhibitors (PPIs) as part of the therapy. PPIs, such as esomeprazole (Nexium) and pantoprazole (Protonix), suppress acid production by halting the mechanism that

when to see a doctor

If you experience stomach pain or a burning sensation, usually in the middle of the night or between meals. These are the classic signs of an ulcer, says David Peura, MD, professor emeritus of medicine at the University of Virginia in Charlottesville.

If your stools are black or tarry. This may be a sign that an ulcer is causing internal bleeding.

If you're tired all the time for no good reason. It's not uncommon for ulcers to bleed slowly, which can result in fatigue and other symptoms of iron deficiency anemia.

pumps the acid into the stomach. Some treatment plans also include drugs that shield the stomach's mucous lining from acid damage.

Your doctor may also recommend a course with a bismuth compound (Pepto-Bismol) which coats ulcers, protecting them from stomach acid as well as killing *H. pylori*.

Long-Term Solutions

home remedies

Switch pain relievers. People who take a lot of aspirin or other NSAIDs can develop potentially serious ulcers. This can happen to anyone, but it's most common in those 60 years and older.

Your doctor will probably advise you to switch to acetaminophen. It's just as effective as ibuprofen and aspirin, but it's much less likely to cause stomach irritation or ulcers, says Dr. Peura.

Snuff out the cigarette habit. Smoking increases the risk of ulcers, slows the rate at which they heal, and also makes them more likely to come back. There's even evidence to suggest that people who smoke are more likely to get infected with the ulcer-causing bacterium.

Giving up cigarettes isn't easy, of course. (For more information on giving up the habit for good, see Chapter 8.)

urinary incontinence

Women who have gone through pregnancy and childbirth sometimes joke about the frequency of their bathroom stops. What they don't laugh about—or in some cases even discuss with their doctors—are the embarrassing "leaks" that may occur when they sneeze, laugh, or bend over to pick up a sock.

"Women might start noticing small stains or dampness on their underwear," says Gary Lemack, MD, professor of urology at the University of Texas Southwestern Medical Center in Dallas. "The leaks happen suddenly, usually with strenuous activity, such as lifting heavy objects."

As many as 17 million American women suffer from urinary incontinence, which is the inability to completely control the flow of urine. Incontinence often occurs after childbirth or menopause because women may lose strength in the muscles (the pelvic floor muscles) that support the bladder. The muscles that surround the urethra, the tube that carries urine from the body, can also weaken over time. Nerves can also be affected; your bladder may get misfires from your brain so you don't empty it completely, leaving you feeling full and prone to leaking.

If you wonder whether you are incontinent, here is a general rule of thumb: If you use the bathroom 8 or more times in a day, or get up more than once during the night to urinate, you probably are. Similarly, if you feel the need to go to the bathroom but frequently can't make it there in time, you should count yourself incontinent. In both cases, you should see a doctor, especially a urologist who specializes in incontinence.

Incontinence may clear up on its own, but often it doesn't. The good news is that about 80 percent of women can reduce or eliminate incontinence with a combination of medical treatments and home-care strategies.

For Immediate Relief

home remedies

Put your bladder on a schedule. "Go to the bathroom every 2 hours, even if you don't feel like you have to go," says Dr. Lemack. Women who practice "timed voiding" are less likely to leak urine accidentally.

Drink less coffee. Or at least switch to decaf. The caffeine in coffee and other beverages increases the body's output of urine. Caffeine also stimulates bladder contractions, which can lead to unexpected leaks, says Lily A. Arya, MD, assistant professor of urogynecology at the University of Pennsylvania in Philadelphia. She advises limiting caffeine intake to 200 mg daily, which is the equivalent of two 6-ounce cups of coffee.

Limit fluids. "You need 32 ounces of fluid a day and get half of that from food," says urologist Larrian Gillespie, MD, former medical director of the Pelvic Pain Treatment Center in Beverly Hills and author of *You Don't Have to Live with Cystitis*. So if you have stress incontinence, you may want to limit yourself to drinking two 8-ounce glasses of water a day.

Use a tampon. If you find that you frequently leak urine when you cough, sneeze, or

---

THREE THINGS I TELL EVERY FEMALE PATIENT

GARY LEMACK, MD, *professor of urology at the University of Texas Southwestern Medical Center in Dallas, gives the following advice for coping with incontinence.*

1 **KEEP A VOIDING DIARY.** For several weeks, record your bladder habits. Write down how often (and how much) you drink, how many times you urinate, and how many accidents you have. The diary will help your doctor determine the best course of treatment.

DO KEGEL EXERCISES DAILY. "I advise people to do Kegels in conjunction with the voiding

diary in order to measure progress," Dr. Lemack says.

2 **CONSIDER YOUR GOALS.** For some women, the treatments used to control incontinence are more inconvenient than the symptoms themselves. If your goal is complete dryness, you may need to consider surgery or other medical treatments. On the other hand, if the leaks only happen once or twice a week, you might want to stick with simpler treatments, such as Kegel exercises or the occasional use of pads. ■ 3

exercise, you might want to use a tampon even when you're not having your period. Tampons provide extra support for the bladder, which can prevent urine from escaping, says Mary Jane Minkin, MD, clinical professor of obstetrics and gynecology at Yale University School of Medicine. Follow the package insert guidelines for how long you can safely wear a tampon without increasing your risk of toxic shock syndrome—usually 4 to 8 hours.

Use pads as necessary. You don't want to depend on absorbent pads, such as sanitary napkins, because they don't solve the underlying problem. But if you find that you're nervous about having accidents, absorbent pads can give you the confidence you need to get out and about, Dr. Lemack says. They're also helpful as an interim measure when you're working with your doctor to get your bladder under control.

Control allergies. Women who suffer from hay fever or other allergies may have flare-ups of incontinence resulting from coughing or sneezing. It's worth trying OTC antihistamines during allergy season, says Dr. Lemack.

medical options

Cap the leaks. For stress incontinence, bulking agents, such as collagen, may be injected into the urethra to create resistance against the flow of urine. The injections are effective, but they may have to be repeated over time, says Dr. Lemack. A number of medications are also available for urge incontinence. Your doctor may also prescribe anticholinergic medications to control muscle spasms in the bladder.

Discuss medications with your doctor. If you're taking diuretics (water pills) for high blood pressure or other conditions, you may have more trouble controlling your bladder. "Changing to a different drug or changing the timing of drug administration may be helpful," says Dr. Lemack.

Long-Term Solutions

home remedies

Squeeze in some muscle training. One of the most effective strategies both for treating and preventing incontinence is to strengthen the pelvic floor muscles, says Dr. Morse. These are the same muscles you use when stopping urine flow in midstream.

All you have to do is clench and relax the muscles about 10 times, and repeat the series 3 times daily. The great thing about these exercises, called Kegel exercises, is that you can do them anytime: when you're lying in bed, watching TV, or standing in line at the grocery store.

Tighten at the right time. Kegel exercises are used mainly to prevent incontinence, but you can also use them to stop leaks before they start. "That means contracting your pelvic floor muscles in anticipation of a cough, laugh, or sneeze to prevent urine from leaking out, says Linda Brubaker, MD, a urogynecologist at Loyola University Health System in Chicago.

Practice with vaginal weights. The tricky part about Kegels is figuring out which muscles you need to contract. Your doctor may recommend vaginal weights, which slip inside the vagina, as a training tool. If you aren't clenching the right muscles, the weights will slip out, Dr. Minkin explains.

Maintain a healthful weight. Women who have too much padding around the middle may have excessive pressure on the bladder. Losing weight—by exercising regularly, reducing the amount of fat in the diet, and eating more fruits and vegetables—may reduce the pressure and improve urinary control, says Dr. Lemack.

medical options

Consider electrical stimulation. There's some evidence that applying mild doses of electrical stimulation can strengthen muscles and improve the bladder's holding ability. A probe is temporarily placed in the vagina or rectum and precise amounts of electricity are applied to stimulate the nearby muscles, including those surrounding the urethra, explains Abraham N. Morse, MD, an instructor at Harvard Medical School and urogynecologist at Brigham and Women's Hospital in Boston. You'll learn how to use the device at the doctor's office, then you'll be able take it home to use on a daily basis.

Take muscle-tightening medications. OTC medications that include alpha-agonists (such as Sudafed) tighten muscles in the neck of the bladder and also in the urethra, which can make it easier to control urine flow. The drugs aren't always effective, however, and they may cause side effects, so it's important to use them under the supervision of your doctor, Dr. Lemack adds.

when to see a doctor

If the leaks are accompanied by sudden, uncontrollable urges to urinate, see your family doctor. You could have a urinary tract infection that's irritating the bladder, says Abraham N. Morse, MD, an instructor at Harvard Medical School and urogynecologist at Brigham and Women's Hospital in Boston.

If you're leaking urine and you also have pelvic pressure or lower back pain. You could have a condition called cystocele, which occurs when weakened pelvic floor muscles allow the bladder to sag into the vagina.

Supplement your body's estrogen. The reductions in estrogen that occur at menopause can result in weakness in the urethra or bladder. "I will often start patients on an estrogen suppository or cream if they have evidence of vaginal weakness," says Dr. Lemack.

Talk about surgery. If your bladder has slipped from its normal position—such as after childbirth—there are several operations that will help put it back and help suspend it. Anywhere from half to two-thirds of women are cured after surgery, though there can be side effects such as more urinary tract infections and voiding problems.

For more information on urinary incontinence. Visit the Simon Foundation for Continence Web site at www.simonfoundation.org.

urinary tract infections

About the only good thing you can say about urinary tract infections is that they're easy to treat and rarely serious.

The bad news is that they're extremely common. One in five women will get a urinary tract infection (UTI) at some time in her life, and women get them again and again. If you've already had three, you're at extremely high risk of chronic infections. Pregnant women are particularly vulnerable.

UTIs that occur in the bladder are called cystitis. Those that affect the urethra (the tube through which urine leaves the body) are called urethritis, and infections in the kidneys (the most serious kind) are called pyelonephritis.

UTIs usually occur when bacteria that live around the anus gain entry to the urethra and begin to multiply. Sexual intercourse is a common cause of UTIs, but women who aren't sexually active get them too. The risk of infections rises after menopause, when declines in the body's estrogen levels make tissues in the vagina and urethra more vulnerable to bacterial assaults.

If you suspect that you have a UTI, you'll want to call or see your doctor right away. You can diagnose some UTIs based on symptoms alone; typical symptoms for cystitis, for example, include a burning sensation while urinating and a powerful urge to urinate even after you've used the bathroom. But your doctor may need to perform tests to ensure that the infection hasn't spread to other parts of the body, explains Sanjay Saint, MD, professor of medicine at the University of Michigan Medical School in Ann Arbor.

Once you start taking antibiotics, the discomfort will usually disappear within a day or two, Dr. Saint adds. After that, you can plan a strategy to prevent infections from coming back.

For Immediate Relief

home remedies

Ease discomfort with heat. Placing a hot-water bottle or heating pad on your lower abdomen will relieve uncomfortable cramps or pressure while you're waiting for antibiotics to take effect, says urologist Larrian Gillespie, MD, former medical director of the Pelvic Pain Treatment Center in Beverly Hills and author of *You Don't Have to Live with Cystitis*.

Avoid coffee or alcohol for a few days. They can irritate the urinary tract when you have an infection. Coffee and other beverages with caffeine also stimulate urination, which can increase discomfort, says Dr. Gillespie.

Drink lots of water. If your infection is mild, water may be enough to wash bacteria away.

alternative therapies

Avoid acidic foods. Orange juice, strawberries, vinegar, and other foods with a high acid content may create a more favorable environment for bacteria in the bladder, says Dr. Gillespie. "Eating these foods when you have an infection can increase the irritation," she adds.

Put aside the soy sauce. Along with bananas,

nuts, cheese, and wine, it contains biogenic amines, amino acids that affect sensory nerve fibers in the bladder. Eating these foods when you have an infection may increase urinary urgency, says Dr. Gillespie.

Ask your doctor about supplemental hormones. If you're past menopause and have been getting frequent infections, you may be a good candidate for hormone replacement therapy. Taking low doses of estradiol, a form of estrogen, strengthens tissues in the urethra and vagina and helps prevent infections, says Dr. Gillespie.

Long-Term Solutions

Wash away bacteria. Removing bacteria from the area around the urethra is among the best strategies for preventing UTIs, says Mary Jane Minkin, MD, clinical professor of obstetrics and gynecology at Yale University School of Medicine. Wash the genital area before having sex, and remember to urinate before and after intercourse. After using the bathroom, wipe from front to back. This helps ensure that anal bacteria don't get moved toward the urethral opening.

Consider alternative forms of birth control. Women who use diaphragms have a higher risk of UTIs. If you use a diaphragm and have recurrent infections, discuss alternative forms of birth control with your doctor.

Drink eight glasses of water daily. Water dilutes the urine and reduces the concentration of infection-causing bacteria, says Dr. Gillespie. Drinking water also promotes urination, which helps remove bacteria from the bladder.

Stay clean naturally. The use of douches, deodorant sprays, and other feminine products

---

THREE THINGS I TELL EVERY FEMALE PATIENT

LARRIAN GILLESPIE, MD, *urologist, former medical director of the Pelvic Pain Treatment Center in Beverly Hills and author of* You Don't Have to Live with Cystitis, *gives the following advice for dealing with urinary tract infections.*

DON'T WAIT TO TAKE ANTIBIOTICS. They're extremely effective at stopping UTIs. Most women can be treated with a single triple dose, which is more convenient than the older, weeklong regimens.

DRINK BAKING SODA MIXED WITH WATER. "It makes the urine more alkaline for about 24

hours, which takes away the acid environment that bacteria need to multiply," says Dr. Gillespie. When you first notice symptoms, mix $1/4$ teaspoon of baking soda in a glass of water and drink it once daily until your symptoms are improved, she advises.

EASE DISCOMFORT WITH THE ORANGE PILL. An over-the-counter medication called phenazopyridine (such as Pyridium or Urobiotic) is a dye that turns the urine orange. It decreases bladder irritability and can be taken along with antibiotics to ease discomfort. ■

can irritate the urethra and promote infections. Washing with soap and water is more effective and less irritating.

alternative therapies

Drink a glass of cranberry juice daily. Cranberry juice contains chemical compounds called proanthocyanidins, which help prevent bacteria from sticking to cells in the urinary tract. Blueberries contain the same helpful substances, says Dr. Minkin.

medical options

Arrange a plan with your doctor. UTIs respond quickly to antibiotics, but you can get them only with a prescription, which means that you have to put up with symptoms until you can see your doctor. Women who get frequent UTIs sometimes arrange for their doctors to prescribe antibiotics over the telephone when symptoms first appear. This is a reasonable approach if the infections are uncomplicated and your doctor is familiar with your health history, says Dr. Saint.

when to see a doctor

If you have flank pain, difficulty urinating, a burning sensation when you urinate, or frequent urges to urinate, call a doctor right away. These are classic symptoms of urinary tract infections, says Sanjay Saint, MD, professor of medicine at the University of Michigan Medical School in Ann Arbor.

If you have a flank pain, fever, chills, or nausea that accompanies the typical symptoms of a UTI. You could have a potentially serious kidney infection called pyelonephritis and must see a doctor right away.

If you feel pressure in the lower abdomen and the urine has a strong smell. The infection could be in the bladder, a condition called cystitis.

Dr. Saint led a study that looked at nearly 4,000 women with uncomplicated UTIs. The researchers found that those who had phone consultations with their doctors did just as well as those who came into the office for examinations.

vaginal dryness

One of the downsides of menopause is vaginal dryness, which makes sex anything but pleasurable. Once a woman's ovaries stop making estrogen, the vaginal glands that produce lubricating moisture lose their trigger and the vaginal tissues become thinner—an equation that can add up to painful intercourse.

"In addition to discomfort during intercourse, a woman who's menopausal may have a higher risk of vaginal infections because the natural vaginal environment changes," adds Debra Papa, MD, assistant professor of obstetrics/gynecology at the University of Massachusetts Medical School in Worcester. Also, the thinning of vaginal tissues makes women more susceptible to irritation or trauma, which may provide a gateway for an infection.

Here are some good ways to enhance moisture and maintain your natural lubrication.

For Immediate Relief

Use a water-based lubricant. Available over the counter, lubricants such as Astroglide and Replens help prevent dryness by replenishing moisture in the vagina. This reduces irritation and itching and decreases friction during intercourse, says Dr. Papa. They're also safe to use with condoms.

Product ingredients vary, so it's best to follow instructions on the package on how to apply.

Switch tampons. Many premenopausal women find that vaginal dryness makes the use of tampons difficult or painful. You may want to try a brand that uses a cardboard or plastic applicator. Or use one that has a slimmer shape or a rounder tip, suggests Mary Jane Minkin, MD, clinical professor of obstetrics and gynecology at Yale University School of Medicine.

To reduce irritation, it's fine to dab the tampon with a small amount of a water-based lubricant, Dr. Minkin adds.

Long-Term Solutions

Stay sexually active. Having sex regularly maintains the elasticity of the vaginal tissues, which get dry at menopause.

Put out the cigarettes. Smoking constricts blood vessels and reduces vaginal circulation, which can cause a decrease in lubrication, says Dr. Papa.

Use an estrogen cream. Available by prescription, estrogen creams are applied directly to the vagina. They relieve dryness by strengthening vaginal tissue and promoting the ability of the glands to secrete adequate amounts of moisture, says Dr. Papa.

The creams initially need to be applied daily for several weeks, Dr. Papa advises. Then they're usually used 2 or 3 times a week. Follow your doctor's instructions or those that come in the package for dosage.

Use an estrogen ring or suppository. Estrogen creams are messy and inconvenient to apply, which is why some women opt for an estrogen ring. A diaphragm-like device, the ring is kept in the vagina for up to 3 months. It releases steady amounts of estrogen, keeping the vaginal environment healthy.

For more information about vaginal dryness and other conditions associated with menopause. Visit the Web site of the North American Menopause Society at www.menopause.org.

when to see a doctor

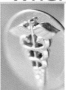

If you're getting recurrent infections, visit your gynecologist. Changes in the vagina's natural acidity can make women more prone to yeast and other infections, says Debra Papa, MD, assistant professor of obstetrics/gynecology at the University of Massachusetts Medical School in Worcester.

If you're experiencing dryness even though you're premenopausal. Vaginal dryness is not a common complaint in younger women. If you're premenopausal and sex is uncomfortable for you, discuss this with your doctor.

vaginal infections

The tropical rain forests are home to more species of life than any other location on earth. There's something about the warm, moist environments that allow many of nature's creatures to thrive.

Closer to home, quite a few organisms also thrive in a hothouse environment—which is why most women will get a vaginal infection at some time in their lives.

"The vaginal environment usually prevents infections by maintaining a balance between normal organisms and those that can cause infection," explains Debra Papa, MD, assistant professor of obstetrics/gynecology at the University of Massachusetts Medical School in Worcester.

A fungus called *Candida albicans*, for example, is often present in the vagina. When the conditions are right, it can multiply out of control and cause a yeast infection. It is estimated that at least 75 percent of women will get at least one yeast infection in their lifetime.

Infections can also be caused by bacteria, viruses, parasites, and species of fungus that are not the *albicans* type. Some infections are transmitted sexually. Others occur when offending germs on the outside of the body manage to get inside. An infection can also be a result of a disturbance in the vaginal environment resulting from antibiotics, douches, hormones, or stress. Regardless of how you get them, vaginal infections often cause a discharge along with intense irritation, itching, and odor.

Most vaginal infections can be treated with antifungal creams, antibiotics, or other medications. In addition, there are things you can do to reduce the discomfort and prevent the infections from coming back.

For Immediate Relief

home remedies

Enjoy an oatmeal bath. Add colloidal oatmeal (such as Aveeno) to a warm bath and soak for a while. "Yeast infections especially can be pretty severe and intense," says Dr. Papa. "An oatmeal bath won't stop the infection, but it will relieve the itching and burning."

Let air circulate. Stay out of tight clothing while the infection is healing, Dr. Papa advises. At home, don't wear underwear under your skirt. "You want to keep the area dry, which will reduce the irritation," she says.

Sleep in just your nightie. Sleeping without underwear under your nightgown allows the area to breathe, which reduces irritation and also makes it more difficult for yeast or other moisture-loving organisms to thrive.

Use a hair-dryer. "When you have an infection, rubbing yourself dry with a towel can be uncomfortable," Dr. Papa says. She advises drying yourself with a hair-dryer—set on low, of course.

medical options

Start with a checkup. If you've never had a vaginal infection before, don't assume that your symptoms are caused by yeast. Studies have shown that women often misdiagnose what they believe to be a yeast infection, which means that you could have a more serious infection that requires medical care.

Choose your medication. If you've had yeast infections in the past and you're sure that's what you have, it's fine to use an over-the-counter medication to treat it. Except in rare cases when yeast infections are caused by resistant organisms in the vagina, OTC products work well, says Meg Autry, MD, an obstetrician and gynecologist at the University of San Francisco Women's Health Center.

There are a number of products to choose from: creams, suppositories, and prefilled syringes. The active ingredient usually will be clotrimazole (such as Gyne-Lotrimin and Mycelex) or miconazole (Monistat). All these products are effective for most *Candida albicans* infections. Just be sure to read the label. Different products may require that you use them for different lengths of time.

For most women, the 3-day treatments work just as well as those that are used for 7 days, Dr. Autry adds. Although, she adds, "a woman might have a species of yeast that can't be killed in 3 days." If your infection doesn't clear up after 3 days, you can try a 7-day product. If that doesn't work, you'll definitely want to see your doctor.

Reduce discomfort with a local steroid cream. The burning and itching sensations of yeast infections sometimes last for a week or more, even after using medication. To ease discomfort in the meantime, you may want to apply an OTC cream containing hydrocortisone (such as Cortaid or Cortizone). Towelettes moistened with hydrocortisone are also available (Massengill Clean Relief). Your doctor may also prescribe a combination medicine, such as Lotrisone or Mycolog II, to treat the infection and relieve symptoms at the same time. These contain a steroid and an antifungal.

Get a prescription. If your infection is caused by a resistant strain of yeast or other organisms, you'll probably need to take a prescription medication. For trichomoniasis, a sexually transmitted infection caused by the parasite *Trichomonas vaginalis,* your doctor may advise you to take oral metronidazole (Flagyl). Bacterial infections can also be treated with metronidazole (MetroGel-Vaginal) or with an antibiotic called clindamycin (Cleocin). Severe yeast infections may call for fluconazole (Diflucan) or itraconazole (Sporanax); less severe infections can be treated with a vaginal tablet or cream such as nystatin (Mycostatin).

For Long-Term Relief
home remedies

Wash with plain water. Nearly everyone enjoys scented soaps and bath oil, but you should avoid using these products even when you don't have an infection. The chemicals in them can irritate the vulvar tissues (the external parts of the genitals) and cause scratching. This may make it easier for infections to establish themselves, says Dr. Papa. Douches, too, can be irritating, so if you feel you must douche, use plain vinegar and water, advises Dr. Papa.

Change into something dry. After swimming or working out, change into dry clothing immediately afterward. It will make the vulvar and vaginal areas less hospitable to yeast.

Wear cotton panties. Unlike nylon and other synthetic fabrics, cotton allows air to get in and moisture to get out, which can reduce your risk of infections. If you wear pantyhose, use the ones with cotton crotches. It's also a good idea to wear comfortable, not tight-fitting, clothing.

Wipe microbes away. Vaginal infections can occur when bacteria that live around the anus migrate into the vaginal area. One way to prevent this is to wipe from front to back after urinating or having a bowel movement, says Dr. Papa.

Keep your blood sugar under control. Women with diabetes have an increased risk of vaginal yeast infections because they may have higher than normal levels of glucose (blood sugar), which can change the vagina's protective balance.

If you have diabetes, keeping your blood sugar levels stable—by eating a healthful diet, controlling your weight, and using medication if necessary—is helpful in preventing infections from getting started, says Dr. Papa.

alternative therapies

Prevent infections with yogurt. Eating yogurt won't stop a yeast infection that's already in progress, but there's some evidence that it may reduce the risk of getting them in the future.

"The acidophilus in yogurt changes the vaginal pH," says Dr. Autry. In addition, when you eat yogurt that contains live bacterial cultures, the good organisms migrate into the vaginal

THREE THINGS I TELL EVERY FEMALE PATIENT

MEG AUTRY, MD, *an obstetrican/gynecology at the University of San Francisco Women's Health Center, gives the following advice to women who suffer from vaginal infections.*

NEVER DOUCHE. "It's always bad," says Dr. Autry. "It changes the vaginal environment and it also increases the risk of upper genital infections. There's some evidence that it may increase the risk of ovarian cancer as well."

BE GENEROUS WITH ANTIFUNGAL CREAMS. It's not uncommon for women with yeast infections to have inflammation outside the vagina. When applying a medicated cream, you may need to put it outside as well as inside the vagina.

GET CHECKED FOR DIABETES IF YOU HAVE FREQUENT INFECTIONS. This is especially true if you have any of the risk factors for diabetes, such as being overweight or having a family history of the disease. ■

canal and inhibit the growth of yeast. It may be especially helpful to eat yogurt when you're taking antibiotics. It replenishes the healthful organisms that are killed by the medication.

One 6-month study found that women who ate 8 ounces of live-culture yogurt daily were much less likely to develop yeast infections than those who didn't eat yogurt. "If you have recurrent infections, including yogurt in your diet is a good approach," says Dr. Autry. You can also take *lactobacillus acidophilus*—one of the bacteria in yogurt—orally.

Munch on mushrooms. In a small study, maitake, a delectable Japanese mushroom with scientifically proven immune-enhancing abilities, significantly eased the uncomfortable symptoms of chronic yeast infections in all but one of the 13 women who participated in the study.

"The real culprit in chronic yeast infections is a depressed immune system, which I find to be a common problem for women who undergo constant stress," says herbalist Douglas Schar, PhD, who conducted the study in his London clinic. "In my experience, raising a woman's immune function makes her less susceptible to chronic yeast infections."

Maitake is well known for its ability to increase immune cell count and activity. In addition, it contains compounds that specifically inhibit or destroy *Candida albicans*, the organism that causes vaginal yeast infections. But watch out for some unwanted side effects: mannitol, the natural sugar found in maitake, causes gas and intestinal discomfort in some people.

when to see a doctor

If you get recurrent infections or have symptoms that don't improve after treatment with over-the-counter products. You may have a strain of yeast that requires treatment with prescription medications, says Debra Papa, MD, assistant professor of obstetrics/gynecology at the University of Massachusetts Medical School in Worcester. You may also have a type of vaginal infection other than that caused by yeast.

If you develop a greenish or yellow discharge or lower abdominal pain. You could have a vaginal infection, one of which is called trichomoniasis, a sexually transmitted disease.

If you get a vaginal infection after having a new sex partner or if you've had multiple partners prior to the infection. Any symptom should be evaluated by your doctor.

medical options

Take care around your period. "The risk of almost all vaginal infections increases around the time of a woman's period because blood is an excellent culture medium," says Dr. Autry. "Sometimes women who get chronic infections may benefit from fluconazole (Diflucan) toward the end of their periods as a preventive measure."

For more information about vaginal infections. Visit the National Women's Health Information Center Web site at www.4women.org.

varicose veins

Women are much more prone to varicose veins than men, possibly because the female hormones estrogen and progesterone gradually weaken the vein walls, eventually reducing their ability to move blood uphill. No one knows the exact cause of this condition, which causes swollen, twisted, disfiguring and sometimes painful veins, but several factors may play a role. Women with a family history of varicose veins are much more likely to get them. Other factors that may cause or aggravate varicose veins include pregnancy, a lack of exercise, standing or sitting for long periods of time, crossing your legs, and obesity.

"By the time they're in their fifties, nearly one out of two women will have to contend with varicose veins," says Luis Navarro, MD, founder and director of the Vein Treatment Center and clinical instructor of surgery at Mount Sinai School of Medicine in New York City.

The veins in the legs are in a constant struggle with gravity. It's easy for venous blood, the blood that's going back to the heart, to circulate from other parts of the body because the route it follows is usually downhill. But the venous blood that travels from the leg veins has to make an arduous uphill journey in order to reach the heart.

Sometimes the trip takes longer. If portions of the leg veins are weaker than they should be, or if tiny valves in the veins malfunction, blood tends to pool in the leg veins, causing them to bulge like little balloons. These areas of stagnant blood are called varicose veins.

Most varicose veins are the small, spider variety. They are blue or red in color and can resemble a tree branch or spider's web. These veins cover areas that range from very small to very large. Located close to the surface of the skin, they are usually found on the legs or face but may occur anywhere on the body and often coincide with larger varicose veins. Although spider veins may be unattractive, they rarely cause discomfort and you can pretty much ignore them.

Larger varicose veins, however, make the legs feel tired and sore. These blue, dark purple, or green veins may be raised above the skin's surface and are found most often on the backs of the calves or on the insides of the legs, anywhere from the groin to the ankle. They may be quite ropy or bulging. In some cases the veins cause swelling in the legs or feet or around the ankles. Excess fluid leaks from the blood vessels into the tissues around the veins. The tissues become fragile, and the skin appears thin and may be inflamed. Open ulcers or sores may form and heal slowly.

Once varicose veins have formed, the only way to get rid of them is with surgery or other medical treatments. Most women don't need to do this because the discomfort of varicose veins, assuming there is any, can easily be managed with home remedies. In addition, there are a number of simple strategies that will help delay the formation of these veins.

For Immediate Relief

home remedies

Change positions often. Varicose veins tend to cause the most discomfort when women have been standing or sitting for a long time, which allows the blood to pool. "Get up from your chair, or just get moving if you're standing, and walk around for a few minutes every 1 to 2 hours," Dr. Navarro suggests. "When you move, the calf muscles flex against the veins, which gets the venous circulation moving again."

Elevate your legs. When you raise your legs above the heart, blood that's pooled in the veins flows back into circulation, says Dr. Navarro. "You can put a couple of bricks or books under the legs at the foot of the bed, which will give some elevation. You can also sleep with a pillow or two under your feet. This will take the pressure off the veins and prevent the blood from pooling in the lower extremities." Putting your legs up while you're reading or watching TV is a good idea, too.

Wear compression stockings. Available from doctors and in pharmacies, stores that carry medical supplies, and department stores, compression stockings put precise amounts of pressure against the leg veins, which can reduce painful swelling. Compression stockings also help prevent varicose veins from getting worse.

"They essentially add an extra layer of muscle to your leg, which helps the calf and foot muscles move blood upward to the heart," says Dr. Navarro.

When buying compression stockings, here are a few things to keep in mind.

- Different stockings provide different amounts of compression, which is measured in millimeters of mercury (mmHg). For spider veins, you'll want stockings with moderate compression (15 to 20 mmHg). If the veins are bulging, use stockings with more compression (20 to 30 mmHg).

- Compression stockings come in different lengths: calf only, which extend to the knee; mid-thigh, which reach to the upper third of the thigh; full-thigh, which extend to the groin; and full-length pantyhose. Choose a length that covers all the veins that you want to compress.

alternative therapies

Take horse chestnut. Available in health food stores, this herb (aesculus hippocastanum) strengthens veins that have lost their elasticity, which can help ease discomfort. A number of studies have shown that women who take 250 to 312.5 mg of the standardized extract of horse chestnut twice daily will have considerable relief from symptoms, including pain, fatigue, itching, water retention, and swelling in the legs.

medical options

Consider injections. If your legs keep hurting no matter what you do or if you're simply tired of looking at the unsightly veins, your doctor may recommend a procedure called sclerotherapy, in which a solution is injected into the varicose veins. The solution irritates the inner lining of the blood vessels, making the veins swell, close, and eventually disappear. This treatment can be used to eliminate both varicose and spider veins, as long as the main leg vein is not involved.

Apart from the prick of the needle, sclerotherapy is almost painless, although you may have some cramping for a day or two afterward. Since new veins may form, sclerotherapy is usually repeated every 2 to 4 years.

Talk to your doctor about other options. Laser treatments are often used to treat spider and smaller varicose veins. The lasers seal and shrink the varicose veins, says Dr. Navarro. "It's done as an in-office procedure, using a local anesthetic," he explains, "and is used, when the main vein of the leg is affected, as a way to avoid surgery."

when to see a doctor

If leg pain wakes you up at night or if the area around varicose veins is swelling, itching, or scaling, make an appointment to see your doctor. It's possible that the tissues around the veins aren't getting enough blood and oxygen, or you may have circulatory or arterial problems. You may need medical treatment to remove or seal the veins, says Luis Navarro, MD, founder and director of the Vein Treatment Center and clinical instructor of surgery at Mount Sinai School of Medicine in New York City.

Varicose veins involving the deeper veins in the leg can also be shut down with the use of radio waves, sometimes with a laser to seal the veins. Surgery is used to treat very large varicose veins. It usually involves small cuts in the skin, though it requires anesthesia and the procedure is done in an operating room. In some case, outpatient procedures called perforate invaginate, or PIN, stripping, and ambulatory phlebectomy can be done under local anesthesia.

For Long-Term Prevention
home remedies

Exercise often. "It's my number one tip for preventing varicose veins," says Dr. Navarro. "Try to exercise for 30 minutes at least three times a week. I recommend walking, running, swimming, bicycling, yoga, dancing, and tai chi. They are all great for circulation and building up the calf muscles."

Do toe raises. It's a good exercise for strengthening muscles in the feet and calves and also for removing pooled blood from the veins. Put your hand on a wall for support, and rise on your toes as far as you can go. Hold the stretch for a moment, then lower yourself back down. "Do this for 5 to 10 minutes every day," suggests Dr. Navarro.

Get plenty of fiber in your diet. Women who eat a lot of whole grains, legumes, and other fiber-rich foods are much less likely to get constipated. This is important because constipation causes straining, which puts extra pressure on the leg veins.

Although some studies have not found a consistent relationship between fiber, constipation, and the presence or severity of varicose veins, other research suggests that the diet of industrialized countries may be a risk factor.

"Studies have shown that in countries where people eat diets that are rich in fiber, the incidence of varicose veins is low," says Dr. Navarro. "When the same people come to Western countries and adopt a low-fiber diet, they have the same risk of developing varicose veins as the rest of the population." The optimal amount of fiber is 25 to 35 grams daily. All plant foods contain fiber. Some of the best include beans, peas, fruits, potatoes (with the skins on), berries, and whole grain breakfast cereals, such as Fiber One.

Eat less salt. The average American consumes more than 3,000 mg of sodium daily, a lot more than the Daily Value of 2,400 mg. "Consuming a lot of high-sodium foods causes inflammation and swelling, which makes the discomfort of varicose veins worse," says Dr. Navarro.

He advises women to buy low-sodium soups and other packaged foods and to avoid high-salt foods such as lunch meat and fast food.

Wear sunscreen. Protecting your skin from the sun will help limit the development of spider veins on the face.

Choose low-heeled shoes. They can help tone your calf muscles to help blood move through your veins.

medical options

Ask your doctor to check your medications. Women who take supplemental hormones—either in the form of birth control or as hormone replacement therapy—sometimes develop varicose veins. Taking a lower dose will often provide the same benefits, but without the side effects, says Dr. Navarro.

For more information about varicose veins. Visit the Web site of the American Society for Dermatologic Surgery at www.asds-net. org. Other helpful Web sites are provided by the American College of Phlebology at www. phlebology.org and the American Academy of Dermatology at www.aad.org.

Guidelines for Safe Use of Supplements

Vitamin and Mineral Supplements

It's rare for anyone to experience serious side effects from vitamin and mineral supplements, but they can happen. These guidelines can help you use the supplements mentioned in this book safely and wisely.

Be sure to talk to your doctor before using any supplement if you have a chronic illness requiring medical supervision or medication. In fact, if you have any type of health problem, your doctor or pharmacist needs to know about any supplements you're taking before treating you with a prescription or over-the-counter medicine. If you are a woman who is pregnant, nursing, or attempting to conceive, do not use supplements unless under the supervision of your physician.

The vitamin and mineral doses listed below are the Daily Values or the suggested daily intakes (noted in italics). Also given below are the safe upper limits for adults, above which harmful side effects can occur. These amounts are the total from both food and supplements. Do not take more than the safe upper limit of any vitamin or mineral without first consulting your physician.

(Note: mg = milligrams; mcg = micrograms; IU = international units.)

Nutrient	Daily Value (DV) or Suggested Daily Intake	Safe Upper Limit	Cautions and Other Information
CALCIUM	1,000 mg; 1,200 mg if over age 50	2,500 mg for adults 19–50; 2,000 mg for adults over 50	Taking more than 2,000–2,500 mg a day can cause side effects such as kidney stones and constipation. Too much calcium can make it harder for the body to absorb iron and zinc. For best absorption, avoid taking more than 500 mg at one time. Look for a formula that contains vitamin D as well as calcium since you may need more vitamin D than is supplied by a multivitamin alone. Choose a brand marked with the USP (United States Pharmacopeia) symbol, which means it's free of lead and other contaminants.
MAGNESIUM	320 mg for adults 31 and over	350 mg from supplements only	Check with your doctor before beginning supplementation in any amount if you have heart or kidney problems. Doses exceeding 350 mg a day can cause diarrhea in some people. Too much magnesium can also lead to kidney failure.

Nutrient	Daily Value (DV) or Suggested Daily Intake	Safe Upper Limit	Cautions and Other Information
PANTOTHENIC ACID	5 mg	None established	A healthy, balanced diet provides enough of this nutrient to meet your body's needs.
SELENIUM	70 mcg	400 mcg	Taking more than 400 mcg a day can cause dizziness, nausea, hair or nail loss, or a garlic odor on the breath or skin.
VITAMIN B$_6$ (pyridoxine)	1.3 mg for adults over 18; 1.5 mg for those 51 and over	100 mg	Taking more than 100 mg a day can cause reversible nerve damage. When selecting a B-complex supplement, check the label for the amount of each ingredient to help you determine its safe use.
VITAMIN C	75mg	2,000 mg	Taking more than 2,000 mg a day can cause diarrhea in some people. To help maintain levels of vitamin C throughout the day, take half of the recommended dose in the morning and half at night.
VITAMIN D	600 IU (the DV), up to 800 IU if over age 70	4,000 IU	Taking more than 4,000 IU a day can cause headache, fatigue, nausea, diarrhea, or loss of appetite, as well as serious heart problems.
VITAMIN E	100 to 400 IU (DV is 22.4 IU) or 15 mg	1,500 IU (natural form, d-alpha- tocopherol) or 1,100 IU (synthetic form, from dl-alpha-tocoph-erol) supplements only	Because it acts like a blood thinner, consult your doctor before taking vitamin E if you are already taking aspirin or a blood-thinning medication such as warfarin (Coumadin).
ZINC	8 mg	40 mg	Taking more than 40 mg a day can cause nausea, dizziness, or vomiting. When levels of zinc are elevated, the absorption of copper can become impaired, reduce your immunity, and lower levels of HDL (good) cholesterol.

Emerging Supplements

Reports of adverse effects from emerging supplements are rare, especially when compared with prescription drugs, and supplement manufacturers are required by law to provide information on labels about reasonably safe recommended dosages for healthy individuals. Be aware that the potency and dosing strategy can vary significantly among products.

You should note, however, that little scientific research exists to assess the safety or long-term effects of many emerging supplements, and some supplements can complicate existing conditions or cause allergic reactions in some people. For these reasons, you should always check with your doctor before taking any supplements.

We recommend that you take supplements with food for best absorption and to avoid stomach irritation, unless otherwise directed. Never take them as a substitute for a healthy diet since they do not provide all the nutritional benefits of whole foods.

And, if you are pregnant, nursing, or attempting to conceive, do not supplement without the supervision of a doctor.

Supplement	Safe-Use Guidelines and Possible Side Effects
COENZYME Q10	Discuss supplementation with your doctor if you are taking the blood thinner warfarin (Coumadin). On rare occasions coenzyme Q10 may reduce the effectiveness of warfarin. Side effects are rare but include heartburn, nausea, or stomach upset, which can be prevented by consuming the supplement with a meal. Recommended if you're on a cholesterol-lowering statin drug, since the medication lowers CoQ-10 levels in the body. Some evidence suggests that it may prevent or lessen statin side effects.
EPA/OMEGA-3 (fish oil)	Do not take if any of the following apply: bleeding disorder, uncontrolled high blood pressure, use of anticoagulants (blood thinners) or regular aspirin, or allergy to any kind of fish. People with diabetes should not take fish oil because of its high fat content. Increases bleeding time, possibly resulting in nosebleeds and easy bruising, and may cause upset stomach. Take fish oil, not fish liver oil, because fish liver oil is high in vitamins A and D, which are toxic in high amounts.
FIBER	Do not take if you are allergic to the source of fiber in the supplement, such as wheat or psyllium. Take under the supervision of your doctor if you have diverticulitis, ulcerative colitis, Crohn's disease, bowel obstruction, or any serious gastrointestinal disorder, or if you are taking any medications. May cause gas or bloating.
FLAXSEED	If you are on medication, check with your doctor before supplementing with flaxseed because it may negatively affect absorption. Do not take if you have a bowel obstruction.
GLUCOSAMINE	May cause stomach upset, heartburn, or diarrhea.
QUERCETIN (bioflavonoid)	Generally safe, though in doses of 1 gram or more you may experience kidney damage. In some people, doses above 100 mg may dilate blood vessels and cause blood thinning. Should be avoided by individuals at risk for low blood pressure or problems with blood clotting. Do not take if you're pregnant or breastfeeding.

Photo Credits

Index

Boldface page references indicate illustrations. <u>Underscored</u> references indicate tables or boxed text.

f